Transplantation Immunology

Transplantation Immunology

Editor: Alex Collins

FOSTER
ACADEMICS
www.fosteracademics.com

www.fosteracademics.com

FOSTER ACADEMICS

Cataloging-in-Publication Data

Transplantation immunology / edited by Alex Collins.
p. cm.
Includes bibliographical references and index.
ISBN 978-1-63242-817-2
1. Transplantation immunology. 2. Transplantation of organs, tissues, etc.
3. Immunology. 4. Surgery. I. Collins, Alex.
RD120.7 .T73 2019
617.954--dc23

Foster Academics,
118-35 Queens Blvd., Suite 400,
Forest Hills, NY 11375, USA

ISBN 978-1-63242-817-2 (Hardback)

Printed and bound in China.

Contents

Preface

The main aim of this book is to educate learners and enhance their research focus by presenting diverse topics covering this vast field. This is an advanced book which compiles significant studies by distinguished experts in the area of analysis. This book addresses successive solutions to the challenges arising in the area of application, along with it; the book provides scope for future developments.

Immunology is a branch of biology that studies immune systems and malfunctions of the immune system such as in immune deficiencies, autoimmune diseases, hypersensitivities and transplant rejection. A key area of medical management is the study of transplant rejection in which the immune system attempts to destroy allografts leading to transplant failure. This results in an immediate need to remove the organ from the recipient. The risk of such a rejection can be determined by measuring the panel reactive antibody level. To prevent this, serotyping is done to determine recipient-donor transplantation suitability and immunosuppressant drugs are used. This book unfolds the innovative aspects of transplantation immunology, which will be crucial for the progress of this field in the future. It strives to provide a fair idea about this discipline and to help develop a better understanding of the latest advances within this field. It is a complete source of knowledge on the present status of this important field.

It was a great honour to edit this book, though there were challenges, as it involved a lot of communication and networking between me and the editorial team. However, the end result was this all-inclusive book covering diverse themes in the field.

Finally, it is important to acknowledge the efforts of the contributors for their excellent chapters, through which a wide variety of issues have been addressed. I would also like to thank my colleagues for their valuable feedback during the making of this book.

Editor

1

Influencing Factors of New-Onset Diabetes after a Renal Transplant and Their Effects on Complications and Survival Rate

Chaoyang Lv[1], Minling Chen[1,4], Ming Xu[2], Guiping Xu[1,5], Yao Zhang[1], Shunmei He[1], Mengjuan Xue[1], Jian Gao[3], Mingxiang Yu[1]*, Xin Gao[1]*, Tongyu Zhu[2]

1 Department of Endocrinology and Metabolism, Zhongshan Hospital, Fudan University, Shanghai, P.R. China, **2** Department of Urology, Zhongshan Hospital, Fudan University, Shanghai Key Laboratory of Organ Transplantation, Shanghai, P.R. China, **3** Evidence Base Medicine Center, Zhongshan Hospital, Fudan University, Shanghai, P.R. China, **4** Department of Endocrinology and Metabolism, People's Hospital Affiliated to Fujian University of Traditional Chinese Medicine (The People's Hospital of Fujian Province), Fuzhou, P.R. China, **5** Department of Cadre's Ward, Fujian Provincial Hospital, Fujian Medical University, Fuzhou, Fujian, P.R. China

Abstract

Objective: To discuss the onset of and relevant risk factors for new-onset diabetes after a transplant (NODAT) in patients who survive more than 1 year after undergoing a renal transplant and the influence of these risk factors on complications and long-term survival.

Method: A total of 428 patients who underwent a renal transplant between January 1993 and December 2008 and were not diabetic before surgery were studied. The prevalence rate of and relevant risk factors for postoperative NODAT were analyzed on the basis of fasting plasma glucose (FPG) levels, and differences in postoperative complications and survival rates between patients with and without NODAT were compared.

Results: The patients in this study were followed up for a mean of 5.65 ± 3.68 years. In total, 87 patients (20.3%) developed NODAT. Patients who converted from treatment with CSA to FK506 had increased prevalence rates of NODAT ($P < 0.05$). Multi-factor analysis indicated that preoperative FPG level (odds ratio [OR] = 1.48), age (OR = 1.10), body mass index (OR = 1.05), hepatitis C virus infection (OR = 2.72), and cadaveric donor kidney (OR = 1.18) were independent risk factors for NODAT (All $P < 0.05$). Compared with the N-NODAT group, the NODAT group had higher prevalence rates ($P < 0.05$) of postoperative infection, hypertension, and dyslipidemia; in addition, the survival rate and survival time of the 2 groups did not significantly differ.

Conclusion: Among the patients who survived more than 1 year after a renal transplant, the prevalence rate of NODAT was 20.32%. Preoperative FPG level, age, body mass index, hepatitis C virus infection, and cadaveric donor kidney were independent risk factors for NODAT. Patients who converted from treatment with CSA to FK506 after a renal transplant had aggravated impairments in glycometabolism. Patients with NODAT were also more vulnerable to postoperative complications such as infection, hypertension, and hyperlipidemia.

Editor: Paolo Fiorina, Children's Hospital Boston/Harvard Medical School, United States of America

Funding: The authors have no support or funding to report.

Competing Interests: The authors have declared that no competing interests exist.

* E-mail: yu.mingxiang@zs-hospital.sh.cn (MXY); gao.xin@zs-hospital.sh.cn (XG)

Introduction

Since the first renal transplant was performed in the United States in 1954, the number of renal transplant recipients has greatly increased along with the continuous promotion and maturation of the renal transplantation technique. In China, the first renal allotransplant was performed in 1960, and more than 5,000 renal transplants are now conducted in this country each year [1,2]. The survival time of renal transplant recipients has gradually increased because of the improved survival rate during the perioperative period and enhancements in treatment with anti-rejection drugs [3–6]; as a result, long-term complications and the quality of life of transplant recipients have recently received more attention.

New-onset diabetes after transplantation (NODAT) is an important complication after a renal transplant and is officially considered a risk factor for patients undergoing a renal transplant according to the 2003 NODAT international consensus guidelines [7]. Although there is evidence that novel glycometabolism and several chronic diabetic complications are improved by kidney transplantation [8–12], NODAT severely affects the quality of life and long-term survival rate of renal transplant recipients [13–16]; NODAT is the major factor leading to dysfunction of the renal graft and patient death and is a risk factor for cardiovascular diseases in these patients [17–19]. Several in-depth clinical and animal studies have been conducted to study the prevalence rate, risk factors, and pathogenesis of NODAT [20,21,34,35]. With the increasing number of patients with extended survival, the long-term influence of NODAT has been gradually emerging; thus, in recent years, the focus of research has shifted to long-term complications and their influences on continuing human/renal survival.

Our clinical investigation was based on detailed and accurate data from renal transplant cases at Zhongshan Hospital as well as their standardized and orderly postoperative management. Using relevant data from renal allotransplant recipients from January 1993 to December 2008 who survived more than 1 year after surgery, combined with data in the literature on the prevalence rate, outcome, and relevant risk factors for NODAT, this study evaluated the influence of NODAT on complications and long-term survival of these patients and provides a new clinical basis for the prevention and treatment of NODAT.

Subjects and Methods

1. Subjects

We retrospectively analyzed the records of 709 patients who underwent a renal transplant at Zhongshan Hospital, Fudan University, from January 1993 to December 2008. The following patients were excluded: 162 patients with unclear data on preoperative medical history and missing postoperative follow-up information, 75 patients whose renal graft survived less than 1 year after surgery, 10 patients with a combined liver-kidney transplant or other multi-organ transplant, 16 patients who underwent 2 or more renal transplants, and 18 patients who were diabetic before surgery. The remaining 428 non-diabetic patients who underwent a renal transplant for the first time and had a renal graft survival time of more than 1 year and complete data were included for analysis. This study was approved by the institutional review board of Zhongshan Hospital, Fudan University, and all participants provided written informed consent.

2. Methods

(1) Collection of data. Hospitalization and outpatient data from patients who underwent a renal transplant at Zhongshan Hospital, Fudan University, between January 1993 and December 2008 were collected. Basic preoperative data included general data (gender, age, BMI), preoperative examination, history of smoking and family history of diabetes, primary renal diseases and source of donor kidney, and preoperative biochemical indicators. Data on the patient's condition during the perioperative period included intraoperative immune induction, initial immunosuppressant regimen, acute rejection (AR), and recovery of renal function. Postoperative follow-up data included postoperative fasting plasma glucose (FPG) level, blood lipid level, glycated hemoglobin level, renal function, hepatitis B virus/hepatitis C virus/cytomegalovirus markers, postoperative immunosuppressant maintenance regimen, drug dosage and concentration, complications (AR, history of major infections, tumor), renal graft (normal function, dysfunction), and patient survival or death. Endpoints were defined as death of patients or dysfunction of renal grafts.

(2) Immunosuppressant treatment regimen after a renal transplant. A triple regimen of cyclosporin (CSA) plus mycophenolate mofetil/azathioprine plus glucocorticoids or tacrolimus (FK506) plus mycophenolate mofetil/azathioprine plus glucocorticoids was used for postoperative immunosuppressant treatment. Primary CSA-treated patients were converted to treatment with FK506 or rapamycin if adverse reactions such as liver and kidney poisoning, insensitivity to CSA, significant gingival hyperplasia, chronic rejection, or malignant tumors were observed. Drug concentrations were monitored during follow-up, and drug dosages were adjusted on the basis of the plasma drug concentrations and the particular conditions of the patients. Peak concentration was monitored for CSA and trough concentration was monitored for FK506; plasma drug concentrations were maintained within the therapeutic window (Table 1).

(3) Blood sugar management regimen. All patients underwent periodic follow-up after surgery as required by the follow-up system at our medical center. FPG and blood lipid levels were measured, and the immunosuppressant regimen was adjusted according to the particular conditions of the patients during follow-up. Patients who were diabetic before a transplant and patients with NODAT were treated and monitored according to the 2005 guidelines for treatment and management of NODAT [22].

(4) Criteria of relevant indexes. Patients were considered to have NODAT if they were not diabetic before surgery and did not have an acute glycometabolism disorder after surgery but met the diagnostic criteria for diabetes with a sustained high hyperglycemic state or normal blood sugar level and were currently being treated with insulin or an oral anti-diabetic drug. The diagnosis of NODAT was based on the following diagnostic criteria for diabetes proposed by the American Diabetes Association in 2007: typical symptoms of diabetes with a random blood glucose level $\geq$11.1 mmol/L, an FPG level $\geq$7.0 mmol/L, and a 2-hour blood glucose level after glucose load (75 g anhydrous glucose) $\geq$11.1 mmol/L on an oral glucose tolerance test (OGTT); an FPG level between 5.6 and 6.9 mmol/L is considered impaired fasting glucose (IFG), and a 2-hour blood glucose level between 7.8 and 11.0 mmol/L is considered impaired glucose tolerance (IGT) [23].

Patients may have significantly different recovery of early renal function after a renal transplant. For the purposes of our research, all patients in this study were divided into 4 categories: (1) immediate recovery of renal function: serum creatinine level decreased to less than 140 μmol/L within 7 days after surgery; (2) slow recovery of renal function: serum creatinine level decreased to less than 140 μmol/L after 1 week, but hemodialysis was not needed; (3) delayed recovery of renal function: serum creatinine level decreased to less than 140 μmol/L after 1 week, but postoperative oliguria or anuria was observed and dialysis transition was needed; and (4) impaired recovery of renal function: serum creatinine level was greater than 140 μmol/L 30 days after surgery. Delayed recovery of renal function was not included in the cases of impaired recovery of renal function.

On the basis of the time of NODAT, patients were considered to have early NODAT (new-onset diabetes within 1 year after a renal transplant), late NODAT (new-onset diabetes more than 1 year after a renal transplant), or no NODAT (N-NODAT) (no NODAT was observed after surgery and until the endpoint of follow-up). According to whether NODAT existed continuously, the patients were considered to have transient NODAT (T-NODAT) (NODAT persisted for at least 3 months and returned to normal during follow-up) or persistent NODAT (P-NODAT) (NODAT existed during follow-up and to the endpoint).

(5) Statistical analysis. SPSS 16.0 and SAS 8.2 software packages were used for statistical analysis. Measurement data are expressed as mean ± standard deviation, and count data are expressed as values and percentages. Intergroup comparisons of measurement data that are in accordance with normal distribution and show homogeneity of variance were performed using the *t* test or single-factor analysis of variance; otherwise, the grouped Wilcoxon test was used. Count data were analyzed using chi-

Table 1. Reference plasma drug concentration (ng/ml) of immunosuppressor in different periods after transplantation.

Drug	1 month after transplantation	2–3 months after transplantation	4–6 months after transplantation	7–12 months after transplantation	1 year after transplantation
Cmin of FK506	6–15	8–15	7–12	5–10	7–9
Cmax of CSA	1200–1500	1000–1200	800–1100	700–1000	650–900

square test or Fisher exact probability test. $P < 0.05$ was considered to be a statistically significant difference. Analysis of the influences of immunosuppressant therapy on FPG and blood lipid levels before and after immunosuppressant conversion was performed using *t* test. Logistic multivariate stepwise regression analysis was used for multi-factor analysis of risk factors for NODAT. The Kaplan–Meier method was used for survival analysis to estimate the survival rate, and the stratified log-rank test was used to compare the 2 survival curves. The Cox proportional hazards model was used to analyze factors that affect the survival of renal transplant recipients.

Results

1. General preoperative conditions of patients with and without NODAT

After eliminating 281 of the 709 renal transplant recipients on the basis of the exclusion criteria, 428 non-diabetic patients who underwent a renal transplant for the first time and had a renal graft survival time of more than 1 year and complete data were included for analysis. Patients were divided into the NODAT and N-NODAT groups according to their postoperative FPG levels; the general preoperative condition of the patients is shown in Table 2. Compared with the N-NODAT group, the NODAT group was older, had higher body mass index (BMI) values, and had higher proportions of patients with a preoperative history of smoking and a family history of diabetes in first-degree relatives. HCV and CMV infection rates were higher in the NODAT group than in the N-NODAT group, whereas there was no significant difference in hepatitis B virus infection rates between the 2 groups. Preoperative total cholesterol (TC) and triglyceride (TG) levels were both higher in the NODAT group than in the N-NODAT group.

2. Prevalence and outcome of NODAT

The 428 patients who were non-diabetic before surgery (including 45 patients with IFG and 383 patients with normal fasting glucose levels) had an average follow-up time of 5.65 ± 3.68 years until the endpoints of follow-up. Eighty-seven (20.32%) of these patients had onset of NODAT, and 57 of these cases occurred within 1 year (accounting for 65.5% of all cases of NODAT). Among all patients with NODAT, 72 had persistent NODAT and 15 (17.2%) shifted to normal fasting glucose or IFG (Figure 1).

3. Risk factors for NODAT

(1) Risk factors for NODAT. Risk factors that might be involved in postoperative onset of NODAT were analyzed using single factor analysis, and the results are shown in Table 3. The proportion of patients with a cadaveric donor kidney was higher in the NODAT group than in the N-NODAT group. The early postoperative FPG level 7 days after surgery was higher in the NODAT group than in the N-NODAT group. The proportion of patients treated with basic CSA or FK506 immunosuppressant regimens at discharge was not statistically significant between the 2 groups. However, during the course of disease, 19 patients (21.8%) in the NODAT group and 30 patients (8.8%) in the N-NODAT group converted from treatment with CSA to FK506, which was significantly different between the 2 groups. In the NODAT group, some of the patients experienced onset of NODAT after adjustment of their immunosuppressant regimen (conversion from CSA to FK506). In terms of the comparison of anti-rejection drug dosage and plasma drug concentration, the daily dosage of corticosteroid maintenance therapy was not significantly different between the 2 groups. CSA peak concentrations in the NODAT group at 6 months and 1 year were greater than those of the N-NODAT group, and the difference was statistically significant; however, differences in FK506 trough concentrations at each period were not statistically significant.

Risk factors for NODAT (multi-factor analysis). Logistic multivariate regression analysis was performed to analyze age, BMI, history of smoking, family history of diabetes, source of donor kidney, HCV infection and CMV infection, preoperative TC and TG levels, postoperative immunosuppressant regimen, daily dosage of corticosteroid maintenance for different times of year, and plasma concentration of CSA and FK506. As shown in Table 4, age, BMI, HCV infection, preoperative FPG level, and a cadaveric donor kidney can increase the risk of NODAT.

(2) Comparison of risk factors between P-NODAT and T-NODAT. As shown in Table 5, compared with T-NODAT, the P-NODAT group was older, had higher BMI values, had greater proportions of patients with a family history of diabetes and a cadaveric donor kidney, and had higher preoperative and 1-year postoperative FPG, TC, and TG levels; these differences were statistically significant, whereas the concentrations of immunosuppressants showed no significant differences between the 2 groups. It is noteworthy that the prevalence rate of AR in the T-NODAT group was higher than that in the P-NODAT group ($P = 0.043$).

(3) Influence of immunosuppressant conversion on FPG level and NODAT. Single factor analysis indicated that adjustment of immunosuppressant therapy (conversion from CSA to FK506) is a risk factor for onset of NODAT. Hence, for the 51 patients who converted from treatment with CSA to FK506 and the 32 patients who converted from treatment with CSA to rapamycin, the FPG levels and the number of cases of NODAT before and after drug adjustment were matched separately to analyze the influence of adjustment of immunosuppressant therapy. As shown in Figures 2A and 2B, the FPG levels and the NODAT prevalence rate for the patients who converted from treatment with CSA to FK506 were significantly elevated, and both were statistically significant. However, the FPG levels and the number of cases of NODAT for patients who converted from treatment with CSA to rapamycin showed no significant changes. These results indicate that the impairment of glycometabolism was aggravated in patients who converted from treatment with CSA to FK506, but the glycometabolism of patients who converted from treatment with CSA to rapamycin was not significantly affected.

Table 2. Characteristics of patients with NODAT versus N-NODAT before transplantation.

Clinical index	NODAT (n = 87)	N-NODAT (n = 341)	P-Value
Gender (Male)	60(69.0%)	228(66.9%)	0.798
Age (year)	45.61±9.86	38.89±12.67	0.004
BMI (kg/m^2)	24.84±4.12	20.97±2.81	0.010
History of smoking	25(28.7%)	37(10.9%)	<0.001
History of diabetes	20(23.0%)	20(5.9%)	<0.001
Type of dialysis			
Hematodialysis	68(78.2%)	277(81.3%)	0.505
Peritoneal dialysis	5(5.7%)	30(8.8%)	
Without dialysis	14(16.1%)	34(10%)	
Duration of dialysis	423.67±536.42	344.65±439.45	0.154
HBV infection	11(12.6%)	28(8.2%)	0.212
HCV infection	18(20.7%)	27(7.9%)	0.001
CMV infection	15(17.2%)	27(7.9%)	0.020
FPG (mmol/L)	5.48±0.79	4.39±0.55	0.002
TC (mmol/L)	4.58±1.26	4.05±0.96	0.045
TG (mmol/L)	1.86±1.06	1.43±0.76	0.024

Abbreviations: NODAT: new onset diabetes after transplantation; N-NODAT: no NODAT; BMI: body mass index; HBV: hepatitis B virus; HCV: hepatitis C virus; CMV: cytomegalovirus; FPG: fasting plasma glucose; TC: cholesterol; TG: triglyceride.

4. Influence of NODAT on complications and survival rate

(1) Influence of NODAT on complications after a renal transplant. As shown in Table 6, compared with the N-NODAT group, the NODAT group had statistically significant higher prevalence rates of postoperative infection, hypertension, and lipid metabolism disorder, whereas the prevalence rate of malignant tumors was not significantly different.

(2) Influence of NODAT on the survival rate of renal transplant recipients. As of December 2009, 34 renal graft recipients who did not have preoperative diabetes had died (7.9%); the major causes of death were cardiovascular diseases, malignant tumors, infections, bone marrow suppression, gastrointestinal bleeding ulcers and other hemorrhagic diseases, and renal insufficiency (Figure 3). Survival analysis showed that the 5-year survival rate of the NODAT group was not significantly different from that of the N-NODAT group, and the 10-year survival rate of the NODAT group was lower than that of the N-NODAT group with no statistical difference (Table 7). The previously mentioned results suggest that after an average follow-up time of 5.65 ± 3.68 years, there were no significant differences in the postoperative survival rate and survival time between the NODAT group and the N-NODAT group. Potential risk factors that might affect the death of renal transplant recipients were analyzed using Cox regression analysis (Table 8) after calibrating for age, year of transplant, postoperative onset of tumor, postoperative infection, and other risk factors that might affect the death of patients. The mortality hazard ratio of NODAT was 1.216 (95% confidence interval, 0.804–1.840), but it was not statistically significant (P = 0.354).

Discussion

1. Prevalence and outcome of NODAT

The prevalence rate of diabetes in patients with NODAT is significantly elevated compared with the normal population [24]. In a recent study [25] in which 209 renal transplant recipients underwent OGTT, the prevalence rates of NODAT, impaired glucose tolerance, and IFG were 19%, 14%, and 17%, respectively. The prevalence rate of NODAT in our study was 20.32%, which is close to the prevalence rate reported in the literature. In this study, 15 patients (17.2% of all cases of NODAT) regained a normal FPG level during follow-up. It has been reported [26,27]

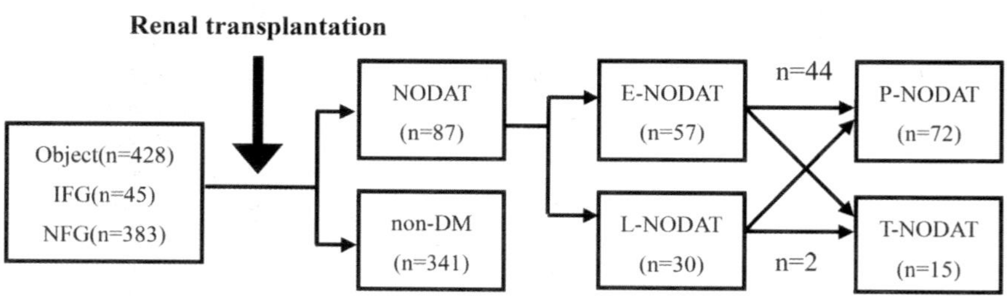

Figure 1. Prevalence and outcome of NODAT. Abbreviations: IFG: impaired fasting glucose; NFG: normal fasting glucose; NODAT: new onset diabetes after transplantation; E-NODAT: early-NODAT; L-NODAT: late NODAT; N-NODAT: no NODAT; T-NODAT: transient-NODAT; P-NODAT: persistent-NODAT.

Table 3. Comparison of risk factors between NODAT and N-NODAT (single factor analysis).

Risk factors	NODAT (n = 87)	N-NODAT (n = 341)	P-value
Graft type (cadaveric)	79(90.8%)	249(73.0%)	<0.001
Recovery of graft function			
Immediately	52(59.8%)	232(68.0%)	0.258
Slowly	23(26.4%)	62(18.2%)	
Delayed	8(9.2%)	24(7.0%)	
Difficult to recover	4(4.6%)	23(6.7%)	
Induction therapy (antiCD25)	38(43.7%)	171(50.1%)	0.337
Acute rejection	14(16.1%)	45(13.2%)	0.488
FPG 1week after transplant (mmol/L)	6.46±4.24	5.12±1.14	0.005
FK506/CSA on discharge	11/76	31/310	0.317
AZA/MMF	13/74	44/297	0.156
CSA convert to FK506	19(21.8%)	30(8.8%)	0.020
CSA convert to rapamycin	6(6.9%)	25(7.3%)	1.000
Daily dose of glucocorticoid (mg)			
On discharge	26.26±4.77	26.73±5.00	0.435
3 months after transplantation	17.42±4.75	16.13±3.26	0.132
6 months after transplantation	13.51±2.70	13.91±3.45	0.573
1 year after transplantation	12.74±3.78	11.47±3.26	0.061
Cmax of CSA (ng/ml)			
On discharge	1284.80±282.44	1276.80±367.74	0.853
3 months after transplantation	1016.50±251.64	1002.30±328.35	0.861
6 months after transplantation	1030.80±332.04	906.38±304.97	0.012
1 year after transplantation	929.81±278.86	785.51±226.02	0.006
Cmin of FK506 (ng/ml)			
On discharge	11.03±3.39	9.04±3.93	0.144
3 months after transplantation	10.60±7.26	7.79±2.57	0.054
6 months after transplantation	7.85±2.48	7.52±2.01	0.808
1 year after transplantation	7.44±2.28	7.20±2.76	0.836

Abbreviations: NODAT: new onset diabetes after transplantation; N-NODAT: no NODAT; FPG: fasting plasma glucose; AZA: azathioprine; MMF: mycophenolate mofetil; FK506: tacrolimus; CSA: cyclosporin.

that one-third to one-half of patients will spontaneously remit with time. However, clinical observation indicates that impaired glycometabolism cannot be reversed in all patients with NODAT [27]. Our study found that patients with P-NODAT have more recognized adjustable or nonadjustable risk factors, whereas patients with T-NODAT have a higher prevalence rate of AR compared with patients with P-NODAT ($P = 0.043$), indicating that AR might be a risk factor for the onset of T-NODAT. The outcome is similar to the results reported in previous literature [28].

2. Risk factors for NODAT

The meta-analysis by Montori [29] showed that nonadjustable risk factors clearly related to NODAT include age, black or Hispanic ethnicity, and HCV infection. Seventy-four percent of

Table 4. Logistic regression analysis of risk factors for NODAT (multiple-factor analysis).

Risk factors	OR	95% confidence interval	P-value
Age	1.10	1.02–1.23	0.044
BMI	1.05	1.04–1.14	0.029
HCV infection	2.72	1.20–6.34	0.008
Cadaveric graft	1.58	1.43–1.90	0.035
Preoperative FPG level	1.48	1.02–1.57	0.036

Abbreviations: NODAT: new onset diabetes after transplantation; BMI: body mass index; HCV: hepatitis C virus.

Table 5. Comparison of risk factors between P-NODAT and T-NODAT.

Risk factors	P-NODAT (n = 72)	T-NODAT (n = 15)	P-value
Age (year)	42.58±9.21	38.73±12.91	0.046
BMI (kg/m^2)	25.98±3.32	22.17±6.92	0.036
Gender (male)	51(21%)	9(60%)	0.540
History of diabetes	19(26.4%)	1(6.7%)	0.045
History of smoking	23(31.9%)	2(13.3%)	0.213
HBV infection	10(13.9%)	1(6.7%)	0.681
HCV infection CMV infection	16(22.2%)	2(13.3%)	0.526
CMV infection	5(6.9%)	0	0.582
FK506/CSA on discharge	9/63	2/13	1.000
AZA/MMF	11/61	2/13	1.000
CSA convert to FK506	17(23.6%)	2(13.3%)	0.506
CSA convert to rapamycin	4(5.6%)	2(13.3%)	0.275
Cmax of CSA (ng/ml)			
3 months after transplantation	1231.90±262.03	1272.10±243.19	0.875
1 year after transplantation	962.19±289.08	816.47±224.28	0.042
Cmin of FK506 (ng/ml)			
3 months after transplantation	8.56±2.52	8.90±2.30	0.419
1 year after transplantation	8.68±1.29	7.00±0.71	0.103
Graft type (cadaveric)	67(93.1%)	12(80.0%)	0.046
Acute rejection	9(12.5%)	5(33.3%)	0.043
FPG (mmol/L)			
Pretransplantation	5.55±0.81	4.55±0.62	0.040
1 year after transplantation	8.66±4.12	5.85±1.69	0.032
TC (mmol/L)			
Pretransplantation	5.65±1.27	3.86±1.06	0.041
1 year after transplantation	6.36±1.10	5.74±1.72	0.022
TG (mmol/L)			
Pretransplantation	1.81±1.13	0.94±0.32	0.002
1 year after transplantation	2.39±0.88	2.20±0.63	0.526

Abbreviations: P-NODAT: persistent-new onset diabetes after transplantation; T-NODAT: transient-new onset diabetes after transplantation; BMI: body mass index; HBV: hepatitis B virus; HCV: hepatitis C virus; CMV: cytomegalovirus; AZA: azathioprine; MMF: mycophenolate mofetil; FK506: tacrolimus; CSA: cyclosporine; FPG: fasting plasma glucose; TC: cholesterol; TG: triglyceride.

the difference in the prevalence rate of NODAT occurring within the first year after a transplant can be explained by the type of immunosuppressant used.

(1) Glucocorticoids. There is evidence that treatment with glucocorticoids is the greatest risk factor for NODAT [30]. In this study, there were no differences in the daily doses at each time point within 1 year after surgery between the NODAT group and the N-NODAT group. Although postoperative withdrawal of corticosteroid therapy is still controversial in clinical studies of a renal transplant, it is commonly recognized that postoperative short-term pulsed therapy and low-dose maintenance therapy are not only safe but also reduce the risk of NODAT [31].

(2) Calcineurin inhibitors. CSA and FK506 are both calcineurin inhibitors (CNIs) with similar mechanisms. Studies have shown that CNI is closely correlated with glucometabolic disorders and diabetic complications in organ transplantation [32–35,37–42]. Animal and clinical studies have demonstrated that CSA has toxic effects on pancreatic β cells [34–36], especially CSA formulations improved by micro-emulsion technology to achieve better oral absorbability and a higher level of drug exposure [37]. The application of CSA micro-emulsion helps explain our finding that the prevalence rate of AR significantly decreased but the prevalence rate of NODAT did not decrease correspondingly. Studies have shown that NODAT is positively correlated with CSA concentration [38,39]. Single factor analysis in this study showed that the patient's CSA peak concentrations 6 months and 12 months after surgery are risk factors for NODAT, indicating that exposure to a high concentration of CSA in the early postoperative stages after a renal transplant is a risk factor for NODAT. Similarly, there are also animal and clinical studies which have demonstrated that FK506 has toxic effects on pancreatic β cells [36,40,41]. Many studies pointed out that FK506's effect on glucose metabolism was dose-dependent. With the increased use of FK506, the occurrence of NODAT was on the rise [42]. Another study [43] showed that the prevalence rate of NODAT was 20.2% higher when using FK506 instead of CSA. In our study, due to the risk of NODAT with FK506 therapy and economic concerns, our center tends to use CSA as an immunosuppressant regimen. Conversion from treatment with CSA to FK506 is a risk factor for NODAT. This also indicates

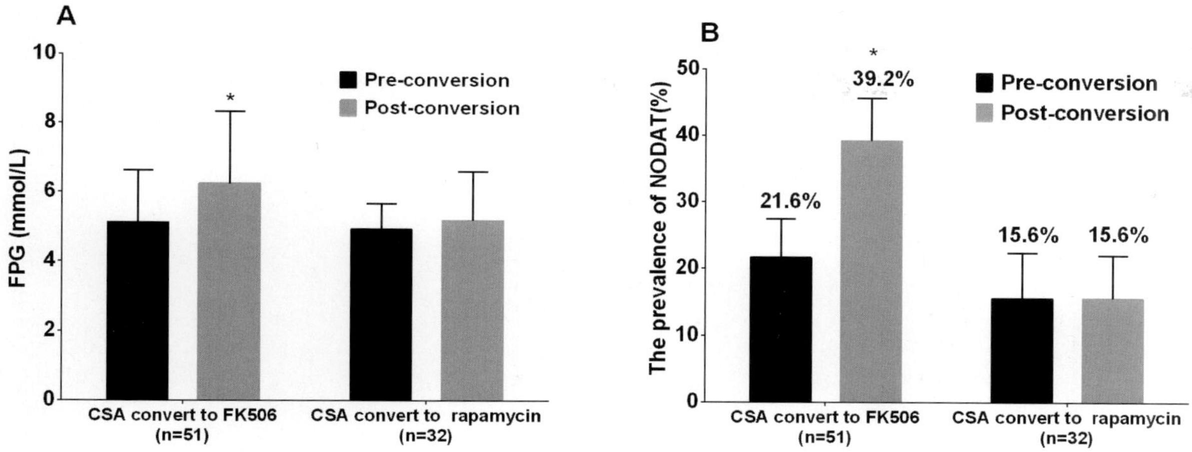

Figure 2. A: FPG before and after immunosuppressor conversion. B: Prevalence of NODAT before and after immunosuppressor conversion. Abbreviations: NODAT: new onset diabetes after transplantation; FPG: fasting plasma glucose; FK506: tacrolimus; CSA: cyclosporine; *$P<0.05$ compared with pre-conversion.

Table 6. Comparison of complications after transplantation between NODAT and N-NODAT.

Complications	NODAT (n = 87)	N-NODAT (n = 341)	P-value
Malignancy	5(5.7%)	11(3.2%)	0.337
Frequency of hospitalization for infection	0.77±1.227	0.48±0.754	0.036
Days of hospitalization for infection	16.67±30.25	7.42±13.23	0.006
Antihypertensive agents	1.98±1.26	1.26±1.05	<0.001
TC (mmol/L)			
3 months after transplantation	5.78±0.85	5.31±0.91	0.012
6 months after transplantation	5.93±1.06	5.35±1.01	0.015
1 year after transplantation	5.75±1.23	5.20±1.01	0.004
TG (mmol/L)			
3 months after transplantation	2.26±0.86	2.07±0.84	0.275
6 months after transplantation	2.50±1.12	1.92±0.81	0.023
1 year after transplantation	2.35±0.82	1.87±0.99	0.004

Abbreviations: NODAT: new onset diabetes after transplantation; N-NODAT: no NODAT; TC: cholesterol; TG: triglyceride.

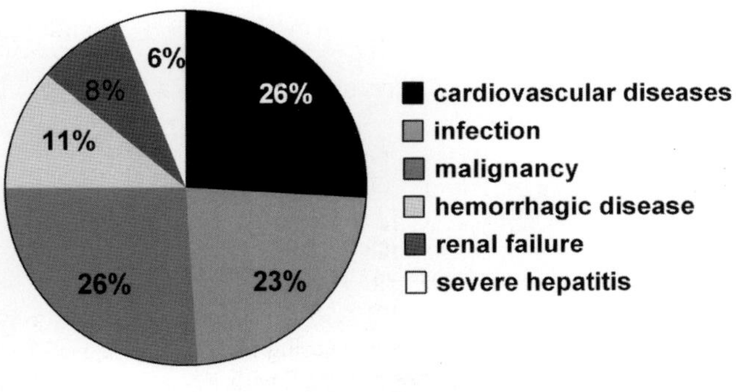

Figure 3. Proportion of death causes in renal transplant recipients.

that FK506 is a risk factor for NODAT, which is consistent with reports in the literature [40–43]. The FK506 trough concentrations in the NODAT group at each time point within 1 year after surgery showed no statistically significant difference compared with the N-NODAT group. This might be because our center followed the guidelines for the treatment and management of NODAT, closely monitored FK506 concentrations at postoperative follow-up visits, and reduced the dosage as much as possible.

(3) Conversion of immunosuppressant therapy. Patients had a high conversion rate of immunosuppressant regimens at our situation. In our investigation, after converting patients who were initially treated with CSA to FK506, their glycometabolism disorder was exacerbated. However, another study [44] showed that conversion in late stages from CSA to FK506 had no significant influence on glycometabolism. Patients who were converted from treatment with CSA to rapamycin in this study showed no significant changes in glycometabolism before and after conversion; however, in a study conducted by Teutonico [45], who observed the influence of CNI withdrawal with conversion to

Table 7. Comparison of risk survival rateand survival time between NODAT and N- NODAT (P = 0.959).

Group	N	5-year survival rate	10-year survival rate	Mean survival time (month)	95% confidence interval
NODAT	87	93%	81%	171.800±8.010	156.106–187.511
N-NODAT	341	93%	85%	172.160±5.130	162.090–182.232

Abbreviations: N: number;NODAT: new onset diabetes after transplantation; N-NODAT:no NODAT.

rapamycin on glycometabolism, showed that the prevalence rate of impaired glucose tolerance increased by 30%, with 4 new cases of NODAT.

(4) Preoperative and early-stage postoperative glycometabolism disorders. Both single factor analysis and multi-factor analysis (OR [odds ratio] = 1.48) suggested that preoperative FPG level is clearly correlated with NODAT. International studies have also shown that preoperative glycometabolism disorder is an independent risk factor for NODAT [46]. Patients with end-stage renal disease did not show improvements in glycometabolism as renal function recovered after a renal transplant and developed NODAT. This can be explained by the "second strike" theory. Single factor analysis in our study also found that elevation of the FPG level in the first week after surgery is a risk factor for NODAT; similar results have also been reported by relevant international studies [47]. Early postoperative hyperglycemia can be used to predict postoperative glycometabolism disorder (OR = 5.4); this is thought to be related to accumulated doses of corticosteroids after surgery.

(5) Others. Both single factor analysis and multi-factor analysis (OR = 1.58) suggest that recipients of cadaveric donor kidneys are at higher risk for NODAT; this has also been reported in a related study [48]. In clinical practice, recipients of living donor kidneys are usually treated with lower doses of immunosuppressants compared with recipients of cadaveric donor kidneys, so this could be the main reason. Our investigation found that HCV and CMV are related to NODAT and that HCV infection is an independent risk factor for NODAT (OR = 2.72), which has also been reported in related studies [49,50]. The mechanism of diabetes caused by virus infection is unclear, but it has been speculated that insulin resistance and defects in islet cell secretion are both involved.

3. Influence of NODAT on patients' complications and survival rate

In our investigation, the frequency and days of hospitalization due to infections in patients with NODAT are both higher than those of patients with N-NODAT. Use of immunosuppressants after an organ transplant reduces the resistance of the body to exogenous infections, and recipients with concomitant NODAT are more vulnerable to infections. This is considered to be related to the lower chemotaxis, migration, and phagocytic function of neutrophil granulocytes in diabetic patients compared with healthy people [51]. In this study, patients in the NODAT group had more severe postoperative concomitant hypertension and lipid metabolism disorder compared with the N-NODAT group, that is, an increased prevalence rate of metabolic syndrome (MS). Another study showed that MS and NODAT were significantly correlated after a renal transplant [52]. A study by Porrini et al [53] found that patients with NODAT after a renal transplant were more likely to have MS during follow-up, with a lower human/renal survival rate. Several studies have shown the adverse effects of NODAT on renal transplantation, which is considered the second most influential factor of long-term survival after acute and chronic rejections [53–55]. In this study, the 5-year survival rates of the NODAT and N-NODAT groups were both 93%, and the 10-year survival rates were 81% and 85%, respectively. The difference between the 2 groups was not statistically significant (P = 0.959). This is slightly different from the results reported in the literature [28,56]. We consider the differences may be due to different inclusion criteria and duration of follow-up [57].

We recognize limitations of our study. First, the early preoperative OGTT data from renal transplant recipients at our hospital were not complete. The postoperative diagnosis of NODAT was only based on FPG level, so the prevalence rate of NODAT might be biased. On the one hand, diabetic patients with normal preoperative FPG but high 2-hour postprandial blood glucose levels, who met the diabetes diagnostic criteria, were not excluded, which may have caused bias and increased the prevalence rate of NODAT. On the other hand, the prevalence rate of glycometabolism disorders in our patients might have been underestimated, especially impaired glucose tolerance. Second, blood glucose, FPG, 2-hour postprandial blood glucose, and glycosylated hemoglobin levels should be routinely tested postop-

Table 8. Cox regression analysis of risk factors affecting death.

Parameter	HR	P-value	95% confidence interval
Age	**1.040**	**0.017**	**1.007–1.075**
NODAT	**1.216**	**0.354**	**0.804–1.840**
Malignancy	**3.463**	**0.003**	**1.518–7.899**
Days of hospitalization for infection	**1.019**	**0.001**	**1.008–1.031**
Cadaveric graft	1.650	0.647	0.193–14.112

Abbreviations: NODAT: new onset diabetes after transplantation.

eratively and monitored on follow-up. Third, we believe that the homeostasis model of insulin resistance should be used to assess the insulin resistance level of patients; however, relevant data were only available from a small number of patients. Fourth, this was a single-center study and thus we are unable to reach a general conclusion. Fifth, due to the significantly extended survival time of renal transplant recipients, sample sizes should be enlarged and follow-up time should be extended as much as possible. Sixth, although the influence of NODAT on the long-term survival of patients has not emerged, its influence on the cardiovascular system might have already appeared, so extensive cardiovascular examinations should be performed to evaluate cardiovascular influences on NODAT.

In conclusion, NODAT is a severe metabolic complication after an organ transplant and has many adverse, long-term influences on the patient's life. Certain issues still need further study. First, the pathogenesis of NODAT is still unknown. Inflammation, dimethylarginines and homocysteine are recently reported to participate in the pathogenesis of diabetes, while few studies focus on pathogenesis of NODAT [51,58,59,60]. Deep researches on pathogenesis of NODAT are needed. Second, more optimized immunosuppressant regimens need to be studied and developed to reduce the effects of risk factors for NODAT and thus reduce the prevalence of NODAT. At last, transplant recipients treated with long-term immunosuppressant therapy should be strictly followed up to assess the prevalence rate, type, and risk factors for long-term complications of diabetes.

Author Contributions

Conceived and designed the experiments: MXY XG. Performed the experiments: CYL MLC MX. Analyzed the data: CYL GPX YZ SH. Contributed reagents/materials/analysis tools: MJX JG. Wrote the paper: CYL MXY XG TYZ.

References

1. Huang J (2007) Ethical and legislative perspectives on liver transplantation in the People's Republic of China. Am J Transplant 13: 193–196.
2. Hanto DW (2008) Ethics committee oversight of living related donor kidney transplantation in China. Am J Transplant 8: 1765–1766.
3. Aktas A (2014) Transplanted kidney function evaluation. Semin Nucl Med 44: 129–145.
4. D'Addio F, Vergani A, Di Fenza R, Tezza S, Bassi R, et al. (2012) Novel immunological aspects of pediatric kidney transplantation. G Ital Nefrol 29: 44–48.
5. Del Carro U, Fiorina P, Amadio S, De Toni Franceschini L, Petrelli A, et al. (2007) Evaluation of polyneuropathy markers in type 1 diabetic kidney transplant patients and effects of islet transplantation: neurophysiological and skin biopsy longitudinal analysis. Diabetes Care 30: 3063–3069.
6. Orsenigo E, Socci C, Fiorina P, Cristallo M, Castoldi R, et al. (2004) Simultaneous pancreas-kidney transplantation: short- and long-term results. Transplant Proc 36: 568–588.
7. Davidson J, Wilkinson A, Dantal J (2003) New-onset diabetes after transplantation: 2003 International Consensus Guidelines. Transplantation 75: SS3–SS24.
8. Folli F, Guzzi V, Perego L, Coletta DK, Finzi G, et al. (2010) Proteomics reveals novel oxidative and glycolytic mechanisms in type 1 diabetic patients' skin which are normalized by kidney-pancreas transplantation. Plos one 5: e9923.
9. Fiorina P, Vezzull P, Bassi R, Gremizzi C, Falautano M, et al. (2012) Near normalization of metabolic and functional features of the central nervous system in type 1 diabetic patients with end-stage renal disease after kidney-pancreas transplantation. Diabetes Care 35: 367–374.
10. Salonia A, D'Addio F, Gremizzi C, Briganti A, Deho F, et al. (2011) Kidney-pancreas transplantation is associated with near-normal sexual function in uremic type 1 diabetic patients. Transplantation 92: 802–808.
11. Orsenigo E, Socci C, Fiorina P, Zuber V, Secchi A, et al. (2005) Cardiovascular benefits of simultaneous pancreas-kidney transplant versus kidney alone transplant in diabetic patients. Transplant Proc 37: 3570–3571.
12. Fiorina P, Folli F, D'Angelo A, Finzi G, Pellegatta F, et al. (2004) Normalization of multiple hemostatic abnormalities in uremic type 1 diabetic patients after kidney-pancreas transplantation. Diabetes 53: 2291–2300.
13. Valderhaug TG, Hjelmesaeth J, Hartmann A, Roislien J, Bergrem HA, et al. (2011) The association of early post-transplant glucose levels with long-term mortality. Diabetologia 54: 1341–1349.
14. Fiorina P, Bassi R, Gremizzi C, Vergani A, Caldara R, et al. (2012) 31P-magnetic resonance spectroscopy (31P-MRS) detects early changes in kidney high-energy phosphate metabolism during a 6-month Valsartan treatment in diabetic and non-diabetic kidney-transplanted patients. Acta Diabetol 49: 133–139.
15. Fiorina P, Perseghin G, De Cobelli F, Gremizzi C, Petrelli A, et al. (2007) Altered kidney graft high-energy phosphate metabolism in kidney-transplanted end-stage renal disease type 1 diabetic patients: a cross-sectional analysis of the effect of kidney alone and kidney-pancreas transplantation. Diabetes Care 30: 597–603.
16. Fiorina P, Venturini M, Folli F, Losio C, Maffi P, et al. (2005) Natural history of kidney graft survival, hypertrophy, and vascular function in end-stage renal disease type 1 diabetic kidney-transplanted patients: beneficial impact of pancreas and successful islet cotransplantation. Diabetes Care 28: 1303–1310.
17. Ducloux D, Kazory A, Chalopin JM (2005) Post-transplant diabetes mellitus and atherosclerotic events in renal transplant recipients: A prospective study. Transplantation 79: 438–443.
18. Astorri E, Fiorina P, Gavaruzzi G, Astorri A, Magnati G (1997) Left ventricular function in insulin-dependent and in non-insulin-dependent diabetic patients: radionuclide assessment. Cardiology 88: 152–155.
19. Perseghin G, Fiorina P, De Cobelli F, Scifo P, Esposito A, et al. (2005) Cross-sectional assessment of the effect of kidney and kidney-pancreas transplantation on resting left ventricular energy metabolism in type 1 diabetic-uremic patients: a phosphorous-31 magnetic resonance spectroscopy study. J Am Coll Cardiol 46: 1085–1092.
20. Hecking M, Werzowa J, Haidinger M, Horl WH, Pascual J, et al. (2013) Novel views on new-onset diabetes after transplantation: development, prevention and treatment. Nephrol Dial Transplant 28: 1–15.
21. Hagen M, Hjelmesaeth J, Jenssen T, Morkrid L, Hartmann A (2003) A 6-year prospective study on new onset diabetes mellitus, insulin release and insulin sensitivity in renal transplant recipients. Nephrol Dial Transplant 18: 2154–2159.
22. Wilkinson A, Davidson J, Dotta F, Home PD, Keown P, et al. (2005) Guidelines for the treatment and management of new-onset diabetes after transplantation. Clin Transplant 19: 291–298.
23. Amer Diabet, Assoc (2007) Diagnosis and classification of diabetes mellitus. Diabetes Care 30: S42–S47.
24. Wyzgal J, Paczek L, Sanko-Resmer J, Ciszek M, Nowak M, et al. (2007) Insulin resistance in kidney allograft recipients treated with calcineurin inhibitors. Ann Transplant 12: 26–29.
25. Brzezinska B, Junik R, Kaminska A, Wlodarczyk Z, Adamowicz A (2013) Factors associated with glucose metabolism disorder after kidney transplantation. Endokrynol Pol 64: 21–25.
26. Xu Y, Liang JX, Liu B, Yao B, Pokharel S, et al. (2011) Prevalence and long-term glucose metabolism evolution of post-transplant diabetes mellitus in Chinese renal recipients. Diabetes Res Clin Pract 92: 11–18.
27. Hur KY, Kim MS, Kim YS, Kang ES, Nam JH, et al. (2007) Risk factors associated with the onset and progress of post transplantation diabetes in renal allograft recipients. Diabetes care 30: 609–615.
28. Marin M, Renoult E, Bondor CI, Kessler M (2005) Factors influencing the onset of diabetes mellitus after kidney transplantation: A single french center experience. Transplant Proc 37: 1851–1856.
29. Montori VM, Basu A, Erwin PJ, Velosa JA, Gabriel EK, et al. (2002) Posttransplantation diabetes: a systematic review of the literature. Diabetes Care 25: 583–592.
30. Luan FL, Steffick DE, Ojo AO (2011) New-onset diabetes mellitus in kidney transplant recipients discharged on steroid-free immunosuppression. Transplantation 91: 334–341.
31. Knight SR, Morris PJ (2010) Steroid avoidance or withdrawal after renal transplantation increases the risk of acute rejection but decreases cardiovascular risk. A Meta-Analysis. Transplantation 89: 1–14.
32. Fernandez LA, Lehmann R, Luzi L, Battezzati A, Angelico MC, et al. (1999) The effects of maintenance doses of FK506 versus Cyclosporin A on glucose and lipid metabolism after orthotopic liver transplantation. Transplantation 68: 1532–1541.
33. Maffi P, Bertuzzi F, De Taddeo F, Magistretti P, Nano R, et al. (2007) Kidney function after islet transplant alone in type 1 diabetes: impact of immunosuppressive therapy on progressive of diabetic nephropathy. Diabetes Care 30: 1150–1155.
34. Ozbay LA, Smidt K, Mortensen DM, Carstens J, Jorgensen KA, et al. (2011) Cyclosporin and tacrolimus impair insulin secretion and transcriptional regulation in INS-1E beta-cells. Br J pharmacol 162: 136–146.
35. Heit JJ, Apelqvist AA, Gu X, Winslow MM, Neilson JR, et al. (2006) Calcineurin/NFAT signaling regulates pancreastic bata-cell growth and function. Nature 443: 345–349.
36. Polastri L, Galbiati F, Bertuzzi F, Fiorina P, Nano R, et al. (2002) Secretory defects induced by immunosuppressive agents on human pancreatic beta-cells. Acta Diabetol 39: 229–233.

37. Neumayer HH, Farber L, Haller P, Kohnen R, Maibucher A, et al. (1996) Substitution of conventional cyclosporine with a new microemusion formulation in renal transplant patients: result after 1 year. Nephrol Dial Transplant 11: 165–172.
38. Mathew JT, Rao M, Job V, Ratnaswamy S, Jacob CK (2003) Post-transplant hyperglycaemia: a study of risk factors. Nephrol Dial Transplant 18: 164–171.
39. Cotovio M, Neves L, Rodrigues R, Alves R, Bastos M, et al. (2013) New-onset diabetes after transplantations: assessment of risk factors and clinical outcomes. Transplant Proc 45: 1079–1083.
40. Duijnhoven EM, Boots JM, Christiaans MH, Wolffenbuttel BH, Van Hooff JP (2001) Influence of tacrolimus on glucose metabolism before and after transplantation: a prospective study. J Am Soc Nephrol 12: 583–588.
41. Tamura K, Fujimura T, Tsutsumi T, Nakamura K, Ogawa T, et al. (1995) Transcriptional inhibition of insulin by FK506 and possible involvement of FK506 binding protein-12 in pancreatic beta-cell. Transplantation 59: 1606–1613.
42. Davidson JA, Wilkinson A (2004) New-onset diabetes after transplantation 2003 international consensus guidelines - An endocrinologist's view. Diabetes Care 27: 805–812.
43. Borda B, Lengyel C, Szederkenyi E, Eller J, Keresztes, et al. (2012) Post-transplantation diabetes mellitus-Risk factors and effects on the function and morphology of the allograft. Acta Physiol Hung 99: 206–215.
44. Luan FL, Zhang H, Schaubel DE, Miles CD, Cibrik D, et al. (2008) Comparative risk of impaired glucose metabolism associated with cyclosporine versus tacrolimus in the late post-transplant period. Am J Transplant 8: 1871–1877.
45. Teutonico A, Schena PF, Di Paolo S (2005) Glucose metabolism in renal transplant recipients: Effect of calcineurin inhibitor withdrawal and conversion to sirolimus. J Am Soc Nephrol 16: 3128–3135.
46. Bergrem HA, Valderhaug TG, Hartmann A, Bergrem H, Hjelmesaeth J, et al. (2010) Glucose tolerance before and after renal transplantation. Nephrol Dial Transplant 25: 985–992.
47. Maldonado F, Tapia G, Ardiles L (2009) Early Hyperglycemia: A risk factor for posttransplant diabetes mellitus among renal transplant recipients. Transplant Proc 41: 2664–2667.
48. Kuo HT, Poommipanit N, Sampaio M, Reddy P, Cho YW, et al. (2010) Risk factors for development of New-Onset Diabetes Mellitus in pediatric renal transplant recipients: an analysis of the OPTN/UNOS Database. Transplantation 89: 434–439.
49. Baid-Agrawal S, Frei U, Reinke P, Schindler R, Kopp MA, et al. (2009) Impaired insulin sensitivity as an underlying mechanism linking hepatitis C and posttransplant diabetes mellitus in kidney recipients. Am J Transplant 9: 2777–2784.
50. Zelle DM, Corpeleijn E, VanRee RM, Stolk RP, van der Veer E, et al. (2010) Markers of the hepatic component of the metabolic syndrome as predictors of mortality in renal transplant recipient. Am J Transplant 10: 106–114.
51. Neetha S, Biju T, Amita R (2008) Comparison of neutrophil function in diabetic and healthy subjects with chronic generalized periodontitis. J Indian Soc Periodontol 12: 41–44.
52. Luan FL, Langewisch E, Ojo A (2010) Metabolic syndrome and new onset diabetes after transplantation in kidney transplant recipients. Clin Transplant 24: 778–783.
53. Porrini E, Delgado P, Bigo C, Alvarez A, Cobo M, et al. (2006) Impact of metabolic syndrome on graft function and survival after cadaveric renal transplantation. Am J Kidney Dis 48: 134–142.
54. Wiesbauer F, Heinze G, Regele H, Horl WH, Schernthaner GH, et al. (2010) Glucose control is associated with patient survival in diabetic patients after Renal transplantation. Transplantation 89: 612–619.
55. Sezer S, Akgul A, Altunoglu A, Arat Z, Ozdemir FN, et al. (2012) Posttransplantation diabetes mellitus: Impact of blood glucose regulation on renal transplant recipient outcome. Transplant Proc 44: 2893–2893.
56. Orsenigo E, Fiorina P, Cristallo M, Scocci C, La Rocca E, et al. (2004) Long-term survival after kidney and kidney-pancreas transplantation in diabetic patients. Transplant Proc 36: 1072–1075.
57. Elmagd MM, Bakr MA, Metwally AH, Wahab AM (2008) Clinicoepidemiologic study of posttransplant diabetes after living-donor renal transplant. Exp Clin Transplant 6: 42–47.
58. Huang T, Ren J, Huang J, Li D (2013) Association of homocysteine with type 2 diabetes: a meta-analysis implementing Mendelian randomization approach. BMC Genomics 14: 1471–2164.
59. Paroni R, Fermo I, Fiorina P, Cighetti G (2005) Determination of asymmetric and symmetric dimethylarginines in plasma of hyperhomocysteinemic subjects. Amino acids 28: 389–394.
60. Cighetti G, Fermo I, Aman CS, Ferraroni M, Secchi A, et al. (2009) Dimethylarginines in complicated type 1 diabetes: roles of insulin, glucose, and oxidative stress. Free Radic Biol Med 47: 307–311.

Killer Immunoglobulin-like Receptor (KIR) and *HLA* Genotypes Affect the Outcome of Allogeneic Kidney Transplantation

Izabela Nowak[1], Maria Magott-Procelewska[2], Agnieszka Kowal[1], Maciej Miazga[1], Marta Wagner[1], Wanda Niepiekło-Miniewska[1], Małgorzata Kamińska[3], Andrzej Wiśniewski[1], Edyta Majorczyk[1], Marian Klinger[2], Wioleta Łuszczek[1], Andrzej Pawlik[4], Rafał Płoski[5], Ewa Barcz[6], David Senitzer[7], Piotr Kuśnierczyk[1]*

1 Laboratory of Immunogenetics and Tissue Immunology, Department of Clinical Immunology, Ludwik Hirszfeld Institute of Immunology and Experimental Therapy, Polish Academy of Sciences, Wrocław, Poland, **2** Department and Clinic of Nephrology and Transplant Medicine, Faculty of Medicine, Medical University of Wroclaw, Wrocław, Poland, **3** Health Care Center at the Ludwik Hirszfeld Institute of Immunology and Experimental Therapy, Wrocław, Poland, **4** Department of Pharmacokinetics and Therapeutic Drug Monitoring, Pomeranian Medical University, Szczecin, Poland, **5** Department of Medical Genetics, Centre of Biostructure Research, Medical University of Warsaw, Warsaw, Poland, **6** 1st Chair and Clinic of Obstetrics and Gynecology, Medical University of Warsaw, Warsaw, Poland, **7** City of Hope Comprehensive Cancer Center, Duarte, California, United States of America

Abstract

Background: Recipient NK cells may detect the lack of recipient's (i.e., self) HLA antigens on donor renal tissue by means of their killer cell immunoglobulin-like receptors (KIRs). *KIR* genes are differently distributed in individuals, possibly contributing to differences in response to allogeneic graft.

Methodology/Principal Findings: We compared frequencies of 10 *KIR* genes by PCR-SSP in 93 kidney graft recipients rejecting allogeneic renal transplants with those in 190 recipients accepting grafts and 690 healthy control individuals. HLA matching results were drawn from medical records. We observed associations of both a full-length *KIR2DS4* gene and its variant with 22-bp deletion with kidney graft rejection. This effect was modulated by the *HLA-B,-DR* matching, particularly in recipients who did not have glomerulonephritis but had both forms of *KIR2DS4* gene. In contrast, in recipients with glomerulonephritis, *HLA* compatibility seemed to be much less important for graft rejection than the presence of *KIR2DS4* gene. Simultaneous presence of both *KIR2DS4* variants strongly increased the probability of rejection. Interestingly, *KIR2DS5* seemed to protect the graft in the presence of *KIR2DS4fl* but in the absence of *KIR2DS4del*.

Conclusions/Significance: Our results suggest a protective role of *KIR2DS5* in graft rejection and an association of *KIR2DS4* with kidney rejection, particularly in recipients with glomerulonephritis.

Editor: Antonio Perez-Martinez, Hospital Infantil Universitario Niño Jesús, Spain

Funding: This work was supported by the Ministry of Science and High Education grant No. N401077 31/1819 and by the Ludwik Hirszfeld Institute of Immunology and Experimental Therapy grant no. 14/2011. The funders had no role in study design, data collection and analysis, decision to publish, or preparation of the manuscript.

Competing Interests: The authors have declared that no competing interests exist.

* E-mail: pkusnier@iitd.pan.wroc.pl

Introduction

Acute or chronic rejection of solid organ grafts such as kidney is mediated by alloreactive T lymphocytes recognizing major (HLA) and minor histocompatibility antigens by means of antigen-specific T cell receptors (TCR) [1,2]. However, a contribution of natural killer (NK) cells has also been postulated. Thus, infiltration of renal allografts by NK cells [3–5], increased numbers of NK cells in peripheral blood of patients acutely rejecting kidney graft [6], and increased cytotoxicity of recipient NK cells against donor peripheral blood cells in vitro were described [7].

NK cells recognize the presence of HLA class I (HLA I) molecules on the surface of potential target cells using several types of the receptors, among them polymorphic killer cell immunoglobulin-like receptors (KIRs). Normal cells of an individual are spared by his or her NK cells because they express normal level of cell surface HLA I molecules detected by NK cell inhibitory receptors. However, virus-infected or neoplastic cells tend to lose HLA I expression, and may be eliminated by NK cells [8].

Due to HLA and KIR polymorphism, in some combinations of the graft donor and recipient, recipient NK cell's inhibitory KIRs may not bind HLA I molecules present on donor cells, leading to NK cell alloreactivity against the transplanted organ, similarly to the reaction in opposite direction in hematopoietic cell transplantation [9–11]. In addition, KIRs are expressed also on some T lymphocytes, particularly on special subpopulation of CD4+CD28− cytotoxic T cells involved in autoimmune vasculitis [12–14], potentially influencing their activity in graft rejection.

Human KIRs are encoded by genes located in the chromosomal region 19q14. KIR genetics is characterized by both allelic (up to more than 50 alleles for some *KIRs*) and haplotypic (i.e., different numbers of inhibitory and activating genes on individual chromosomes) polymorphism [8,15]. As a result, above 97% of unrelated persons differ by their *KIR* genotype [16–17]. Two categories of *KIR* haplotypes were described: A-type haplotypes containing mostly inhibitory *KIRs*, and only *KIR2DS4* and *KIR2DL4* as activating ones, and B-type haplotypes, characterized by one or more of other activating *KIRs* in addition to inhibitory ones. For this reason, people may differ substantially in their NK and T cell responses, depending on *KIR* genotype. We have recently published results showing a contribution of *KIR2DS5* gene to a tolerance of kidney graft as well as to other clinical situations [18]. Here, we focused on kidney graft rejection and compared frequencies of 10 *KIR* genes in recipients rejecting the allogeneic renal transplant with those in recipients accepting such a graft. Our study is the first report on different HLA and KIR genetic associations of kidney graft acute rejection in recipients whose pre-transplant renal failure resulted from glomerulonephritis versus those whose renal failure was a result of other disease.

Materials and Methods

Kidney graft recipients and controls

All individuals, including kidney graft recipients, donors, and healthy controls, were Polish Caucasians. Two hundred eighty-three kidney patients (clinical data presented in **Table 1**) underwent first transplantation and received deceased donor kidney between 1989 and 2008 (166 patients after 2000). All patients were treated with triple-therapy (**Figure 1**) as initial immunosuppression that incorporated cyclosporine (n = 219) or tacrolimus (n = 64, beginning in 2000) in combination with azathioprine (n = 129) or mycofenolate mofetil (n = 154, since 1998) (**Figure 2**) and steroids. No induction with antibodies was used. During the follow up (mean time was 7 years) there were 246 (87%) patients who were treated with the same calcineurin inhibitor. Among 29 patients who changed the type of calcineurin inhibitor, 20 patients were converted from CsA to tacrolimus after an episode of rejection treated with methylprednisolone. Calcineurin inhibitor was withdrawn in 8 individuals. There were 233 patients who received the same type of purine metabolism inhibitor during follow up: azathioprine (n = 84) and mycofenolate mofetil (n = 149). Azathioprine was replaced by mycofenolate mofetil in 33 patients (in 20 patients after an episode of acute rejection) or stopped in 12 patients. The frequency of a change in treatment regimen was almost 2-fold higher in patients who suffered a rejection (refers to 38% and 21% of patients with and without rejection, respectively, p = 0.0063).

93 recipients exhibited symptoms of acute graft rejection based on clinical criteria (an increase in serum creatinine level of at least 20% above the baseline measurements not attributable to another cause) confirmed by histopathological examination according to Banff criteria [19]. Apart from three patients, all had a biopsy-confirmed acute rejection episode. Remaining 190 recipients experienced stable graft function during long-term follow-up. 31 (33%) patients who suffered acute rejection subsequently lost their grafts in comparison to 22 (12%) patients without an episode of rejection. During the follow-up, 5 out of 93 (5.4%) patients with AGR and 13 out of 190 (6.8%) patients without AGR died for different reasons.

Six hundred and ninety unrelated healthy volunteers, constituting a basic control group in KIR studies performed in our laboratory, were recruited in the years 2001–2008 by the Regional Center of Blood Transfusion, Wroc^{3}aw, as well as by clinics of the Wroc^{3}aw Medical University, the Medical University of Warsaw, and the Pomeranian Medical University, Szczecin.

The same cohorts of patients and controls have already been used to describe a protective effect of *KIR2DS5* gene on kidney graft rejection and some other clinical situations [18].

The Bioethics Committee of the Wroc^{3}aw Medical University specifically approved this study. Signed written informed consent was given by all participants.

DNA isolation and KIR typing

DNA was isolated from venal blood as described [20,21]. The presence or absence of *KIR* genes was detected by either individual [20–22] or multiplex [23] polymerase chain reactions (PCR) which, when tested on the same samples, gave virtually identical results. Our *KIR* typing has been validated three times per year by the International KIR Exchange program organized by the Immunogenetics Center of the University of California at Los Angeles.

HLA-A, *-B*, and *-DR* typing of donors and recipients has been routinely done before transplantation either in Non-Public Tissue Typing Facility at our Institute or in other transplant centers in Poland, and it was drawn from the clinical histories of the patients. Tissue samples were available for only 42 donors, therefore their *HLA-C* typing was possible only in these instances, had statistically insufficient power, and therefore its results are not presented here. Recipient *HLA-C* variants encoding C1 and C2 epitopes were described and discussed earlier [18].

Statistical analysis

General linear model (GLM) with binomial errors was used to investigate relationship between clinical and genetic variables and probability of rejecting the transplanted kidney (**Table 2**). Frequencies of *KIR* genes in recipients and *HLA* matching between donors and recipients were explanatory variables. Clinical characteristics (age, sex, creatinine, course of transplantation and time of observation) was concomitant variables. Akaike's information criterion (AIC) was used as a measure of fit of models. *Bootstrap* approach was employed to estimate model's coefficients and 95% confidence intervals. Chi-squared test with Yates' continuity correction was used to test hypothesis that rejection and type of genotype were independent. To test differences in *KIR*'s distribution among patients and control, a group permutation test was employed. This procedure was based on Mahalanobis distance (D_M) between two groups and test performed in 10 000 permutations. *Odds ratio* (OR) was computed as a measure of effect size. Probability that graft is not rejected at a given time, S(t), was computed according to the Kaplan-Meier method, comparing *KIR* genotypes. Haplotype frequencies (HFs) among two *KIRs*: *2DS4* (full-length or deletion variant) and *2DS5* were estimated with *maximum likelihood* function [24].

Measures for the estimation of linkage disequilibrium (LD) were the correlation of two alleles frequencies, r, global squared correlation between two loci, R^2 and Kullback-Leibler divergency two loci from LE [24,25]. For two loci *2DS4* and *2DS5*, r and R^2 obtained as: $r = \frac{D_{ij}}{\sqrt{p_i q_j}}$, where p_i and q_j are the population allele frequencies of the ith allele on locus 2DS4 and the jth allele on locus *2DS5*, $D_{ij} = x_{ij} - p_i q_j$, and x_{ij} is the frequency of the haplotype with alleles i and j on loci *2DS4* and *2DS5*, respectively. $R^2 = \sum_i^3 \sum_j^2 \frac{D_{ij}^2}{p_i q_j}$. Kullback-Leibler divergence [26,27], D_{KL}, is a measure of distance between the observed haplotype distribution

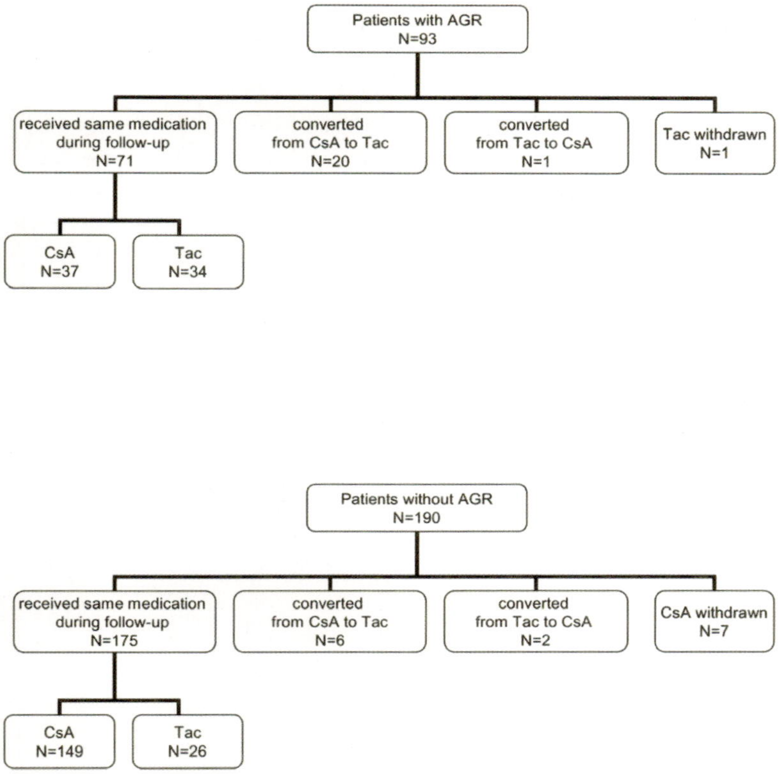

Figure 1. Patient disposition according to initial calcineurine inhibitor use. AGR, acute graft rejection; CsA, cyclosporine A; Tac, Tacrolimus.

and the expected distribution assuming LE: $D_{KL} = \sum_i^3 \sum_j^2 x_{ij} log \frac{x_{ij}}{p_i q_j}$. Chi-square statistic was calculated to test that all of the D_{ij}'s between 2DS4 and 2DS5 are zeros: $\chi^2_{df=2} = \sum_i^3 \sum_j^2 \frac{nD_{ij}^2}{p_i q_j}$. Likelihood ratio statistic, LRS, was used to test for differences in haplotype frequencies between rejectors, non-rejectors and controls.

$LRS_{df=5} = 2(LL_{\text{Rejectors}} + LL_{\text{Non-rejectors}} - LL_{\text{Combined}})$, where log likelihoods were produced based on haplotype frequencies and LRS is approximately a χ^2. Results were regarded as statistically significant at $p<0.05$. All data were analyzed using R version 2.2.1.

Results

HLA and *KIR2DS4* gene effects on acute kidney graft rejection

Frequencies of *KIR* genes were not different between patients and controls (**Table 3**). However, there were some differences between patients with acute graft rejection (AGR) (determined by Banff criteria) and patients without AGR. First, the frequency of the *KIR2DS5* gene in patients with AGR was two times lower than in control individuals (p = 0.0056). This protective effect of *KIR2DS5* gene on kidney graft rejection has already been published recently on the same cohorts of patients and controls [18]. Multivariate analysis indicated significant protective effect of *HLA-B,-DR* matching (**Table 2**) but HLA-A did not affect graft fate (data not shown). We also observed that the presence of both *KIR2DS4* full-length (*KIR2DS4fl*) and 22-base pair deletion variant (*KIR2DS4del)* gene was increasing a probability of rejection at least twofold (**Table 2**). This effect was amplified to a great extent by the *HLA-B,-DR* mismatching (matching = 0, **Figure 3**).

Effects of *KIR2DS4* gene variants and *KIR2DS5* gene on the probability of graft rejection

Probability that graft was not rejected at a given time, S(t), was computed for the presence or absence of *KIR2DS4fl*, *KIR2DS4del* or both (**Figure 4**). Simultaneous presence of both gene variants strongly increased the probability of graft rejection, whereas the presence of only *KIR2DS4fl*, only *KIR2DS4del*, or none of them gave much lower probability of rejection. Interestingly, the two variants of *KIR2DS4* gene had opposite influence on the effect of *KIR2DS5* gene: *KIR2DS5* seemed to protect the graft stronger in the presence of *KIR2DS4fl* than in its absence (**Figure 5**), but stronger in the absence than presence of *KIR2DS4del* (**Figure 6**).

Combinations of *KIR* genes gave 133 different genotypes present in patients and/or controls (data not shown). These genotypes were divided into AA and BX genotypes, containing two A haplotypes or at least one B haplotype, respectively (for a definition of A and B haplotypes, see Introduction). Two individual AA genotypes were distributed significantly differently between patient subgroups: among patients with the genotype No. 1 acute graft rejection (AGR) was nearly four times less frequent than lack of AGR (21.9% vs 78.1%), whereas in those with the genotype No. 2 the ratio of AGR and non-AGR was 1:1 (**Table 4**). Interestingly, these two genotypes differed only by the absence of full-length *KIR2DS4* gene in the genotype No. 1 and its presence in the genotype No. 2, and both were devoid of *KIR2DS5* by definition, as AA genotypes. An additional AA genotype containing *KIR2DS4fl* but no *KIR2DS4del* gene was extremely rare

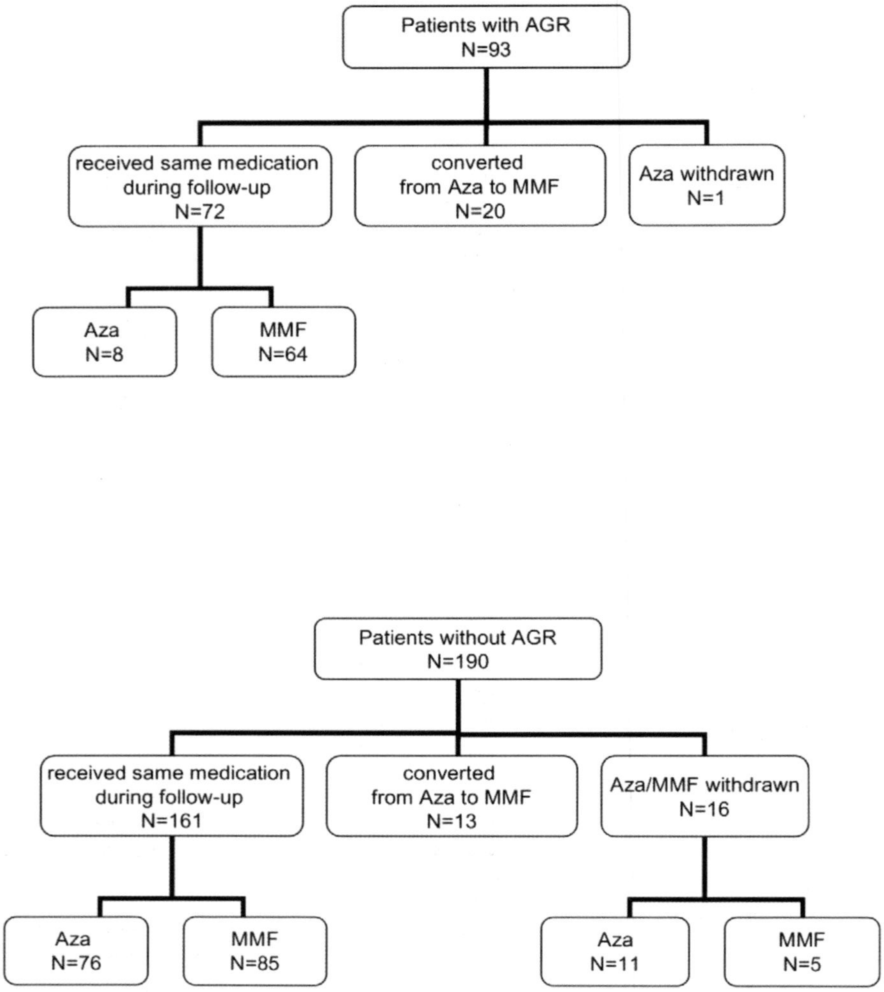

Figure 2. Patient disposition according to purine metabolism inhibitor use. AGR, acute graft rejection; Aza, azathioprine; MMF, mycophenolate mofetil.

Table 1. Clinical characteristics of patients.

		Patients with AGR	Patients without AGR	P	OR	95%CI
		N = 93	**N = 190**			
Age	Mean +/− SD	43.65±11.31	43.36±11.46	0.8		
	min-max	15–67	16–72			
Sex	Females/Males	32/61	92/98	0.03	0.56	0.33–0.93
	% of Females	34.4%	48.4%			
		N (%)	N (%)			
Cause	Glomerulonephritis	58 (62.4)	74 (39.0)	0.0002	2.60	1.56–4.33
of	Interstitial nephritis	10 (10.7)	27 (14.2)	0.46	0.73	0.34–1.58
renal	Cystic kidney	10 (10.7)	24 (12.6)	0.7	0.83	0.38–1.82
failure	Hypertensive nephropathy	3 (3.2)	13 (6.8)	0.28	0.45	0.13–1.63
	Diabetic nephropathy	5 (5.4)	7 (3.7)	0.54	1.49	0.46–4.81
	Other	7 (7.6)	45 (23.7)	0.0009	0.26	0.11–0.61

Table 2. Variables significantly associated with probability of graft rejection.

Variable	OR	95% CI		P
HLA-B+DR match	0.46	0.30	0.70	0.0003
KIR2DS4fl	2.02	1.05	3.90	0.03
KIR2DS4del	2.61	1.19	5.75	0.02
HLA-B+DR match×GN	2.01	1.46	2.76	0.0000

Abbreviations: CI, confidence interval; GN, glomerulonephritis; HLA, human leukocyte antigen; KIR, killer immunoglobulin-like receptor; *KIR2DS4fl*, *KIR2DS4* full length gene; *KIR2DS4del*, *KIR2DS4* 22-base pair deletion variant of the *KIR2DS4* gene; OR, odds ratio.

(one individual among patients and 8 in controls), therefore it could not play any role in rejection and was omitted from our calculations. Within BX (i.e., non-AA) genotype group, fraction of patients with AGR was nearly two times less frequent than these without AGR. These differences between genotype groups were not accidental ($\chi^2 = 6.675$, df = 2, p = 0.035).

KIR2DS4 and *KIR2DS5* are in negative linkage disequilibrium (LD) in all populations tested so far [28]. **Table 5** shows that they are in negative LD also in our population. *KIR2DS4/KIR2DS5* haplotype frequencies for non-rejectors and controls were very similar, and these two groups were combined in the following calculations. Likelihood ratio statistics (LRS) for patients with AGR versus combined group of patients without AGR and controls was high, which suggests that haplotype frequencies in the former were different from those in the latter (p = 0.05). We see, for example, that a haplotype *KIR2DS4−/KIR2DS5+* (*−/2DS5*) was three times less frequent in patients with AGR than in other groups. This seems to confirm a protective role of *KIR2DS5* in graft rejection shown above.

Difference between patients with glomerulonephritis and those with other kidney diseases in association of acute graft rejection with *KIR2DS4* and *HLA* genotype

Multivariate analysis revealed also a difference between patients whose end stage renal failure was caused by glomerulonephritis and those with other nephropathies. Namely, in the non-glomerulonephritis group, *HLA-B,-DR* matching seemed to be much more important for acute graft rejection than the presence or absence of *KIR2DS4* gene variants (**Figure 7**, right panel). Thus, in the case of perfect *HLA-B,-DR* matching (matching = 4), the presence or absence of *KIR2DS4fl* and *KIR2DS4del* genes only very weakly influenced graft fate. Recipients of completely *HLA-B,-DR* incompatible grafts (matching = 0) possessing both forms of *KIR2DS4* gene had only 6 times higher chance of kidney rejection than recipients of similarly *HLA-B,-DR*-incompatible grafts negative for *KIR2DS4* (**Figure 7**, right panel).

In contrast, in recipient group with glomerulonephritis, *HLA* incompatibility seemed to be much less important than *KIR2DS4* for graft rejection. For example, completely *HLA*-mismatched *KIR2DS4*-negative recipients had only about 1.4 times higher chance of acute rejection than perfectly *HLA*-matched *KIR2DS4*-negative recipients (**Figure 7**, left panel). On the other hand, the presence of both forms of *KIR2DS4* gene had strong effect on graft rejection in glomerulonephritis group, as even perfect HLA matching did not reduce a chance of rejection below odds ratio of 85 (**Figure 7**, left panel). Individuals from the glomerulonephritis group possessing both variants of *KIR2DS4* and perfect *HLA-B,-DR* matching had about 15 times higher chance of rejection than analogous persons from the non-glomerulonephritis group (see **Figure 7**, both panels).

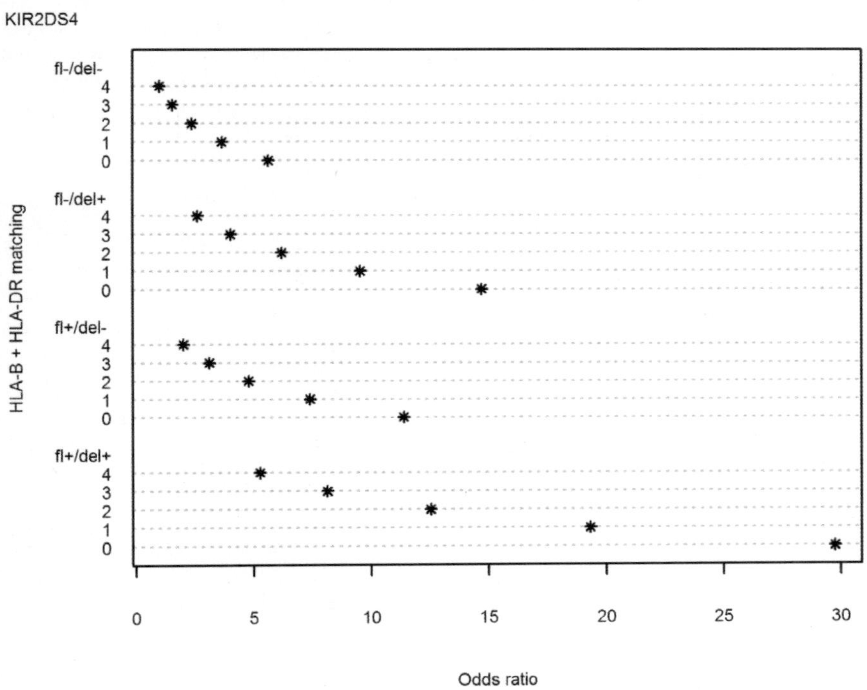

Figure 3. Dependence of odds ratio for kidney graft rejection on *HLA-B,-DR* matching, *KIR2DS4* full length (*KIR2DS4fl*) and/or *KIR2DS4* deletion variant (*KIR2DS4del*) gene presence. For odds ratio calculations, the recipient group with complete (n = 4) *HLA-B,-DR* match with the donor and a lack of any *KIR2DS4* variant (*KIR2DS4fl* and *KIR2DS4del* negative: fl-/del-) was taken as 1.

Table 3. *KIR* gene frequencies in controls and patients.

							KIR					
Group		**2DL1**	**2DL2**	**2DL3**	**2DS1**	**2DS2**	**2DS3**	**2DS4fl**	**2DS4del**	**2DS5**	**3DL1**	**3DS1**
Patients	Present	268	142	257	105	143	81	82	236	65	256	93
N = 283	%	94.70	50.18	90.81	37.10	50.53	28.62	28.97	83.39	22.97	90.46	32.86
Control	Present	665	374	623	299	369	214	194	561	205	642	264
N = 690	%	96.38	54.20	90.29	43.33	53.48	31.01	28.12	81.30	29.71	93.04	38.26
	p	0.3	0.3	0.9	0.07	0.4	0.5	0.8	0.5	0.03	0.2	0.1
	OR	0.67	0.85	1.06	0.77	0.89	0.89	1.04	1.55	0.71	0.71	0.79
	95%CI	0.35–1.29	0.65–1.12	0.66–1.71	0.58–1.03	0.67–1.17	0.66–1.21	0.77–1.42	0.80–1.67	0.51–0.97	0.43–1.16	0.59–1.06

Abbreviations: CI, confidence interval; KIR, killer immunoglobulin-like receptor; *KIR2DS4fl, KIR2DS4* full length gene; *KIR2DS4del, KIR2DS4* 22-base pair deletion variant of the *KIR2DS4* gene; OR, odds ratio.

Discussion

We compared the distribution of *KIR* genes in patients rejecting and non-rejecting kidney graft as well as in healthy controls. Among individual *KIR* genes, only *KIR2DS4* (both full-length and deletion variants) was remarkably more frequent in patients with AGR than in patients with stable graft function and controls. Moreover, this effect was particularly strong in the absence of *KIR2DS5* gene which exerted opposite effect, i.e., its presence decreased the chance of graft rejection as published already on the same cohorts of patients and controls [18]. It is interesting in this context that KIR2DS4 molecule was expressed on remarkable proportion of CD4+CD28− T cell clones isolated from an acute coronary syndrome patient [29]. Also, dialyzed patients exhibited an increased number of circulating CD4+CD28− T cells [30]. In addition, CMV positivity is universal in our transplant population (data not shown), and the association of CMV infection and the presence of CD4+CD28− cells is well documented (ref.30 and references therein). CD4+CD28− T cells, virtually absent from peripheral blood of healthy individuals but present in acute coronary syndrome and rheumatoid vasculitis [29], multiple sclerosis [14] and, most important here, in end-stage renal disease [30,31], were found to be resistant to immunoregulation [14] and therefore postulated to play a role in autoimmune diseases and aging [12]. *KIR2DS4fl* encodes an activating receptor which might possibly be involved in stimulation of effector cells (e.g., CD4+CD28− T cells) contributing to transplant rejection, whereas *KIR2DS4del* potentially codes for a soluble molecule [32]. It might be that, in kidney graft recipients, this soluble KIR2DS4 molecule is masking a ligand for membrane-bound KIR2DS4 or another receptor of some regulatory cells (T, NK, or other). The ligand for KIR2DS5 receptor is not known, however it has been observed that the simultaneous presence of *KIR2DS5* gene and *HLA-C*-encoded epitopes for both KIR2DL1 and KIR2DL2/3 receptors significantly decreased leukemia-free survival of hematopoietic stem cell-transplanted patients [33], which could suggest KIR2DS5 interaction with HLA-C. Thus, in the case of renal transplant recipients, soluble KIR2DS4 might block interaction of KIR2DS5 with its ligand which otherwise would protect a graft from rejection. In recipients negative for *KIR2DS4del* gene the presence of *KIR2DS5* seems to favor the

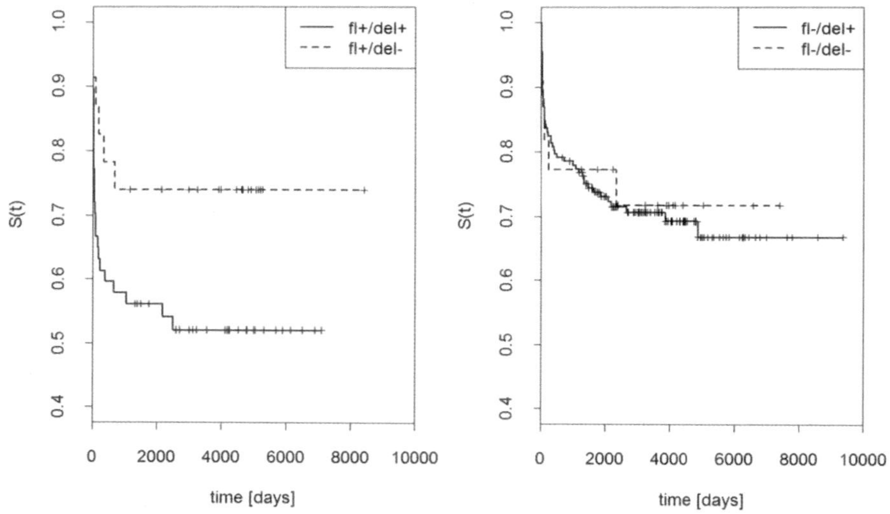

Figure 4. Effects of full-length *KIR2DS4* gene (fl) and its deletion variant (del) on the outcome of renal transplantation. Kaplan Kaplan-Meier estimations of probability that graft is not rejected at a given time, S(t). Left panel: *KIR2DS4fl* present, *KIR2DS4del* present or absent; right panel: *KIR2DS4fl* absent, *KIR2DS4del* present or absent.

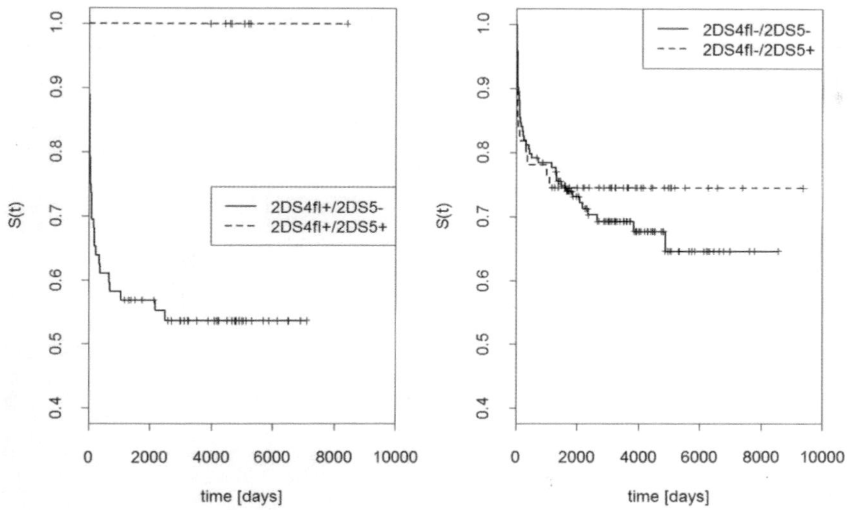

Figure 5. Effects of *KIR2DS5* and full-length (fl) *KIR2DS4* gene on the outcome of renal transplantation. Kaplan Kaplan-Meier estimations as in Figure 4. Left panel: *KIR2DS4fl* present, *KIR2DS5* present or absent; right panel: *KIR2DS4fl* absent, *KIR2DS5* present or absent.

acceptance of the graft, particularly in the presence of *KIR2DS4fl* gene. The reason for the latter effect is not clear; either both KIR2DS5 and KIR2DS4fl act in the same direction, e.g. expressed on the same or on two different regulatory cells, or, alternatively, the presence of *KIR2DS4fl* gene, by excluding the presence of its allele, *KIR2DS4del*, from the same chromosome, decreases its frequency in *KIR2DS4fl*-positive patient population.

KIR2DS4 molecule differs from KIR2DS1 and KIR2DS2/3 by weaker interaction with HLA-C and by binding to HLA-A*11 [34]. As mentioned in Material and Methods section, blood, lymphoid tissue or DNA samples of majority of donors were not available for our study, and their *HLA-C* typing was not possible here. However, in a recent study, Hanvesakul and coworkers [35] have not detected any association between **donor** *HLA-C*-encoded KIR ligand and acute rejection of kidney allograft. On the other hand, these authors have reported an effect of **recipient** *HLA-C* on the kidney graft rejection, i.e., a protective effect of C2 on allograft survival. They observed donor-derived NK cells in the allograft at the time of transplantation. These NK cells could stimulate maturation of dendritic cells which would then be capable of indirect stimulation of adaptive immune system for alloreactivity. *In vitro* studies of Hanvesakul et al. [35] have shown that donor-derived, interleukin-15-activated NK cells promoted efficiently the maturation of recipient dendritic cells only when these were C2-negative. They propose that, after kidney transplantation, donor NK cells interacting with recipient C2-positive dendritic cells do not stimulate them for maturation as efficiently as in C2-negative recipients, and this is beneficial for graft survival. In our earlier study, we have not observed such an effect of recipient C2 on graft survival; on the contrary, we have rather seen some, albeit weak and non-significant, association of C2 with kidney rejection [18]. The reason for this discrepancy may lie in numbers: our sample (283 patients) was 2.7 times less numerous than that of the British group (760 individuals). Alternatively, the

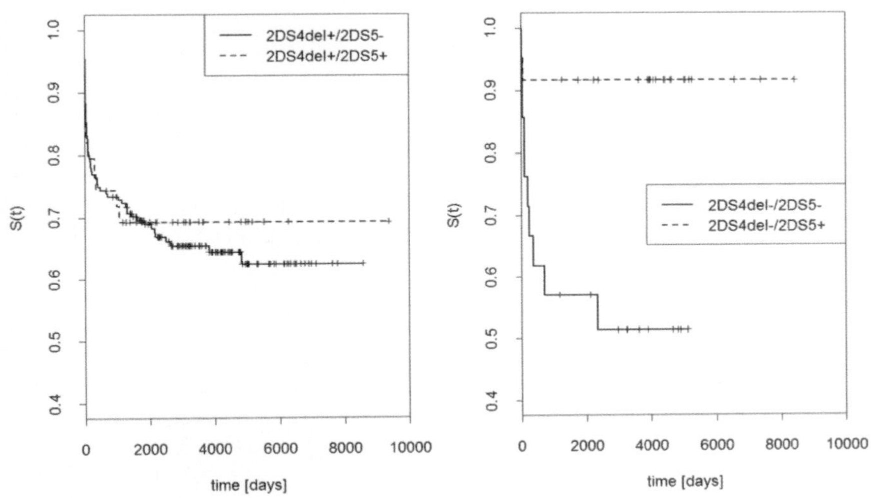

Figure 6. Effects of *KIR2DS5* and *KIR2DS4* deletion variant (*KIR2DS4del*) gene on the outcome of renal transplantation. Kaplan Kaplan-Meier estimations as in Figure 4. Left panel: *KIR2DS4del* present, *KIR2DS5* present or absent; right panel: *KIR2DS4del* absent, *KIR2DS5* present or absent.

Table 4. Distribution of *KIR* genotype groups in patients with and without acute graft rejection.

No.	Genotype	KIR 2DL1	2DL2	2DL3	2DS1	2DS2	2DS3	2DS4 fl	2DS4 del	2DS5	3DL1	3DS1	Pts with AGR N	Pts with AGR %	Pts without AGR N	Pts without AGR %
1	**AA/2DS4fl−**	+	−	+	−	−	−	−	+	−	+	−	14	21.9	50	78.1
2	**AA/2DS4fl+**	+	−	+	−	−	−	+	+	−	+	−	11	50.0	11	50.0
3	**BX**												68	34.5	129	65.5

Differences between frequencies of three genotype groups: $\chi^2 = 6.675$, df = 2, p = 0.035.
Abbreviations: AA, homozygote for the killer immunoglobulin-like receptor A haplotype (for a definition of A and B haplotypes, see Introduction); AGR, acute graft rejection; BX, a group of the killer immunoglobulin-like receptor genotypes containing at least one B haplotype; as they contain different combinations of KIR genes, the presence or absence of particular genes could not been shown here; KIR, killer immunoglobulin-like receptor; *KIR2DS4fl*, *KIR2DS4* full length gene; *KIR2DS4del*, *KIR2DS4* 22-base pair deletion variant of the *KIR2DS4* gene; Pts, patients.

British and our patients might have differed in a cause of renal failure: we have found a substantial genetic difference between recipients with glomerulonephritis and those with other conditions, whereas Hanvesakul et al. [35] did not show a clinical status of their patients before transplantation.

*HLA-A*11* allele (a KIR2DS4 ligand, see above) frequency in the Polish population is 6.239%, as established by Schmidt and colleagues [36]; therefore, its effect on kidney graft survival, if any, could not be strong. Nevertheless, we have noticed that a majority of *HLA-A11*-positive graft-rejecting recipients (4 out of 5) possessed *KIR2DS4fl* gene, whereas only one fifth of A11-positive patients with stable graft function (4 out of 20) typed positive for *KIR2DS4fl* (p = 0.02). However, the numbers were far too small for any conclusion. No difference between distribution of *KIR2DS4del* variant in A11-positive patients with and without AGR was seen (data not shown).

So far, only few publications dealt with *KIR* gene associations with kidney graft rejection. Tran et al. [37] studied an effect of KIR ligand (i.e., C1, C2, and Bw4) matching on graft survival in 1416 recipients of cadaver kidney (both first grafts and regrafts) from all inhabited continents, but did not detect any effect. Similarly negative result was obtained by Kreijveld et al. [38] who tested not only KIR ligands, but also *KIR* genes themselves as well as combinations of both in Dutch population. On the other hand, upon testing a *KIR* polymorphism in *HLA*-identical recipient-donor pairs from U.S.A., Cirocco et al. [39] obtained a result suggesting protective effect of *KIR2DL2* and *KIR2DS2* genes; however, their study was based on extremely low number of individuals (only 12 recipient-donor pairs). Nevertheless, this finding was confirmed by Kunert et al. [40] on 105 graft recipients and 119 controls in Germany. Finally, van Bergen et al. [41] observed an effect of KIR-KIR ligand mismatch between recipient and donor in Dutch population, but only in *HLA-A,-B,-DR*-compatible donor-recipient pairs, i.e., when *HLA*-identical partners differed in their *KIR* gene repertoire, resulting in lack of a ligand in donor for a KIR present in recipient. Notably, the effect of *KIRs* in *HLA*-matched pairs was as strong as that of *HLA-A,-B* mismatch in pairs matched only for *HLA-DR* [41,42]. In our study, we observed a strong effect of *KIR2DS4* variants in patients with glomerulonephritis, where *HLA-B,-DR* mismatch exerted much weaker influence on the graft fate, whereas in recipients without glomerulonephritis the effect of HLA-mismatch was predominant. The striking finding of this study was the stronger association of *KIR2DS4* polymorphism than *HLA* incompatibility in GN patients. We can speculate that engagement of KIRs in inflammatory pathway activation defined by their polymorphism may represent a common link between autoimune and alloimmune response. The possibility that KIR-ligand interaction may aggravate both the natural history of glomerulonephritis sustaining immune injury leading to end-stage renal disease and influence alloimmune

Table 5. Linkage disequilibrium between *KIR2DS4* gene variants and *KIR2DS5* gene in patients and controls.

Group	Haplotypes	2DS4full/2DS5	2DS4del/2DS5	—/DS25	2DS4full/—	2DS4del/—	—/—
Controls	HFs	0.000	0.006	0.155	0.152	0.558	0.129
	r	−0.157	−0.282	0.512	0.069	0.123	−0.224
	$R^2 = 0.436$	$D_{KL} = 0.306$	$\chi^2 = 300$	*df* = 2	p<0.00001		
Patients with AGR	HFs	0.000	0.041	0.048	0.214	0.636	0.061
	r	−0.138	−0.079	0.39	0.043	0.025	−0.122
	$R^2 = 0.194$	$D_{KL} = 0.102$	$\chi^2 = 17.49$	*df* = 2	p = 0.00016		
Patients without AGR	HFs	0.005	0.000	0.136	0.131	0.586	0.142
	r	−0.138	−0.287	0.489	0.042	0.116	−0.198
	$R^2 = 0.395$	$D_{KL} = 0.278$	$\chi^2 = 77.06$	*df* = 2	p<0.00001		

Abbreviations: AGR, acute graft rejection; HFs, haplotype frequencies; D_{KL}, Kullback-Leibler divergence from linkage equilibrium; KIR, killer immunoglobulin-like receptor; *KIR2DS4fl*, *KIR2DS4* full length gene; *KIR2DS4del*, *KIR2DS4* 22-base pair deletion variant of the *KIR2DS4* gene; R^2, global squared correlation coefficient for two loci; r, correlation coefficient for alleles frequencies. *Likelihood ratio statistics* (LRS): {Pts with AGR} *vs* {Controls+Pts without AGR}; LRS = 11.01; *df* = 5; p = 0.0513.

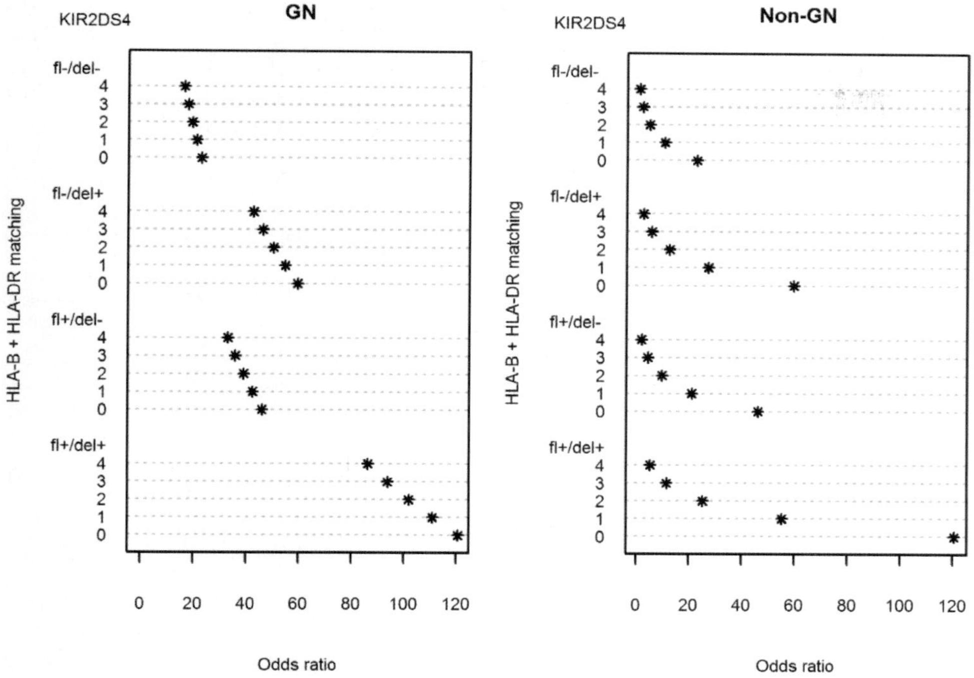

Figure 7. Effect of glomerulonephritis on the dependence of odds ratio for kidney graft rejection on *HLA-B,-DR* matching, *KIR2DS4* full length (*KIR2DS4fl*) and/or *KIR2DS4* deletion variant (*KIR2DS4del*) gene presence. For odds ratio calculations, the non-GN group with complete (n = 4) *HLA-B,-DR* match and lack of any *KIR2DS4* variant (*KIR2DS4fl* and *KIR2DS4del* negative: fl-/del) was taken as 1.

response causing acute rejection cannot be ruled out. In this setting, *KIR2DS4* polymorphism can provoke the immune response as it can modulate autoimmunity. We can hypothesize that GN and non-GN patients may differ in KIR2D receptor expression on NK and T cells, particularly in those rejecting vs. non-rejecting the graft, as it has recently been shown in liver transplantation [43].

In summary, our results suggest that typing of the recipient for *KIR2DS4* and *KIR2DS5* genes may help to predict the outcome of renal transplantation. We show here, for the first time, that the effect of *KIR* genotype on the fate of kidney graft in recipients with glomerulonephritis seems to be stronger than that of *HLA* matching, whereas opposite is true for patients with other causes of end-stage renal disease. The lack of strong association of graft rejection with *HLA-B,-DR* mismatching in recipients with glomerulonephritis could not have been observed in earlier studies done without stratification for the presence or absence of *KIR2DS4* gene. However, a small number of data that was collected over a long time period is a limitation to the reliability of our findings. Therefore, more definitive studies would require data input from much higher number of patients and, preferably, from more than one institution.

Acknowledgments

We wish to thank our patients for blood donation and agreement to participate in this study. We are also grateful to Mr. Maciej Sobczyñski, M. Sci., from the Faculty of Biotechnology, University of Wroc[3]aw, for statistical analysis.

Author Contributions

Conceived and designed the experiments: PK IN MM-P. Performed the experiments: IN EM AW WŁ MM AK MW WN-M M. Kaminska. Analyzed the data: PK IN MM-P. Contributed reagents/materials/analysis tools: MM-P AP RP EB M. Klinger DS. Wrote the paper: PK IN MM-P.

References

1. Womer KL, Kaplan B (2009) Recent developments in kidney transplantation – a critical assessment. Am J Transplant 9: 1265–1271.
2. Nankivell BJ, Alexander SI (2010) Rejection of the kidney allograft. N Engl J Med 363: 1451–1462.
3. Andersen CB, Ladefoged SD, Larsen S (1994) Acute kidney graft rejection. A morphological and immunohistochemical study on 'zero-hour' and follow-up biopsies with special emphasis on cellular infiltrates and adhesion molecules. APMIS 102: 23–37.
4. Hancock WW, Gee D, De Moerloose P, Rickles FR, Ewan VA, et al. (1985) Immunohistological analysis of serial biopsies taken during human renal allograft rejection. Changing profile of infiltrating cells and activation of the coagulation system. Transplantation 39: 430–438.
5. Totterman TH, Hanas E, Bergstrom R, Larsson E, Tufveson G (1989) Immunologic diagnosis of kidney rejection using FACS analysis of graft-infiltrating functional and activated T and NK cell subsets. Transplantation 47: 817–823.
6. Cooksey G, Robins RA, Blamey RW (1984) Natural killer cells in renal allograft rejection. Br J Surg 71: 874–877.
7. Vampa ML, Norman PJ, Burnapp L, Vaughan RW, Sacks SH, et al. (2003) Natural killer-cell activity after human renal transplantation in relation to killer immunoglobulin-like receptors and human leukocyte antigen mismatch. Transplantation 76: 1220–1228.
8. Parham P (2005) MHC class I molecules and KIRs in human history, health and survival. Nature Rev Immunol 5: 201–214.
9. Moretta L, Locatelli F, Pende D, Marcenaro E, Mingari MC, et al. (2011) Killer Ig-like receptor-mediated control of natural killer cell alloreactivity in haploidentical hematopoietic stem cell transplantation. Blood 117: 764–771.
10. Velardi A, Ruggeri L, Mancusi A, Aversa F, Christiansen FT (2009) Natural killer cell allorecognition of missing self in allogeneic hematopoietic transplantation: a tool for immunotherapy of leukemia. Curr Opin Immunol 21: 525–530.
11. Pegram HJ, Ritchie DS, Smyth MJ, Wiernik A, Prince HM, et al. (2011) Alloreactive natural killer cells in hematopoietic stem cell transplantation. Leuk Res 35: 14–21.

12. Weng N-p, Akbar AN, Goronzy J (2009) CD28− T cells: their role in the age-associated decline of immune function. Trends Immunol 30: 306–312.
13. Snyder MR, Nakajima T, Leibson PJ, Weyand CM, Goronzy JJ (2004) Stimulatory killer Ig-like receptors modulate T cell activation through DAP12-dependent and DAP12-independent mechanisms. J Immunol 173: 3725–3731.
14. Thewissen M, Somers V, Hellings N, Fraussen J, Damoiseaux J, et al. (2007) CD4+CD28^{null} T cells in autoimmune disease: Pathogenic features and decreased susceptibility to immunoregulation. J Immunol 179: 6514–6523.
15. Middleton D, Meenagh A, Moscoso J, Arnaiz-Villena A (2008) Killer immunoglobulin receptor gene and allele frequencies in Caucasoid, Oriental and Black populations from different continents. Tissue Antigens 71: 105–113.
16. Middleton D, Gonzelez F (2009) The extensive polymorphism of KIR genes. Immunology 129: 8–19.
17. Shilling HG, Young N, Guethlein LA, Cheng NW, Gardiner CM, et al. (2002) Genetic control of human NK repertoire. J Immunol 169: 239–247.
18. Nowak I, Majorczyk E, Wiśniewski A, Pawlik A, Magott-Procelewska M, et al. (2010) Does the KIR2DS5 gene protect from some human diseases? PLoS ONE 5: e12381.
19. Racusen LC, Solez K, Colvin RB, Bonsib SM, Castro MC, et al. (1999) The Banff 97 working classification of renal allograft pathology. Kidney International 55: 713–723.
20. Majorczyk E, Pawlik A, Łuszczek W, Nowak I, Wiśniewski A, et al. (2007) Associations of killer cell immunoglobulin-like receptor genes with complications of rheumatoid arthritis. Genes Immunity 8: 678–683.
21. Łuszczek W, Mańczak M, Cisło M, Nockowski P, Wiśniewski A, et al. (2004) Gene for the activating natural killer cell receptor, KIR2DS1, is associated with susceptibility to psoriasis vulgaris. Hum Immunol 65: 758–766.
22. Vilches C, Castaño J, Gómez-Lozano N, Estefanía E (2007) Facilitation of KIR genotyping by a PCR-SSP method that amplifies short DNA fragments. Tissue Antigens 70: 415–422.
23. Sun JY, Gaidulis L, Miller MM, Goto RM, Rodriguez R, et al. (2004) Development of a multiplex PCR-SSP method for killer cell immunoglobulin-like receptor genotyping. Tissue Antigens 64: 462–468.
24. Excoffier L, Slatkin M (1995) Maximum-likelihood estimation of molecular haplotype frequencies in a diploid population. Mol Biol Evol 12: 921–927.
25. Abdallah JM, Goffinet B, Cierco-Ayrolles C, Pérez-Enciso M (2003) Linkage disequilibrium fine mapping of quantitative trait loci: a simulation study. Genet Sel Evol 35: 513–532.
26. Bhasi K, Zhang L, Brazeau D, Zhang A, Ramanathan M (2006) Information-theoretic identification of predictive SNPs and supervised visualization of genome-wide association studies. Nucleic Acids Res 34: e101.
27. Liu Z, Lin S (2005) Multilocus LD measure and tagging SNP selection with generalized mutual information. Genet Epidemiol 29: 353–364.
28. Single RM, Martin MP, Meyer D, Gao X, Carrington M (2008) Methods for assessing gene content diversity of KIR with examples from a global set of populations. Immunogenetics 60: 711–725.
29. Yen JH, Moore BE, Nakajima T, Scholl D, Schaid DJ, et al. (2001) Major histocompatibility complex class I-recognizing receptors are disease risk genes in rheumatoid arthritis. J Exp Med 193: 1159–1167.
30. Yadav AK, Jha V (2011) CD4^{+}CD28^{null} cells are expanded and exhibit a cytolytic profile in end-stage renal disease patients on peritoneal dialysis. Nephrol Dial Transplant 26: 1689–1694.
31. Betjes MGH, Huisman M, Weimar W, Litjens NHR (2008) Expansion of cytolytic CD4+CD28− T cells in end-stage renal disease. Kidney International 74: 760–767.
32. Middleton D, Gonzalez A, Gilmore PM (2007) Studies on the expression of the deleted KIR2DS4*003 gene product and distribution of KIR2DS4 deleted and nondeleted versions in different populations. Hum Immunol 68: 128–134.
33. van der Meer A, Schaap NPM, Schattenberg AVMB, van Cranenbroek B, Tijssen HJ, Joosten I (2998) KIR2DS5 is associated with leukemia free survival after HLA identical stem cell transplantation in chronic myeloid leukemia patients. Molec Immunol 45: 3631–3638.
34. Graef T, Moesta AK, Norman PJ, Abi-Rached L, Vago L, et al. (2009) KIR2DS4 is a product of gene conversion with KIR3DL2 that introduced specificity for HLA-A*11 while diminishing avidity for HLA-C. J Exp Med 206: 2557–2572.
35. Hanvesakul R, Kubal C, Moore J, Neil D, Cook M, Ball S, et al. (2011) KIR and HLA-C interactions promote differential dendritic cell maturation and is a major determinant of graft failure following kidney transplantation. PLoS ONE 6: e23631.
36. Schmidt AH, Solloch UV, Pingel J, Baier D, Böhme I, et al. (2011) High resolution human leukocyte antigen allele and haplotype frequencies of the Polish population based on 20,653 stem cell donors. Hum Immunol 72: 558–565.
37. Tran TH, Mytilineos J, Scherer S, Laux G, Middleton D, et al. (2005) Analysis of KIR ligand incompatibility in human renal transplantation. Transplantation 80: 1121–1123.
38. Kreijveld E, van der Meer A, Tijssen HJ, Hilbrands LB, Joosten I (2007) KIR gene and KIR ligand analysis to predict graft rejection after renal transplantation. Transplantation 84: 1045–1051.
39. Cirocco RE, Mathew JM, Burke GW 3rd, Esquenazi V, Miller J (2007) Killer cell immunoglobulin-like receptor polymorphisms in HLA-identical kidney transplant recipients: lack of 2DL2 and 2DS2 may be associated with poor graft function. Tissue Antigens 69 (Suppl 1): S123–S124.
40. Kunert K, Seiler M, Mashreghi MF, Klippert K, Schönemann C, et al. (2007) KIR/HLA ligand incompatibility in kidney transplantation. Transplantation 84: 1527–1533.
41. van Bergen J, Thompson A, Haasnoot GW, Roodnat JI, de Fijter JW, et al. (2011) KIR-ligand mismatches are associated with reduced long-term graft survival in HLA-compatible kidney transplantation. Am J Transplant 11: 1959–1964.
42. Rajalingam R, Gebel HM (2011) KIR-HLA mismatching in human renal allograft transplantation: Emergence of a new concept. Am J Transplant 11: 1771–1772.
43. López-Álvarez MR, Campillo JA, Legaz I, Blanco-García RM, Salgado-Cecilia G, et al. (2011) Divergences in KIR2D+ natural killer and KIR2D+ CD8+ T-cell reconstitution following liver transplantation. Hum Immunol 72: 229–237.

3

Promoting Long-Term Survival of Insulin-Producing Cell Grafts That Differentiate from Adipose Tissue-Derived Stem Cells to Cure Type 1 Diabetes

Shuzi Zhang, Hehua Dai, Ni Wan, Yolonda Moore, Zhenhua Dai*

Department of Microbiology and Immunology, Center for Biomedical Research, University of Texas Health Science Center, Tyler, Texas, United States of America

Abstract

Background: Insulin-producing cell clusters (IPCCs) have recently been generated in vitro from adipose tissue-derived stem cells (ASCs) to circumvent islet shortage. However, it is unknown how long they can survive upon transplantation, whether they are eventually rejected by recipients, and how their long-term survival can be induced to permanently cure type 1 diabetes. IPCC graft survival is critical for their clinical application and this issue must be systematically addressed prior to their in-depth clinical trials.

Methodology/Principal Findings: Here we found that IPCC grafts that differentiated from murine ASCs in vitro, unlike their freshly isolated islet counterparts, did not survive long-term in syngeneic mice, suggesting that ASC-derived IPCCs have intrinsic survival disadvantage over freshly isolated islets. Indeed, β cells retrieved from IPCC syngrafts underwent faster apoptosis than their islet counterparts. However, blocking both Fas and TNF receptor death pathways inhibited their apoptosis and restored their long-term survival in syngeneic recipients. Furthermore, blocking CD40-CD154 costimulation and Fas/TNF signaling induced long-term IPCC allograft survival in overwhelming majority of recipients. Importantly, Fas-deficient IPCC allografts exhibited certain immune privilege and enjoyed long-term survival in diabetic NOD mice in the presence of CD28/CD40 joint blockade while their islet counterparts failed to do so.

Conclusions/Significance: Long-term survival of ASC-derived IPCC syngeneic grafts requires blocking Fas and TNF death pathways, whereas blocking both death pathways and CD28/CD40 costimulation is needed for long-term IPCC allograft survival in diabetic NOD mice. Our studies have important clinical implications for treating type 1 diabetes via ASC-derived IPCC transplantation.

Editor: Matthias G. von Herrath, La Jolla Institute for Allergy and Immunology, United States of America

Funding: This work was supported by a research grant from Juvenile Diabetes Research Foundation International (JDRF 1-2008-583, www.jdrf.org). The funders had no role in study design, data collection and analysis, decision to publish, or preparation of the manuscript.

Competing Interests: The authors have declared that no competing interests exist.

* E-mail: zhenhua.dai@uthct.edu

Introduction

Pancreatic islet transplantation holds much promise for the cure of type 1 diabetes as transplantation of cadaveric islets is already conducted in the clinic to treat patients with type 1 diabetes. However, the scarcity of human donor islets remains a major obstacle to widespread islet transplantation. It is therefore compelling to search for alternative sources of islets. Embryonic stem cells originally have been exploited as a source for β cells due to their tremendous differentiation potential. Previous studies have shown that insulin-secreting cells are indeed generated from embryonic stem cells [1,2,3,4,5,6,7]. However, their application in translational medicine could be limited because of ethical and legal concerns. Therefore, adult mesenchymal stem cells have recently been studied to generate β cells. Previous studies have shown that insulin-producing cells can be generated from bone marrow cells [8], hepatic [9] and pancreatic stem cells [10]. Nevertheless, the limited sources and invasive procedures have hampered their progress.

Adipose tissue has recently gained much attention as a prime source of mesenchymal stem cells that can differentiate into the cells of mesodermal origin, including insulin-producing cell clusters (IPCCs) [11]. The simple surgical procedure, easy accessibility, uncomplicated isolation and tissue abundance make adipose tissue a most attractive source of mesenchymal stem cells for researchers [11,12,13]. Indeed, recent studies have shown that IPCCs can differentiate from both human and murine adipose tissue-derived stem cells (ASCs) [14,15,16,17]. Moreover, transplantation of ASCs over-expressing Pdx1 gene [18,19] or IPCCs generated from ASCs in vitro [16,17] restored normoglycemia in chemical-induced diabetic mice, although it was not known how long IPCC graft survival could last, suggesting that ASCs or ASC-derived IPCCs may be potentially utilized to treat human type 1 diabetes. However, it remains unknown how long IPCC grafts survive upon transplantation and how their long-term survival can be induced in diabetic recipients.

In this study, we generated IPCCs that differentiated from murine ASCs in vitro and investigated their survival after transplantation in diabetic mice. The aim of this study is to induce long-term IPCC graft survival in a preclinical animal model, because their long-term survival is critical for the cure of type 1 diabetes. Previous studies have focused on other important issues at the early stage of IPCC studies, including the generation of IPCCs in vitro, their temporary functions in vivo, and their immunogenicity. The novelty of this study lies in the first induction of long-term IPCC graft survival in diabetic mice, including autoimmune-prone NOD mice, by blocking both IPCC cell death and T cell costimulation.

Results

In vitro differentiation of ASCs into IPCCs

ASCs were isolated from the fat pads of C57BL/6 mice as described previously [16,20]. Although newly isolated ASCs had a heterogeneous phenotype in the initial culture, a single fibroblastoid cell population was expanded following the subsequent cultures. The homogeneity of ASCs at passages 4–6 was confirmed by FACS analysis showing that they highly expressed CD29, CD44, CD90, CD105 and Sca-1 surface markers [16], as shown in Figure 1. They also expressed low MHC-class-I while lacking MHC-class-II, CD45 and CD80. Day-10 IPCCs highly expressed many genes related to pancreatic endocrine development and glucose sensing (Figure 2). The IPCCs were stained positively for DTZ, a zinc-chelating agent that specifically stains pancreatic β cells (Figure 3A). RT-PCR also showed that IPCCs and islets express insulin mRNA while undifferentiated ASCs do not (Figure 3B). Immunofluorescence staining demonstrated that both IPCCs (Figure 3C) and freshly isolated islets (Figure 3D) abundantly express insulin and C-peptide before transplantation. Moreover, IPCC grafts also highly expressed insulin and C-peptide (Figure 3E) compared to isotype control (Figure 3F) five days after they were transplanted under the kidney capsule of recipient mice. These findings confirmed that IPCCs express both insulin and C-peptide at both gene and protein levels. Finally, IPCCs, just like their islet counterparts, released significant amount of insulin upon in vitro-stimulation with high glucose, as shown in the supporting information (Figure S1), suggesting that ASC-derived IPCCs are fully functional.

Blocking Fas and TNF signaling promotes IPCC graft survival in syngeneic recipients

It remains unclear whether IPCC grafts, like freshly isolated islets, can survive forever in a syngeneic recipient. Either islets or ASC-derived IPCCs from B6 donors (H-2^b) were transplanted to B6.Rag1-/- or WT B6 recipients. Surprisingly, we found that most IPCC syngrafts did not survive for long-term in both Rag1-/- and WT B6 recipients (Median survival time, MST = 37 and 22 days) while almost all of islet syngrafts survived for long-term in both recipients (Figure 4A), suggesting that ASC-derived IPCC grafts have a survival disadvantage over their freshly isolated islet counterparts, perhaps because of their passive cell death even in the absence of alloimmunity. We therefore retrieved IPCCs or islets and determined their cell apoptosis one week after their transplantation in syngeneic mice. As shown in Figure 4B, IPCC cells underwent much faster apoptosis than islet cells (percentage of TUNEL-positive cells: 25±3 or 26±4 vs. 9±2 or 10±3, both $P<0.05$).

We then investigated how to prevent the failure of IPCC grafts in syngeneic mice by transplanting IPCCs derived from either WT B6 or B6.Fas-/- donors to WT B6 recipients or treating recipients with anti-FasL or anti-TNFα blocking Ab. As shown in Figure 5A, most IPCC syngrafts (63%), which differentiated from Fas-/- ASCs, achieved long-term survival (MST>100 days) whereas 88% of IPCC syngrafts that differentiated from WT-derived ASCs failed to do so (MST = 22 days, Figure 4A). IPCCs that differentiated from Fas-/- ASCs were confirmed to be Fas-negative by FACS analysis (data not shown). Moreover, treatments with either anti-FasL or anti-TNFα blocking Ab in recipients that received Fas-replete IPCCs significantly prolonged IPCC syngraft survival compared with isotype Ab control (MST = 79 vs. 21 or 60 vs. 21 days, both $P<0.05$, Figure 5A). Importantly, blocking both Fas and TNF death pathways via anti-TNFα Ab treatment plus transplantation of Fas-

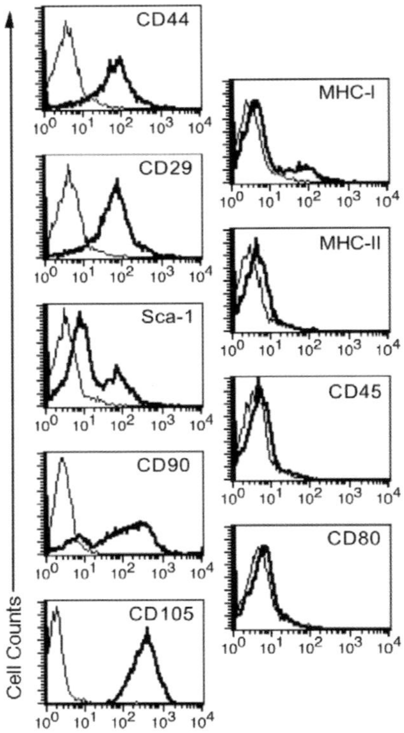

Figure 1. In vitro characterization of ASCs for their markers. Expanded ASC clone at passage 4 was assessed by flow cytometric analysis. Expanded ASCs highly expressed CD29, CD44, CD90, CD105 and Sca-1 while their MHC class-I expression was low. They did not express MHC class-II, CD45 and CD80 at all. One representative of three separate experiments is shown.

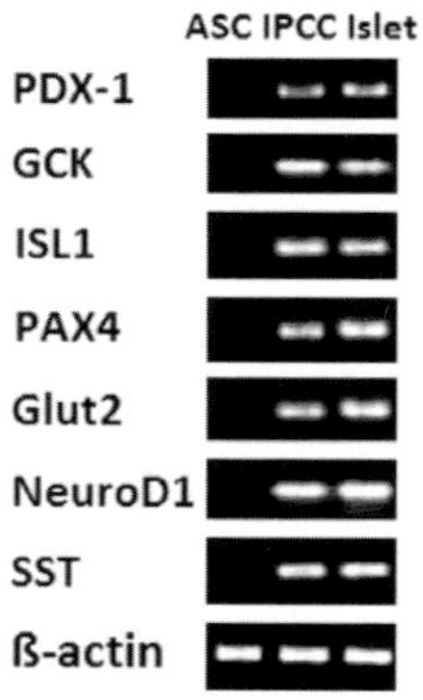

Figure 2. Gene expression of pancreatic endocrine and development markers by ASC-derived IPCCs. Expression of genes by day-10 IPCCs that are related to pancreatic development, hormones and glucose sensing was analyzed by RT-PCR. One representative of three independent experiments is shown.

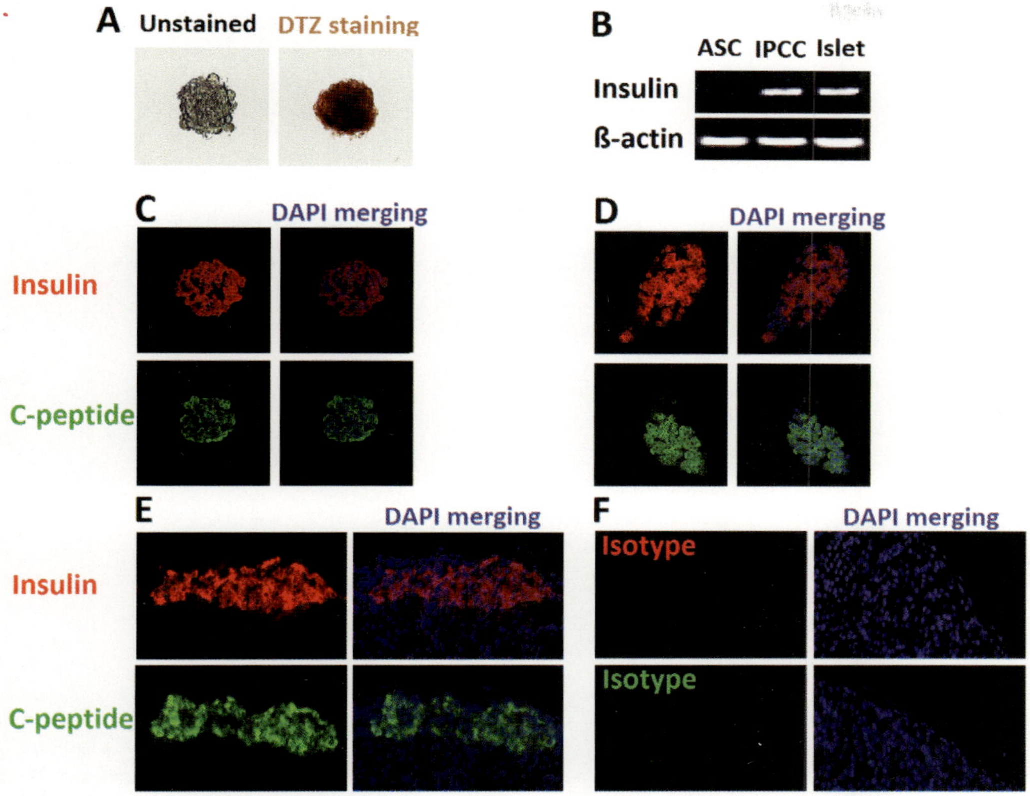

Figure 3. DTZ staining, gene expression and immunofluorescence analysis of IPCCs. (**A**): Day-10 IPCCs were stained with dithizone (DTZ), a agent that selectively stains pancreatic β cells because of their high zinc content. (**B**): Insulin and C-peptide gene expression by RT-PCR. (**C**): Day-10 IPCCs were stained for insulin and C-peptide without transplantation. (**D**) Fresh islets were stained for insulin and C-peptide without transplantation. (**E**): IPCC grafts under the kidney capsule were stained with insulin and C-peptide five days after their transplantation. (**F**): Isotype Ab staining for IPCC grafts. Cell nuclei were stained with DAPI. One representative of three separate experiments is shown.

deficient IPCCs induced long-term IPCC syngraft survival in 7 of 8 recipients. TUNEL analyses confirmed that either Fas deficiency or neutralizing TNFα significantly inhibited IPCC graft cell apoptosis in syngeneic recipients (Figure 5B). These data indicate that blocking Fas death signaling alone is capable of inducing long-term IPCC graft survival in majority of syngeneic recipients while blocking both Fas and TNF death pathways induces long-term IPCC graft survival in nearly all recipients.

Blocking CD40-CD154 (CD40L) costimulation and death pathways induces long-term IPCC allograft survival

Since IPCC recipients likely needs fat tissues from allogeneic donors as a source of ASCs, we investigated whether IPCC allografts would be quickly rejected. To minimize the passive cell death, IPCCs that differentiated from Fas-deficient ASCs isolated from B6.Fas-/- donors were transplanted to WT Balb/C recipients. Recipient mice were then treated with either MR1 (anti-CD154 Ab) or CTLA4-Ig to block CD40-CD154 or B7-CD28 costimulation. As shown in Figure 6A, all Fas-deficient IPCC allografts were rejected within 40 days (MST = 20 days), compared with 63% of Fas-deficient IPCC syngrafts that achieved long-term survival (Figure 5A), suggesting that IPCCs, like intact islets from donors, are immunogenic and subject to acute rejection. However, blocking CD40-CD154 costimulation induced long-term survival of Fas-deficient IPCC allografts in 63% of recipients (Figure 6A), indicating that CD40 blockade is sufficient to prevent IPCC allograft rejection mediated by alloimmune responses. Moreover, blocking CD28 also significantly prolonged IPCC allograft survival (MST = 55 vs. 20 days, $P<0.05$), albeit less effective than CD40 blockade (MST = 55 vs. >100 days, $P<0.05$). Blocking CD40 plus neutralizing TNFα further suppressed Fas-deficient IPCC allograft rejection with 88% of recipients achieving long-term survival. Finally, blocking CD40 and death pathways with triple Abs (MR1+ anti-FasL+ anti-TNFα) was confirmed to induce long-term Fas-replete IPCC allograft survival in most recipients (71%). As controls, isotype Abs did not alter IPCC allograft survival and Fas-replete IPCC allografts without any treatment were acutely rejected within 30 days (data not shown). The kidneys harboring IPCC grafts from some recipients with long-term graft survival were removed to confirm IPCC graft function in diabetic recipients. On the other hand, H&E staining demonstrated massive cell infiltration surrounding IPCC allografts in control group (Fig. 6B), but nearly no infiltration in MR1+anti-TNFα treated recipients (Fig. 6C) two weeks after IPCC transplantation. Taken together, these findings suggest that blocking CD40 and Fas/TNF-receptor death signaling is capable of inducing long-term IPCC allograft survival.

Blocking CD40 or CD28 costimulatory pathway suppresses allograft-infiltrating T cell proliferation in vivo

To further determine how the costimulatory blockade inhibits alloimmunity or IPCC allograft rejection, graft-infiltrating cells were isolated one week after IPCC transplantation and alloreactive T cell proliferation in vivo was measured by BrdU uptakes. As

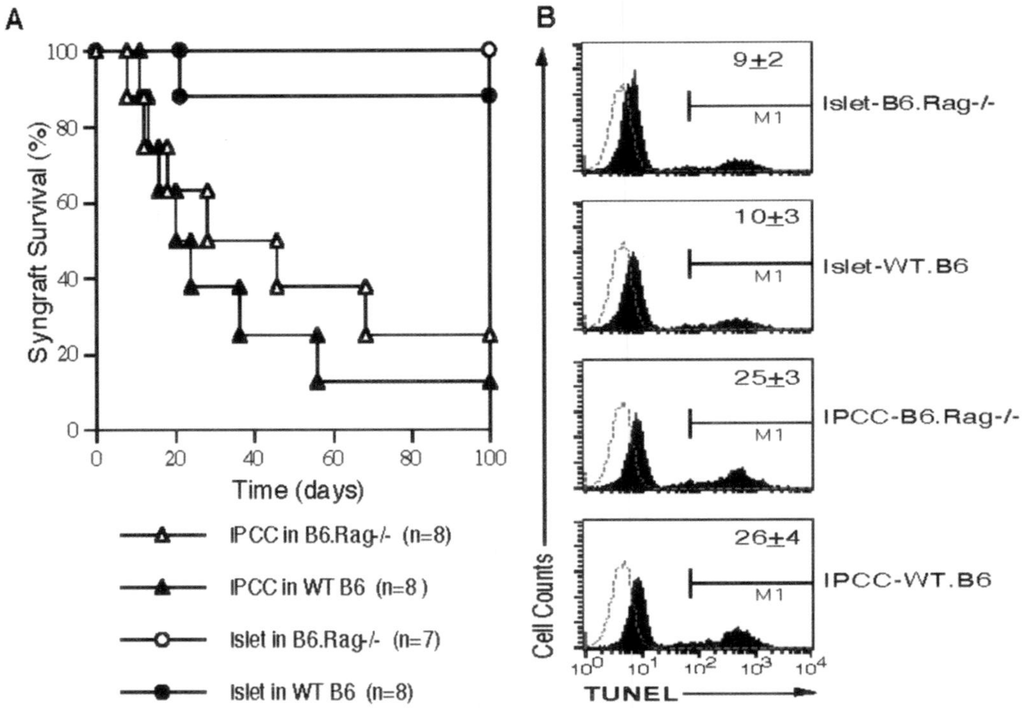

Figure 4. Impaired IPCC, but not islet, graft survival in syngeneic recipient mice. Islets freshly isolated from B6 donors or IPCCs that differentiated from B6-derived ASCs were transplanted under kidney capsule of either B6.Rag-/- or WT B6 recipient mice that were rendered diabetic by a single injection of streptozotocin before transplantation. Islet and IPCC syngraft rejection was observed (**A**). In separate groups, transplanted islets or IPCCs were retrieved and dissociated with trypsin-EDTA one week after transplantation. Cells were then stained with PE-conjugated PDX-1 and their apoptosis was measured by a TUNEL method (**B**). Histograms are gated on PDX-1-positive β cell population. One representative of three separate experiments is shown.

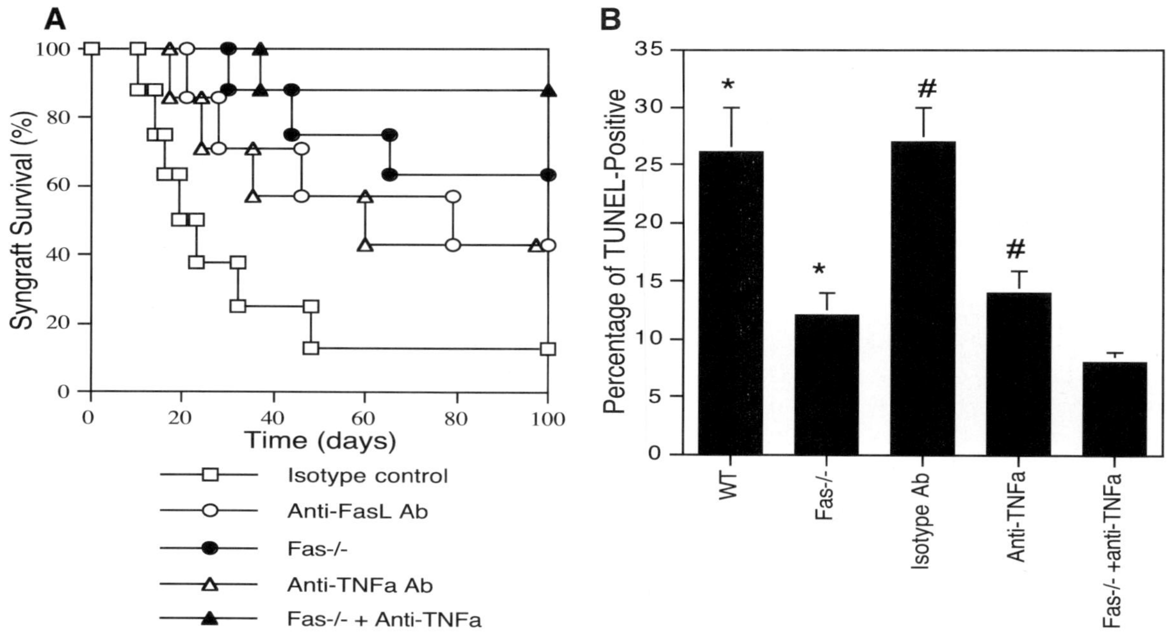

Figure 5. Blocking Fas and TNF receptor death pathways induces long-term IPCC graft survival in syngeneic WT mice. WT.B6-derived IPCCs were transplanted to WT B6 recipients that were treated with isotype Ab (Open square, n = 8), anti-FasL (Open circle, n = 7), or anti-TNFα Ab (Open triangle, n = 7). IPCCs derived from B6.Fas-/- ASCs also were transplanted to WT B6 recipients that were either untreated (Filled circle, n = 8) or treated with anti-TNFα Ab (Filled triangle, n = 8). IPCC syngraft rejection was then observed (**A**). IPCC graft cell apoptosis was determined by PDX-1 staining and a TUNEL method (**B**), as described in Figure 3. One representative of three separate experiments is shown.

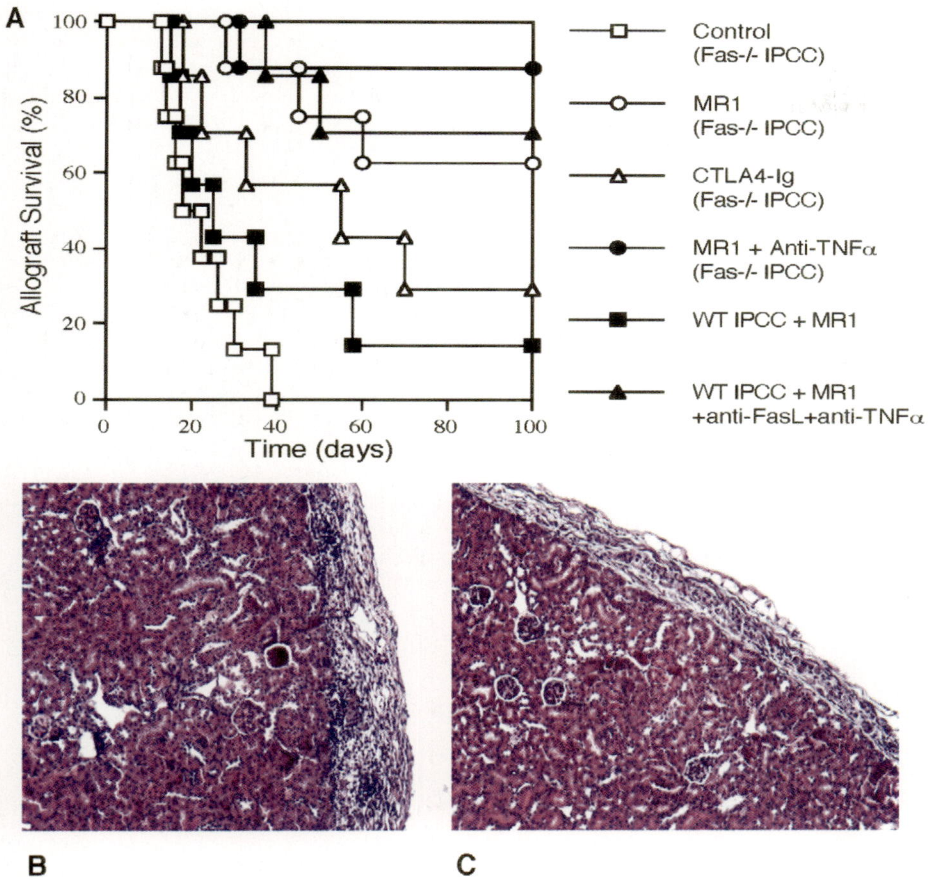

Figure 6. Blocking CD40-CD154 costimulation and Fas/TNF-receptor death pathways induces long-term IPCC allograft survival. IPCCs derived from B6.Fas-/- ASCs were transplanted to Balb/C recipients that were untreated (Open square, n = 8) or treated with MR1 (Open circle, n = 8), CTLA4-Ig (Open triangle, n = 7) or both MR1 and anti-TNFα Ab (Filled circle, n = 8). As a control, WT.B6-derived IPCCs also were transplanted to Balb/C recipients that were treated with MR1 alone (Filled square, n = 7) or MR1 + anti-FasL + anti- TNFα to block both CD154 costimulation and death pathways (Filled triangle, n = 7). IPCC allograft survival was observed (**A**). H&E staining of kidneys harboring Fas-/- IPCC allografts derived from an untreated control (**B**) or MR1+anti-TNF treated recipient (**C**) was performed two weeks after IPCC transplantation. (Magnification ×100).

shown in Figure 7, treatment with either MR1 or CTLA4-Ig significantly reduced the percentage of BrdU-positive T cells (BrdU+: 11±2 vs. 51±5% or 22±3 vs. 51±5%, both P<0.05) although MR1 was more effective in the suppression of graft-infiltrating T cell proliferation than CTLA4-Ig (BrdU+: 11±2 vs. 22±3, P<0.05). Neutralizing TNFα plus MR1 did not further decrease the percentage of BrdU+ T cells compared with MR1 alone. Our data suggest that CD40 or CD28 costimulatory blockade suppresses IPCC allograft rejection by inhibition of alloreactive T cell proliferation.

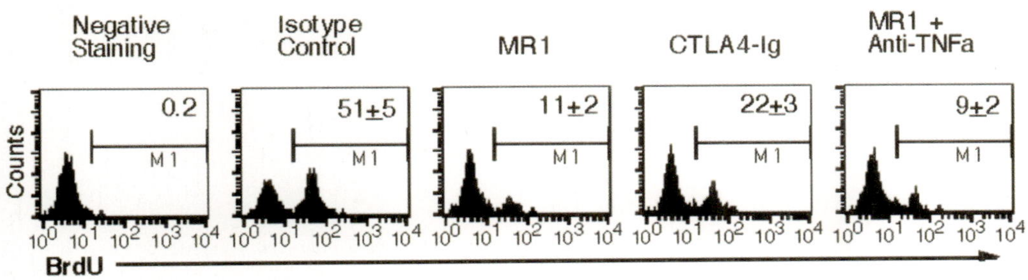

Figure 7. CD154 or CD28 costimulatory blockade inhibits the proliferation of T cells that infiltrate IPCC allografts. B6-derived IPCCs were transplanted to Balb/C recipients that were pulsed i.p. with 0.8 mg of BrdU six days after transplantation. 24 hours later, renal graft-infiltrating cells were isolated, stained with anti-CD3-PE and anti-BrdU-FITC Abs, and analyzed by FACS. Recipients were treated with MR1, CTLA4-Ig or anti-TNFα Ab. Histograms shown are gated on CD3+ cell population. One representative of three independent experiments is shown.

Blocking both CD40-CD154 and B7-CD28 costimulatory pathways is required for long-term IPCC allograft survival in diabetic NOD mice

To promote long-term IPCC allograft survival in diabetic NOD mice, both alloimmunity and autoimmunity must be suppressed. We determined whether T cell costimulatory blockade prevents IPCC allograft rejection in NOD recipients. IPCCs or islets derived from MRL.MpJ.Fas-/- mice (H-2^k) were transplanted to diabetic NOD mice that were then treated with MR1 and/or CTLA4-Ig. As shown in Figure 8, a treatment with either MR1 or CTLA4-Ig significantly prolonged IPCC allograft survival (MST = 46 vs. 16 or 31 vs. 16 days, both $P<0.05$) although neither MR1 nor CTLA4-Ig alone induced long-term IPCC allograft survival. Importantly, combined treatments with both MR1 and CTLA4-Ig induced long-term IPCC allograft survival in six of eight NOD recipients (75%). In contrast, the combined treatments failed to prevent rejection of islet allografts in most NOD recipients (MST = 56 days, Figure 8). Moreover, blocking CD40 with MR1 was more effective in suppression of IPCC than islet allograft rejection in NOD mice (MST = 46 vs. 32 days, $P<0.05$). There was no cellular infiltration in IPCC grafts from MR1+CTLA4-Ig treated recipient versus massive infiltration in control grafts (Fig. 8B & 8C). These results indicate that blocking both CD40 and CD28 costimulatory pathways is required to abrogate alloimmunity and autoimmunity in NOD mice and that it is easier to suppress the rejection of ASC-derived IPCCs than islet allografts in diabetic NOD recipients.

Discussion

Recently, several elegant studies have shown that IPCCs are generated in vitro from both human and murine ASCs [14,15,16,17], suggesting that ASC-derived IPCCs may circumvent worldwide shortage of donor islets and eventually provide a cure for human type 1 diabetes. In this study, we found that ASC-derived IPCCs have the intrinsic survival disadvantage over freshly isolated islets in syngeneic recipients. Nevertheless, IPCC allografts exhibited certain immune privilege and enjoyed long-term survival in diabetic NOD mice in the presence of CD28/CD154 and Fas blockade. Therefore, long-term survival of ASC-derived IPCCs in syngeneic recipients requires only blocking Fas and TNF death pathways whereas blocking both death pathways and CD28/CD154 costimulation is needed for long-term IPCC allograft

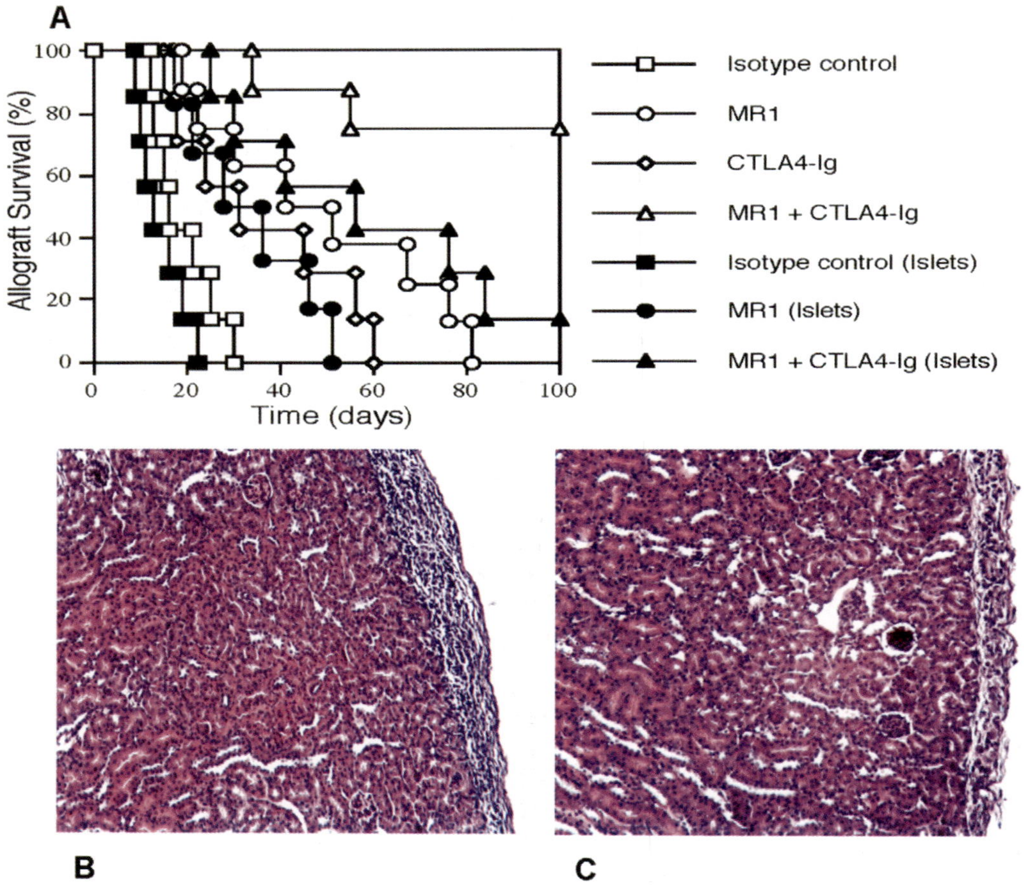

Figure 8. CD154/CD28 blockade induces long-term IPCC, but not freshly isolated islet, allograft survival in diabetic NOD mice. IPCCs that differentiated from Fas-deficient ASCs derived from MRL.MpJ.Fas-/- (H-2^k) mice were transplanted to diabetic NOD mice that were treated with isotype Ab (Open square, n = 7), MR1 (Open circle, n = 8), CTLA4-Ig (Open diamond, n = 7), or MR1 plus CTLA4-Ig (Open triangle, n = 8). As controls, freshly isolated islets from MRL.MpJ.Fas-/- donor mice were also transplanted to NOD mice that were treated with isotype Ab (Filled square, n = 7), MR1 (Filled circle, n = 6), or MR1 plus CTLA4-Ig (Filled triangle, n = 7). Graft survival was observed (**A**). H&E staining of kidneys harboring IPCC allografts derived from a control (**B**) or MR1+CTLA4-Ig treated recipient (**C**) was performed either at the time of graft rejection or 100 days after IPCC transplantation and survival.

survival in diabetic NOD mice. Thus, our studies suggest that ASC-derived IPCCs may provide an effective cell replacement therapy in human type 1 diabetes.

Using IPCCs that differentiated in vitro from murine ASCs based on a recent protocol [16], we first compared their survival to that of freshly-isolated intact islets in syngeneic recipients. Surprisingly, we found that overwhelming majority of IPCC grafts did not survive for long-term in syngeneic WT or Rag1-/- mice whereas nearly all of syngeneic islet grafts survived for long-term (>100 days). Our findings suggest that freshly isolated islets have a survival advantage over in vitro-generated IPCCs upon transplantation. Therefore, IPCC syngrafts die out in vivo even in the absence of alloimmune responses, although exact mechanisms responsible for their shortened survival in syngeneic hosts remain to be defined. Our results are consistent with a previous study showing that IPCC grafts, derived from murine embryonic stem cells, have survived for only a average of two to three weeks in syngeneic Rag-/- hosts [7], implying that IPCC grafts generated from stem cells are incapable of surviving for long-term even in the absence of alloimmune-based rejection. However, our findings differ from a recent study showing that human ASC-derived IPCC grafts have survived beyond 60 days in 50% of xenogeneic recipient mice without immunosuppression [17]. It is unclear how IPCC xenografts survived for such a long time without immunosuppression.

We then investigated how to prevent IPCC graft dysfunction in the absence of alloimmunity or any immune-based rejection, which is an important step prior to in-depth IPCC allotransplantation. Since Fas or TNF signaling mediates apoptosis in most cell types, including β cells [21,22,23,24], we asked whether blocking their signaling pathways would enhance IPCC graft survival or restore their function in syngeneic recipient mice. Indeed, blocking either Fas or TNF signaling significantly prolonged IPCC graft survival and inhibited IPCC cell apoptosis in syngeneic recipients while blocking both pathways induced long-term IPCC syngraft survival in overwhelming majority, if not all, of recipient mice. Our findings suggest that IPCC graft dysfunction due to passive cell death, which is mediated by Fas and TNF signal pathways but independent of alloimmune-based rejection, must also be overcome upon IPCC allotransplantation.

We next examined IPCC allograft survival in alloimmune-competent WT recipient mice. We found that IPCC allografts derived from both Fas-replete and Fas-deficient ASCs were acutely rejected in allogeneic WT recipient mice, suggesting that ASC-derived IPCCs are highly immunogenic and can evoke acute allograft rejection. Blocking CD40-CD154 costimulation induced Fas-deficient IPCC allograft survival for long-term in 63% of recipient mice. Given that the same percentage of Fas-deficient IPCC grafts survived in syngeneic recipients without CD154 costimulatory blockade, we conclude that blocking CD40-CD154 costimulation is sufficient to suppress IPCC allograft rejection mediated by alloimmune responses. Furthermore, simultaneously blocking CD154, Fas and TNF-receptor signaling induced long-term IPCC allograft survival in overwhelming majority, if not all, of recipient mice. Taken together, both death signaling of β cells and alloreactivity of recipients need to be suppressed in order to achieve long-term IPCC allograft survival.

In this study, we determined whether costimulatory blockade promotes long-term IPCC allograft survival in NOD mice that are closely relevant to human type 1 diabetes. Costimulatory blockade has been shown to suppress alloimmune responses and induce long-term allograft survival [25,26,27]. Previous studies have also shown that blocking both CD28 and CD154 costimulatory pathways prevents autoimmune diabetes induced by transfer of transgenic T cells in NOD.SCID mice [28] but fails to induce long-term islet allograft survival in NOD recipients [29], suggesting that CD28/CD154 blockade is sufficient to suppress autoimmunity but insufficient to simultaneously suppress both alloimmunity and autoimmunity in NOD recipients. In contrast, another study has shown that ICOS/CD154 blockade is capable of inducing islet allograft tolerance and preventing autoimmune diabetes in NOD mice [30]. Here we found that CD28/CD154 blockade induces long-term Fas-/- IPCC, but not Fas-/- islet, allograft survival in diabetic NOD recipients. We utilized Fas-deficient IPCCs because Fas-replete IPCC grafts died out over time even in syngeneic recipients due to Fas-mediated cell death. Our data have further confirmed that CD28/CD154 blockade does not induce long-term islet allograft survival in diabetic NOD recipients. On the other hand, we have demonstrated for the first time that blocking CD28 and CD154 costimulatory signaling is capable of inducing long-term survival of ASC-derived IPCC allografts in diabetic NOD mice, although a recent study has shown that blocking CD28/CD154/LFA-1 enhances engraftment of allogeneic ESC-derived endothelial cells in non-diabetic environment [31].

It is unclear whether CD154 costimulatory blockade can be translated to the clinic in the future, although it prolongs IPCC allograft survival. Clinical trials using anti-CD154 Ab were halted due to its thromboembolic side effects [32,33]. The progress in its clinical application, hence, has been hampered. Recently, Abs against its counter receptor, CD40, have been sought as an alternative to blocking CD40/CD154 costimulatory pathway. These promising Abs have been shown to potently suppress allograft rejection in both mice and non-human primates [34,35]. However, it remains to be defined whether they will also cause the same side effects in the future clinical trials.

Our finding indicates that it is easier to suppress the rejection of ASC-derived IPCC allografts than freshly isolated islet allografts in NOD recipient mice once passive cell death is blocked. This is consistent with previous studies showing that ESC-derived IPCCs or tissues exhibit a certain degree of immune privilege [6,7,36]. Therefore, ASC-derived IPCCs enjoy at least two advantages over freshly isolated islets: relatively immune privilege and unlimited sources while displaying an intrinsic survival disadvantage that is unrelated to alloimmune-based rejection. A recent study has demonstrated that transplantation of IPCCs derived from human umbilical cord mesenchymal stem cells alleviates hyperglycemia in diabetic NOD mice without any immunosuppressive treatment [37], although it was not observed how long IPCC xenografts survived and how their rejection could be suppressed. Taken together, previous and our current studies indicate that clinical application of ASC-derived IPCCs for treating type 1 diabetes is no longer elusive.

Materials and Methods

Ethics Statement

All animal experiments were approved by the Animal Care and Use Committee of the University of Texas Health Science Center (animal approval ID: 463B), Tyler, TX.

Mice

Wild-type BALB/c (H-2^d) and C57BL/6 (H-2^b) mice were purchased from National Cancer Institute (NIH, Bethesda, MD, USA). B6.Rag1-/-, NOD, B6.MRL.Fas-/- (H-2^b) and MRL/MpJ.Fas-/- (H-2^k) were purchased from the Jackson Laboratory. All mice were aged 6–8 weeks when experiments were initiated. They were housed in a specific pathogen-free environment.

Adipose-derived stem cell isolation and culture

Adipose tissues from epididymal fat and subcutaneous fat of anterior abdominal wall of donor mice were minced and digested with 0.1% type II collagenase (Invitrogen) in phosphate-buffered saline (PBS) for 30 minutes at 37°C with gentle stirring. Cell suspensions were cultured in Dulbecco's modified Eagle's medium (DMEM)/Ham's F-12 with 10% FBS and 100 U/ml penicillin, 0.1 mg/ml streptomycin (Invitrogen) at 5% CO2, 37°C. Cells were passaged under maintenance culture conditions. All experiments were performed using ASCs at 4–6 passages.

In vitro differentiation of ASCs into IPCCs

ASCs at p4-p6 were suspended in medium M (DMEM/F12 at 1:1) with 17.5 mM glucose, 1% BSA and 5 mg/l insulin-transferrin-selenium, plated on ultralow attachment tissue culture plates (Fisher Scientific) at 1×10^6 cells per well, and then cultured in medium MA (M with 4 nM activin A, R&D System) for two days, medium MB (M with 0.3 mM taurine) for two days, and medium MC (M with 100 nM glucagon-like peptide-1, 1 mM nicotinamide and 1× nonessential amino acids) for five days as described previously [16]. All chemicals and supplements were purchased from Sigma Aldrich unless otherwise indicated.

Flow cytometric analysis for phenotyping

Immunophenotyping of ASCs were performed using fluorescent-conjugated antibodies against mouse antigens MHC I (H-$2K^b$), MHC II (I-A^b), CD44, CD45, CD29, CD80, CD90, CD105 and Sca-1 (Biolegend). ASCs at the fourth passage were released by 0.25% trypsin-EDTA. A total of 1×10^6 cells were incubated with fluorescent-conjugated Abs for 30 min at room temperature. Cells finally were analyzed using FACSCalibur.

RT-PCR detection of pancreatic gene expression by IPCCs

Total RNA was isolated from undifferentiated ASCs, IPCCs and islets using TRIzol extraction method (TRIzol Reagent, Invitrogen). The extracted RNA was subject to cDNA synthesis using the Superscript III First-Strand Synthesis system for RT-PCR (Invitrogen). The PCR cycling conditions varied depending on different pancreatic genes and primers, which were listed in the supporting information (Table S1).

Transplantation of islets or IPCCs

~400 donor islets or 800 IPCCs that differentiated from ASCs were transplanted under the kidney capsule of recipient mice as described in our previous studies [38,39]. Previous studies and our preliminary data have determined that at least 800–900 IPCCs are required to reverse hyperglycemia. Recipient mice were rendered diabetic by a single injection of streptozotocin (Sigma) (180 mg/kg for WT mice and 200 mg/kg for Rag-/- recipients) 8–10 days before transplantation. Primary graft function was defined as blood glucose under 200 mg/dl for 48 hours after transplantation. Graft rejection was defined as a rise in blood glucose to >300 mg/dl for three consecutive days after primary function. Rejection was also confirmed by histology showing cellular infiltration. In some recipients that survived for long-term, the kidney harboring IPCC grafts was removed to confirm that normalizing hyperglycemia in diabetic mice was caused by IPCC transplantation.

Treatments of recipient mice with Abs

Recipient mice were treated with MR1 (anti-CD40L), CTLA4-Ig, or anti-TNFα Ab (Bio-Express Inc, West Lebanon, NH) at 0.25 mg on days 0, 2, 4, and 6 while anti-FasL blocking Ab (BD Biosciences) was administered at 0.1 mg on days 0, 2, 4, and 6 after transplantation.

Histology and immunofluorescence staining

Kidney samples containing IPCC grafts from transplanted mice were harvested, fixed in 10% formalin, embedded in paraffin, sectioned with a microtome at 4 μm thickness, stained with haematoxylin/eosin (H&E), and observed for cell infiltration under the light microscope. Moreover, both IPCCs and kidneys harboring IPCC grafts were fixed, embedded and sectioned as described above. Sections were used for immunofluorescence staining of murine insulin and c-peptide. Briefly, slides were deparaffinized in xylene, rehydrated in descending grades of alcohol, immersed in citrate buffer in a microwave oven with heating for 20 min at 95°C, and treated with 0.3% hydrogen peroxide in methanol for 10 min. Sections were then placed in diluted (10%) normal serum for 20 min, covered with primary antibody (Cell Signaling) overnight at 4°C and incubated with 1:500-diluted Alexa Fluor 488- or 568-conjugated secondary Ab solution (Invitrogen) at room temperature for 1 hour. They were finally visualized under a fluorescence microscope.

Isolation of tissue-infiltrating cells

Tissue-infiltrating cells were isolated as described in our previous publications [40,41]. Briefly, the kidneys harboring islet grafts were perfused *in situ* with heparinized 0.9% saline. They were then minced and digested at 37°C for 30 min in 20 ml RPMI-1640 medium containing 5% FCS and 350 u/ml collagenase (Sigma, St. Louis, MO). To clear the debris, cell suspensions were rapidly passed down 70 μm cell strainer, then mixed with Percoll solution (Sigma) to a concentration of 30%, and centrifuged at 2000 rpm for 15 minutes at room temperature. The pellet was re-suspended and stained before analysis.

Analysis of T cell proliferation in vivo by 5-Bromo-2′-Deoxyuridine (BrdU) labeling

Recipient mice were pulsed i.p. with 0.8 mg of BrdU (Sigma) six days after transplantation. 24 hours later, renal graft-infiltrating cells were isolated and first stained with anti-CD3-PE Ab. Cells were then fixed in 70% ethanol followed by 1% paraformaldehyde and incubated with 50 Units/ml of DNase I (Sigma). Cells were finally stained with anti-BrdU-FITC (BD Biosciences) and analyzed by a FACSCalibur as described previously [40,41].

Analysis of insulin-producing cell apoptosis in vivo by a TUNEL method

IPCCs or islets were retrieved and dissociated with 0.25% trypsin-EDTA (Sigma-Aldrich) at 37°C for 10 minutes. To detect cell apoptosis, cells were fixed in 2% paraformaldehyde, permeabilized with 0.1% Triton X-100 solution, and labeled with fluorescein-tagged deoxyuridine triphosphate (dUTP) by the terminal deoxynucleotidyl transferase-mediated dUTP nick-end labeling (TUNEL) method according to the manufacture's instructions (Roche Applied Science, Mannheim, Germany) [40,42].

Statistical Analysis

Data are presented as mean ± SEM and represent an average of at least three independent experiments. Comparisons of the mean among different groups were done using the Student t test and ANOVA. The analysis of graft survival data was performed using the Kaplan-Meier method (log-rank test). A value of $P<0.05$ was considered statistically significant.

Supporting Information

Figure S1 Insulin release by IPCCs and islets in vitro. Day-10 IPCCs or freshly isolated islets were cultured in DMEM-LG (low glucose) containing 0.5% BSA for 10 hours, washed and then stimulated or incubated in DMEM-HG (high glucose) media at 37°C for two hours. Insulin released into the media was measured using ELISA kit (Mercodia, Winston Salem, NC) according to the manufacturer's instructions. Undifferentiated ASCs were also utilized as a control. Both IPCCs and islets produced significant amount of insulin in high-glucose condition in vitro while undifferentiated ASCs did not. One of three separate experiments is shown.

Table S1 Primers for RT-PCR. The primer sequences, including the sense and anti-sense, for RT-PCR for pancreatic gene expression are listed.

Author Contributions

Conceived and designed the experiments: SZ ZD. Performed the experiments: SZ HD. Analyzed the data: SZ ZD. Contributed reagents/materials/analysis tools: NW YM. Wrote the paper: SZ ZD.

References

1. Assady S, Maor G, Amit M, Itskovitz-Eldor J, Skorecki KL, et al. (2001) Insulin production by human embryonic stem cells. Diabetes 50: 1691–1697.
2. Lumelsky N, Blondel O, Laeng P, Velasco I, Ravin R, et al. (2001) Differentiation of embryonic stem cells to insulin-secreting structures similar to pancreatic islets. Science 292: 1389–1394.
3. Soria B, Roche E, Berna G, Leon-Quinto T, Reig JA, et al. (2000) Insulin-secreting cells derived from embryonic stem cells normalize glycemia in streptozotocin-induced diabetic mice. Diabetes 49: 157–162.
4. D'Amour KA, Bang AG, Eliazer S, Kelly OG, Agulnick AD, et al. (2006) Production of pancreatic hormone-expressing endocrine cells from human embryonic stem cells. Nat Biotechnol 24: 1392–1401.
5. Jiang J, Au M, Lu K, Eshpeter A, Korbutt G, et al. (2007) Generation of insulin-producing islet-like clusters from human embryonic stem cells. Stem Cells 25: 1940–1953.
6. Boyd AS, Wood KJ (2010) Characteristics of the early immune response following transplantation of mouse ES cell derived insulin-producing cell clusters. PLoS One 5: e10965.
7. Wu DC, Boyd AS, Wood KJ (2008) Embryonic stem cells and their differentiated derivatives have a fragile immune privilege but still represent novel targets of immune attack. Stem Cells 26: 1939–1950.
8. Tang DQ, Cao LZ, Burkhardt BR, Xia CQ, Litherland SA, et al. (2004) In vivo and in vitro characterization of insulin-producing cells obtained from murine bone marrow. Diabetes 53: 1721–1732.
9. Yang L, Li S, Hatch H, Ahrens K, Cornelius JG, et al. (2002) In vitro trans-differentiation of adult hepatic stem cells into pancreatic endocrine hormone-producing cells. Proc Natl Acad Sci U S A 99: 8078–8083.
10. Seaberg RM, Smukler SR, Kieffer TJ, Enikolopov G, Asghar Z, et al. (2004) Clonal identification of multipotent precursors from adult mouse pancreas that generate neural and pancreatic lineages. Nat Biotechnol 22: 1115–1124.
11. Schaffler A, Buchler C (2007) Concise review: adipose tissue-derived stromal cells–basic and clinical implications for novel cell-based therapies. Stem Cells 25: 818–827.
12. Zuk PA, Zhu M, Ashjian P, De Ugarte DA, Huang JI, et al. (2002) Human adipose tissue is a source of multipotent stem cells. Mol Biol Cell 13: 4279–4295.
13. Kim SC, Han DJ, Lee JY (2010) Adipose tissue derived stem cells for regeneration and differentiation into insulin-producing cells. Curr Stem Cell Res Ther 5: 190–194.
14. Timper K, Seboek D, Eberhardt M, Linscheid P, Christ-Crain M, et al. (2006) Human adipose tissue-derived mesenchymal stem cells differentiate into insulin, somatostatin, and glucagon expressing cells. Biochem Biophys Res Commun 341: 1135–1140.
15. Lee J, Han DJ, Kim SC (2008) In vitro differentiation of human adipose tissue-derived stem cells into cells with pancreatic phenotype by regenerating pancreas extract. Biochem Biophys Res Commun 375: 547–551.
16. Chandra VGS, Phadnis S, Nair PD, Bhonde RR (2009) Generation of pancreatic hormone-expressing islet-like cell aggregates from murine adipose tissue-derived stem cells. Stem Cells 27: 1941–1953.
17. Kang HM, Kim J, Park S, Kim H, Kim KS, et al. (2009) Insulin-secreting cells from human eyelid-derived stem cells alleviate type I diabetes in immunocompetent mice. Stem Cells 27: 1999–2008.
18. Lin G, Wang G, Liu G, Yang LJ, Chang LJ, et al. (2009) Treatment of type 1 diabetes with adipose tissue-derived stem cells expressing pancreatic duodenal homeobox 1. Stem Cells Dev 18: 1399–1406.
19. Kajiyama H, Hamazaki TS, Tokuhara M, Masui S, Okabayashi K, et al. (2010) Pdx1-transfected adipose tissue-derived stem cells differentiate into insulin-producing cells in vivo and reduce hyperglycemia in diabetic mice. Int J Dev Biol 54: 699–705.
20. Di Rocco G, Iachininoto MG, Tritarelli A, Straino S, Zacheo A, et al. (2006) Myogenic potential of adipose-tissue-derived cells. J Cell Sci 119: 2945–2952.
21. Pearl-Yafe M, Yolcu ES, Yaniv I, Stein J, Shirwan H, et al. (2006) The dual role of Fas-ligand as an injury effector and defense strategy in diabetes and islet transplantation. Bioessays 28: 211–222.
22. Giannoukakis N, Rudert WA, Ghivizzani SC, Gambotto A, Ricordi C, et al. (1999) Adenoviral gene transfer of the interleukin-1 receptor antagonist protein to human islets prevents IL-1beta-induced beta-cell impairment and activation of islet cell apoptosis in vitro. Diabetes 48: 1730–1736.
23. Silva DG, Petrovsky N, Socha L, Slattery R, Gatenby P, et al. (2003) Mechanisms of accelerated immune-mediated diabetes resulting from islet beta cell expression of a Fas ligand transgene. J Immunol 170: 4996–5002.
24. Judge TA, Desai NM, Yang Z, Rostami S, Alonso L, et al. (1998) Utility of adenoviral-mediated Fas ligand gene transfer to modulate islet allograft survival. Transplantation 66: 426–434.
25. Larsen C, Elwood E, Alexander D, Ritchie S, Hendrix R, et al. (1996) Long-term acceptance of skin and cardiac allografts after blocking CD40 and CD28 pathways. Nature 381: 434–438.
26. Wekerle T, Kurtz J, Bigenzahn S, Takeuchi Y, Sykes M (2002) Mechanisms of transplant tolerance induction using costimulatory blockade. Curr Opin Immunol 14: 592–600.
27. Li XC, Rothstein DM, Sayegh MH (2009) Costimulatory pathways in transplantation: challenges and new developments. Immunol Rev 229: 271–293.
28. Rigby MR, Trexler AM, Pearson TC, Larsen CP (2008) CD28/CD154 blockade prevents autoimmune diabetes by inducing nondeletional tolerance after effector t-cell inhibition and regulatory T-cell expansion. Diabetes 57: 2672–2683.
29. Demirci G, Strom TB, Li XC (2003) Islet allograft rejection in nonobese diabetic mice involves the common gamma-chain and CD28/CD154-dependent and -independent mechanisms. J Immunol 171: 3878–3885.
30. Nanji SA, Hancock WW, Luo B, Schur CD, Pawlick RL, et al. (2006) Costimulation blockade of both inducible costimulator and CD40 ligand induces dominant tolerance to islet allografts and prevents spontaneous autoimmune diabetes in the NOD mouse. Diabetes 55: 27–33.
31. Pearl JI, Lee AS, Leveson-Gower DB, Sun N, Ghosh Z, et al. (2011) Short-term immunosuppression promotes engraftment of embryonic and induced pluripotent stem cells. Cell Stem Cell 8: 309–317.
32. Kanmaz T, Fechner JJ, Jr., Torrealba J, Kim HT, Dong Y, et al. (2004) Monotherapy with the novel human anti-CD154 monoclonal antibody ABI793 in rhesus monkey renal transplantation model. Transplantation 77: 914–920.
33. Kawai T, Andrews D, Colvin RB, Sachs DH, Cosimi AB (2000) Thromboembolic complications after treatment with monoclonal antibody against CD40 ligand. Nature medicine 6: 114.
34. Gilson CR, Milas Z, Gangappa S, Hollenbaugh D, Pearson TC, et al. (2009) Anti-CD40 monoclonal antibody synergizes with CTLA4-Ig in promoting long-term graft survival in murine models of transplantation. Journal of immunology 183: 1625–1635.
35. Aoyagi T, Yamashita K, Suzuki T, Uno M, Goto R, et al. (2009) A human anti-CD40 monoclonal antibody, 4D11, for kidney transplantation in cynomolgus monkeys: induction and maintenance therapy. American journal of transplantation : official journal of the American Society of Transplantation and the American Society of Transplant Surgeons 9: 1732–1741.
36. Lui KO, Boyd AS, Cobbold SP, Waldmann H, Fairchild PJ (2010) A role for regulatory T cells in acceptance of ESC-derived tissues transplanted across an major histocompatibility complex barrier. Stem Cells 28: 1905–1914.
37. Wang HS, Shyu JF, Shen WS, Hsu HC, Chi TC, et al. (2011) Transplantation of Insulin-Producing Cells Derived From Umbilical Cord Stromal Mesenchymal Stem Cells to Treat NOD Mice. Cell Transplant 20: 455–466.
38. Liu ZW, Dai H, Wan N, Wang T, Bertera S, et al. (2007) Suppression of memory CD8 T cell generation and function by tryptophan catabolism. J Immunol 178: 4260–4266.
39. Wan N, Dai H, Wang T, Moore Y, Zheng XX, et al. (2008) Bystander central memory but not effector memory CD8+ T cells suppress allograft rejection. J Immunol 180: 113–121.
40. Dai Z, Li Q, Wang Y, Gao G, Diggs LS, et al. (2004) CD4+CD25+ regulatory T cells suppress allograft rejection mediated by memory CD8+ T cells via a CD30-dependent mechanism. J Clin Invest 113: 310–317.
41. Wang Y, Dai H, Liu Z, Cheng X, Tellides G, et al. (2006) Neutralizing IL-7 promotes long-term allograft survival induced by CD40/CD40L costimulatory blockade. Am J Transplant 6: 2851–2860.
42. Wang T, Dai H, Wan N, Moore Y, Dai Z (2008) The role for monocyte chemoattractant protein-1 in the generation and function of memory CD8+ T cells. J Immunol 180: 2886–2893.

4

Tolerance Induction by Exosomes from Immature Dendritic Cells and Rapamycin in a Mouse Cardiac Allograft Model

Xiao Li[1]ⓘ, Jun-Jie Li[1]ⓘ, Jing-Yue Yang[2]ⓘ, De-Sheng Wang[1], Wei Zhao[1], Wen-Jie Song[1], Wei-Min Li[1], Jian-Feng Wang[1], Wei Han[1], Zhuo-Chao Zhang[1], Yong Yu[1], Da-Yong Cao[1]*, Ke-Feng Dou[1]*

1 Department of Hepatobiliary Surgery, Xijing Hospital, Fourth Military Medical University, Xi'an, Shaanxi Province, China, **2** Department of Clinical Oncology, Xijing Hospital, Fourth Military Medical University, Xi'an, Shaanxi Province, China

Abstract

Background: Dendritic cells (DCs) release bioactive exosomes that play an important role in immune regulation. Because they express low levels of class I major histocompatibility complex (MHC) and co-stimulatory molecules, exosomes derived from donor immature DCs (imDex) prolong allograft survival by inhibiting T-cell activation. However, this effect is limited and does not induce immunological tolerance when imDex are administered alone. Thus, we tested the effect of combined treatment with donor imDex and low-dose rapamycin on inducing tolerance in a mouse cardiac transplantation model.

Methods: ImDex were obtained from the culture supernatant of immature DCs derived from donor mouse (C57BL/6) bone marrow and were injected with suboptimal doses of rapamycin into recipient mouse (BALB/c) before and after transplantation. The capacity of this treatment to induce immune tolerance was analyzed in vitro and in vivo using the mouse cardiac transplantation model.

Results: Donor imDex expressed moderate levels of MHC class II and low levels of MHC class I and co-stimulatory molecules, but neither imDex nor subtherapeutic rapamycin dose alone induced cardiac allograft tolerance. Combined treatment with imDex and rapamycin, however, led to donor specific cardiac allograft tolerance. This effect was accompanied by decreased anti-donor antigen cellular response and an increased percentage of spleen $CD4^{+}CD25^{+}$ T cells in recipients. Furthermore, this donor specific tolerance could be further transferred to naïve allograft recipients through injection of splenocytes, but not serum, from tolerant recipients.

Conclusion: Combined with immunosuppressive treatment, donor imDex can prolong cardiac allograft survival and induce donor specific allograft tolerance.

Editor: George Kassiotis, MRC National Institute for Medical Research, United Kingdom

Funding: The study was supported by grants from National High Technology Research and Development Program of China (2012AA021000). The funders had no role in study design, data collection and analysis, decision to publish, or preparation of the manuscript.

Competing Interests: The authors have declared that no competing interests exist.

* E-mail: gdwkgwx@fmmu.edu.cn (K-FD); caody777@sina.com (D-YC)

ⓘ These authors contributed equally to this work.

Introduction

Organ transplantation is almost the only hope of complete cure for patients with organ failure. In addition to organ shortage, immune rejection is the biggest obstacle to the development of organ transplantation [1]. Although non-specific immunosuppressants can suppress immune rejection and prolong allograft survival, long-term use of these drugs causes serious adverse reactions, such as increased occurrence of opportunistic infections or increased cancer recurrence rate [2]. Thus, donor specific tolerance must be established and maintained to reduce the dosage of immunosuppressants [3].

Dendritic cells (DCs) are the professional antigen-presenting cells (APCs) that present donor alloantigen to recipient T cells. The view that immature and mature DCs mediate different functional T-cell responses (i.e., tolerance versus priming) is very common, and the effect of immature DCs (imDCs) on inducing transplantation tolerance has been tested in many different animal transplantation models. However, this DC-based technology has some deficiencies that limit its application in the clinic, including potential maturation and short-term lifetime in vivo, the requirement of 7 days (d) for production, and short-term preservation in vitro [4,5]. Thus, donor imDCs cannot be used repeatedly and do not induce sufficient immune tolerance.

Exosomes are small membrane vesicles (diameter 50–100 nm) of late endocytic compartment origin secreted by a variety of cell types [6]. DC-derived exosomes (Dex) present antigen-major histocompatibility complex (MHC) and co-stimulatory molecules to T lymphocytes and therefore have strong immunological regulatory activities [7,8]. Depending on the maturation state of

DCs producing exosomes, Dex induces T-cell tolerance or priming. Mature DC-derived exosomes (mDex) trigger effector T-cell response and lead to fast skin allograft rejection [9], whereas imDC-derived exosomes (imDex) display a certain degree of immunosuppressive activity in autoimmune diseases [10–12] and animal models of allogenetic organ transplantation [13–15]. Moreover, as imDex are stable and can be easily stored in vitro, they may be a good substitute for imDCs in inducing immune tolerance. However, there are few reports on the utility of imDex as an immunosuppressant, and only two findings show that treatment with imDex alone induces limited immunosuppressant activity without inducing tolerance [13,14].

In this study, we analyzed the effect of allogenetic donor imDex, purified from mouse bone marrow (BM), on tolerance induction in a mouse model of heart transplantation. We found that low doses (10 μg) of donor imDex could significantly prolong cardiac allograft survival, but this was limited. To increase graft survival, therefore, we used imDex together with a subtherapeutic regimen (1 mg/kg/d) of rapamycin. Impressively, the combination of imDex and rapamycin led to donor specific cardiac allograft tolerance, and this effect was accompanied by decreased anti-donor antigen cellular response and an increased percentage of spleen $CD4^{+}CD25^{+}$ T cells in recipients. These findings demonstrate that donor imDex in combination with an immunosuppressant can induce donor specific allograft tolerance and thus prolong cardiac allograft survival.

Results

Characterization of Exosomes Derived from DCs

Eight days after culturing in the presence of granulocyte macrophage colony-stimulating factor (GM-CSF) and recombinant interleukin-4 (IL-4), murine BM cells developed a typical DC profile as reported by Lutz *et al.* [16]. Phenotypic profiles of mature DCs (lipopolysaccharide (LPS)-treated) and imDCs (untreated) analyzed by fluorescence-activated cells sorting (FACS). Mature DCs (mDCs) expressed high levels of MHC class I, class II, and co-stimulatory CD80 and CD86 compared with imDCs. The DC marker NLDC-145 showed exclusive staining in mDCs but was reduced in imDCs, whereas CD11c was moderately expressed in both mDCs and imDCs. These data proved that DCs were immature throughout the culture period in the presence of GM-CSF and IL-4. Exosomes were purified from culture supernatants of mDCs and imDCs by ultrafiltration and ultracentrifugation [17]. We obtained about 0.35±0.1 μg and 0.94±0.2 μg of exosome proteins (as measured by Bradford assay) from one million mDCs and imDCs, respectively. The morphology of exosomes observed by electron microscopy. The purified exosomes showed typical heterogeneous vesicle structures ranging from 60 to 90 nm in diameter. A typical phenotypic profile of imDex and mDex is shown in Figure 1A. Lower levels of MHC class I and co-stimulatory CD80 and CD86 were expressed in imDex than mDex. MHC class II, which was highly expressed in mDex, was slightly down-modulated in imDex. Additionally, we analyzed the expression of HSP70, HSP90, MFG-E8, and ICAM-1 by western blotting (Figure 1B). HSP70 and HSP90 were present in similar amounts in imDex and mDex, but ICAM-1 expression was relatively higher and MFG-E8 was relatively lower in mDex.

Administration of Donor imDex in Combination with Low-Dose Rapamycin Prolongs Survival of Cardiac Allografts

Some reports have shown that administration of donor imDex before transplantation significantly prolongs allograft survival of heart or intestine in rat transplantation models [13,14]. However, transplant immunological tolerance or long-term graft survival was not achieved, and the role of imDex treatment in allograft transplantation was not completely clear. Thus, we treated recipients with donor imDex alone or in combination with low-dose rapamycin and analyzed the effects on survival of cardiac allografts. First, we tested the effects of different doses of donor imDex. We established a murine model of cardiac allotransplantation, and treated BALB/c recipients with 0.1, 1, 10, 25, or 50 μg imDex derived from a C57BL/6 donor. The imDex were injected via caudal vein 7 d before, the day of, and 7 d after transplantation. As shown in Table 1 and Figure 2A, treatment with 0.1 or 1 μg of donor imDex (median survival time (MST): 8 d for 0.1 μg, n = 7; 12.5 d for 1 μg, n = 8) did not prolong allograft survival compared with the untreated recipients (MST: 7.5 d, n = 8); treatment with 10 μg imDex (MST: 27 days, n = 8), however, significantly prolonged allograft survival ($P<0.001$). Notably, allograft survival decreased when the dose of donor imDex increased above 10 μg. We found that treatment with 25 μg imDex (MST: 14 d, n = 8) also prolonged allograft survival compared with untreated recipients ($P = 0.042$), but the effect was significantly weaker than for treatment with 10 μg imDex ($P = 0.001$). Finally, treatment with 50 μg imDex (MST: 12 d, n = 7) did not affect allograft survival compared with the untreated recipients ($P = 0.192$). Thus, treatment of the recipient mice with a low-dose (10 μg) of donor imDex before and after transplantation inhibited the immunological rejection of the cardiac allograft and significantly prolonged allograft survival.

To determine whether this effect was donor specific, we injected 10 μg imDex derived from BALB/c (recipient) or CBA/H (third-party) mice into BALB/c recipient mice, but we found that neither prolonged cardiac allograft survival (MST: 8 d for BALB/c imDex and 9.5 d for CBA/H imDex; Figure 2B and Table 1), indicating that the effect was donor specific. Notably, increased doses of donor imDex did not induce accelerated rejection despite the negative effect on allograft survival, suggesting that administration of donor imDex via caudal vein before transplantation does not sensitize the recipients.

Although a low dose (10 μg) donor imDex significantly prolonged cardiac allograft survival in our experiments, this effect was limited and merely yielded MST of 27 d and a maximum survival of 51 d. To improve allograft survival, we used 10 μg donor imDex together with a short course of immunosuppression intended to develop tolerance in the immunological microenvironment in vivo. Rapamycin–the mammalian target of rapamycin (mTOR) inhibitor -blocks DC maturation [18,19], inhibits capacity of DC to stimulate T cells even following exposure to LPS [20], and prolongs organ allograft survival [21]. Thus, we hypothesized that 10 μg donor imDex combined with a short course of minimally effective rapamycin could induce immunological tolerance and effectively promote allograft survival. To test this hypothesis, we treated recipient mice with a subtherapeutic regimen of 1 mg/kg/d rapamycin injected via caudal vein for 11 consecutive days (days -3 to 7) with or without donor imDex. We found that this combination dramatically induced long-term cardiac allograft survival (MST: 92 d, n = 7; Table 1 and Figure 2C), whereas the subtherapeutic regimen of rapamycin alone did not significantly prolong allograft survival (MST: 19 d, n = 6; Table 1 and Figure 2C). We also confirmed that this effect was specific for donor antigen by combining injection of the subtherapeutic regimen of rapamycin with 10 μg imDex derived from either recipient or third-party mice and found that these treatments had no significant effect on allograft survival (MST: 21 d for imDex/rapamycin-cotreatment, n = 6; 17 d for third-

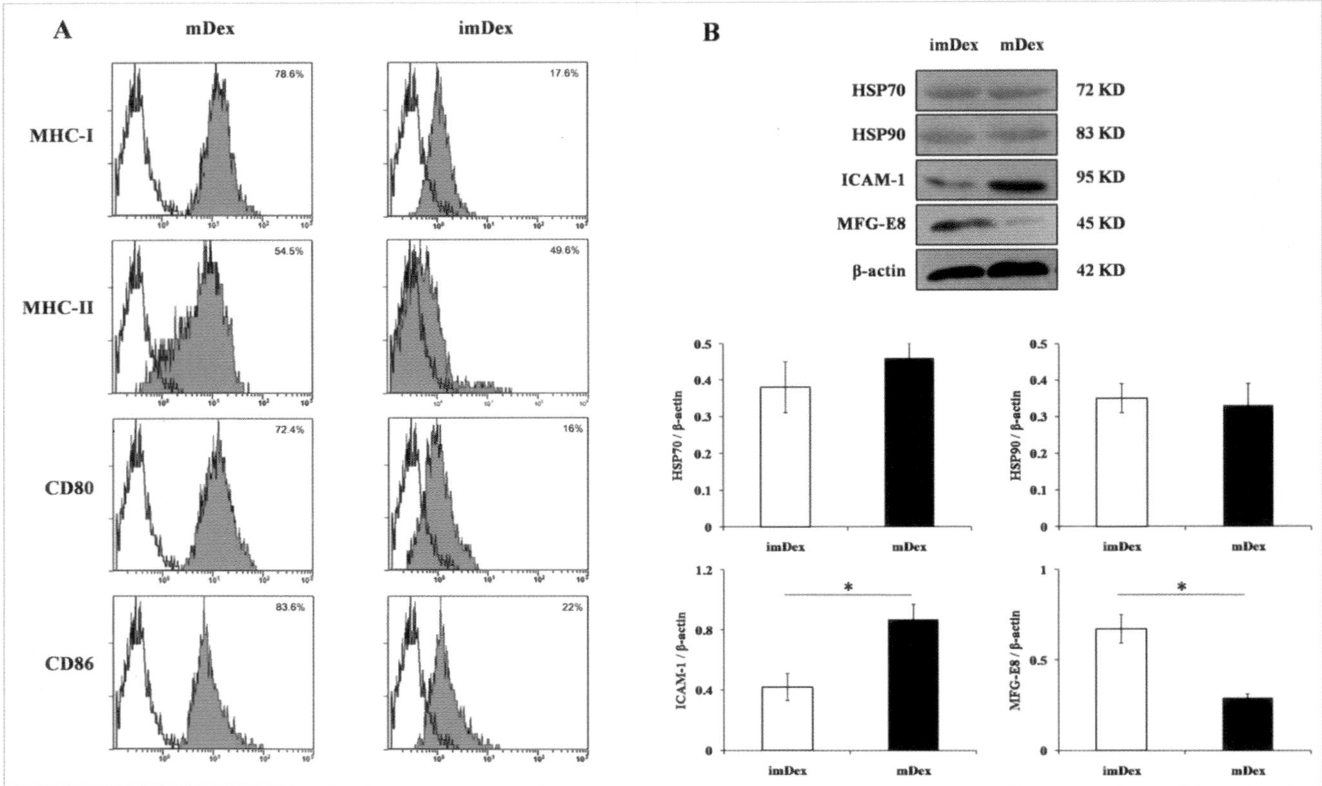

Figure 1. Characterization of exosomes derived from DCs. (A) The phenotypic profile of imDex and mDex were analyzed by cytofluorometry. The two kinds of the exosomes were coated on surfactant-free white aldehyde sulfate latex beads, then stained with FITC-coupled monoclonal antibodies against MHC class I, II and CD80, CD86. The isotype monoclonal antibody of IgG was used as control. The results are representative of four independent experiments. (B) Western blotting analysis of imDex and mDex using monoclonal antibodies specific for HSP70, HSP90, ICAM-1, and MFG-E8. The signal intensities in the blot were assessed by densitometry and are represented in the graphs. One representation of three independent experiments is shown. * $P<0.01$.

party imDex/rapamycin-cotreatment, n = 6; Figure 2C and Table 1).

The Combination of Rapamycin and Donor imDex Decreases the Cellular Response against Donor Antigen Post-Transplantation

To determine the mechanism of the cardiac allograft tolerance induced by imDex/rapamycin-cotreatment, we assessed the anti-donor cellular response in recipients after transplantation; at 5 or 10 d post-transplantation, total splenocytes and purified splenic T lymphocytes were separated from different recipients, which included untreated recipients (n = 6, 3 mice each for d5 and d10), recipients of donor imDex (n = 5, 3 mice for d5 and 2 mice for d10) or rapamycin (n = 6, 3 mice each for d5 and d10) alone, and imDex/rapamycin-cotreated recipients (n = 6, 3 mice each for d5 and d10). These splenocytes and splenic T lymphocytes were responder cells. Stimulator cells were splenocytes from donor (C57BL/6) or third party (CBA/H) treated with mitomycin C for 24 hours (h). Responder cells (5×10^4) were co-cultured with stimulator cells (2×10^4) for 72 h. Cell proliferation was quantified by incubating the cells with 1 μCi [^{3}H]-thymidine during the last 18 h of co-culture. Total splenocytes from imDex/rapamycin-cotreated recipients induced a significant decrease in proliferation against donor splenocytes compared with responder cells from untreated recipients (d5: $P<0.001$, d10: $P<0.001$). Total splenocytes from recipients treated with donor imDex or rapamycin alone also negatively affected the anti-donor antigen cellular response compared with splenocytes from untreated recipients (d5: $P=0.164$, d10: $P=0.008$, for donor imDex; d5: $P=0.004$, d10: $P<0.001$, for rapamycin), but splenocytes from recipients treated with donor imDex or rapamycin alone were 4- to 5-fold less efficient than those from recipients co-treated with imDex and rapamycin (Figure 3A). However, splenocytes from the four groups proliferated equivalently against the third-party CBA/H splenocytes (Figure 3B). These results were also observed in proliferation of purified T lymphocytes against donor or third-party splenocytes (Figure 3C–D). Furthermore, we assessed activation of T lymphocytes by measuring upregulation of the early activation marker CD69 after splenic T lymphocytes purified from different recipients (10 d after transplantation) were co-cultured with stimulator cells for 24 h. T lymphocytes of imDex/rapamycin-cotreated recipients expressed lower levels of CD69 compared with those of untreated recipients (Figure 3E, $P<0.001$). The levels of CD69 were also downregulated on T lymphocytes of donor imDex-treated or rapamycin-treated recipients compared with those of untreated recipients, but were significantly different than those of imDex/rapamycin-cotreated recipients ($P=0.013$ for rapamycin; $P=0.025$ for imDex). However, CD69 was expressed similarly on splenocytes of the four groups against third-party CBA/H lymphocytes (Figure 3F). We concluded that activation and proliferation of T

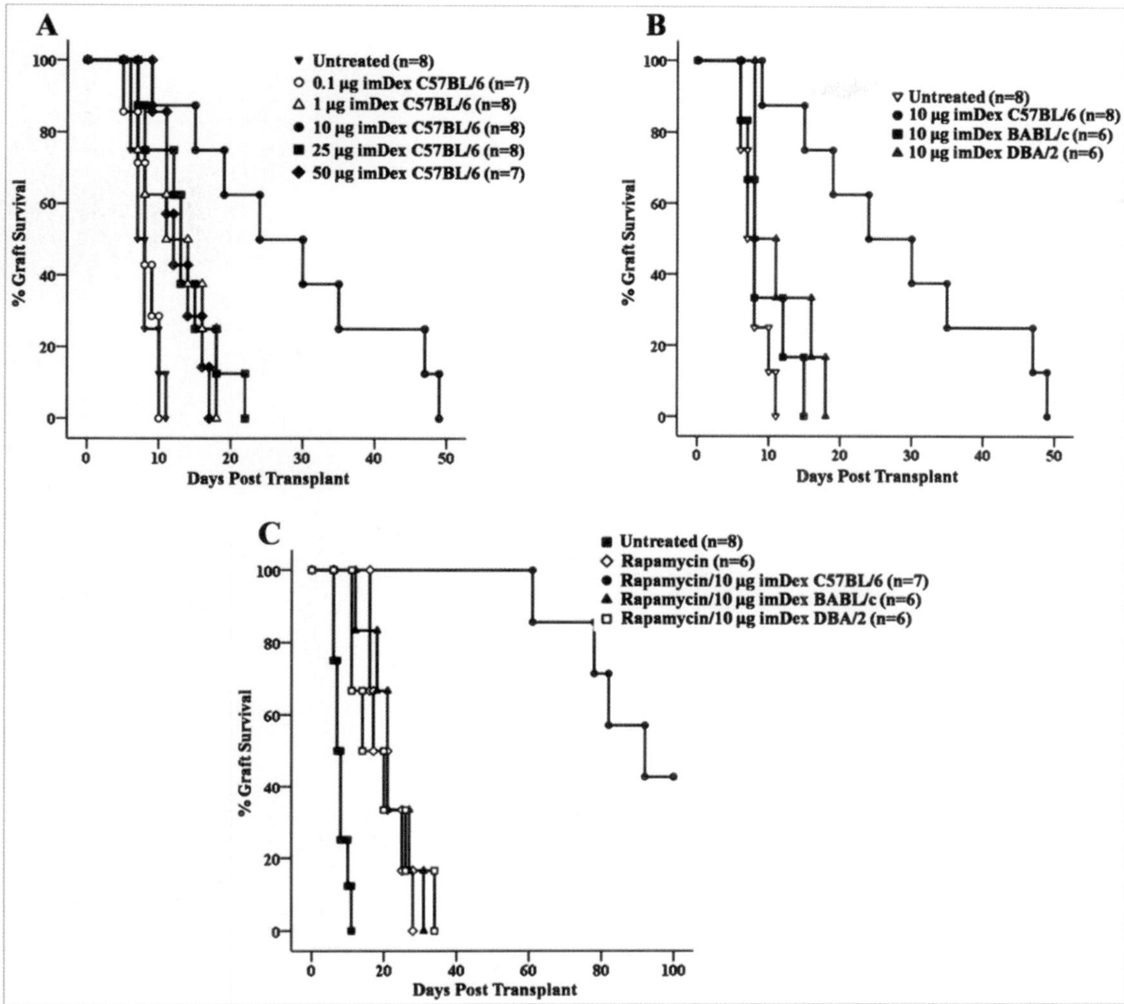

Figure 2. Administration of low-dose donor imDex with a subtherapeutic rapamycin promotes cardiac allograft survival. Different imDex concentrations were injected via caudal vein 7 d before, the day of, and 7 d after transplantation, and 1 mg/kg/d rapamycin was injected via caudal vein for 11 consecutive days (days −3 to 7) with or without imDex. (A) The cardiac allograft survival for different donor imDex concentrations in the absence of rapamycin. (B) ImDex (10 µg) of the donor (C57BL/6), recipient (BALB/c), or third-party (CBA/H) were injected into recipient mice. (C) The allograft survival following rapamycin treatment alone or with 10 µg donor, recipient, or third-party imDex.

lymphocytes against donor antigen are more efficiently inhibited by rapamycin/imDex-cotreatment than by donor imDex treatment alone.

Treatment with Donor imDex and Rapamycin Induces Spleen $CD4^+CD25^+$ T Cells in Recipient Mice

The inhibition of T lymphocyte activation and proliferation against donor antigen suggested that treatment with imDex plus rapamycin may favor expansion of the percentage of $CD4^+CD25^+Fox3^+$ regulatory T (Treg) cells. To this end, purified splenic T lymphocytes were collected from untreated recipients (n = 6), recipients of donor imDex (n = 6) or rapamycin (n = 6) treatment alone, and imDex/rapamycin-cotreated recipients (n = 6) 5 or 10 d after transplantation. The percent of $CD4^+CD25^+$ T cells was analyzed by FACS, and the Foxp3 expression level was analyzed by western blotting. As shown in Figure 4A, treatment with imDex/rapamycin resulted in a notable increase in the proportion of $CD4^+CD25^+$ T cells compared with that of the untreated group (d5: 12% ±0.9% versus 2% ±0.4%, $P<0.001$; d10: 11% ±1.4% versus 3% ±0.2%, $P<0.001$). Treatment with donor imDex or rapamycin alone also increased the proportion of $CD4^+CD25^+$ T cells, but neither treatment was as efficient as imDex/rapamycin-cotreatment (d5: $P<0.001$, d10: $P<0.001$, for donor imDex; d5: $P=0.001$, d10: $P<0.001$, for rapamycin). Western blotting showed enhanced production of Foxp3 in purified splenic T lymphocytes from imDex/rapamycin-cotreated recipients as compared with untreated recipients (d5: $P=0.007$, d10: $P<0.001$; Figure 4B). Moreover, we found a striking 1.7- to 1.9-fold decrease in Foxp3 expression in recipients treated with donor imDex or rapamycin alone as compared with recipients cotreated with imDex and rapamycin. These data indicated that the combination of imDex and rapamycin may inhibit proliferation and activation of alloreactive T lymphocytes, which is closely related to increased proportion of the spleen $CD4^+CD25^+$ T cells in recipients.

Table 1. Cardiac allograft survival after treatment with imDex or imDex+rapamycin.

Treatment	Median (days)	Graft survival days	*P* value
Untreated*	7.5	6×2, 7×2, 8×2, 10, 11	
0.1 μg imDex C57BL/6	8	5, 7, 8×2, 9, 10×2,	>0.05[a]
1 μg imDex C57BL/6	12.5	7×2, 8, 11, 14, 16, 18×2	>0.05[a]
10 μg imDex C57BL/6	27	9, 15, 19, 24, 30, 35, 47, 49	<0.001[a]
25 μg imDex C57BL/6	14	7, 8, 12, 13, 15, 18, 22, 29	<0.05[a], <0.01[b]
50 μg imDex C57BL/6	12	9, 11×2, 12, 14, 16, 17	>0.05[a]
10 μg imDex BALB/c	8	6, 7, 8×2, 12, 15,	>0.05[a], <0.001[b]
10 μg imDex CBA/H	9.5	8×3, 11, 16, 18	>0.05[a], <0.01[b]
Rapamycin	19	16×2, 17, 21, 25, 28	<0.05[a], <0.001[c]
Rapamycin/10 μg imDex C57BL/6	92	61, 78, 82, 92, >100×3	<0.001[a]
Rapamycin/10 μg imDex BALB/c	21	12, 18, 21×2, 27, 31	<0.05[a], <0.001[c]
Rapamycin/10 μg imDex CBA/H	17	11×2, 14, 20, 26, 34	<0.05[a], <0.001[c]

BALB/c recipients were transplanted with a C57BL/6 heart. Recipients were treated with imDex or imDex/rapamycin.
*Treated with physiological saline.
[a]Compared with untreated mice.
[b]Compared with 10 μg imDex C57BL/6-treated mice.
[c]Compared with 10 μg imDex C57BL/6/rapamycin-treated mice.

Administration of Donor imDex in Combination with Low-Dose Rapamycin Prevents Acute Cardiac Allograft Rejection Lesions

To determine the degree of the benefit of the combination of donor imDex with rapamycin for preventing acute cardiac allograft rejection lesions, we harvested hearts of untreated (n = 3) and imDex/rapamycin-cotreated (n = 3) recipients 7 d post-transplantation and examined the histology of these allografts. A heart of syngenetic transplantation (BALB/c to BALB/c) was used as a control. Upon gross examination, the heart of the untreated recipient was obviously congestive and edematous, but the imDex/rapamycin-cotreated recipient's heart was similar to the control (Figure 5A). As compared with the control (Figure 5F and 5G), microscopic examination of allografts of the untreated group showed severe lymphocyte infiltration and interstitial edema, which are signs of acute graft rejection (Figure 5B and 5C). By contrast, the allografts of imDex/rapamycin-cotreated recipients displayed minor pathological changes of acute graft rejection (Figure 5D and 5E). These results indicated that administration of donor imDex in combination with rapamycin can efficiently prevent acute cardiac allograft rejection.

Tolerance Induced by Cotreatment with imDex and Rapamycin Is Donor Specific and Transferable

To assess whether the recipients cotreated with imDex and rapamycin displayed donor specific tolerance, these mice had a second heart from donor mice (C57BL/6, n = 3) or third-party mice (CBA/H, n = 3) transplanted in the neck. Three naïve BALB/c mice that received hearts from C57BL/6 mice were used as controls. As shown in Table 2, the cardiac allografts from donor mice survived longer than the hearts from third-party mice and control mice (MST: >100 d for donor hearts; 21 d for third-party hearts; 9 d for control group).

To determine whether the tolerance in imDex/rapamycin-cotreated recipients was transferable, we injected serum or splenocytes from tolerant recipients (n = 3) or naïve mice (n = 3) into naïve irradiated BALB/c mice via the caudal vein and then transplanted C57BL/6 mouse hearts into them. As shown in Table 3, the administration of splenocytes derived from tolerant mice significantly prolonged the cardiac allograft survival (MST: 83 d), but the splenocytes derived from naïve BALB/c mice did not exhibit this effect (MST: 16 d). We also found that the transfer of serum derived from the tolerant recipients prolonged the allograft survival to a limited extent compared with the splenocytes of tolerant recipients (MST: 44 d). These data suggested that tolerance induced by imDex/rapamycin-cotreatment is donor specific and transferable, and it may be mediated by recipient immunoregulatory cells but not by recipient serum.

Discussion

The principle method for generating immature BM-DCs with GM-CSF plus IL-4 was first reported by Inaba *et al.* [22] and Sallusto *et al.* [23]. So, we applied this conventional method to obtain imDCs that expressed lower MHC class I and co-stimulatory CD80 and CD86 than DCs stimulated with LPS, and this is consistent with many reported data [16,24]. Next, we extracted exosomes from the culture supernatant of imDCs or mDCs and comparatively analyzed the differences in morphology and protein composition between the two kinds of Dex. Although there were no significant differences in morphology, there was a large difference in protein composition. Similar to imDCs, imDex expressed the "tolerance" phenotype with low levels of MHC class I, CD80, and CD86 and moderate levels of MHC class II molecules. Meanwhile, imDex expressed lower levels of ICAM-1 than mDex, which is necessary for the immune activity of mDex and as a major exosomal protein for inducing immune rejection to skin allografts [9]. These results suggest that imDex have the potential to induce immune tolerance. Thus, we injected donor imDex into recipients before and after transplantation, and found that treatment with 10 μg of donor imDex significantly prolonged cardiac allograft survival, but this effect decreased when imDex dose was increased. This effect was donor specific because imDex from syngenetic mice or third-party mice had no such effect.

The above results indicate that, compared with imDCs, use of imDex to induce immune tolerance has several advantages. First, as a source of donor antigens, imDex can be frozen long-term in

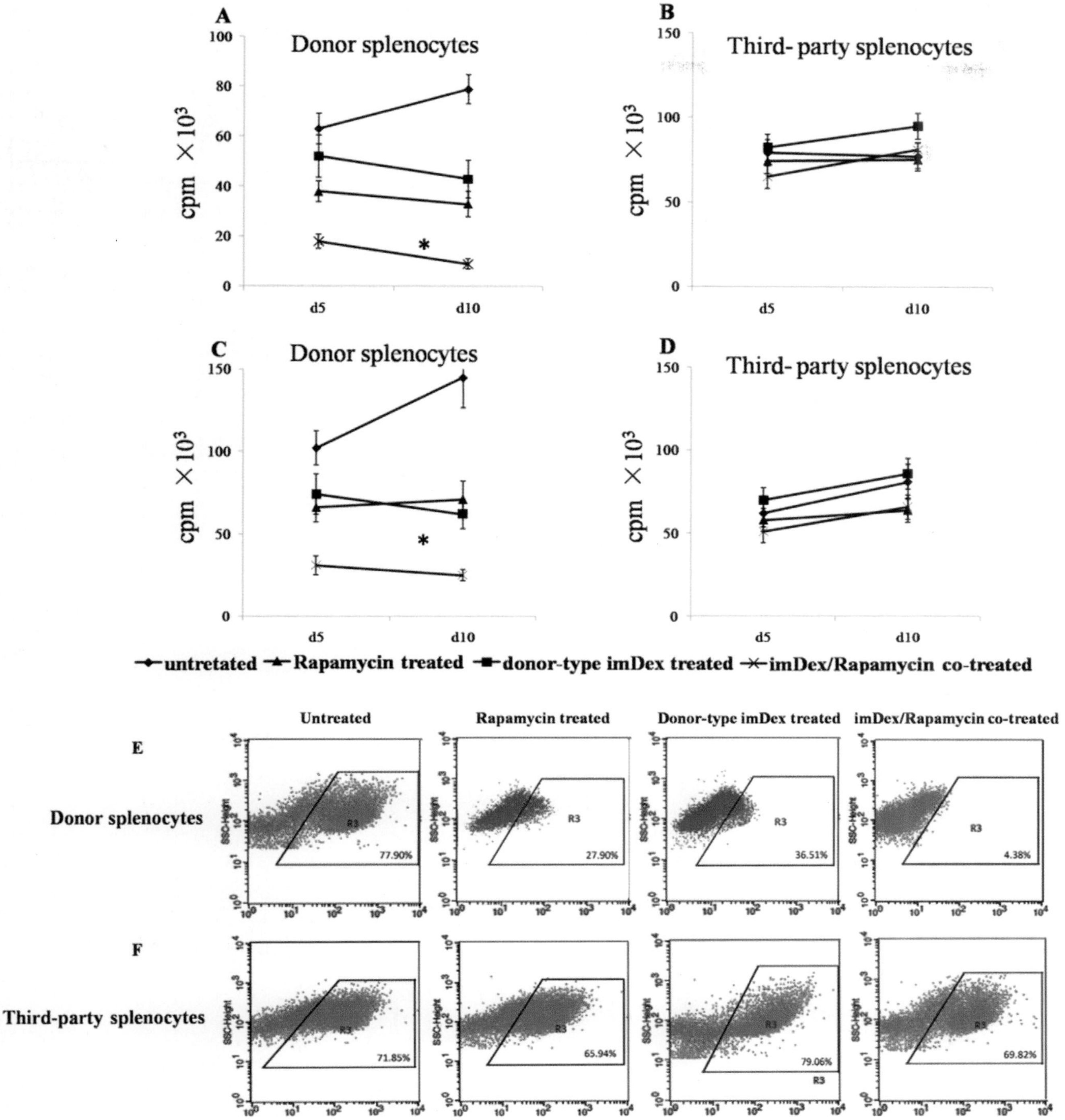

Figure 3. Donor imDex combined with rapamycin inhibits proliferation and activation of alloreactive T lymphocytes against donor antigen. At 5 or 10 d post-transplantation, 5×10^4 total splenocytes (A-B) or purified T lymphocytes (C-D) from untreated, donor imDex-treated, rapamycin-treated or imDex/rapamycin-cotreated recipients (responder cells) were incubated with 2×10^4 donor or third-party splenocytes (stimulator cells) for 72 h. Label (1 μCi [^{3}H]-thymidine) was added for the last 18 h of culture, and incorporation was determined using a liquid scintillation counter. Upregulation of CD69 on the four groups of responder cells (10 d after transplantation) was measured by FACS 24 h after simulator cell addition (E-F). One representation of four independent experiments is shown. * $P<0.01$.

vitro without affecting biological activity [25], so imDex can be prepared quickly and used immediately when necessary. Second, because only a small amount of imDex is needed to prolong allograft survival, it can be used repeatedly on recipients if necessary. Third, imDex do not undergo maturation in vivo, which is a crucial drawback in current DC-based therapies for tolerance induction. Finally, large doses of donor imDex (50 μg) do not accelerate immune rejection, so it is safe to treat recipients

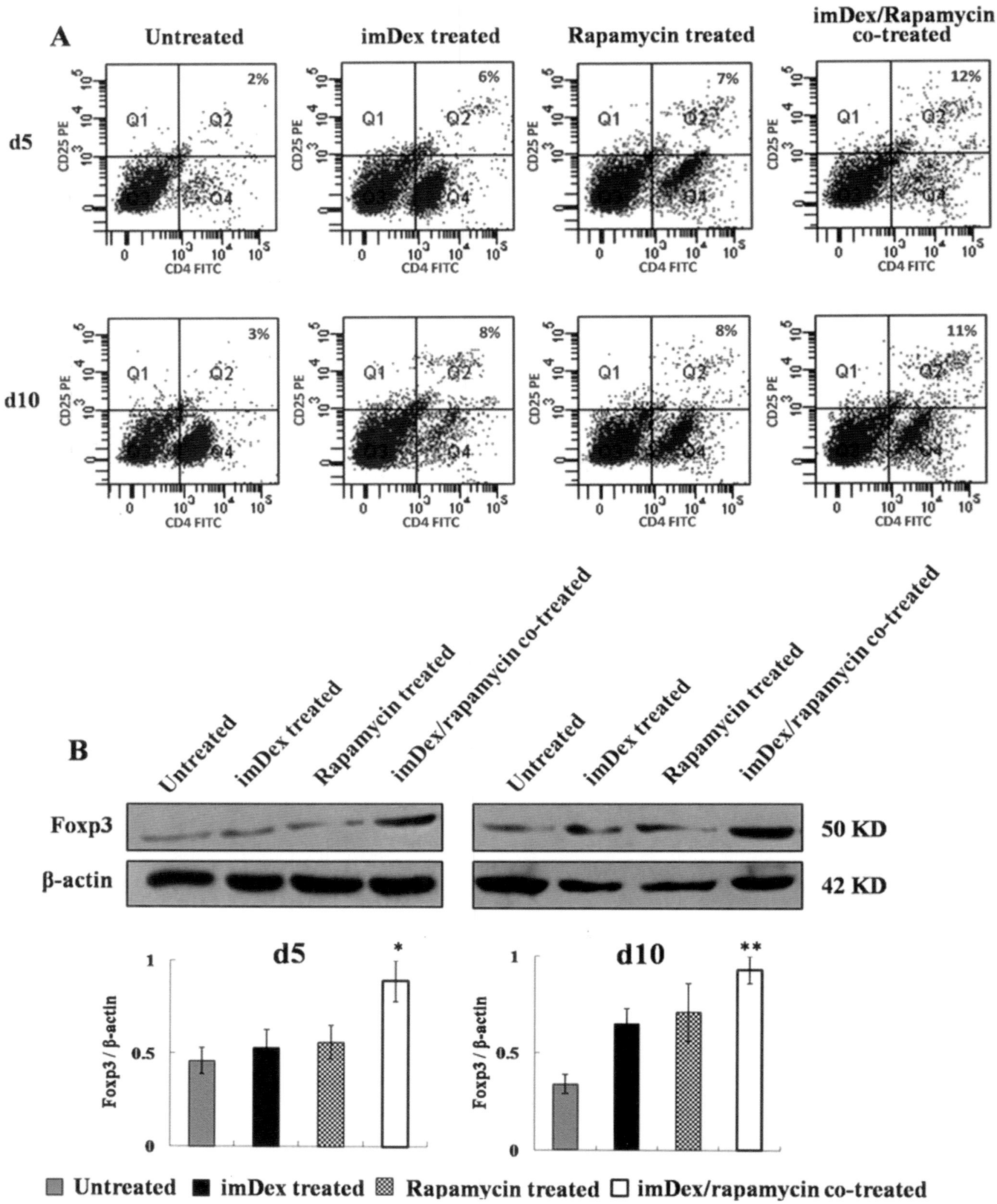

Figure 4. FACS and western blotting analysis of splenic CD4$^+$CD25$^+$Foxp3$^+$ T cells. Splenic T lymphocytes were isolated from untreated recipients (n = 6), recipients treated with donor imDex (n = 6) or rapamycin (n = 6) alone, and imDex/rapamycin-cotreated (n = 6) recipients at d5 or d10 after transplantation. (A) The percentages of splenic CD4$^+$CD25$^+$ T cells from the four groups of recipient mice were calculated from flow cytometric analysis. The number in the upper-right quadrant of each histogram indicates the percentage of CD4$^+$CD25$^+$ T cells. Results were obtained from three mice per condition, and one representative of four independent experiments is shown. (B) Foxp3 versus β-actin western blotting analysis

of splenic T lymphocytes from the groups of recipients upper. Densitometry shows fold induction of Foxp3:β-actin ratio. Bars = mean ± SD (n = 3), * $P<0.01$, ** $P<0.001$. One representation of three independent experiments is shown.

with donor imDex through the veins before transplantation, and the donor imDex do not sensitize recipients against donor antigens.

Previous reports showed that the role of exosomes in developing tolerance or immunity depends not only on the stage and type of the secreting cells but also on the state of the immune microenvironment where the exosome-APC interaction takes place [11,26]. In our study, although a low dose of donor imDex significantly prolonged cardiac allograft survival, this effect was limited and was insufficient to induce immune tolerance. We considered that donor imDex should be combined with non-specific immunosuppressive therapy to develop a tolerance microenvironment in vivo. Rapamycin was thus used to favor the presentation of alloantigens in a tolerogenic fashion because it blocks T-cell activation, inhibits DCs maturation, and selectively allows for proliferation while fostering the suppressive function of $Foxp3^+$ Treg cells [27,28]. We observed that the combination of low-dose rapamycin and donor imDex induced long-term cardiac allograft survival, but rapamycin alone did not have this effect. This result suggests that, in a steady and tolerogenic state, imDex-delivered donor antigens will prevent immune rejection and promote immune tolerance.

Although the exact mechanism remains unclear, there is increasing evidence that donor APC-derived exosomes administered intravenously might participate in induction and maintenance of peripheral T-cell tolerance. Morelli *et al.* [29] reported that circulating allogeneic exosomes are efficiently captured by recipient splenic DCs without triggering their activation, and they deliver donor MHC molecules to host T cells, which induce donor specific T-cell tolerance in recipients. In this study, we found that total splenocytes and splenic T cells from imDex/rapamycin-cotreated recipients showed a significant decrease in proliferation and activation response against donor splenocytes. These data suggest that combined treatment with donor imDex and rapamycin inhibits T-cell activation and may induce anergy of alloreactive T cells for donor antigen.

We also observed that the combination of imDex and rapamycin notably increased the percentage of $CD4^+CD25^+$ T cells and up-regulated Foxp3 expression in recipient splenic T cells. Furthermore, we found that the tolerance in imDex/rapamycin-cotreated recipients could be transferred to naïve syngenetic mice by injecting the recipients' splenocytes but not serum. These results suggest that the tolerance may be mediated by immunoregulatory cells of recipients. But on the other hand, we did not confirm whether these $CD4^+CD25^+$ T cells are Treg cells or not. We didn't analyze their alloantigen-specificity and regulatory functions experimentally either. Because of this, we cannot confirm the immune tolerance we induced are directly related to the $CD4^+CD25^+Foxp3^+$ Treg cells. However, only a few studies have focused on the effect of exosomes on Treg cells. Wang *et al.* reported that exosomes derived from thymus can induce Treg cell proliferation in vivo [30]. Cai *et al.* described utilizing exosomes that were derived from TGF-β1 gene-modified BM-DCs to induce $Foxp3^+$ Treg cells and decrease the proportion of Th17 cells in a mouse model of inflammatory bowel disease [31]. In the future, we will do more study on the number, phenotype and function of splenic $CD4^+CD25^+$ T cells in the tolerant recipients to find the relation between these cells and Treg cells.

Taken together, our study demonstrates that the combination of donor imDex and low-dose rapamycin treatment can induce donor specific immune tolerance in a murine heterotopic cardiac transplantation model and prolong allograft survival. The tolerance can persist long term and be transferred to naïve syngenetic recipients by injecting tolerific immunocytes. Our study reports a novel therapeutic approach for inducing transplant immune tolerance, but mechanisms such as inter-regulation among imDex, DCs, and Treg cells should be examined in future studies.

Materials and Methods

Ethnics Statements

All animals experiments were performed in accordance with a guideline from the Administration of Animal Experiments for Medical Research Purposes issued by the Ministry of Health of China. The protocol was approved by the Animal Experiment Administration Committee of Fourth Military Medical University. All surgery was performed under sodium pentobarbital anesthesia and accomplished in a clean surgery room with sterilized instruments. All efforts were made to minimize the suffering of the mice during the experiments.

Mice

Six- to twelve- week-old male C57BL/6 (H-2b), male BALB/c (H-2d) and male CBA/H (H-2k) mice were obtained from the Experimental Animal Center of The Fourth Military Medical University and housed in specific pathogen-free conditions.

Antibodies

The monoclonal antibodies used for cytofluorometric analysis were fluorescein isothiocyanate (FITC)-conjugated anti-MHC class I, anti-MHC class II, anti-CD80, anti-CD86, anti-CD4, anti-CD69 were purchased from Bioscience (San Diego, CA, USA), and FITC-conjugated anti-CD11c, FITC-conjugated anti-NLDC-145, and phycoerythrin (PE)-conjugated anti-CD25 were purchased from Abcam (Cambridge, UK). The corresponding isotype antibodies were control. Western blotting utilized monoclonal antibodies (all from Santa Cruz Biotechnology, Santa Cruz, CA) against HSP70, HSP90, ICAM-1, MFG-E8, and Foxp3; horseradish peroxidase (HRP)-conjugated secondary antibodies (Santa Cruz Biotechnology) were used.

Cultivation of BMDCs in vitro

DCs were generated from BM progenitor cells as described by Muthana *et al.* [32]. In brief, BM cells were collected from femurs and tibias of mice. To remove the adherent macrophages, the BM cells then were cultured for 24 h in complete RPMI 1640 medium (Invitrogen, Carlsbad, CA, USA) supplemented with 10% endotoxin-free fetal bovine serum (Gibco, Carlsbad, CA, USA) that had been centrifuged (110,000×g overnight) to deplete contaminating vesicles and protein aggregates. The non-adherent cells were culture for 8 d in fresh complete medium containing recombinant mouse GM-CSF and IL-4 (10 ng/mL, Peprotech, Rocky Hill, NJ). The cells and supernatant of culture medium were harvested. Then, part of the harvested cells were re-cultured in fresh complete medium containing LPS (10 µg/mL, Sigma, St. Louis, M.O.) for 48 h, and the cells and supernatant were also harvested.

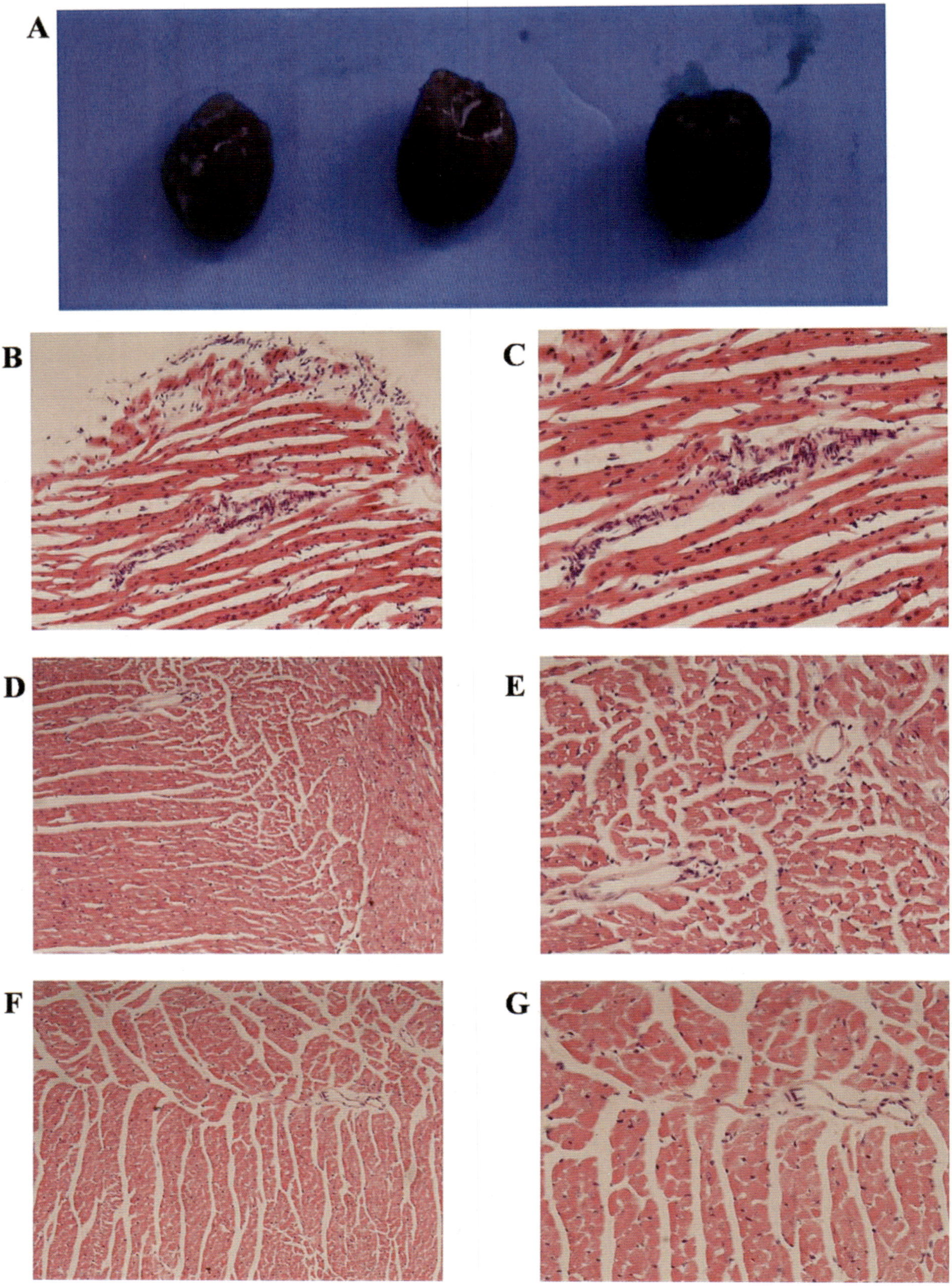

Figure 5. Signs of acute rejection in cardiac allografts. Cardiac allografts of untreated and imDex/rapamycin-cotreated recipients were harvested at 7 d post-transplantation, and transplantation of a syngenetic heart (BALB/c to BALB/c) was used as control. (A) The left heart is from the syngenetic transplantation recipient, the middle heart is from the imDex/rapamycin-cotreated recipient, and the right heart is from the untreated

recipient. Paraffin sections were stained with hematoxylin-eosin and observed by optical microscope. Representative allografts of untreated recipients (B and C), allografts of imDex/rapamycin-cotreated recipients (D and E), and control specimens from syngenetic transplantation recipients (F and G) are shown.

Exosomes Preparation

Exosomes were purified from the culture supernatant of mDCs and imDCs by ultrafiltration and ultracentrifugation as described by Lamparski *et al.* [17]. In brief, the supernatants were first centrifuged at 300×g for 10 min and then at 1,200×g for 30 min, each at 4°C. The clarified supernatant was concentrated by centrifugation for 30 min at 4,000×g, at 4°C, in a pre-rinsed Centricon Plus-80 capsule filter (MW 100 KDa, Millipore, Danvers, MA). The ultrafiltrate was underlayed with 30% sucrose/D_2O density cushion, followed by ultracentrifugation at 110,000×g and 4°C for 1 h. The cushion was collected and diluted in Dulbecco's phosphate-buffered saline (DPBS), and then concentrated by centrifugation for 30 min at 4,000×g at 4°C in a pre-rinsed 100 KDa MWCO Millipore Centricon Plus-80 capsule filter. The protein amounts were quantified by Bradford assay (Bio-Rad, Hercules, CA, USA).

Electron Microscopy

The sample of exosomes was loaded onto a copper grid at room temperature. After the exosomes precipitated for 3 min, the sample liquid was sucked up slowly with filter paper from the side of the copper mesh. The sample was then counterstainded with 2% phosphotungstic acid solution (30 μL, pH 6.8) for 10 min at room temperature. The sample liquid was sucked up again, and the sample was placed under an incandescent lamp for 5 min. Finally, the exosomes sample was examined with a CM20 Twin Philips electron microscope (Phillips Electronic Instruments, Mahway, NJ).

Flow Cytometry

The two kinds of DCs were harvested, washed, and resuspended in PBS, 1% bovine serum albumin, 5% heat-inactivated normal rabbit serum, and 0.1% sodium azide. Cells were incubated for 45 min at 4°C with FITC-conjugated anti-MHC class I, anti-MHC class II, anti-CD80, anti-CD86, anti-CD11c, or anti-NLDC-145. The two kinds of exosomes were incubated with aldehyde/sulfate latex beads (Interfacial Dynamics, Portland, OR, USA) at 4°C overnight. The reaction was stopped with 100 mM glycine for 30 min. The beads were washed three times in flow buffer (3% fetal bovine serum in PBS) and stained with FITC-conjugated anti-MHC class I, anti-MHC class II, anti-CD80, or anti-CD86. The beads and cells were analyzed by flow cytometry using a FACSCalibur (BD Immunocytometry Systems, Franklin Lakes, NJ, USA).

Western Blotting

Proteins (10 μg) from the two kinds of exosomes were separated by 10% SDS-PAGE, transferred onto PVDF membranes (Millipore, USA). After blocking with 5% nonfat dry milk in PBS, the membrane was incubated with anti-HSP70, anti-HSP90, anti-ICAM-1, and anti-MFG-E8 followed by HRP-conjugated secondary antibodies and detected by enhanced chemiluminescence using X-ray films.

Transplantation

Celiac heart transplants were performed using a modified technique as described by Niimi [33]. C57BL/6 mice served as heart donors and BALB/c mice as allograft recipients. After the donor mice were anesthetized, the inferior vena cava, azygos vein, superior vena cava, ascending artery and pulmonary artery were ligated with 7-0 silk sutures and cut in order. An end-to-side anastomosis was performed with 10-0 surgical sutures between the donor ascending artery with the recipient abdominal artery and between the donor pulmonary artery with the recipient inferior vena cava. Cervical heterotopic heart transplants were performed according to the Chen technique [34]. The donor ascending artery was sutured end-to-side to the recipient right common carotid artery, and the donor pulmonary artery was anastomosed to the recipient right external jugular vein. Cardiac graft function was tested daily by transabdominal palpation. Rejection was defined as a complete cessation of palpable beating. Cardiac allografts that stopped beating within 2 d were regarded as technical failures and excluded from further analysis.

In vitro T-Cell Stimulation Assay

Five or ten days after transplantation, total splenocytes of recipient BABL/c mice were sterilely extracted, and T cells were isolated from the splenocytes using nylon wool columns (Fenwall Laboratories, Lake Zurich, IL, USA); the two kind of cells were responder cells. Responder cells (5×10^4) were seeded into 96-well round-bottom plates (Costar, Santa Fe Springs, CA, USA) with stimulatory cells that were donor (C57BL/6) or third-party (CBA/H) splenocytes treated with mitomycin C 24 h. [^{3}H]-thymidine (1 μCi/well) was added 72 h later for 18 h, and [^{3}H]-thymidine incorporation was countered by liquid scintillation. Additionally, the T cells were harvested after co-cultured with stimulatory cells and stained with anti-CD69. T cells were then analyzed by flow cytometry.

Table 2. Survival of the second cardiac allograft for tolerant imDex/rapamycin-cotreated recipients.

Recipients	Second graft	Median (days)	Graft survival days	*P* value
Naïve BALB/c	C57BL/6	9	7, 9, 12	
Tolerant imDex/rapamycin- cotreated BALB/c	C57BL/6	>100	75, >100×2	<0.001[a, b]
Tolerant imDex/rapamycin- cotreated BALB/c	CBA/H	21	11, 21, 24	>0.05[a]

Donor imDex/rapamycin-cotreated recipients were transplanted with a secondary C57BL/6 or CBA/H heart in the neck. Naïve BALB/c recipients that received C57BL/6 hearts were used as controls.
[a]Compared with naïve BALB/c group.
[b]Compared with cardiac allograft of CBA/H.

Table 3. Cardiac allograft survival for BALB/c recipients injected with splenocytes or serum from tolerant imDex/rapamycin-cotreated recipients.

Treatment	Median (days)	Graft survival days	*P* value
Untreated*	15	12, 15, 21	
Splenocytes from naïve BALB/c	16	15, 16, 19	>0.05 [a]
Splenocytes from imDex/rapamycin- cotreated recipients	83	83, 88, >100	<0.001 [a, b]
Serum of naïve BALB/c	19	14, 19, 20	>0.05 [a]
Serum of imDex/rapamycin-cotreated recipients	44	38, 44, 57	<0.001 [a]

All naïve BALB/c mice were irradiated with 3 Gy before transfer of 5×10^7 splenocytes or 0.8 mL serum.
*Treated with physiological saline.
[a]Compared with untreated group.
[b]Compared with serum of imDex/rapamycin-cotreated recipients.

Spleen CD4$^+$CD25$^+$ T Cells and Foxp3 Protein Quantification

Five or ten days after transplantation, splenic T cells were purified from recipient mice and stained with FITC-conjugated anti-CD4 and PE-conjugated anti-CD25, and then analyzed by flow cytometry. Foxp3 protein of splenic T cells was measured by western blotting.

Assessment of Histological and Morphometric Changes

Seven days after transplantation, specimens of cardiac allografts from different recipients were obtained and fixed with paraformaldehyde and then embedded in paraffin. Sections (5 μm) were stained with hematoxylin-eosin to assess morphological changes. Transplantation of a syngenetic heart (BALB/c to BALB/c) was used as a control.

Statistics Analysis

One-way analysis of variance was used for analysis within groups. The Kaplan and Meier method was used to calculate the survival curves, and the log-rank test was used to compare animal survival in different groups of mice using SPSS for Windows 17.0 software. $P<0.05$ was considered significant.

Acknowledgments

We thank Xia Li and Fu-Qin Zhang for raising mice and ultracentrifugation.

Author Contributions

Conceived and designed the experiments: K-FD D-YC. Performed the experiments: XL D-SW WZ W-JS W-ML J-FW WH Z-CZ YY. Analyzed the data: J-JL J-YY. Wrote the paper: K-FD.

References

1. Wood KJ, Goto R (2010) Mechanisms of rejection: current perspectives. Transplantation 93: 1–10.
2. Schonder KS (2011) Pharmacology of immunosuppressive medications in solid organ transplantation. Crit Care Nurs Clin North Am 23: 405–423.
3. Mendieta-Zerón H (2011) Developing immunologic tolerance for transplantation at the fetal stage. Immunotherapy 3: 1499–1512.
4. Morelli AE (2006) The immune regulatory effect of apoptotic cells and exosomes on dendritic cells: its impact on transplantation. Am J Transplant 6: 254–261.
5. van Kooten C, Lombardi G, Gelderman KA, Sagoo P, Buckland M, et al. (2011) Dendritic cells as a tool to induce transplantation tolerance: obstacles and opportunities. Transplantation 91: 2–7.
6. Chaput N, Théry C (2011) Exosomes: immune properties and potential clinical implementations. Semin Immunopathol 33: 419–440.
7. Admyre C, Johansson SM, Paulie S, Gabrielsson S (2006) Direct exosome stimulation of peripheral human T cells detected by ELISPOT. Eur J Immunol 36: 1772–1781.
8. Montecalvo A, Shufesky WJ, Stolz DB, Sullivan MG, Wang Z, et al. (2008) Exosomes as a short-range mechanism to spread alloantigen between dendritic cells during T cell allorecognition. J Immunol 180: 3081–3090.
9. Segura E, Nicco C, Lombard B, Véron P, Raposo G, et al. (2005) ICAM-1 on exosomes from mature dendritic cells is critical for efficient naive T cell priming. Blood 106: 216–223.
10. Bianco NR, Kim SH, Ruffner MA, Robbins PD (2009) Therapeutic effect of exosomes from indoleamine 2, 3-dioxygenase-positive dendritic cells in collagen-induced arthritis and delayed-type hypersensitivity disease models. Arthritis Rheum 60: 380–389.
11. Kim SH, Bianco NR, Shufesky WJ, Morelli AE, Robbins PD (2007) Effective treatment of inflammatory disease models with exosomes derived from dendritic cells genetically modified to express IL-4. J Immunol 179: 2242–2249.
12. Yang X, Meng S, Jiang H, Chen T, Wu W (2010) Exosomes derived from interleukin-10-treated dendritic cells can inhibit trinitrobenzene sulfonic acid-induced rat colitis. Scand J Gastroenterol 45: 1168–1177.
13. Yang X, Meng S, Jiang H, Zhu C, Wu W (2011) Exosomes derived from immature bone marrow dendritic cells induce tolerogenicity of intestinal transplantation in rats. Surg Res 171: 826–832.
14. Pêche H, Heslan M, Usal C, Amigorena S, Cuturi MC (2003) Presentation of donor major histocompatibility complex antigens by bone marrow dendritic cell-derived exosomes modulates allograft rejection. Transplantation 76: 1503–1510.
15. Pêche H, Trinite B, Martinet B, Cuturi MC (2005) Prolongation of heart allograft survival by immature dendritic cells generated from recipient type bone marrow progenitors. Am J Transplant 5: 255–267.
16. Lutz MB, Kukutsch N, Ogilvie AL, Rössner S, Koch F, et al. (1999) An advanced culture method for generating large quantities of highly pure dendritic cells from mouse bone marrow. J Immunol Methods 223: 77–92.
17. Lamparski HG, Metha-Damani A, Yao JY, Patel S, Hsu DH, et al. (2002) Production and characterization of clinical grade exosomes derived from dendritic cells. J Immunol Methods 270: 211–226.
18. Hackstein H, Taner T, Zahorchak AF, Morelli AE, Logar AJ, et al. (2003) Rapamycin inhibits IL-4-induced dendritic cell maturation in vitro and dendritic cell mobilization and function in vivo. Blood 101: 4457–4463.
19. Taner T, Hackstein H, Wang Z, Morelli AE, Thomson AW (2005) Rapamycin-treated, alloantigen-pulsed host dendritic cells induce Ag-specific T cell regulation and prolong graft survival. Am J Transplant 5: 228–236.
20. Turnquist HR, Cardinal J, Macedo C, Rosborough BR, Sumpter TL, et al. (2010) mTOR and GSK-3 shape the CD4+ T-cell stimulatory and differentiation capacity of myeloid DCs after exposure to LPS. Blood 115: 4758–4769.
21. Pliszczynski J, Kahan BD (2011) Better actual 10-year renal transplant outcomes of 80% reduced cyclosporine exposure with sirolimus base therapy compared with full cyclosporine exposure without or with concomittant sirolimus treatment [J]. Transplant Proc 43: 3657–3668.
22. Inaba K, Inaba M, Romani N, et al. (1992) Generation of large numbers of dendritic cells from mouse bone marrow cultures supplemented with granulocytermacrophage colonystimulating factor. J Exp Med 176: 1693–1702.
23. Sallusto F, Lanzavecchia A (1994) Efficient presentation of soluble antigen by cultured human dendritic cells is maintained by granulocytermacrophage colony-stimulating factor plus interleukin 4 and downregulated by tumor necrosis factor alpha. J Exp Med 179: 1109–1118.
24. Hume PS, He J, Haskins K, Anseth KS (2012) Strategies to reduce dendritic cell activation through functional biomaterial design. Biomaterials 33: 3615–3625.
25. Morse MA, Garst J, Osada T, Khan S, Hobeika A, et al. (2005) A phase I study of dexosome immunotherapy in patients with advanced non-small cell lung cancer. J Transl Med 3: 9–9.

26. Kim SH, Lechman ER, Bianco N, Menon R, Keravala A, et al. (2005) Exosomes derived from IL-10-treated dendritic cells can suppress inflammation and collagen-induced arthritis. J Immunol 174: 6440–6448.
27. Battaglia M, Stabilini A, Roncarolo MG (2005) Rapamycin selectively expands CD4+CD25+FoxP3+ regulatory T cells. Blood 105: 4743–4748.
28. Monti P, Scirpoli M, Maffi P, Piemonti L, Secchi A, et al. (2008) Rapamycin monotherapy in patients with type 1 diabetes modifies CD4+CD25+FOXP3+ regulatory T-cells. Diabetes 57: 2341–2347.
29. Morelli AE, Larregina AT, Shufesky WJ, Sullivan ML, Stolz DB, et al. (2004) Endocytosis, intracellular sorting, and processing of exosomes by dendritic cells. Blood 104: 3257–3266.
30. Wang GJ, Liu Y, Qin A, Shah SV, Deng ZB, et al. (2008) Thymus exosomes-like particles induce regulatory T cells. J Immunol 181: 5242–5248.
31. Cai Z, Zhang W, Yang F, Yu L, Yu Z, et al. (2012) Immunosuppressive exosomes from TGF-β1 gene-modified dendritic cells attenuate Th17-mediated inflammatory autoimmune disease by inducing regulatory T cells. Cell Res 22: 607–610.
32. Muthana M, Fairburn B, Mirza S, Slack LK, Pockley AG (2004) Systematic evaluation of the conditions required for the generation of immature rat bone marrow-derived dendritic cells and their phenotypic and functional characterization. J Immunol Methods 294(1–2): 165–179.
33. Niimi M (2001) The technique for heterotopic cardiac transplantation in mice: experience of 3000 operations by one surgeon. J Heart Lung Transplant 20: 1123–1128.
34. Chen ZH (1991) A technique of cervical heterotopic heart transplantation in mice. Transplantation 52: 1099–1101.

5

Evaluation of the Therapeutic Potential of Bone Marrow-Derived Myeloid Suppressor Cell (MDSC) Adoptive Transfer in Mouse Models of Autoimmunity and Allograft Rejection

Lucile Drujont[1]⁹, Laura Carretero-Iglesia[1]⁹, Laurence Bouchet-Delbos[1], Gaelle Beriou[1], Emmanuel Merieau[1], Marcelo Hill[¤1], Yves Delneste[2], Maria Cristina Cuturi[1], Cedric Louvet[1]*

1 ITUN, Inserm UMR_S 1064, Center for Research in Transplantation and Immunology, Nantes, France, **2** UMR Inserm 892 CNRS 6299, Université d'Angers, CHU Angers, Laboratoire d'Immunologie et Allergologie, Angers, France

Abstract

Therapeutic use of immunoregulatory cells represents a promising approach for the treatment of uncontrolled immunity. During the last decade, myeloid-derived suppressor cells (MDSC) have emerged as novel key regulatory players in the context of tumor growth, inflammation, transplantation or autoimmunity. Recently, MDSC have been successfully generated in vitro from naive mouse bone marrow cells or healthy human PBMCs using minimal cytokine combinations. In this study, we aimed to evaluate the potential of adoptive transfer of such cells to control auto- and allo-immunity in the mouse. Culture of bone marrow cells with GM-CSF and IL-6 consistently yielded a majority of $CD11b^{+}Gr1^{hi/lo}$ cells exhibiting strong inhibition of $CD8^{+}$ T cell proliferation in vitro. However, adoptive transfer of these cells failed to alter antigen-specific $CD8^{+}$ T cell proliferation and cytotoxicity in vivo. Furthermore, MDSC could not prevent the development of autoimmunity in a stringent model of type 1 diabetes. Rather, loading the cells prior to injection with a pancreatic neo-antigen peptide accelerated the development of the disease. Contrastingly, in a model of skin transplantation, repeated injection of MDSC or single injection of LPS-activated MDSC resulted in a significant prolongation of allograft survival. The beneficial effect of MDSC infusions on skin graft survival was paradoxically not explained by a decrease of donor-specific T cell response but associated with a systemic over-activation of T cells and antigen presenting cells, prominently in the spleen. Taken together, our results indicate that in vitro generated MDSC bear therapeutic potential but will require additional in vitro factors or adjunct immunosuppressive treatments to achieve safe and more robust immunomodulation upon adoptive transfer.

Editor: Ryan M. Teague, Saint Louis University School of Medicine, United States of America

Funding: This work has been carried out thanks to the support of the Labex IGO project (n° ANR-11-LABX-0016-01) funded by the «Investissements d'Avenir» French Government program, managed by the French National Research Agency (ANR). This work was also supported by funds from IHU-Cesti (Investissement d'Avenir ANR-10-IBHU-005, région Pays de la Loire et Nantes Métropole). LD was supported by an Inserm-Région Pays de la Loire fellowship. CL was supported by an Inserm "young researcher" CDD. The funders had no role in study design, data collection and analysis, decision to publish, or preparation of the manuscript.

Competing Interests: The authors have declared that no competing interests exist.

* E-mail: cedric.louvet@univ-nantes.fr

⁹ These authors contributed equally to this work.

¤ Current address: Laboratorio de Inmunorregulacion e inflamación, Institut Pasteur de Montevideo, Departamento de Inmunobiologia, Facultad de Medicina, Universidad de la Republica, Montevideo, Uruguay

Introduction

Myeloid-derived suppressor cells (MDSC) comprise a heterogeneous population of myeloid cells at various stages of differentiation accumulating during pathological situations, such as tumor development or inflammation, and with the ability to suppress T-cell responses [1,2,3]. In mice, MDSC are broadly defined as $CD11b^{+}$ $Gr1^{+}$ cells and have been shown to exhibit a variety of suppressor mechanisms [4,5].

Growing evidence indicate a central role of MDSC in diverse models of autoimmune diseases [6] including type 1 diabetes [7,8], arthritis [9], colitis [10], alopecia areata [11], myocarditis [12] or experimental autoimmune encephalomyelitis (EAE) [13,14,15]. A protective role of MDSC has also been documented in the context of allogenic transplantation [4,16,17,18,19,20,21]. Interestingly, a recent report linked the accumulation of MDSC with $FoxP3^{+}$ regulatory T cells (Tregs) in kidney-transplanted patients [22].

Thus, similarly to Tregs [23], MDSC represent a novel regulatory cell type that could be manipulated to achieve immune tolerance in the context of autoimmunity or transplantation. Although injections of G-CSF [24], LPS [18] or IL-33 [25] have been shown to favor the generation of endogeneous MDSC in allograft recipient mice, a promising and clinically applicable approach would consist in the adoptive transfer of in vitro-generated MDSC. In this regard, the study by Rossner et al. initially paved the way towards MDSC generation from bone marrow (BM) cells using GM-CSF [26]. Alternatively, Zhou et al. demonstrated the development of MDSC from mouse stem cells

[27]. Other studies reported that BM cells co-cultured with hepatic stellate cells could lead to the production of MDSC effectively preventing murine islet allograft rejection [28] or colitis [29]. Generally, GM-CSF, in conjunction with tumor cells conditioned culture medium, appeared as a pivotal cytokine for the generation of MDSC [30,31]. IL-6 has subsequently been identified as a potent complement to GM-CSF for the generation of both mouse and human MDSC [32,33]. Importantly, Marigo et al. showed that mouse bone marrow-derived MDSC generated with GM-CSF and IL-6 exhibit a stronger immunosuppressive activity in vivo and could induce long-term survival of pancreatic islet allograft upon repeated adoptive transfer [32]. This latter study opened an avenue to the generation of these cells in great numbers and in a controlled manner for their use in cellular immunotherapy.

In the current study, we investigated and compared the suppressive potential of BM-derived MDSC generated in vitro with GM-CSF and IL-6, without combination treatment, in different mouse models of auto- and allo-immunity.

Results

Based on the method described by Marigo et al. [32], we cultured BM cells from naive mice with GM-CSF and IL-6 and examined their phenotype after 4 days. We routinely obtained > 90% of $CD11b^+$ cells that could be subdivided in $Gr1^{hi}$ and $Gr1^{low}$ cells (Figure 1A and B). $Gr1^{low}$ cells, which contain the majority of $CD11c^+$ cells (Figure 1C), were shown to exhibit the highest suppressive activity [32]. Attributing the term MDSC to immature myeloid cells requires the demonstration of an immunosuppressive function, at least in vitro. As shown in Figure 2A and B, BM cells cultured with GM-CSF and IL-6 efficiently prevented $CD8^+$ T cell proliferation in a dose-dependent manner, reaching >80% inhibition at a ratio of 2:1 (MDSC:T cells).

We then examined the suppressive potential of these MDSC in vivo. In order to best reproduce a T cell response triggered by a cellular antigen, we immunized mice with COS cells transfected with a plasmid encoding a non-secreted fusion protein linking the ovalbumin peptide SIINFEKL ($OVA_{257-264}$) to GFP. In this system, the OVA peptide is presented to $CD8^+$ T cells by recipient APCs on their MHC class I molecules through the processes of phagocytosis and antigen cross-presentation. The injection of $CD8^+$ T cells from TCR-transgenic OT-1 mice then allows the monitoring of an antigen-specific T cell reponse in vivo, as depicted in Figure 3A and C. Immunization with OVA-expressing COS cells resulted in a strong $CD8^+$ T cell proliferation while control COS cells did not. Concomitant adoptive transfer of MDSC and immunization did not prevent this proliferation (Figure 3B). We then hypothesized that, rather than significantly altering proliferation, MDSC could influence their differentiation into CTLs. However, as shown in Figure 3D, MDSC failed to impact antigen-specific T cell cytoxicity.

To assess the effect of MDSC adoptive transfer in a more physiological context, we made use of a model of type 1 diabetes [34,35] in which autoimmunity is induced by the injection of $CD8^+$ OT-1 T cells in conjunction with a polyclonal anti-OVA antibody (Ab) into RIP-mOVA transgenic mice (membrane OVA is expressed as a neo-antigen by the pancreatic beta cells under the rat insulin promoter). In our hands, and as previously established [34], virtually all mice become diabetic within 5 to 12 days. Single adoptive transfer of MDSC on the day of OT-1 and Ab injection did not prevent diabetes development (Figure 4A). We reasoned that MDSC might benefit from an inflammatory milieu to stably exert their suppressive function on T cells. However, neither two consecutive adoptive transfers of MDSC, 2 and 5 days after OT-1 and Ab injection (Figure 4B), nor a single injection at day 5 using twice as much cells (data not shown) significantly impinged on the progression of the disease. Finally, we tested whether the loading of MDSC with the antigenic peptide before injection could potentiate the suppression by promoting their interaction with the diabetogenic T cells. Strikingly, this approach seemed to rather exacerbate the development of the disease, since treated mice developed accelerated diabetes compared to control mice (Figure 4C).

Next, we tested whether adoptive transfer of MDSC could modulate a polyclonal response in the context of allograft rejection. As shown in Figure 5A, while male skin grafts transplanted onto female recipients were rejected within 19 to 28 days, two injections of syngenic (female) MDSC, the day before transplantation and at day 6 post-transplantation, were sufficient to prolong graft survival. A single injection of LPS-activated MDSC (LPS was added to the MDSC culture for the last 5 hours) on the day of transplantation similarly achieved a significant outcome (Figure 5B). However, this effect was markedly and reproducibly enhanced with five weekly consecutive injections, leading to graft survival up to 40 days (Figure 5C).

To understand the beneficial effect of MDSC adoptive transfers on skin graft survival, we investigated the immune cell composition directly in the graft as well as in the draining lymph nodes and in the spleen, two weeks post-transplantation (after three weekly injections of MDSC). Few or no injected MDSC were detected (using the congenic marker Ly5.1) suggesting that these cells are rapidly eliminated or preferentially home to a distinct location than the skin graft, the draining lymph nodes or the spleen. Surprisingly, we found that skin grafts from both untreated and MDSC-treated mice showed similar numbers of total infiltrated leucocytes (data not shown). In fact, the proportion of $CD4^+$ T cells was even increased in MDSC-treated mice (Figure 6A) whereas no difference was observed for $CD8^+$ T cells (Figure 6B). In addition, donor-specific $CD8^+$ T cells were found in similar numbers both in skin grafts (Figure 6C) and in the periphery (Figure 7A). The proportions of $CD19^+$ B cells, $CD3^-$ $NK1.1^+$ NK cells, $CD3^+$ $CD4^+$ or $CD3^+$ $CD8^+$ T cells were not altered by MDSC adoptive transfers (data not shown). $FoxP3^+$ cell numbers among $CD4^+$ T cells were increased in skin-grafted mice compared to naive mice but no significant differences were observed between untreated and MDSC-treated mice (Figure 7B). As expected, increased numbers of $CD25^+$ and $CD69^+$ T cells were detected mostly in the draining lymph nodes of skin graft recipients compared to naive mice (Figure 7C and D). However, MDSC adoptive transfers did not prevent this activation phenotype. On the contrary, we observed a dramatic increase of $CD25^+$ and $CD69^+$ T cell numbers in MDSC-treated mice, almost exclusively in the spleen (Figure 7C and D), a phenomenon that was also associated with increased numbers of MHC II^+ and $CD86^+$ cells (Figure 8A and B). Thus, MDSC adoptive transfers, rather than specifically suppressing the allogenic immune response, appears to induce a state of systemic activation that correlates with prolongation of skin graft survival.

Discussion

Compelling evidence from animal models suggest a great potential of MDSC adoptive transfer for preventing graft rejection or treating autoimmune disorders. For example, MDSC from tumor-bearing mice have been shown to prevent the onset of type 1 diabetes when co-transferred with diabetogenic $CD4^+$ T cells [7]. Similarly, MDSC purified from LPS-treated mice are capable

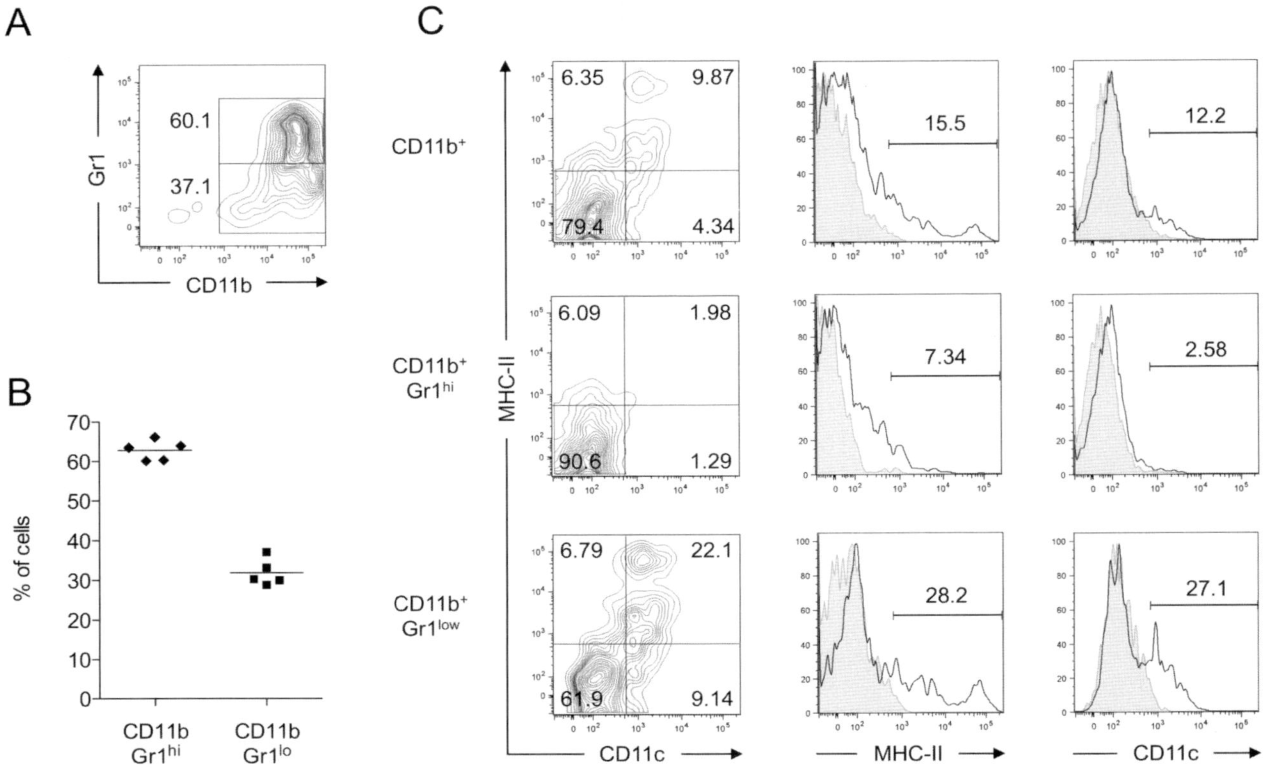

Figure 1. Phenotype of BM-derived MDSC. (A) BM cells from naive mice were cultured in the presence of GM-CSF and IL-6 for 4 days. Surface expression of CD11b and Gr1 was measured by flow cytometry. (B) Quantification of the relative proportions of CD11b$^+$ Gr1^{hi} and CD11b$^+$ Gr1^{low} populations in independent preparations. (C) Expression of CD11c and MHC II on total CD11b$^+$ cells or in Gr1^{hi} and Gr1^{low} populations. Gray areas represent fluorescence minus one (FMO) controls. Data show representative results from at least four independent experiments.

of prolonging skin allograft survival [18]. These findings prompted us to embark on a study to assess their therapeutic potential in mouse models of autoimmunity and transplant rejection. A translational view implicates the development of a clinically acceptable method for the production of these cells. Marigo et al. provided convincing data highlighting the high suppressive activity of MDSC generated from BM cells using GM-CSF supplemented with IL-6, for the in vivo inhibition of T cell responses as well as the prevention of allogenic islet rejection [32].

While we succeeded in producing in vitro suppressive CD11b$^+$ cells using this approach, we did not observe any alteration of in vivo antigen-specific CD8$^+$ T cell responses or autoimmune diabetes development after adoptive transfer of these cells. It is important to note that this stringent in vivo experimental procedure involves a high number of strongly reactive monoclonal (OT-1 TCR transgenic) T cells. Furthermore, the expansion of diabetogenic CD8$^+$ T cells is not the result of homeostatic proliferation since RIP-mOVA mice are non-irradiated lymphosufficient hosts, but strictly depends on robust Fc receptor-mediated OVA cross-presentation by DCs [34].

Surprisingly, we found that loading MDSC with the neo-antigen OVA peptide rather exacerbated than dampened the development of the disease. This observation was reproduced using in vivo cytotoxicity assay (data not shown). The culture of whole BM cells with GM-CSF and IL-6 results in an heterogeneous mixture of myeloid cells, a fraction of them likely bearing the potential to differentiate into highly immunogenic DCs. Additional factors, such as PGE_2 [36] or subset separation before injection, may help to maintain a suppressive homogeneity. The use of few markers expressed at the surface of MDSC obviously does not satisfy the requirement of a pure and stable suppressive population. In this regard, CD11b$^+$ Gr1$^+$ cells have also been described as immunostimulatory during tumor growth [37] or autoimmunity [38]. Taken together, these observations could raise doubts over the safety of BM-derived myeloid cell transfer, potentially detrimental in specific inflammatory situations.

The transplantation of male skin onto female recipients mounts a progressive expansion of low frequency polyclonal T cell clones leading to graft rejection. In this model, in contrast to type 1 diabetes, we found that multiple injections of MDSC significantly prolonged graft survival. It is tempting to speculate that a continuous treatment could result in long-term acceptance of the graft, as shown by Marigo et al. in pancreatic islet transplantation [32]. Of note, two injections of MDSC were not sufficient to prevent or delay rejection of complete mismatch skin grafts (Balb/c onto C57BL/6 mice, data not shown) pointing to the limit of these in vitro generated MDSC to impinge, by themselves, on a strong allogenic response, yet in the same manner as in vitro expanded Tregs, alone, failed to provide significant graft prolongation in a complete mismatch setting, in lymphosufficient mice [39].

These results also emphasize the need for identifying strategies to increase and preserve the suppressive ability of MDSC after transfer in order to reduce the frequency of injections. Indeed, MDSC have been shown to rapidly differentiate into mature myeloid cells in the absence of tumor-derived factors or sustained inflammation [40,41]. In this regard, Greifenberg et al. originally demonstrated that LPS + IFN-γ combination considerably

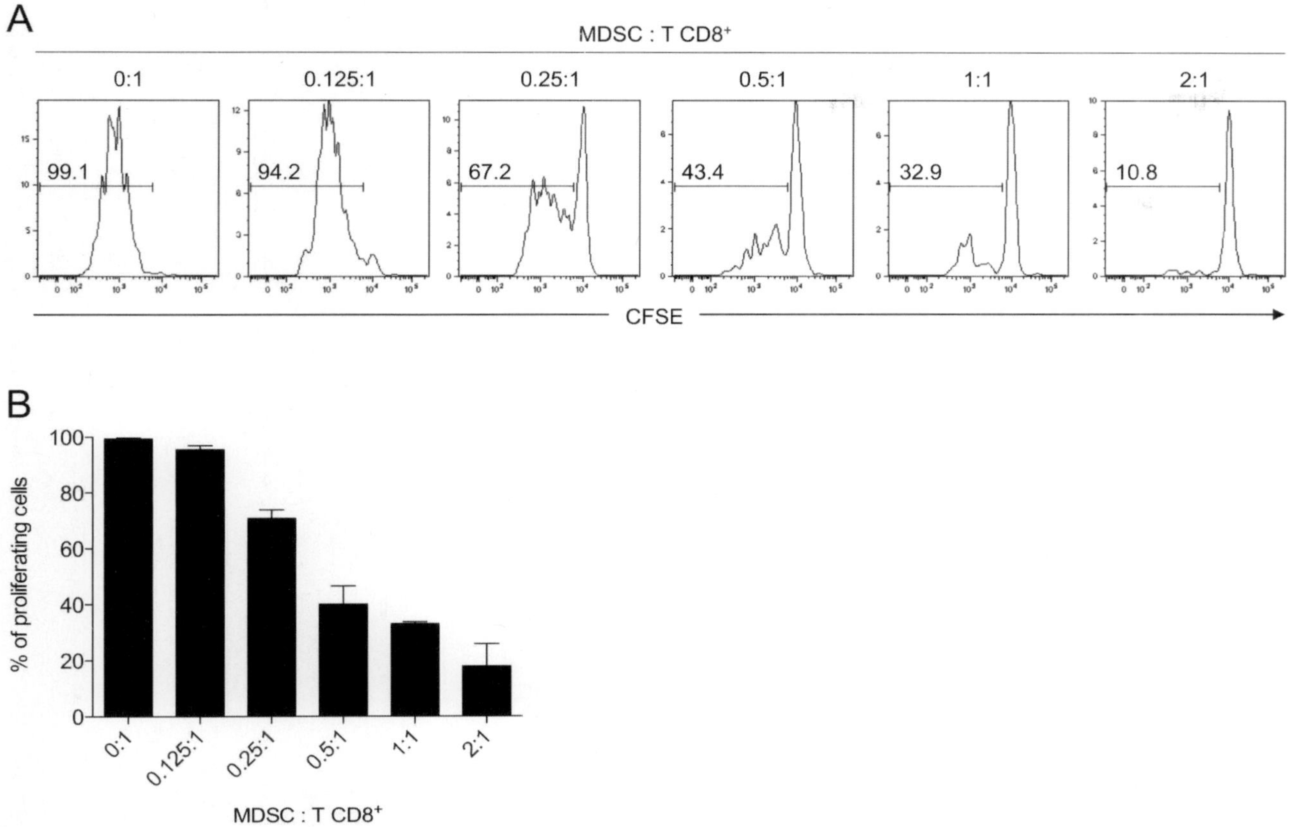

Figure 2. BM-derived MDSC efficiently inhibit T cell proliferation *in vitro.* $CD8^+$ T cells were purified from OT-1 transgenic mice and labeled with CFSE before anti-CD3/CD28 bead stimulation. MDSC generated in vitro with GM-CSF and IL-6 were added to T cells at different ratios. After three days of culture, the percentage of proliferating cells ($CFSE^{low}$) in $CD8^+$ cells was assessed by flow cytometry. Representative histograms of CFSE dilution (A) and quantification of triplicates for each condition are shown (B). Data are representative of three independent experiments.

augmented the suppressive capacity of MDSC by impairing DC differentiation [42]. Similarly, Highfill et al. showed that addition of IL-13 in BM cells cultured with GM-CSF and G-CSF resulted in the production of potently suppressive MDSC that efficiently inhibited graft-versus-host disease [43]. Thus, amongst other strategies that have been reported to promote MDSC activation/expansion [5], our results support the relevance of this approach since a single injection of LPS-activated MDSC was sufficient to induce a significant prolongation of graft survival. It remains to be evaluated whether additional injections of these activated cells will reinforce this beneficial effect and if the addition of IFN-γ (or other cytokines) could further boost their suppressive function in vivo.

Mechanistically, we have found that the beneficial effect of MDSC infusions on skin graft survival was paradoxically not explained by a decrease of donor-specific T cell response but rather associated with an over-activation of T cells and antigen presenting cells. The fact that this observation was prominently made in the spleen suggests that MDSC transfers could create a window of systemic exhaustion in the immune system allowing the allogenic graft to survive, a phenomenon that would terminate immediately after cessation of the therapy, then excluding any mechanism of long term tolerance. Thus, while this effect is associated with delayed graft rejection in the setting of transplantation, it appears inefficient or rather detrimental during the developpement of a fast and potent autoimmune response. These differential outcomes stress the need to carefully evaluate MDSC adoptive transfer therapies, or any other approaches, by using carefully chosen models in relation with the clinical aim.

Interestingly, Treg therapy alone in lymphosufficient hosts, even in an antigen-specific fashion, similarly fails to induce a long-term protection from allograft rejection [39,44]. The combination of MDSC and Treg cell therapies could result in a synergistic effect. Indeed, numerous reports have shown that MDSC promote the development and homeostasis of Tregs over $CD4^+$ T effector cells [45], notably in the context of type 1 diabetes [7,8]. Moreover, MDSC can capture and present exogenous antigens to their MHC class II molecules which can be drastically upregulated upon IFN-γ stimulation [46]. Treg accumulation has also been attributed to monocytic suppressive cells [19]. Thus, in spite of a recent study that challenged this view concerning granulocytic MDSC [47], these results generally argue for a beneficial interplay between Tregs and MDSC that could be relevant in the context of cellular therapy. Athough similar levels of $FoxP3^+$ Treg were found in the draining lymph nodes or spleen of MDSC-treated mice, the detection of a potential beneficial effect of MDSC on these cells in the periphery will probably require the examination of the (donor) antigenic specificity. Moreover, it will be interesting to determine whether the increase of $CD4^+$ T cells that we observed in the skin grafts of MDSC-treated mice could reflect an influx of Treg that would be mostly specific for the donor antigens.

In summary, in the present study, we have compared the potential of in vitro generated MDSC adoptive transfer in relevant and distinct in vivo models of immune response. Our data

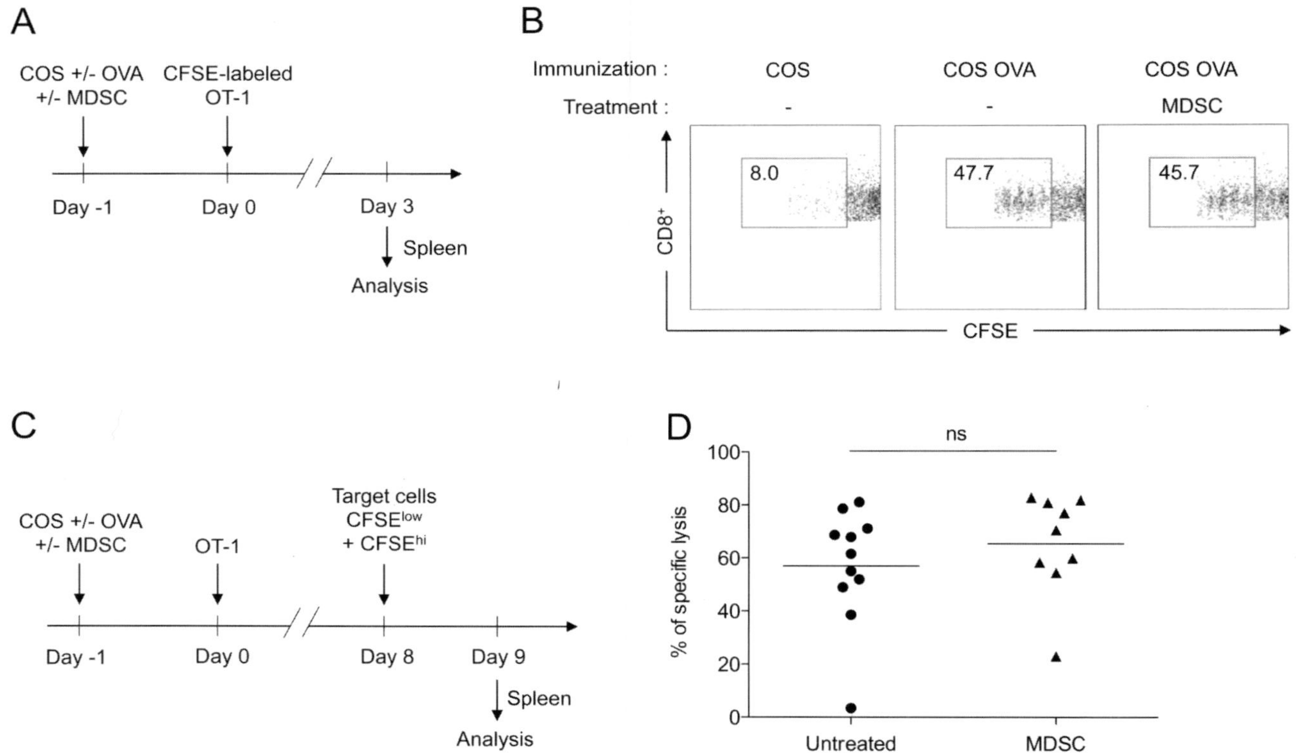

Figure 3. Adoptive transfer of BM-derived MDSC does not alter antigen-specific CD8$^+$ T cell responses. (A–B) In vivo proliferation assay: COS cells transfected with a plasmid coding for GFP fused to the $OVA_{257-264}$ peptide (COS OVA) or GFP alone (COS) were injected i.v. into mice with or without MDSC generated in vitro with GM-CSF and IL-6. Responder CD8$^+$ T cells purified from OT-1 TCR-transgenic mice were labeled with CFSE and injected i.v. the following day. After 3 days, spleens of recipient mice were harvested to assess CFSE dilution by flow cytometry. Data are representative of two experiments. (C–D) In vivo cytotoxicity assay: CD8$^+$ T cells purified from OT-1 TCR-transgenic mice (non labeled with CFSE) were injected in COS GFP/OVA-immunized mice as described above. After 8 days, CFSE-labeled CD45.1$^+$ target cells either loaded with $OVA_{257-264}$ (CFSE^{hi}) or control (CFSE^{low}) peptides were injected. Specific lysis was determined the next day by flow cytometry by measuring the relative proportion of each population in the spleen of MDSC-treated or untreated mice compared to non-immunized mice. Data show results from four independent experiments with 9 to 11 mice per group.

highlight the need to refine the in vitro generation of homogeneous, stable and strongly suppressive myeloid cells before considering a therapeutic approach, most likely with combination treatments.

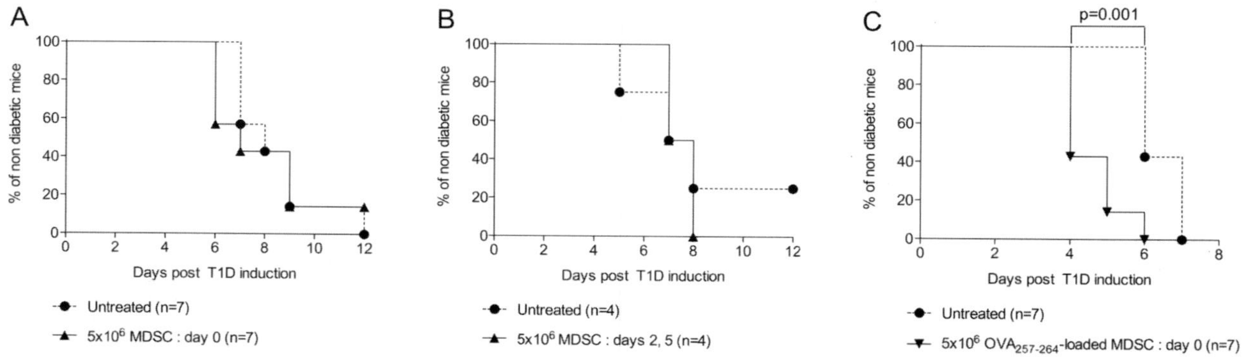

Figure 4. Adoptive transfer of BM-derived MDSC does not prevent the development of autoimmune diabetes. Type 1 diabetes was induced in RIP-mOVA mice by injecting (i.v.) naive CD8$^+$ T cells from OT-1 TCR-transgenic mice together with an anti-OVA polyclonal antibody (i.p.). Blood glycemia was monitored every day during at least 12 days. Indicated numbers of MDSC generated in vitro with GM-CSF and IL-6 were adoptively transferred at day 0 (A) or at days 2 and 5 (B). Alternatively, MDSC were loaded with the $OVA_{257-264}$ peptide before injection at day 0 (C). In each experiment, MDSC-treated mice were compared to a group of untreated mice.

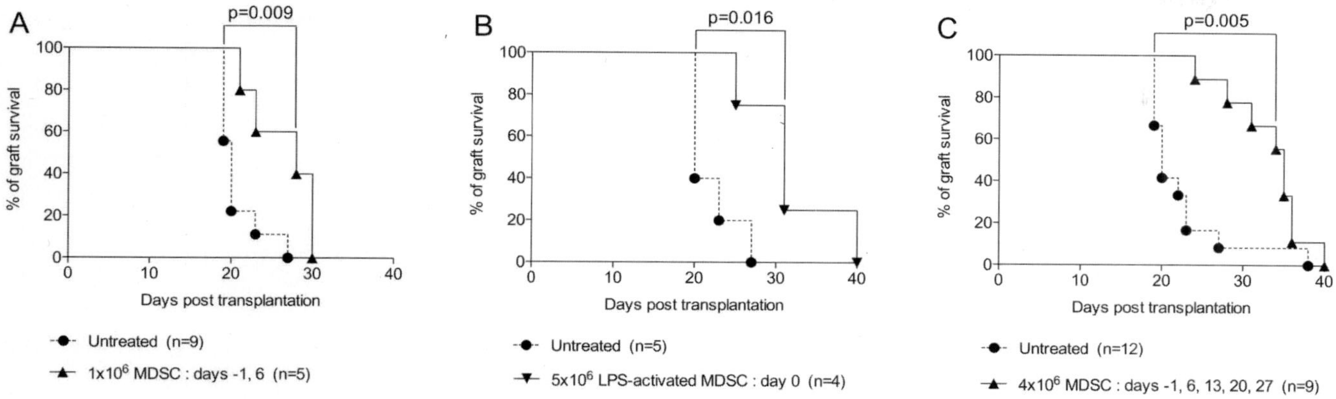

Figure 5. Adoptive transfer of BM-derived MDSC prolongs skin allograft survival. (A) Male skin grafts were transplanted onto females recipients treated or not at days −1 and 6 post-transplantation, with one million autologous (female) MDSC generated in vitro with GM-CSF and IL-6. (B) Alternatively, LPS was added in vitro for the last 5 hours of the MDSC culture and five million cells were injected at day 0. (C) Male skin grafts were transplanted onto females recipients treated or not at days −1, 6, 13, 20 and 27 post-transplantation, with four million autologous (female) MDSC generated in vitro with GM-CSF and IL-6. Graft survival was monitored every other day from day 7 post-transplantation.

Materials and Methods

Ethics Statement

This study was carried out in strict accordance with the protocol approved by the Commitee on the Ethics of Animal Experiments of Pays de la Loire (Ref: CEEA.2012.211 and CEEA.2013.9).

Mice

C57BL/6 mice were purshased from Janvier (France). RIP-mOVA (C57BL/6-Tg(Ins2-TFRC/OVA)296Wehi/WehiJ) transgenic mice [48] were purchased from The Jackson Laboratory (Bar Harbor, ME, USA). For this line, hemizigous mice were maintained in the laboratory by breeding transgenic mice, selected by PCR genotyping, with wild-type C57BL/6 mice. OT-1 TCR-transgenic mice (C57BL/6-Tg(TcraTcrb)1100Mjb/Crl) [49] and Ly5.1 congenic mice (B6.SJL-*Ptprc*^{a} *Pepc*^{b}/BoyCrl) were purshased from Charles Rivers (France).

Reagents

Murine GM-CSF was from Peprotech (Neuilly-sur-Seine, France). IL-6 and LPS were from Sigma-Aldrich (Saint-Quentin Fallavier, France). CFDA-SE (CFSE) was from Molecular Probes (Montluçon, France). OVA (SIINFEKL) and Smcy (KCSRNRQYL) peptides were from PolyPeptide (Strasbourg, France). Anti mouse CD11b biotin (M1/70) (used with streptavidin APC or streptavidin APC-Cy7), CD11b APC-Cy7 (M1/70), CD11c PE-Cy7 (HL3), I-A^b FITC (AF6-120.1), Gr1 PE (Ly6C/G, RB6-8C5), CD45.1 APC (A20), CD45.2 APC-Cy7 (104), CD45.2 PerCP-Cy5.5 (104), CD19 APC (1D3), NK1.1 PE (PK136), CD3ε PerCP-Cy5.5 (145-2C11), CD3ε Pacific Blue (500A2), CD3ε FITC (145-2C11), CD4 PE-Cy7 (RM4-5), CD8α Pacific blue (53-6.7), CD8α APC-Cy7 (53-6.7), CD8α PerCP-Cy5.5 (53-6.7), FoxP3 Alexa Fluor647 (MF23), CD25 PE (704), CD69 FITC (H1.2F3), and CD86 FITC (B7.2, GL1) were from BD PharMingen (Le Pont de Claix, France). Male antigen UTY-specific CD8$^+$ T cells were detected using a PE labelled Pro5 MHC Pentamer (H-2D^b, WMHHNMDLI) (ProImmune Limited, Oxford, UK).

Generation of BM-derived MDSC

MDSC were generated as previously described [32]. Tibias and femurs from C57BL/6 mice were removed and BM was flushed. Red blood cells (RBCs) were lysed with ammonium chloride. To obtain BM-derived MDSC, 2.5×10^6 cells were plated into dishes with 100 mm diameter in 10 mL of complete medium, which consisted of 10% heat-inactivated fetal bovine serum (Lonza, Levallois, France), nonessential amino acids, 1 mM sodium

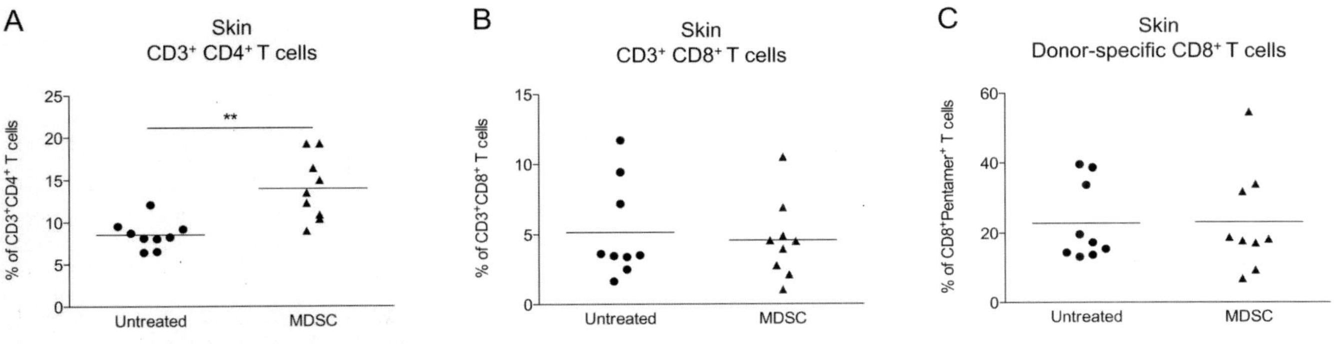

Figure 6. Adoptive transfer of BM-derived MDSC does not prevent lymphocyte infiltration in skin allografts. Male skin grafts were transplanted onto females recipients treated or not at days −1, 6 and 13 post-transplantation with four million autologous (female) MDSC generated in vitro with GM-CSF and IL-6. Skin grafts were harvested 14 days after transplantation and infiltrated leukocytes were analyzed by flow cytometry. Results are expressed in percentages of CD3$^+$ CD4$^+$ T cells (A), CD3$^+$ CD8$^+$ T cells (B) and donor-specific Pentamer$^+$ cells among CD8$^+$ T cells (C). Data show results from two independent experiments with 4 to 9 mice per group. **$p<0.01$.

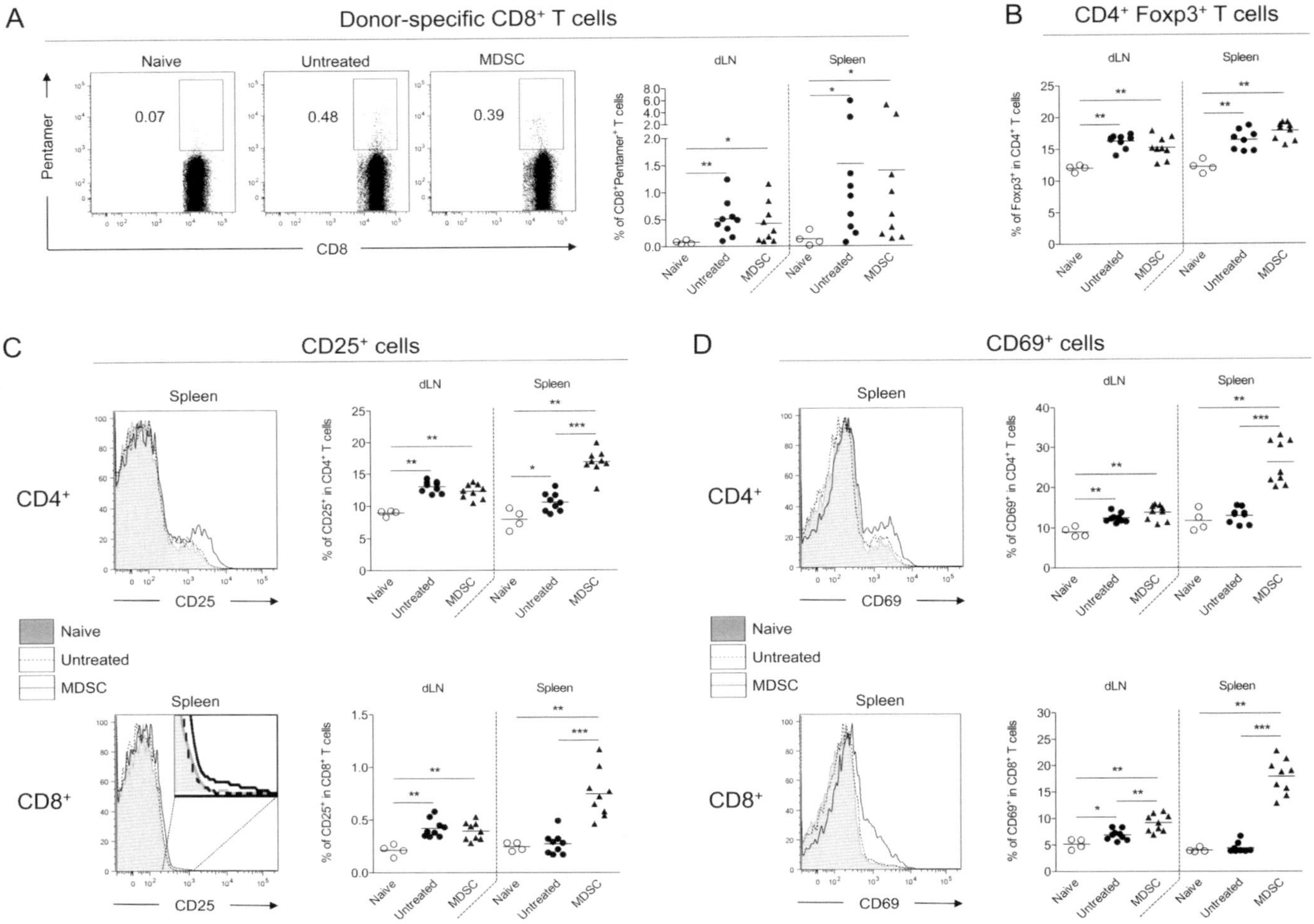

Figure 7. Adoptive transfer of BM-derived MDSC is associated with increased numbers of CD25⁺ and CD69⁺ cells, mainly in the spleen. Male skin grafts were transplanted onto females recipients treated or not at days −1, 6 and 13 post-transplantation with four million autologous (female) MDSC generated in vitro with GM-CSF and IL-6. Draining lymph nodes and spleen were harvested from skin-grafted mice 14 days after transplantation or from naive mice for flow cytometry analysis. (A) Representative staining and quantification of donor-specific Pentamer⁺ CD8⁺ T cells in naive or skin-grafted mice. (B) Quantification of FoxP3⁺ cells among CD3⁺ CD4⁺ T cells. (C, D) Representative stainings and quantifications of CD25⁺ (C) and CD69⁺ (D) among CD3⁺ CD4⁺ or CD3⁺ CD8⁺ T cells. Data show results from two independent experiments with 4 to 9 mice per group. *$p<0.05$, **$p<0.01$, ***$p<0.001$.

pyruvate, 10 mM HEPES (all from Gibco, Saint Aubin, France), 2 mM glutamine and 50 μM β-mercaptoethanol (both from Sigma-Aldrich) in DMEM base (Gibco). Medium was supplemented with GM-CSF (40 ng/ml) and IL-6 (40 ng/ml) cytokines. Cells were maintained at 37°C in 5% CO_2-humidified atmosphere. After 4 days, cells were washed twice before flow cytometry analysis, in vitro culture or in vivo injection. In some experiments, LPS was added (1 μg/mL final) for the last 5 hours of the culture.

In vitro Proliferation Assay

Responder CD8⁺ T cells were purified (CD8a⁺ T cell Isolation Kit II, Miltenyi Biotec, Paris, France) from spleens of naive C57BL/6 mice, labeled with CFSE and plated at the concentration of 2×10^4 cells/mL in 96-well round bottom plate in 200 μL final of complete medium. Anti-CD3/28 microbeads (Life Technologies, Saint Aubin, France) were used at a 1:1 ratio and increased numbers of BM-derived MDSC were added. After 3 days, CFSE dilution in CD8⁺ T cells was analyzed by flow cytometry.

Immunization with OVA-expressing COS Cells

COS cells were transfected (Lipofectamine Transfection Reagent, Life Technologies) with plasmids (pCI-neo backbone, Promega, Charbonnières-les-Bains, France) coding for GFP alone or GFP fused to $OVA_{257-264}$ sequence (SIINFEKL peptide) at N-terminal. After 48 hours, COS cells expressing GFP alone (control COS) or $OVA_{257-264}$-GFP fusion protein (COS OVA) were trypsinized and washed in PBS before i.v. injection (1×10^5 cells). Transfection efficiency routinely reached 40–50% of GFP⁺ cells.

In vivo Proliferation Assay

Experimental scheme is depicted in Figure 3A. C57BL/6 mice were immunized with control COS or COS OVA cells and co-injected (i.v.) or not with 6.5×10^6 BM-derived MDSC. The next day, 5×10^6 CD8⁺ T cells purified (CD8a⁺ T cell Isolation Kit II, Miltenyi Biotec) from pooled spleens and lymph nodes of OT-1 TCR-transgenic mice were labeled with CFSE and injected (i.v.). After 3 days, spleens were harvested and CFSE dilution in injected CD8⁺ T cells was analyzed by flow cytometry.

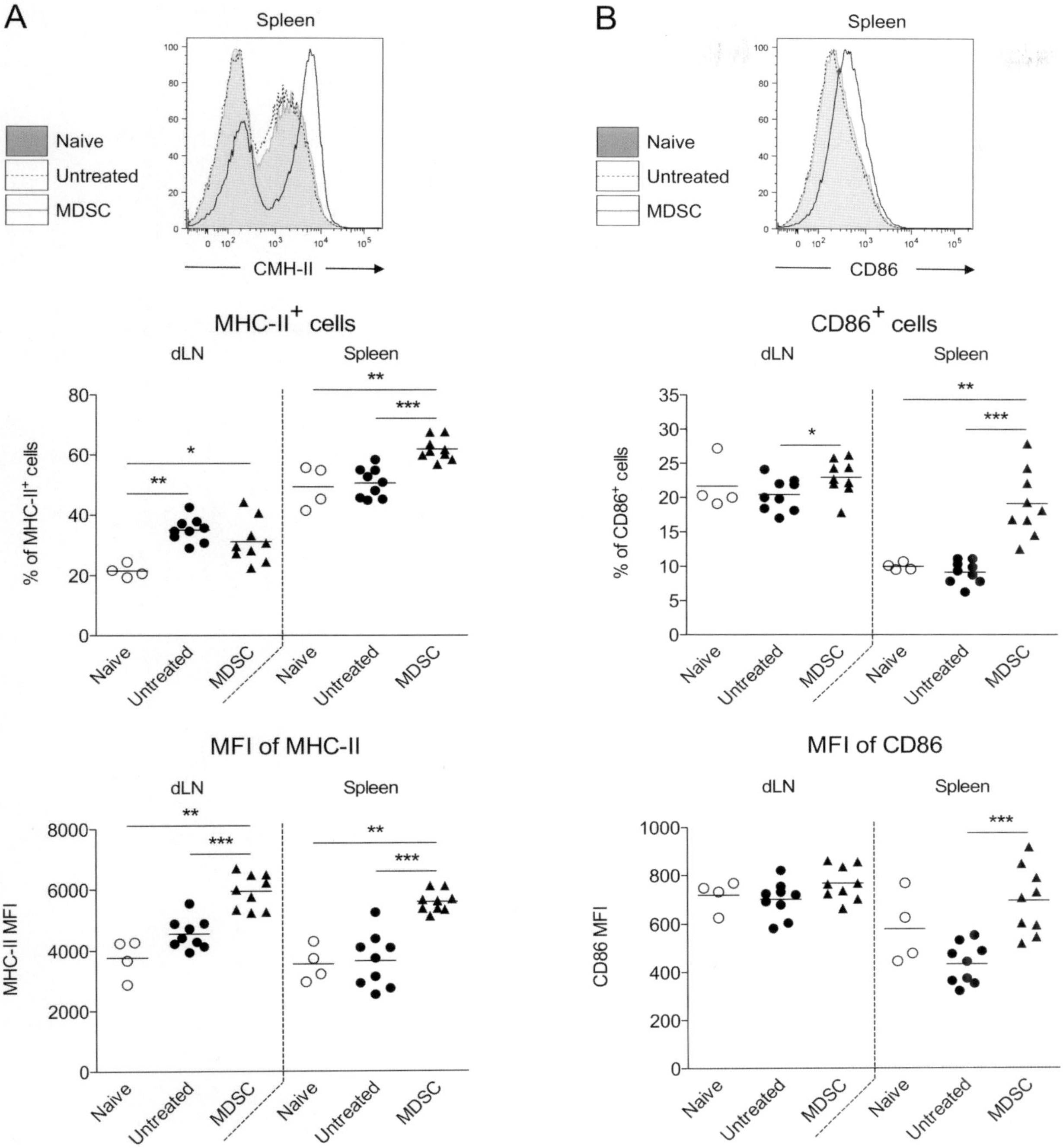

Figure 8. Adoptive transfer of BM-derived MDSC is associated with increased numbers of MHC II$^+$ and CD86$^+$ cells, mainly in the spleen. Male skin grafts were transplanted onto females recipients treated or not at days −1, 6 and 13 post-transplantation with four million autologous (female) MDSC generated in vitro with GM-CSF and IL-6. Draining lymph nodes and spleen were harvested from skin-grafted mice 14 days after transplantation or from naive mice for flow cytometry analysis. Representative stainings and quantifications of MHC II$^+$ (A) and CD86$^+$ (B) cells in naive or skin-grafted mice. Data show results from two independent experiments with 4 to 9 mice per group. *$p<0.05$, **$p<0.01$, ***$p<0.001$.

In vivo Cytotoxicity Assay

Experimental scheme is depicted in Figure 3C. C57BL/6 mice were immunized with control COS or COS OVA cells and co-injected (i.v.) or not with 5×10^6 BM-derived MDSC. The next day, 0.25×10^6 CD8$^+$ T cells purified (CD8a$^+$ T cell Isolation Kit II, Miltenyi Biotec) from pooled spleens and lymph nodes of OT-1 TCR-transgenic mice were injected (i.v.). After 8 days, spleens cells from Ly5.1 mice (CD45.1$^+$ cells) were labeled with 4 µM or 0.2 µM of CFSE to obtain CFSE^{hi} and CFSE^{lo} populations respectively loaded with control Smcy and $OVA_{257-264}$ peptides and were injected (i.v.) at a 1:1 ratio (1.6×10^6 cells for each population). The next day, spleens were harvested to measure the relative proportions of each population within CD45.1$^+$ cells by flow cytometry. Specific lysis was determined by calculating the percentage of decrease of the CFSE^{hi} population in immunized mice compared to non-immunized mice.

Induction of Autoimmune Diabetes

Diabetes was induced in RIP-mOVA mice as previously described [34]. Briefly, 6 to 8 week-old RIP-mOVA mice were injected intravenously with 5×10^6 $CD8^+$ T cells purified ($CD8a^+$ T cell Isolation Kit II, Miltenyi Biotec) from pooled spleens and lymph nodes of OT-1 TCR-transgenic mice together with intraperitoneal administration of 1 mg anti-OVA IgG. Anti-OVA serum was obtained from ovalbumin (OVA)-hyperimmunized rabbits (Covalab, Villeurbanne, France) and IgG were purified by protein A affinity chromatography. Endotoxin-free OVA protein was from Profos (Regensberg, Germany). Blood glucose levels were measured with a StatStrip Xpress Glucose/Ketone Meter monitoring system (Nova Biomedical, Les Ulis, France). Mice were considered diabetic after two consecutive measurements >250 mg/dL.

Skin Transplantation

Mice were anesthetized with a mixture of 5% xylazine (Rompun) and 18% ketamine in PBS (170 µL) injected intraperitoneally (8.5 mg/kg of xylazine and 76.5 mg/kg of ketamine per mouse). Square skin grafts (1 cm^2) were prepared from the tail of male wild-type C57BL/6 donors and transplanted on the shaved left flank of C57BL/6 female recipients. The grafts were fixed to the graft bed with 10–12 interrupted sutures and were covered with protective tape. The first inspection was carried out seven days later and graft survival was monitored every other day. Rejection was defined as complete sloughing or a dry scab.

Analysis of Cellular Populations in Skin Graft Recipients

Fourteen days after skin transplant, mice were sacrificed and draining lymph nodes, spleen and skin graft were harvested. Skin grafts were processed using collagenase D (Sigma-Aldrich) for 45 min at 37°C. Cells were fluorescently labeled and cellular populations were analyzed by flow cytometry.

Statistical Analysis

Statistical analyses were performed with Graphpad Prism 5.0 (La Jolla, CA, USA) using the Mann-Whitney test. Survival rates were compared using the Log-rank (Mantel-cox) test. Statistical significance was defined as $p<0.05$.

Author Contributions

Conceived and designed the experiments: LD LCI GB MH YD MCC CL. Performed the experiments: LD LCI LBD GB EM CL. Analyzed the data: LD LCI GB MCC CL. Wrote the paper: LD YD CL.

References

1. Gabrilovich DI, Nagaraj S (2009) Myeloid-derived suppressor cells as regulators of the immune system. Nat Rev Immunol 9: 162–174.
2. Peranzoni E, Zilio S, Marigo I, Dolcetti L, Zanovello P, et al. (2010) Myeloid-derived suppressor cell heterogeneity and subset definition. Curr Opin Immunol 22: 238–244.
3. Gabrilovich DI, Ostrand-Rosenberg S, Bronte V (2012) Coordinated regulation of myeloid cells by tumours. Nat Rev Immunol 12: 253–268.
4. Dilek N, Vuillefroy de Silly R, Blancho G, Vanhove B (2012) Myeloid-derived suppressor cells: mechanisms of action and recent advances in their role in transplant tolerance. Front Immunol 3: 208.
5. Ochando JC, Chen SH (2012) Myeloid-derived suppressor cells in transplantation and cancer. Immunol Res 54: 275–285.
6. Cripps JG, Gorham JD (2011) MDSC in autoimmunity. Int Immunopharmacol 11: 789–793.
7. Yin B, Ma G, Yen CY, Zhou Z, Wang GX, et al. (2010) Myeloid-derived suppressor cells prevent type 1 diabetes in murine models. J Immunol 185: 5828–5834.
8. Hu C, Du W, Zhang X, Wong FS, Wen L (2012) The role of Gr1+ cells after anti-CD20 treatment in type 1 diabetes in nonobese diabetic mice. J Immunol 188: 294–301.
9. Fujii W, Ashihara E, Hirai H, Nagahara H, Kajitani N, et al. (2013) Myeloid-derived suppressor cells play crucial roles in the regulation of mouse collagen-induced arthritis. J Immunol 191: 1073–1081.
10. Haile LA, von Wasielewski R, Gamrekelashvili J, Kruger C, Bachmann O, et al. (2008) Myeloid-derived suppressor cells in inflammatory bowel disease: a new immunoregulatory pathway. Gastroenterology 135: 871–881, e871–875.
11. Singh V, Mueller U, Freyschmidt-Paul P, Zoller M (2011) Delayed type hypersensitivity-induced myeloid-derived suppressor cells regulate autoreactive T cells. Eur J Immunol 41: 2871–2882.
12. Valaperti A, Marty RR, Kania G, Germano D, Mauermann N, et al. (2008) CD11b+ monocytes abrogate Th17 CD4+ T cell-mediated experimental autoimmune myocarditis. J Immunol 180: 2686–2695.
13. Zehntner SP, Brickman C, Bourbonniere L, Remington L, Caruso M, et al. (2005) Neutrophils that infiltrate the central nervous system regulate T cell responses. J Immunol 174: 5124–5131.
14. Zhu B, Bando Y, Xiao S, Yang K, Anderson AC, et al. (2007) CD11b+Ly-6C(hi) suppressive monocytes in experimental autoimmune encephalomyelitis. J Immunol 179: 5228–5237.
15. Ioannou M, Alissafi T, Lazaridis I, Deraos G, Matsoukas J, et al. (2012) Crucial role of granulocytic myeloid-derived suppressor cells in the regulation of central nervous system autoimmune disease. J Immunol 188: 1136–1146.
16. Zhang W, Liang S, Wu J, Horuzsko A (2008) Human inhibitory receptor immunoglobulin-like transcript 2 amplifies CD11b+Gr1+ myeloid-derived suppressor cells that promote long-term survival of allografts. Transplantation 86: 1125–1134.
17. Dugast AS, Haudebourg T, Coulon F, Heslan M, Haspot F, et al. (2008) Myeloid-derived suppressor cells accumulate in kidney allograft tolerance and specifically suppress effector T cell expansion. J Immunol 180: 7898–7906.
18. De Wilde V, Van Rompaey N, Hill M, Lebrun JF, Lemaitre P, et al. (2009) Endotoxin-induced myeloid-derived suppressor cells inhibit alloimmune responses via heme oxygenase-1. Am J Transplant 9: 2034–2047.
19. Garcia MR, Ledgerwood L, Yang Y, Xu J, Lal G, et al. (2010) Monocytic suppressive cells mediate cardiovascular transplantation tolerance in mice. J Clin Invest 120: 2486–2496.
20. Dilek N, Poirier N, Usal C, Martinet B, Blancho G, et al. (2012) Control of transplant tolerance and intragraft regulatory T cell localization by myeloid-derived suppressor cells and CCL5. J Immunol 188: 4209–4216.
21. Wu T, Sun C, Chen Z, Zhen Y, Peng J, et al. (2012) Smad3-deficient CD11b(+)Gr1(+) myeloid-derived suppressor cells prevent allograft rejection via the nitric oxide pathway. J Immunol 189: 4989–5000.
22. Luan Y, Mosheir E, Menon MC, Wilson D, Woytovich C, et al. (2013) Monocytic Myeloid-Derived Suppressor Cells Accumulate in Renal Transplant Patients and Mediate CD4(+) Foxp3(+) Treg Expansion. Am J Transplant 13: 3123–3131.
23. Leslie M (2011) Immunology. Regulatory T cells get their chance to shine. Science 332: 1020–1021.
24. Adeegbe D, Serafini P, Bronte V, Zoso A, Ricordi C, et al. (2011) In vivo induction of myeloid suppressor cells and CD4(+)Foxp3(+) T regulatory cells prolongs skin allograft survival in mice. Cell Transplant 20: 941–954.
25. Turnquist HR, Zhao Z, Rosborough BR, Liu Q, Castellaneta A, et al. (2011) IL-33 expands suppressive CD11b+ Gr-1(int) and regulatory T cells, including ST2L+ Foxp3+ cells, and mediates regulatory T cell-dependent promotion of cardiac allograft survival. J Immunol 187: 4598–4610.
26. Rossner S, Voigtlander C, Wiethe C, Hanig J, Seifarth C, et al. (2005) Myeloid dendritic cell precursors generated from bone marrow suppress T cell responses via cell contact and nitric oxide production in vitro. Eur J Immunol 35: 3533–3544.
27. Zhou Z, French DL, Ma G, Eisenstein S, Chen Y, et al. (2010) Development and function of myeloid-derived suppressor cells generated from mouse embryonic and hematopoietic stem cells. Stem Cells 28: 620–632.
28. Chou HS, Hsieh CC, Charles R, Wang L, Wagner T, et al. (2011) Myeloid-Derived Suppressor Cells Protect Islet Transplants By B7-H1 Mediated Enhancement of T Regulatory Cells. Transplantation.
29. Guan Q, Moreno S, Qing G, Weiss CR, Lu L, et al. (2013) The role and potential therapeutic application of myeloid-derived suppressor cells in TNBS-induced colitis. J Leukoc Biol 94: 803–811.
30. Nefedova Y, Huang M, Kusmartsev S, Bhattacharya R, Cheng P, et al. (2004) Hyperactivation of STAT3 is involved in abnormal differentiation of dendritic cells in cancer. J Immunol 172: 464–474.
31. Eruslanov E, Daurkin I, Ortiz J, Vieweg J, Kusmartsev S (2010) Pivotal Advance: Tumor-mediated induction of myeloid-derived suppressor cells and M2-polarized macrophages by altering intracellular PGE(2) catabolism in myeloid cells. J Leukoc Biol 88: 839–848.
32. Marigo I, Bosio E, Solito S, Mesa C, Fernandez A, et al. (2010) Tumor-induced tolerance and immune suppression depend on the C/EBPbeta transcription factor. Immunity 32: 790–802.

33. Lechner MG, Liebertz DJ, Epstein AL (2010) Characterization of cytokine-induced myeloid-derived suppressor cells from normal human peripheral blood mononuclear cells. J Immunol 185: 2273–2284.
34. Harbers SO, Crocker A, Catalano G, D'Agati V, Jung S, et al. (2007) Antibody-enhanced cross-presentation of self antigen breaks T cell tolerance. J Clin Invest 117: 1361–1369.
35. Colonna L, Catalano G, Chew C, D'Agati V, Thomas JW, et al. (2011) Therapeutic targeting of Syk in autoimmune diabetes. J Immunol 185: 1532–1543.
36. Obermajer N, Muthuswamy R, Lesnock J, Edwards RP, Kalinski P (2011) Positive feedback between PGE2 and COX2 redirects the differentiation of human dendritic cells toward stable myeloid-derived suppressor cells. Blood 118: 5498–5505.
37. Tomihara K, Guo M, Shin T, Sun X, Ludwig SM, et al. (2010) Antigen-specific immunity and cross-priming by epithelial ovarian carcinoma-induced CD11b(+)Gr-1(+) cells. J Immunol 184: 6151–6160.
38. Yi H, Guo C, Yu X, Zuo D, Wang XY (2012) Mouse CD11b+Gr-1+ myeloid cells can promote Th17 cell differentiation and experimental autoimmune encephalomyelitis. J Immunol 189: 4295–4304.
39. Brennan TV, Tang Q, Liu FC, Hoang V, Bi M, et al. (2011) Requirements for prolongation of allograft survival with regulatory T cell infusion in lymphosufficient hosts. J Surg Res 169: e69–75.
40. Schmidt K, Zilio S, Schmollinger JC, Bronte V, Blankenstein T, et al. (2013) Differently immunogenic cancers in mice induce immature myeloid cells that suppress CTL in vitro but not in vivo following transfer. Blood 121: 1740–1748.
41. Sade-Feldman M, Kanterman J, Ish-Shalom E, Elnekave M, Horwitz E, et al. (2013) Tumor necrosis factor-alpha blocks differentiation and enhances suppressive activity of immature myeloid cells during chronic inflammation. Immunity 38: 541–554.
42. Ribechini E, Greifenberg V, Sandwick S, Lutz MB (2009) Subsets, expansion and activation of myeloid-derived suppressor cells. Med Microbiol Immunol 199: 273–281.
43. Highfill SL, Rodriguez PC, Zhou Q, Goetz CA, Koehn BH, et al. (2010) Bone marrow myeloid-derived suppressor cells (MDSCs) inhibit graft-versus-host disease (GVHD) via an arginase-1-dependent mechanism that is up-regulated by interleukin-13. Blood 116: 5738–5747.
44. Tang Q, Bluestone JA, Kang SM (2011) CD4(+)Foxp3(+) regulatory T cell therapy in transplantation. J Mol Cell Biol 4: 11–21.
45. Nagaraj S, Youn JI, Gabrilovich DI (2013) Reciprocal relationship between myeloid-derived suppressor cells and T cells. J Immunol 191: 17–23.
46. Pan PY, Ma G, Weber KJ, Ozao-Choy J, Wang G, et al. (2010) Immune stimulatory receptor CD40 is required for T-cell suppression and T regulatory cell activation mediated by myeloid-derived suppressor cells in cancer. Cancer Res 70: 99–108.
47. Centuori SM, Trad M, LaCasse CJ, Alizadeh D, Larmonier CB, et al. (2012) Myeloid-derived suppressor cells from tumor-bearing mice impair TGF-beta-induced differentiation of CD4+CD25+FoxP3+ Tregs from CD4+CD25−FoxP3− T cells. J Leukoc Biol 92: 987–997.
48. Kurts C, Heath WR, Carbone FR, Allison J, Miller JF, et al. (1996) Constitutive class I-restricted exogenous presentation of self antigens in vivo. J Exp Med 184: 923–930.
49. Hogquist KA, Jameson SC, Heath WR, Howard JL, Bevan MJ, et al. (1994) T cell receptor antagonist peptides induce positive selection. Cell 76: 17–27.

6

Human Hepatocyte Growth Factor (hHGF)-Modified Hepatic Oval Cells Improve Liver Transplant Survival

Zhu Li[1*§], Juan Chen[1§], Li Li[2], Jiang-Hua Ran[2], Xue-Hua Li[1], Zhi-Heng Liu[1], Gui-Jie Liu[1], Yan-Chao Gao[1], Xue-Li Zhang[1], Hiu-Dong Sun[1]

1 Department of Hepatobiliary Surgery, Liaocheng People's Hospital, Liaocheng, Shandong, China, **2** The First People's Hospital of Kunming, Kunming, Yunnan, China

Abstract

Despite progress in the field of immunosuppression, acute rejection is still a common postoperative complication following liver transplantation. This study aims to investigate the capacity of the human hepatocyte growth factor (hHGF) in modifying hepatic oval cells (HOCs) administered simultaneously with orthotopic liver transplantation as a means of improving graft survival. HOCs were activated and isolated using a modified 2-acetylaminofluorene/partial hepatectomy (2-AAF/PH) model in male Lewis rats. A HOC line stably expressing the HGF gene was established following stable transfection of the pBLAST2-hHGF plasmid. Our results demonstrated that hHGF-modified HOCs could efficiently differentiate into hepatocytes and bile duct epithelial cells *in vitro*. Administration of HOCs at the time of liver transplantation induced a wider distribution of SRY-positive donor cells in liver tissues. Administration of hHGF-HOC at the time of transplantation remarkably prolonged the median survival time and improved liver function for recipients compared to these parameters in the other treatment groups ($P<0.05$). Moreover, hHGF-HOC administration at the time of liver transplantation significantly suppressed elevation of interleukin-2 (IL-2), tumor necrosis factor-α (TNF-α) and interferon-γ (IFN-γ) levels while increasing the production of IL-10 and TGF-β1 ($P<0.05$). HOC or hHGF-HOC administration promoted cell proliferation, reduced cell apoptosis, and decreased liver allograft rejection rates. Furthermore, hHGF-modified HOCs more efficiently reduced acute allograft rejection ($P<0.05$ versus HOC transplantation only). Our results indicate that the combination of hHGF-modified HOCs with liver transplantation decreased host anti-graft immune responses resulting in a reduction of allograft rejection rates and prolonging graft survival in recipient rats. This suggests that HOC-based cell transplantation therapies can be developed as a means of treating severe liver injuries.

Editor: Michael Zimmerman, University of Colorado School of Medicine, United States of America

Funding: The authors have no support or funding to report.

Competing Interests: The authors have declared that no competing interests exist.

* E-mail: lllllzhu@126.com

§ These authors contributed equally to this work.

Introduction

Orthotopic liver transplantation is believed to be the only definitive therapy for patients with end-stage liver diseases; however, severe complications such as acute allograft rejection commonly occur [1,2]. Transplantation of stem cells or progenitor cells, including hepatocytes and hepatic oval cells (HOCs) that have self-renewal and differentiation potential have been utilized as alternative approaches for mediating repair of damaged tissue resulting in liver regeneration [3,4,5]. Nevertheless, loss of transplanted donor cells due to rejection (or other mechanisms) seems to be the major limitation for broader application of liver cell therapy [6]. Therefore, improvements to the efficacy of donor cells and prevention of rejection, is needed as a means of improving transplanted liver survival rates.

Hepatocyte growth factor (HGF) is a multifunctional growth factor which prevents apoptosis, invasion of extracellular matrices, and proliferation [7]. Moreover, it has been demonstrated that the HGF/c-met signaling pathway is required for efficient liver regeneration and repair [8]. Previous studies showed that adenovirus-mediated HGF gene expression could regulate HOC proliferation [9]. In addition, accumulating evidence indicates that HGF can accelerate this proliferation and possibly promote HOC differentiation in the 2-acetylaminofluorene/partial hepatectomy (2-AAF/PH) rat model [10,11]. Moreover, it has been demonstrated that HGF can prevent the development of chronic allograft nephropathy in rats [12]. In a mouse model of cardiac transplantation, HGF suppressed acute and chronic allograft rejection [13]. Based on this evidence, we hypothesized that overexpression of HGF in HOCs may serve to promote graft survival by inhibiting allograft rejection after orthotopic liver transplantation.

In the present study, we investigated the potential effects of combined hHGF-modified HOCs and liver transplantation on the improvement of acute allograft rejection and recipient survival in rats. Our findings suggest that hHGF-modified HOC transplantation may provide a valuable approach for the treatment of patients with severe liver damage.

Results

hHGF-modified HOC characteristics

Enhanced hHGF expression in hHGF-modified HOCs was assessed by Western blot analysis (Fig. 1A). Using ELISA-based assays we detected significantly increased levels of hHGF expression in medium collected from hHGF-modified HOC cultures compared to medium from untreated HOCs (7.324±0.477 ng/ml vs. 0 ng/ml). Unpublished work from our laboratory showed that HOCs modified to express hHGF promoted proliferation, and HOCs stably expressing the hHGF efficiently differentiated into large round-shaped hepatocytes and long, spindle-like bile duct epithelial cells *in vitro* with most HOCs differentiating into bile duct epithelial cells (Fig. 1B). RT-PCR analysis demonstrated that both undifferentiated and differentiated hHGF-HOCs expressed the liver and bile duct markers ALB and CK19 (Table 1). In addition, CK19 mRNA levels in undifferentiated hHGF-HOCs were significantly lower than that in differentiated hHGF-HOCs ($P<0.05$). Immunostaining with specific antibodies for ALB or CK19 further showed the presence of immuno-positive cells in differentiated hHGF-HOCs (Fig. 1C).

Table 1. Quantification of ALB and CK19 mRNA levels using quantitative RT-PCR.

	ALB	CK19
Liver	−1.127±0.486*#	−1.829±0.624*#
Bile duct	−6.534±0.489*#	−1.753±0.692*
Undifferentiated hHGF-HOCs	−1.814±0.603	−3.792±0.953
Differentiated hHGF-HOCs	−1.773±0.538	−1.476±0.615*

Data were quantified from 20 independent experiments and normalized with β-actin. Differences were analyzed using an analysis of variance or an independent sample *t*-test. Negative logs were calculated as described in the Materials and Methods.
*$P<0.05$ *vs.* undifferentiated hHGF-HOCs;
#$P<0.05$ *vs.* differentiated hHGF-HOCs.

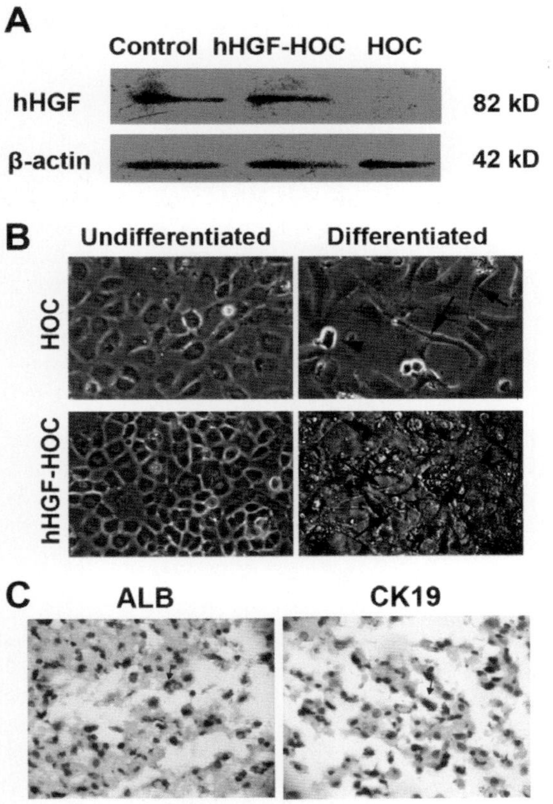

Figure 1. hHGF-modified HOC differentiation potential. LIF was withdrawn from culture medium to induce cell differentiation. (A) Intracellular hHGF protein expression was determined by Western blot analysis. hHGF was used as positive control and β-actin used as an internal control. (B) Undifferentiated or differentiated normal HOCs or hHGF-modified HOCs were monitored under phase contrast microscopy. Arrows indicated long-spindle like bile duct epithelial cells and arrowheads indicat the large, round-shaped hepatocytes. (C) Immunostaining of differentiated cells with specific antibodies for ALB or CK19. Arrows indicated immuno-positive cells (dark brown cells). Sections were double-stained with H&E. Magnification ×200.

Liver transplantation combined with HOC administration

To determine the *in vivo* effects of hHGF-modified HOCs, cells were transplanted into female Lewis rats that also received an orthotopic liver transplant. The outline of the experimental design is presented in Fig. 2. In order to evaluate cell transplantation efficacy, expression of the Y-chromosome-specific SRY gene (present only on male donor HOCs) was assessed by *in situ* hybridization. Following transplantation and administration of untreated HOCs, SRY-positive donor HOCs infiltrated the portal area (Fig. 3). Apoptotic or dead SRY-positive cells were also found in hepatic sinusoids. Compared to the HOC group, hHGF-HOC transplantation induced a wider distribution of donor cells; that is, SRY-positive cells were observed surrounding the portal area, central vein, bile duct, and were diffusely distributed in hepatic lobules (Fig. 3). The percentage of SRY-positive cells was greatly increased over time post transplantation in transplanted rats also treated with hHGF-HOCs compared to transplant rats treated with HOC only ($P<0.05$, Table 2). Moreover, peripheral hHGF levels were somewhat upregulated in hHGF-HOC treated transplant animals ($P<0.05$ compared to other groups, Table 2). Sixteen days post transplantation, gross examination of the control group livers (orthotopic liver transplantation without cell transplantation) revealed that swelling and cirrhosis were accompanied by liver ischemia, congestion and hemorrhage. Localized congestion without cirrhosis or necrosis was observed in HOC-treated, liver transplant rats. In contrast, liver transplant rats treated with hHGF-modified HOCs presented with normal liver morphology.

Effect of HOC administration and transplantation on cytokine levels

We next investigated changes in serum T helper (Th) cells cytokine levels. Two weeks post surgery, transplantation in combination with the administration of HOC or hHGF-HOC significantly suppressed IL-2, TNF-α and IFN-γ production and enhanced the production of IL-10 and TGF-β1 compared to controls ($P<0.05$, Fig. 4). Furthermore, administration of hHGF-modified HOCs resulted in more significant changes to cytokine expression levels ($P<0.05$ compared to the HOC treated transplantation group).

HOC administration prolongs survival of recipients

Liver transplantation combined with the administration of either HOC or hHGF remarkably prolonged the median survival time of recipients compared to transplant control animals not treated with either HOC or hHGF (control, n = 47, median

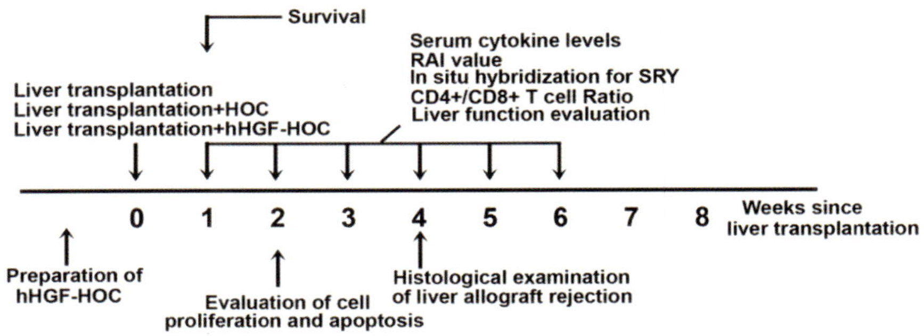

Figure 2. Experimental design outline.

survival time = 21 days; HOC transplantation, n = 33, median survival time = 38 days; hHGF-HOC transplantation, n = 20, median survival time = 48 days; $P<0.05$). In addition, the median survival time of liver transplant rats treated with hHGF-HOC was significantly longer than that of HOC-treated liver transplant rats ($P<0.05$). As demonstrated by the recipient survival curve hHGF-HOC administration greatly prolonged animal survival rates compared to the other 2 treatment groups (Fig. 5).

Transplantation combined with HOC treatment improved host liver function

Liver function indicators, ALT, DBil, ALB, GGT, ALP, and ChE were examined 1, 2, 3, 4, 5 or 6 weeks post transplantation (Table 2). HOC or hHGF-HOC treatment statistically down-regulated ALT levels 2 weeks post transplantation compared to controls ($P<0.05$). Compared to HOC treatment, administration of hHGF-HOC significantly reduced ALT levels 2 weeks post transplantation ($P<0.05$), suggesting that hHGF-HOC treatment prevented liver injury. hHGF-HOC treatment greatly decreased GGT and ALP values 2 weeks post transplantation and DBil levels 3 weeks post transplantation in liver transplant recipient rats ($P<0.05$ compared to HOC+liver transplantation or liver transplantation alone) suggesting that hHGF-HOC treatment promotes the function of intrahepatic bile ducts after transplantation. In addition, administration of hHGF-modified HOCs to transplant recipients also improved liver synthesis function (measured by increased ALB and ChE values) 2 and 3 weeks following transplantation ($P<0.05$ compared to HOC+liver transplantation or liver transplantation alone).

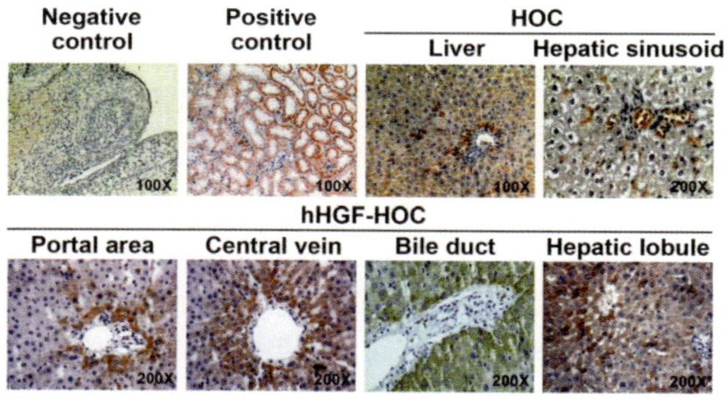

Figure 3. ***In situ*** **hybridization of SRY-positive donor HOCs.** *In situ* hybridization was performed 21 days post transplantation. Ovarian tissue was used as a negative control and renal tissues from male Lewis rats used as positive controls. SRY-positive cells exhibited dark brown staining of their nuclei and/or cytoplasm. Following HOC administration to liver transplant recipients, SRY-positive cells were found in liver tissues and hepatic sinusoids. Additionally, SRY-positive hHGF-HOCs were observed in the surrounding portal area, central vein and bile duct, and were diffusely distributed in hepatic lobules. Magnification is indicated on each image.

Transplantation in the presence of HOCs promotes proliferation and decreased apoptosis

Administration of HOCs or hHGF-modified HOCs to rats significantly promoted the number of proliferating cell nuclear antigen (PCNA)-positive cells 14 days post-transplantation (Fig. 6A). Compared to the HOCs group, rats transplanted with hHGF-HOCs transplantation had significantly elevated numbers of $PCNA^+$ cells. NFκB (nuclear factor kappa-light-chain-enhancer of activated B cells) is an anti-apoptotic factor that regulates expression of a large number of genes critical to the regulation of apoptosis. We therefore examined NFκB expression levels in liver tissues 14 days following transplantation. Increased levels of NFκB were found in the HOCs and hHGF-HOCs groups compared to levels observed in controls (Fig. 6B). hHGF-HOCs significantly elevated the NFκB expression levels compared to levels observed in HOCs, suggesting that hHGF-HOC treatment may promote cell proliferation and decreases apoptosis following transplantation.

Transplantation in the presence of HOCs decreased liver allograft rejection

Administration of hHGF-modified HOCs to rats also receiving liver transplantation presented healthy liver tissues and significantly reduced the rejection activity index scores compared to control liver transplant rats or rats treated with HOCs that received a liver transplant (Fig. 7). In addition, the blood $CD4^+$/$CD8^+$ T lymphocyte ratio gradually increased in liver transplant rats with or without administration of HOC (Table 2). In contrast, transplantation in combination with hHGF-modified HOCs significantly decreased this ratio 2-weeks post transplantation ($P<0.05$ compared to the other groups). In addition, expression levels of ICAM-1, Fas, CD44, and CD40 in liver allografts were evaluated. ICAM-1 expression gradually increased in liver transplant recipient rats. Administration of HOCs or hHGF-modified HOCs greatly decreased ICAM-1 expression (percentage of sections with ICAM-1 positive staining 28 days following transplantation: liver transplantation, n = 55, 94.5%; HOC+liver transplantation, n = 53, 86.8%; hHGF-HOC+liver transplantation, n = 55, 81.8%; $P<0.05$ compared to liver transplantation) (Fig. 8). Combined hHGF-HOC transplantation significantly reduced the number of Fas-positive cells on day 28 post transplantation (liver transplantation, n = 55, 70.61±24.83 cells/

Table 2. Measurement of parameters associated with HOC administration and liver transplantation.

	Weeks since liver transplantation					
	1	2	3	4	5	6
Percentage of SRY-positive cells (%)						
HOC+liver transplantation	14.0±3.7*	18.1±3.4*	21.9±3.7*	29.0±5.5*	31.4±5.9*	30.6±3.8*
hHGF-HOC+liver transplantation	20.9±7.7	33.5±6.8	41.3±4.9	59.7±11.3	63.5±5.1	64.7±8.4
Peripheral hHGF level (ng/ml)						
Liver transplantation	0*	0*	0*	0*	0*	0*
HOC+liver transplantation	0*	0*	0*	0*	0*	0*
hHGF-HOC+liver transplantation	0.80±0.38	1.78±0.59	2.78±0.76	3.88±0.79	4.98±0.68	5.74±0.45
$CD4^+/CD8^+$ T cell Ratio						
Liver transplantation	1.1±0.4	1.8±0.5*#	3.1±0.5*#	4.8±0.9*#	NA	NA
HOC+liver transplantation	1.0±0.3	1.4±0.2*	1.8±0.3*	2.1±0.3*	2.4±0.4*	2.3±0.5*
hHGF-HOC+liver transplantation	0.9±0.5	1.1±0.2	1.4±0.4	1.7±0.5	1.6±0.2	1.5±0.3
ALT level (U/l)						
Liver transplantation	66±19	220±147*#	680±396*#	968±203*#	NA	NA
HOC+liver transplantation	61±15	96±17	121±25	127±19	122±23*	105±32*
hHGF-HOC+liver transplantation	64±21	110±20	115±21	96±27	65±28	41±20
DBil level (μM)						
Liver transplantation	9.4±2.0	22.0±7.0*#	58.6±21.2*#	80.0±21.8*#	NA	NA
HOC+liver transplantation	8.3±3.0	12.2±3.5	19.8±8.2*	22.1±7.9*	25.3±5.5*	21.1±6.2*
hHGF-HOC+liver transplantation	8.6±2.1	11.1±3.3	12.8±1.3	12.8±2.7	13.6±1.7	11.3±3.6
ALB level (g/l)						
Liver transplantation	11.7±3.7*	11.3±2.2*#	9.1±2.5*#	8.2±1.6*#	NA	NA
HOC+liver transplantation	13.3±3.4	13.4±3.3*	14.9±1.9*	14.8±2.4*	15.9±2.4*	15.3±3.4*
hHGF-HOC+liver transplantation	14.5±3.6	16.8±4.1	20.6±3.8	21.0±2.4	23.4±1.5	23.6±1.9
GGT level (U/l)						
Liver transplantation	7.5±3.0	42.2±17.7*#	106±35*#	355±165*#	NA	NA
HOC+liver transplantation	6.2±3.9	24.4±12.0*	36.0±5.1*	65.9±14.4*	70.7±19.4*	71.5±16.6*
hHGF-HOC+liver transplantation	7.0±3.7	16.7±3.3	21.3±8.7	26.5±6.9	25.0±4.4	26.4±8.5
ALP level (U/l)						
Liver transplantation	95±18 295±158	295±158*# 295±158	258±171*# 295±158	680±190*# 295±158	NA	NA
HOC+liver transplantation	88±14	180±41*	196±40*	256±21*	221±41*	209±51*
hHGF-HOC+liver transplantation	93±16	130±46	133±17	100±33	105±17	86±26
ChE level (U/l)						
Liver transplantation	1735±525	1458±255	819±175*#	481±186*#	NA	NA
HOC+liver transplantation	1788±404	1560±166	1800±148*	1838±258*	2104±325*	2147±344*
hHGF-HOC+liver transplantation	1733±176	1558±248	2455±312	2664±206	3092±491	3512±228

Differences were analyzed using an analysis of variance or an independent sample *t*-test.
*$P<0.05$ liver transplantation *vs.* hHGF-HOC+liver transplantation or HOC+liver transplantation vs. hHGF-HOC+liver transplantation;
#P<0.05 liver transplantation vs. HOC+liver transplantation. NA, not available.

mm^2; HOC+liver transplantation, n = 53, 37.02±18.95 cells/mm^2; hHGF-HOC+liver transplantation, n = 55, 12.80±7.54 cells/mm^2; $P<0.05$ compared with liver transplantation only or HOC+liver transplantation). Similar results were obtained in the expression of CD44 and CD40. These results suggest that combined hHGF-HOC transplantation could decrease postoperative liver allograft rejection.

Discussion

Even though liver transplantation is the most efficient means of treating patients with end-stage liver diseases, it is usually associated with postoperative complications, including acute allograft rejection [1,2], chronic renal failure [14], post-transplantation lymphoproliferative disorders [15], and cardiovascular disease [16]. Among these side-effects, liver allograft rejection is considered to be a severe and major complication associated with significant morbidity and reduced life quality in liver transplant recipients [2]. Furthermore, the use of immunosuppressive agents

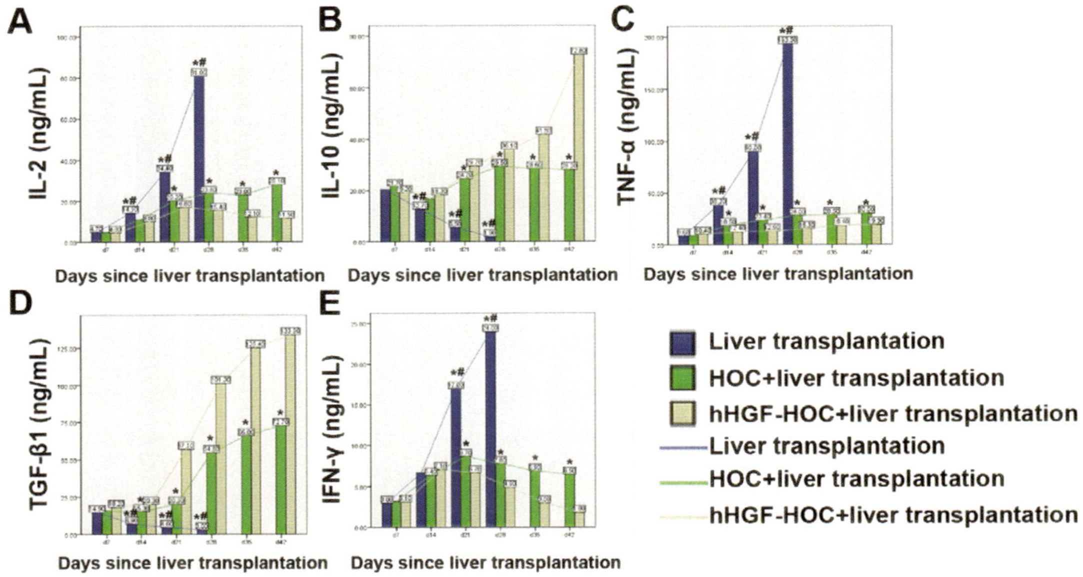

Figure 4. Analysis of serum cytokine levels post transplantation. Serum IL-2, IL-10, TNF-α, TGF-β1, and IFN-γ levels were examined at the indicated time points post transplantation by ELISA. Differences were analyzed using an analysis of variance or an independent sample *t*-test. *$P<0.05$, liver transplantation only vs. hHGF-HOC+liver transplantation or HOC+liver transplantation vs. hHGF-HOC+liver transplantation; #$P<0.05$, liver transplantation vs. HOC+liver transplantation.

may also cause a variety of adverse side effects such as inducing diabetes, hypertension, and nephrotoxicity, and therefore needs careful risk assessments before use [17]. Concomitant stem cell transplantation may induce allograft tolerance by modulating immune cell responses [18,19]. In the present study, administration of HOC following liver transplantation significantly decreased acute liver rejection and prolonged the survival period of recipients.

Previous studies revealed that sustained expression of HGF could accelerate the proliferation of HOCs in a rat 2-AAF/PH model [10,11], suggesting that modification to the HGF gene may promote *in vivo* proliferation and differentiation of HOCs, thereby benefitting liver regeneration post transplantation. In this study, a HOC line stably expressing the hHGF gene (hHGF-HOCs) was successfully established and shown *in vitro* to efficiently differentiate into large, round hepatocytes or into long spindle-like bile duct epithelial cells consistent with previous reports [10,11].

Laboratory tests indicated that combined hHGF-HOC transplantation down-regulated ALT, DBil, GGT, ALP levels but up-regulated ChE, and ALB expression levels, suggesting that transplantation in combination with the administration of HOCs improved liver function, prevented bile duct damage, and protected against development of chronic hepatocyte injury. Since hHGF-modified HOCs are capable of secreting hHGF, it is possible that secreted hHGF may promote the proliferation, differentiation, and migration of HOCs in injured liver tissues

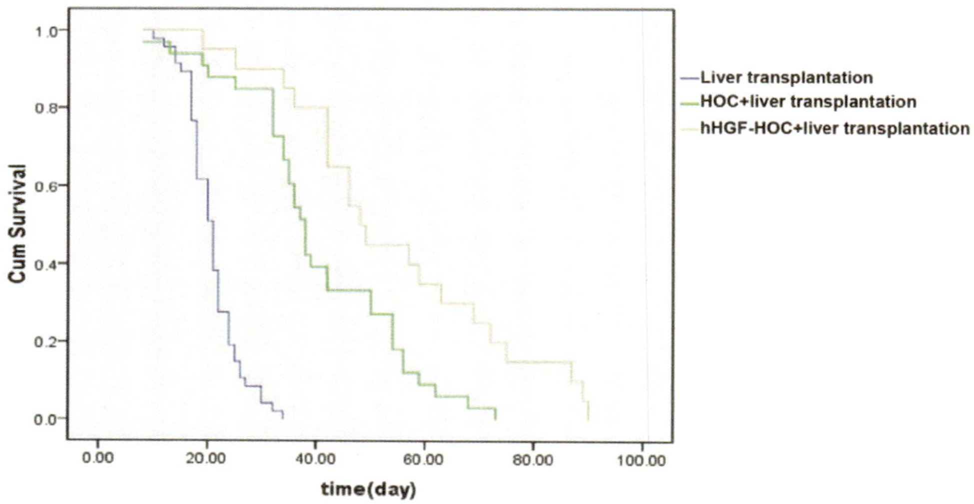

Figure 5. Survival curves of recipients.

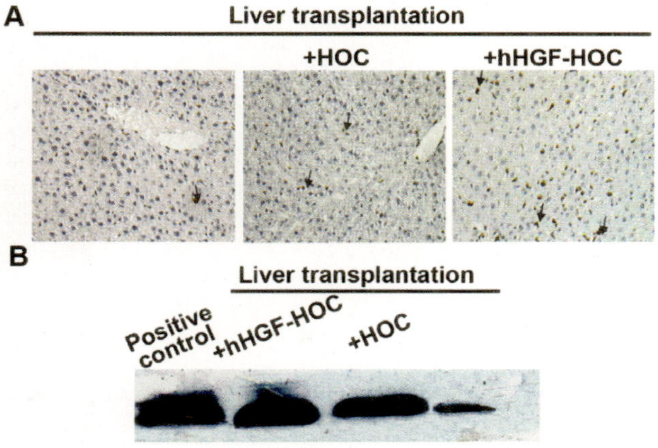

Figure 6. Cell proliferation and apoptosis. The beneficial effects of hHGF-HOCs on liver transplantation were evaluated by measuring cell proliferation and apoptosis. (A) Fourteen days post-transplantation, tissue sections were stained with specific antibodies to PCNA. Arrows indicated immuno-positive cells. Magnification ×100. (B) The protein expression of NFκB was examined by Western blot analysis.

while also enhancing the repair and regeneration of the donor liver. Most of the SRY-positive cells were observed surrounding the portal area, central vein, and bile duct. Therefore, it would be reasonable to suggest that these cells contributed to the protection of intrahepatic biliary epithelial cells.

The rat acute rejection orthotopic liver transplantation model [20] using DA rat livers transplanted into Lewis rats was used to assess the protective effects of HOC cell administration on acute

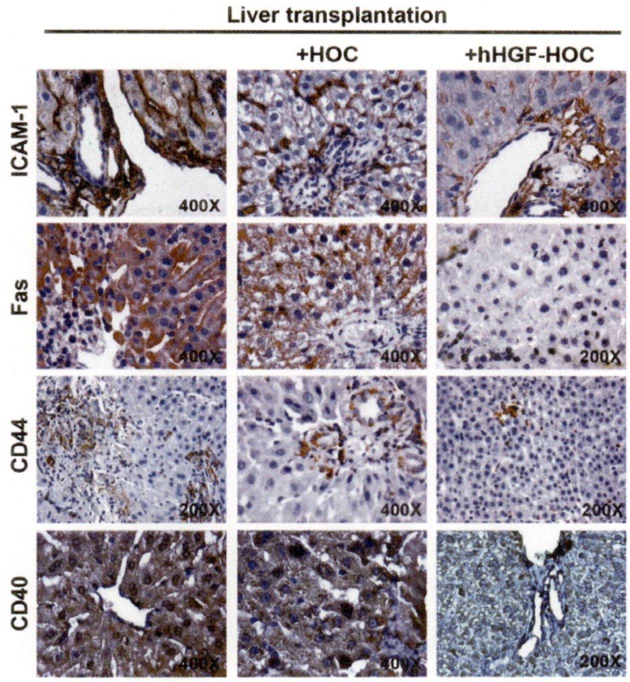

Figure 8. Immunostaining for ICAM-1, Fas, CD44 and CD40 28 days post transplantation. Immunopositive cells exhibited dark-brown staining. Sections were double stained with H&E (blue). Magnification is indicated on each image.

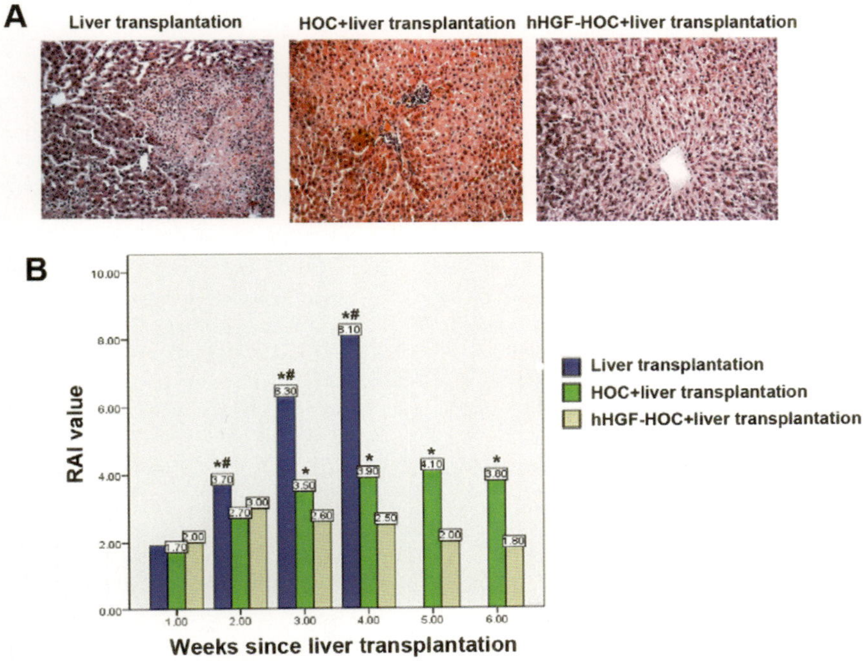

Figure 7. Histological examination of liver allograft rejection. (A) Sections obtained from experimental groups were staining with H&E, magnification ×100. (B) Liver allograft rejection was assessed using the rejection activity index according to the Banff classification of hepatic allograft rejection described in the Materials and Methods. Data were compared with analysis of variance or an independent sample *t*-test. *$P<0.05$ liver transplantation vs. hHGF-HOC+liver transplantation or HOC+liver transplantation vs. hHGF-HOC+liver transplantation; #$P<0.05$, liver transplantation vs. HOC+liver transplantation.

liver rejection. Without interventions, liver recipients would die of acute rejection, postoperative infections, abdominal bleeding, or respiration and circulation failure within one week post surgery [20]. In this study, liver recipients were treated with tacrolimus 1 day prior to surgery until day 13 post surgery. Animals that died within 7 days post surgery were excluded from subsequent examinations.

Acute liver rejection can be triggered by immune responses mediated by different Th cell subtypes *via* redundant or synergistic pathways [21]. Th1 responses initiate allograft rejection by promoting cytotoxic T cell activitiy by producing IFN-γ, TNF-α, and IL-2 [21,22]. By contrast, Th2 responses mediate allograft damage *via* eosinophil recruitment resulting from the production of IL-4, IL-5, IL-6, and IL-10 [22,23]. Th1- and Th2-type cytokines regulate the Th1/Th2 paradigm during allograft responses [24], therefore, decreased levels of IFN-γ, TNF-α, and IL-2 accompanied by increased levels of IL-10 and TGF-β1 resulting from hHGF-HOC administration may reduce immuno-reactivity and subsequently reduce acute liver rejection. Here, we observed a significantly decreased $CD4^+/CD8^+$ ratio in transplant rats also treated with hHGF-HOC, suggesting the induction of transplant tolerance. Furthermore, administration of hHGF-HOC to liver transplant rats significantly decreased expression of CD40, CD44, Fas and ICAM-1 (known bio-indicators for inflammatory cell infiltration and allograft rejection activity [25,26,27,28]) compared to expression levels observed in other groups, suggesting that administration of hHGF-HOC to liver transplant recipients efficiently reduced inflammatory cell infiltration and subsequently decreased allograft rejection. In addition, we found that hHGF-HOCs promoted the number of PCNA positive cells while decreasing the expression of NFκB in liver tissues 14 days following transplantation, indicating that beneficial effects of hHGF-HOCs on liver transplantation might be due to increased cell proliferation and inhibition of apoptosis induced by hHGF-HOCs. Nevertheless, the underlying mechanism needs to be further defined.

In summary, our current study demonstrated that administration of HOCs stably expressing hHGF to liver transplant recipients significantly protected against acute allograft rejection and prolonged animal survival. Although the underlying molecular mechanism of hHGF-mediated prevention of acute liver rejection are unclear, it is possible that hHGF specifically binds to the c-Met tyrosine kinase receptor triggering downstream factors such as phosphatidylinositol 3-kinase (PI3K), phospholipase C (PLC)-γ and mitogen-activated protein kinase (MAPK) [8]. Future studies will be designed to investigate the role of signaling pathways associated with hHGF-mediated prevention of acute liver rejection.

Materials and Methods

Reagents

Fetal bovine serum (FBS) and phosphate buffered saline (PBS) were purchased from Invitrogen (Carlsbad, CA). DMEM (Dulbecco's Minimal Essential Media)/F12 culture medium was obtained from Sigma (St. Louis, MO). Hepatocyte growth factor (HGF), epidermal growth factor (EGF), stem cell factor (SCF) and leukemia inhibitory factor (LIF) were purchased from Millipore (USA). Plasmid pBLAST2-hHGF, blasticidin and lipofectamine 2000 transfection reagent were purchased from Invitrogen. The SRY *in situ* hybridization kit was purchased from the Tianjin Haoyang Biological Manufacture, Co., Ltd. (Tianjin, China). The hematoxylin and eosin (H&E) Staining Kit was purchased from the Shanghai Sangon Biological Engineering Technology and Services Co., Ltd. (Shanghai, China). ELISA kits for hHGF and rat IFN-γ, TGF-β1, TNF-α, IL-2, IL-10 were purchased from Shanghai ExCell Biology (Shanghai, China). Anti-rat CD3-FITC/CD4-PC7/CD8-APC antibodies were obtained from Beckman Coulter, Inc. (Brea, CA). Rat anti-CD44 monoclonal antibody and rat anti-ICAM-1 antibodies were purchased from Millipore (Billerica, MA). Rat anti-Fas and anti-CD40 antibodies were purchased from Stressgen Biotechnologies (San Diego, CA) and Santa Cruz Biotechnology (Santa Cruz, CA), respectively. Tacrolimus was purchased from Fujisawa Pharmaceutical Co. (Fujisawa, Japan).

Animals

All animals were purchased from the Vital River Lab Animal Technology Co., Ltd. (Beijing, China) or the Laboratory Animal Center of Harbin Medical University Harbing, China). Male SPF Lewis rats (n = 10) weighing 200±20 g were used for HOC isolation. For transplantation, 180 female SPF Lewis rats (250–300 g in weight) and 180 female SPF dark agouti (DA) rats (200–350 g in weight) were used. All efforts were made to minimize animal suffering and to reduce the number of animals used. All animal procedures were approved by the Ethics Committee of Liaocheng People's Hospital.

2-AAF/PH model

Male Lewis rats (n = 10) were housed separately for one week prior to use. They were administered 20 mg/kg body weight 2-AAF dissolved in vegetable oil daily by intragastric administration for 6 days. On day 7, ten animals were partially hepatectomized (left lateral lobe excision, 1/2 to 1/3 PH) under general ether anesthesia without 2-AAF administration. 2-AAF feeding commenced on day 8 and the experiment concluded on day14.

Primary HOC cultures

The 2-AAF/PH model was used to generate activated HOCs that were isolated 10 days post operation. Briefly, liver tissues were minced, washed with D-Hank's solution, and digested with 0.1% collagenase IV and 0.025% EDTA at 37°C. Cells were filtered through 100-mesh filters and centrifuged at 500 rpm for 5 min at 4°C. HOCs were separated by Percoll (Amersham Biosciences, Pittsburg, PA) gradient centrifugation. Cells were seeded onto gelatin-coated flasks and maintained in complete DMEM/F12 culture medium containing 10% FBS, 100 U/ml penicillin, 100 μg/ml streptomycin and amphotericin B (1 ng/ml) at 37°C in a 5% CO_2 incubator. Three days after seeding, 20 ng/ml SCF, 10 ng/ml HGF, 10 ng/ml EGF and 10 ng/ml leukemia inhibitory factor (LIF) were added into the culture medium. To induce differentiation, media not containing LIF was added.

Stable transfection of the pBLAST2-hHGF plasmid into HOCs

HOCs were transfected with plasmid pBLAST2-hHGF using the lipofectamine 2000 transfection reagent as previously described [29]. Briefly, for each 25 cm^2 flask, 15 μl DNA was combined with 15 μl lipofectamine 2000 in 150 μl serum- and antibiotic-free DMEM/F12. After a 10–15 min incubation, the mixture was added to cells in the presence of 3 ml serum- and antibiotic-free DMEM/F12 culture medium. The cultures were incubated for 4 h in transfection medium that was then replaced with complete culture medium. Blasticidin-resistant cells were screened and maintained in DMEM/F12, 15% FBS, 20 ng/ml SCF, 10 ng/ml HGF, 10 ng/ml EGF, and 20 ng/ml LIF.

Western blot analysis

Immunoblotting was performed as previously described [29]. Briefly, proteins were extracted from confluent cells using cell lysis buffer. Protein concentrations were determined using the Bradford assay and equal amounts of protein extracts were subjected to SDS-polyacrylamide gel electrophoresis, transferred to a polyvinylidene difluoride (PVDF) membrane, blocked with 5% skim milk in Tris-buffered saline (TBS), and then probed with anti-hHGF (1:50 dilution) or anti-NFκB (1:1000 dilution) at room temperature for 2 h. Secondary antibody was used at a dilution of 1:1000 for 90 min at room temperature. Immunoblotting for β-actin was used as internal control. Proteins were transferred onto PVDF membranes, blocked with 5% skim milk in TBS containing 0.1% Tween-20 (TBST) at 37°C for 1 h, and then probed overnight with anti-β-actin (1:3000 dilution) at 4°C. Goat anti-mouse HRP secondary antibody was used at a dilution of 1:1000. Visualization of immunoreactive bands was carried out using an enhanced chemoluminescence detection method (ECL).

Experimental design

The two-cuff (portal vein and infrahepatic vena cava) technique was used to establish orthotopic liver transplantation in rats as previously described [30]. Female DA rats were used as donors and female Lewis rats as recipients. Recipients were randomly divided into 3 groups: the control group (n = 60), HOC transplantation group (n = 60) and hHGF-modified HOC transplantation group (n = 60). Control group animals received orthotopic liver transplantation and transplantation group animals received either 1 ml of 1×10^6 cells/ml HOCs or hHGF-modified HOCs (passage 4–10) injected into their portal veins and hepatic arteries during orthotopic liver transplantation. Recipients were given tacrolimus one day prior to surgery until 13 days post operation.

Liver function assessment

Liver function indicators, including measurement of alanine aminotransferase (ALT), direct bilirubin (DBil), albumin (ALB), γ-glutamyltransferase (GGT), alkaline phosphate (ALP), and cholinesterase (ChE) levels were determined at the indicated time points after transplantation using a Beckman CX9 automatic biochemical analyzer (Germany).

In situ hybridization

Donor tissues post transplantation were carefully removed and fixed in 10% buffered formaldehyde. Paraffin-embedded sections were rehydrated using a graded ethanol series (95, 80, 60, 30%) with 3–5 min hydration incubations. After a 10 min incubation with 3% H_2O_2 at room temperature, sections were incubated with complex digestive solution for another 10 min at 37°C. After washing with Tris-buffered saline (TBS) and 0.2× SSC, samples were further incubated with the probe working solution at 37°C for 4–8 h. Then, sections were treated with peroxidase (POD) followed by DAB solution, and then stained with H&E. At least 10 images were randomly captured using a phase contrast microscope (Olympus, Japan).

Quantitative RT-PCR

Total RNA was extracted from HOCs, differentiated HOCs, liver tissues, or bile duct tissues using Trizol reagent (Sigma-Aldrich, USA). After purification, the integrity of the purified mRNA was confirmed by agarose gel electrophoresis. The cDNA was then transcribed using the First cDNA Synthesis Kit according to the manufacturer's instructions (Fermentas, CA, USA). The sequences of the specific primers used were as follows: ALB forward primer, 5′-TGTCACGGCGACCTGTTG-3′, reverse primer, 5′-GGAGATAGTGGCCTGGTTCTCA-3′; CK19 forward primer, 5′-GACTTCCGGACCAAGTTTGAG-3′, reverse primer 5′-CGCAGGCCGTTGATGTC-3′; and β-actin forward primer, 5′-ACCGAGCGCGGCTACAGC-3′ and reverse primer, 5′-CTCATTGCCAATGGTGAT-3′. PCR amplification was carried out on a real-time fluorescence quantitative instrument (Roche Diagnostics, Switzerland). The thermocycling conditions were as follows: 60°C for 2 min, 94°C for 10 min, and then 40 cycles at 94°C for 15 s and 60°C for 60 s. The amplified products were analyzed with real-time fluorescence quantitative instrument software. Fold changes in target gene expression were then normalized using the following formula: Fold change = $2^{-\Delta(\Delta Ct)}$. The negative log was calculated and data were analyzed from 20 independent experiments.

Immunohistochemical analysis

Sections were fixed with 4% paraformaldehyde (PFA), dewaxed in xylene, subjected to a graded ethanol series, rinsed with PBS, treated with 3% H_2O_2 and citrate solution, and immunostained with primary antibodies specific for ALB, CK19, PCNA, CD44, Fas, ICAM-1, or CD40 at 37°C for 2 h or at 4°C overnight. After washing with PBS 3 times, sections were stained with goat anti-rabbit biotinylated secondary antibody for 20 min at 37°C. After PBS washing, samples were incubated with SABC solution followed by DAB solution. After double staining with H&E, samples were mounted and fluorescence was detected using a fluorescence microscope (Olympus, Japan).

Evaluation of liver allograft rejection

The severity of acute rejection was assessed using the rejection activity index according to the Banff classification of hepatic allograft rejection [31]. For portal inflammation, 1 = primarily lymphocytic inflammation involving but not noticeably expanding to a minority of the portal triads, 2 = expansion of infiltrates containing a mixture of lymphocytes with occasional blasts, neutrophils and eosinophils into most or all of the portal triad, and 3 = marked expansion of mixed infiltrates containing numerous blasts and eosinophils into most or all of the portal triads with inflammatory spillover into the periportal parenchyma.

For bile duct inflammation damage, 1 = a minority of the ducts are cuffed presenting with inflammatory cells and show only mild reactive changes, and 2 = most or all of the ducts contain inflammatory cell infiltrates. More than an occasional duct shows degenerative changes.

For venous endothelial inflammation, 1 = subendothelial lymphocytic infiltration involving some, but not a majority of the portal and/or hepatic venules, 2 = subendothelial infiltration involving most or all of the portal and/or hepatic venules, 3 = similar to 2 but with moderate to severe perivenular inflammation that extends into the perivenular parenchyma and is associated with perivenular hepatocyte necrosis. The total score is graded as follows: 0–2, no rejection; 3, borderline; 4–5, mild rejection; 6–7, moderate rejection; 8–9, severe rejection.

ELISA

hHGF and cytokine levels were evaluated by ELISA. Primary and secondary antibodies were diluted 1:250 with antibody dilution solution. Biotinylated secondary antibody was added to the 96-well plate wells (100 μl/well) and incubated with samples at 37°C for 90 min. Then, 100 μl of enzyme solution was added to each well and the plate incubated at 37°C for 30 min. After washing, 100 μl of substrate solution was added and plates incubated at 37°C for 15 min in the dark. Stop solution was added (100 μl/well) and the absorbance at 450 nm measured using a plate reader (BioTek, Winooski, VT) immediately after complete mixing.

CD3/CD4/CD8 lymphocyte counting

Anti-rat CD3-FITC/CD4-PC7/CD8-APC antibodies were mixed with the same volume of blood. After a 20 min incubation in the dark at room temperature, lysis buffer was added and percentages of positive cells analyzed using FACS (BD Bioscience).

Statistical analysis

Data were analyzed using SPSS 16.0 software and the data were expressed as the mean ± SD. Comparison of median survival time was carried out using Kaplan-Meier survival analysis. Differences in data measurements were compared with analysis of variance or an independent sample *t*-test. $P<0.05$ was considered as statistically different.

Author Contributions

Conceived and designed the experiments: ZL JC LL JHR. Performed the experiments: ZL JC XHL ZHL GJL. Analyzed the data: ZL JC YCG XLZ HDS. Contributed reagents/materials/analysis tools: ZL JC XHL ZHL GJL. Wrote the paper: ZL JC LL JHR.

References

1. Kaufman DB, Shapiro R, Lucey MR, Cherikh WS, R TB, et al. (2004) Immunosuppression: practice and trends. Am J Transplant 4 Suppl 9: 38–53.
2. Knechtle SJ, Kwun J (2009) Unique aspects of rejection and tolerance in liver transplantation. Semin Liver Dis 29: 91–101.
3. Tosh D, Strain A (2005) Liver stem cells–prospects for clinical use. J Hepatol 42 Suppl: S75–84.
4. Faris RA, Konkin T, Halpert G (2001) Liver stem cells: a potential source of hepatocytes for the treatment of human liver disease. Artif Organs 25: 513–521.
5. Fausto N, Campbell JS (2003) The role of hepatocytes and oval cells in liver regeneration and repopulation. Mech Dev 120: 117–130.
6. Smets F, Najimi M, Sokal EM (2008) Cell transplantation in the treatment of liver diseases. Pediatr Transplant 12: 6–13.
7. Matsumoto K, Nakamura T (1996) Emerging multipotent aspects of hepatocyte growth factor. J Biochem 119: 591–600.
8. Huh CG, Factor VM, Sanchez A, Uchida K, Conner EA, et al. (2004) Hepatocyte growth factor/c-met signaling pathway is required for efficient liver regeneration and repair. Proc Natl Acad Sci U S A 101: 4477–4482.
9. Kato H, Shimomura T, Murai R, Gonda K, Ishii K, et al. (2007) Regulation of hepatic oval cell proliferation by adenoviral mediated hepatocyte growth factor gene transfer and signal transduction inhibitors. Hepatogastroenterology 54: 821–825.
10. Hasuike S, Ido A, Uto H, Moriuchi A, Tahara Y, et al. (2005) Hepatocyte growth factor accelerates the proliferation of hepatic oval cells and possibly promotes the differentiation in a 2-acetylaminofluorene/partial hepatectomy model in rats. J Gastroenterol Hepatol 20: 1753–1761.
11. Shiota G, Kunisada T, Oyama K, Udagawa A, Nomi T, et al. (2000) In vivo transfer of hepatocyte growth factor gene accelerates proliferation of hepatic oval cells in a 2-acetylaminofluorene/partial hepatectomy model in rats. FEBS Lett 470: 325–330.
12. Azuma H, Takahara S, Matsumoto K, Ichimaru N, Wang JD, et al. (2001) Hepatocyte growth factor prevents the development of chronic allograft nephropathy in rats. J Am Soc Nephrol 12: 1280–1292.
13. Yamaura K, Ito K, Tsukioka K, Wada Y, Makiuchi A, et al. (2004) Suppression of acute and chronic rejection by hepatocyte growth factor in a murine model of cardiac transplantation: induction of tolerance and prevention of cardiac allograft vasculopathy. Circulation 110: 1650–1657.
14. Chung H, Kim KH, Kim JG, Lee SY, Yoon YH (2007) Retinal complications in patients with solid organ or bone marrow transplantations. Transplantation 83: 694–699.
15. Patel H, Vogl DT, Aqui N, Shaked A, Olthoff K, et al. (2007) Posttransplant lymphoproliferative disorder in adult liver transplant recipients: a report of seventeen cases. Leuk Lymphoma 48: 885–891.
16. Tamsel S, Demirpolat G, Killi R, Aydin U, Kilic M, et al. (2007) Vascular complications after liver transplantation: evaluation with Doppler US. Abdom Imaging 32: 339–347.
17. Mukherjee S, Mukherjee U (2009) A comprehensive review of immunosuppression used for liver transplantation. J Transplant 2009: 701464.
18. Aggarwal S, Pittenger MF (2005) Human mesenchymal stem cells modulate allogeneic immune cell responses. Blood 105: 1815–1822.
19. Locke JE, Shamblott MJ, Cameron AM (2009) Stem cells and the liver: clinical applications in transplantation. Adv Surg 43: 35–51.
20. Zimmermann FA, Knoll PP, Davies HS, Gokel JM, Schmid T (1983) The fate of orthotopic liver allografts in different rat strain combinations. Transplant Proc 25: 1272.
21. Mosmann TR, Coffman RL (1989) TH1 and TH2 cells: different patterns of lymphokine secretion lead to different functional properties. Annu Rev Immunol 7: 145–173.
22. Chang JT, Reiner SL (2008) Specifying helper T cell fates during immunity. J Pediatr Gastroenterol Nutr 46 Suppl 1: E19–20.
23. VanBuskirk AM, Wakely ME, Orosz CG (1996) Transfusion of polarized TH2-like cell populations into SCID mouse cardiac allograft recipients results in acute allograft rejection. Transplantation 62: 229–238.
24. Strom TB, Roy-Chaudhury P, Manfro R, Zheng XX, Nickerson PW, et al. (1996) The Th1/Th2 paradigm and the allograft response. Curr Opin Immunol 8: 688–693.
25. Marhaba R, Zoller M (2004) CD44 in cancer progression: adhesion, migration and growth regulation. J Mol Histol 35: 211–231.
26. Hubbard AK, Rothlein R (2000) Intercellular adhesion molecule-1 (ICAM-1) expression and cell signaling cascades. Free Radic Biol Med 28: 1379–1386.
27. Strasser A, Jost PJ, Nagata S (2009) The many roles of FAS receptor signaling in the immune system. Immunity 30: 180–192.
28. Chatzigeorgiou A, Lyberi M, Chatzilymperis G, Nezos A, Kamper E (2009) CD40/CD40L signaling and its implication in health and disease. Biofactors 35: 474–483.
29. Yang Y, Fukui K, Koike T, Zheng X (2007) Induction of autophagy in neurite degeneration of mouse superior cervical ganglion neurons. Eur J Neurosci 26: 2979–2988.
30. Xie R, Xu SR (2006) Two-cuff technique was applied in the establishment of orthotopic liver transplantation in rats. Journal of Jiangsu University (Medicine Edition) 16: 392–395.
31. Solez K (2010) History of the Banff classification of allograft pathology as it approaches its 20th year. Curr Opin Organ Transplant 15: 49–51.

7

Role of Donor-Specific Regulatory T Cells in Long-Term Acceptance of Rat Hind Limb Allograft

Yaojun Wang[a], Zhao Zheng[a], Yunchuan Wang, Jiaqi Liu, Na Li, Xiaolong Hu, Fu Han, Yang Liu, Dahai Hu*

Department of Burns and Cutaneous Surgery, Xijing Hospital, Fourth Military Medical University, Xi'an, Shaanxi Province, China

Abstract

Background: Vascularized bone marrow transplantation (VBMT) is widely accepted as an efficient means of establishing chimerism and inducing tolerance. However, the mechanism underlying is poorly understood. Recently, regulatory T cells (Tregs) have been shown to play an important role in regulating immune responses to allogeneic antigens. In this study, we explored the role of Tregs in the induction of tolerance in an allogeneic hind limb transplantation model.

Methodology/Principal Findings: Forty-eight Lewis rats were divided into 6 groups. They received isografts and allografts from Brown-Norway hind limbs. Recipients in groups 1 and 2 received isografts and those in the other groups received allografts. The bone components of donor limbs were kept intact in groups 1, 3, and 5 but removed before transplantation into groups 2, 4, and 6. Tapered cyclosporin A (CsA) was administered to recipients in groups 5 and 6 after transplantation. During the 100-day observation period, all isografts survived, but the allografts in groups 3 and 4 were rejected within 8 to 12 days. CsA-treated intact allografts survived rejection-free for more than 100 days, and CsA-treated allografts lacking bone elements were rejected within 2 months. Stable peripheral chimerism and myeloid chimerism were observed in group 5. Declining peripheral chimerism and a lack of myeloid chimerism were observed in group 6. Donor-specific Tregs were exclusively detected in both peripheral blood and in the spleens of long-term recipient rats in group 5, with an increased FoxP3 mRNA expression in the allografts. This was further demonstrated to be responsible for donor-specific hyporeactivity by *in vitro* one-way mixed lymphocyte reaction (MLR).

Conclusion/Significance: Bone components in the allogeneic hind limbs can induce myeloid chimerism and donor-specific Tregs may be essential to tolerance induction. The bone-removal hind limb model may be a suitable counterpart to the induction of tolerance in the study of limb transplantation.

Editor: Paolo Fiorina, Children's Hospital Boston/Harvard Medical School, United States of America

Funding: Research described in this article was supported by the Academic Support Program Funds of Xijing Hospital, Fourth Military Medical University. The funders had no role in study design, data collection and analysis, decision to publish, or preparation of the manuscript.

Competing Interests: The authors have declared that no competing interests exist.

* E-mail: burns@fmmu.edu.cn

[a] These authors contributed equally to this work.

Introduction

The number of patients undergoing composite tissue defects has increased sharply over the past several years. As of 2005, a total of 1.6 million people are living with the loss of a limb in the U.S. alone, and this number may reach 3.6 million by the year 2050 [1]. People with these defects usually face a number of psychological and social problems, such as social anxiety, lowered self-confidence, negative self-image, depression, and even suicide [2–4]. With the use of immunosuppressants, highly developed composite tissue allotransplantation (CTA) techniques make reconstruction possible. However, the long-term survival of the composite tissue allografts (CTAs) is limited due to both chronic rejection and to the side effects associated with immunosuppressants [5].

The hematopoietic chimerism established by bone marrow cell transplantation leads to condition known as tolerance, in which the recipient's immune system is fundamentally reprogrammed and accepts the donor tissue for long periods without rejection [6–9]. It has been suggested that vascularized bone marrow transplantation (VBMT) may be superior to conventional bone marrow cell transplantation for the induction of tolerance. This phenomenon is thought to be associated with the bone components, which serve as a vascularized method of delivering donor-origin stem and progenitor cells [10,11]. However, the exact mechanism remains poorly understood.

Regulatory T cells (Tregs) are a subset of CD4+ T cells. They express FoxP3, a forkhead/winged helix transcription factor, which is important in the regulation of both Treg development and function. Tregs have been found to be effective in the suppression of autoimmunity and alloimmunity [12]. Recently, they have been approved for peripheral tolerance maintenance and long-term graft acceptance [13,14].

Allogeneic hind limb transplantation, a form of CTA involving different tissues, such as skin, muscle, blood vessels, nerves, and bone, is believed to be more immunogenic than other sets of tissues and that it therefore requires intense immunosuppression [15]. However, the fact that the majority of recipients maintain their transplants on immunosuppression regimens similar to those used in solid organ transplantation suggests that this may not be true [16–18]. We speculate that bone components within the allogeneic limbs may be responsible for this. To assess this speculation and explore the mechanism, we utilized a modified hind limb transplantation model to investigate the role of donor bone components in host immunologic responses. We assessed their contributions to the development of chimerism and allograft survival. Given their known activity on tolerance maintenance, the role of FoxP3$^+$ Tregs in this model was also investigated. We found that the inclusion of bone components promoted stable myeloid chimerism and prolonged allograft survival was achieved. Donor-specific Tregs were found to be associated with long-term allograft survival, as confirmed by *in vitro* one-way mixed lymphocyte reaction (MLR).

Results

Results of the operation

The mean operation time was 150 min in groups 1, 3, and 5 and 180 min in groups 2, 4, and 6. Both groups showed a mean ischemia time of 35 min. No signs of graft versus host disease (GVHD) were observed in all recipient rats during the 100-day observation period. Isografts in groups 1 and 2 survived without signs of rejection (Figs. 1a-A and B). All allografts in groups 3 and 4 showed typical signs of rejection at postoperative days (POD) 4–6. Signs of rejection included bulla formation followed by exudation, epidermolysis, crust formation, and stiffness of limb tissues. Allografts were completely rejected during POD 8–12 (Figs. 1a-C and D). Allografts in group 5 survived rejection-free during the entire observation period (Figs. 1a-E). All bone-removal (B–R) allografts in group 6 showed signs of rejection, including loss of hair, ulceration, epidermolysis, exudation, and stiffness at POD 38–42. Allografts were completely rejected at POD 46–51 (Fig. 1a-F).

Quantification of hind limb graft perfusion

All grafts showed considerable blood supply during the first 7 days after operation (Fig. 2a). In groups 1 and 2, the blood perfusion in the transplanted grafts were assessed at 2.12±0.22 versus 2.21±0.33 at POD 1 and 1.78±0.19 versus 1.75±0.16 at POD 4, respectively. When it came to POD 7, the perfusion value paralleled with the contralateral hind limb with a perfusion ratio 1.14±0.11 versus 1.14±0.15. Groups 1 and 2 showed no significant differences in perfusion ($^*P>0.05$). In groups 3 and 4, the mean blood perfusion of the allografts at POD 1 were 1.9±0.13 versus 2.1±0.24. These values increased more than 3 fold at POD 4 (3.04±0.32 versus 3.27±0.3) and decreased sharply thereafter (0.81±0.14 versus 0.85±0.03). No significant differences were observed between groups 3 and 4 ($^*P>0.05$). In contrast, allograft blood perfusion in groups 5 and 6 remained low at all points in time, with the most marked decrease occurring at POD 4 (0.81±0.10 versus 0.74±0.11) and a tendency toward increase at POD 7 (0.88±0.09 versus 0.95±0.12). There were no significant differences between these two groups ($^*P>0.05$). However, the rejection and experimental groups showed statistically significant differences in blood perfusion at POD 4 ($^\#P<0.05$) (Fig. 2b).

Histopathological evaluation

In the isograft groups (groups 1 and 2), skin biopsy at POD 30 and 100 showed normal epidermis and dermis (Fig. 1b-A). In contrast, allograft skin samples from recipients in groups 3 and 4 showed grade 3 rejection (Fig. 1b-B). Skin biopsy from transplanted allografts in groups 5 and 6 showed grade 1 rejection characterized by focal epidermal mononuclear cell infiltration at POD 30 (Figs. 1b-C, 1D). A mild increase in the number of lymphocytic infiltrates in the upper dermis of POD 100 tissue sections from group 5 was observed (Fig. 1 b-E). In group 6, signs of grade 3 rejection were confirmed by microscopic evaluation in all allografts on the day of rejection (Fig. 1 b-F).

Donor-specific chimerism in the peripheral blood of recipients

We quantified the donor-specific cells in the peripheral blood of LEW recipients in groups 3 and 4 by flow cytometry at POD 1 and 7. We quantified it in groups 5 and 6 at POD 7, 21, 42, and 100. The percentage of donor-origin cells in groups 3 and 4 peaked at POD 1 (7.4%±0.3% and 6.8%±0.9%, respectively). However, this chimerism declined swiftly. At POD 7, only 1.8%±0.8% and 1.6%±0.7% donor origin cells were detected in the peripheral blood in groups 3 and 4. In group 5, peripheral chimerism at POD 7 was assessed at 8%±0.9%, which was similar to the level observed in groups 3 and 4 at POD 1. A higher degree of chimerism was observed at POD 21 among 15.9%±1.6% of donor cells. Levels plateaued at 8.7%±0.6%. In group 6, the relative number of donor cells reached 7.5%±0.3%, 6.9%±0.6%, and 1.4%±0.3% at POD 7, 21, and 42, respectively. No differences in chimerism were observed at POD 7. At POD 21, the chimerism in group 5 peaked, but it showed moderate decreases in group 6. Differences between these two groups were found to be significant ($P<0.05$). At POD 42, chimerism in group 5 stabilized, but chimerism in group 6 decreased sharply down to nearly background levels. Differences between groups 5 and 6 were again found to be significant ($P<0.05$) (Fig. 3a). Dynamic changes in the peripheral chimerism of one representative recipient in group 5 are shown in Fig. 4.

Myeloid chimerism in the bone compartments of recipients

Myeloid engraftment was a result of the homing of primitive donor-origin cells. This contributes to a constant chimerism in peripheral blood. Background noise analysis was performed in isograft recipients, which was not detected (N.D.). The proportion of RT1^n cells in the contralateral femurs of recipients in groups 3 and 4 on the day of rejection and in group 6 on POD 30 and on rejection day were also N.D (Fig. 5a-A). The proportion of donor-origin cells observed from 2 representative recipients at POD 30 and from the other 6 recipients at POD 100 were 5.7%, 5.5% (Figs. 5 a-B, C) and 6.3%±0.5%, respectively (Fig. 3b).

Immunocytochemical staining confirmed myeloid engraftment

Donor-origin RT1^n-FITC positive cells were detectable in the bone marrow cells of the contralateral innate femur from recipients in group 5 at POD 30 and 100. However, they did not appear in any other group. This confirmed that myeloid engraftment occurred solely in CsA-treated intact allogeneic hind limb recipients (Figs. 5b, 5c).

Engraftment and tolerance to allografts accompanied by increased Foxp3$^+$ Tregs with donor property

To determine whether Foxp3$^+$ Tregs contribute to the allograft survival in our model, we analyzed their locations in the peripheral blood and the spleen and the levels of mRNA expression in the graft of CsA-treated rats in groups 5 and 6 at the end of the observation period (i.e., at POD 100 or at the allograft rejection day). FoxP3$^+$ Tregs in the peripheral blood were also analyzed at POD 30. These analyses showed that the frequency of Foxp3$^+$

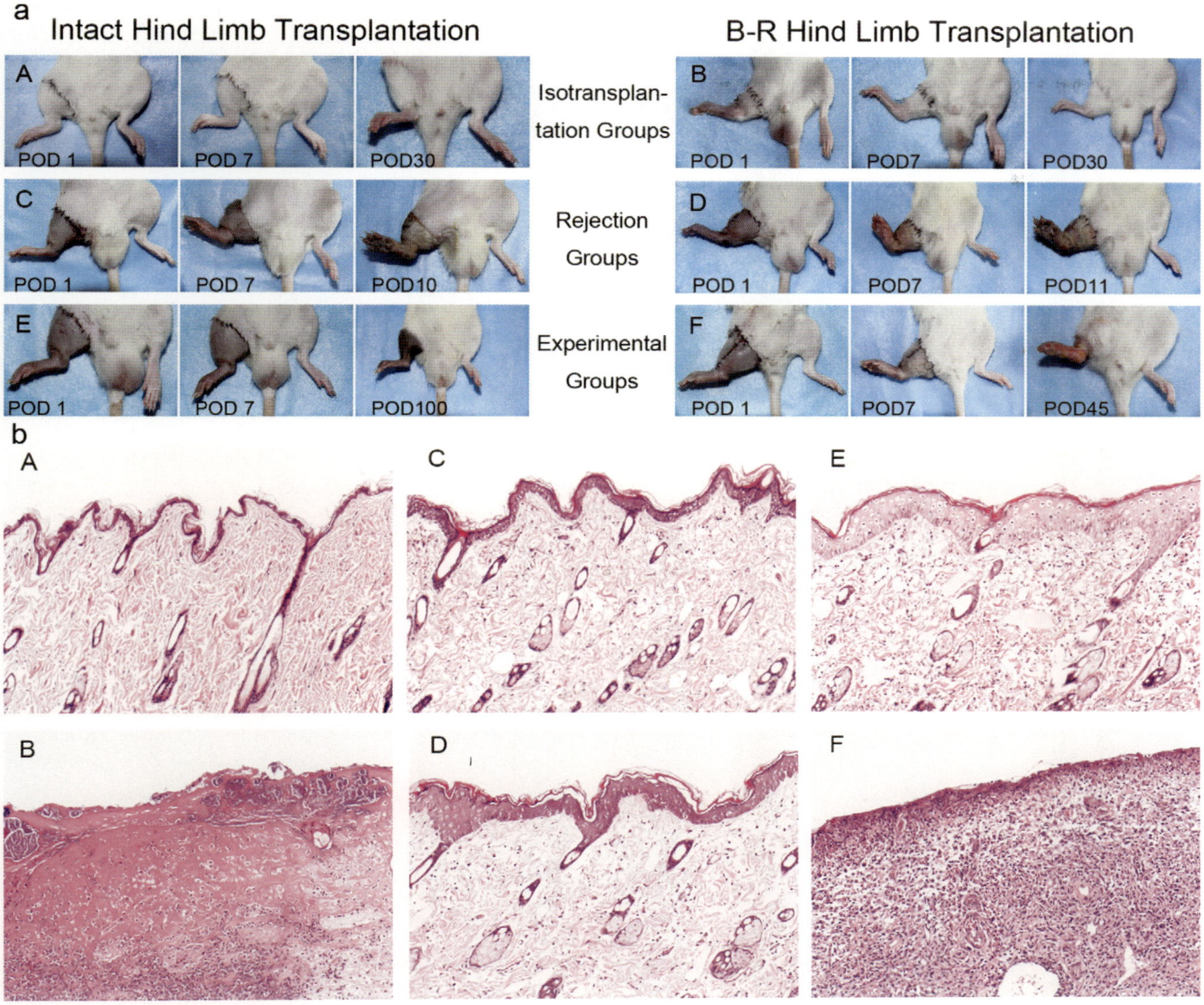

Figure 1. Evaluation of tissue viability and pathological changes of transplanted grafts. (a-A, B): Isografts in groups 1 and 2 survived well. (a-C, D): Allografts in groups 3 and 4 that received N.S showed obvious rejection profiles at 10–12 days postoperatively. (a-E): Allografts in group 5 survived rejection-freely for up to 100 days. With the same CsA protocol, the B–R hind limbs in group 6 were all rejected within 2 months (a-F). (b-A): Skin histologic sections from isograft groups showed normal epidermis and dermis. (b-B): Skin histologic sections from rejection control groups showed necrotic epidermis features of grade 3 rejection reaction at POD 11. (b-C, D): Skin biopsies from CsA treatment groups 5 and 6 at POD 30 showed grade 1 rejection reaction with focal epidermal mononuclear cell infiltration, respectively. (b-E): At POD 100, skin biopsies from recipients in group 5 showed grade 1 rejection and a mild increase in the number of lymphocytes infiltrating the upper dermis at POD 100. (b-F): Skin biopsy from group 6 when the allograft was rejected showed necrotic features of grade 3 rejection reaction in the epidermis and a marked increase in the number of lymphocytes infiltrating all tissues from the dermis down to the muscles (H&E, ×20).

Tregs in the peripheral blood in groups 5 and 6 at POD 30 were both at the background levels obtained from the naïve LEW rats (data not shown). At POD 100, the proportion of Foxp3$^+$ Tregs increased in both the peripheral blood and the spleens of recipient rats in group 5, with a high degree of FoxP3 mRNA expression in the allografts (Figs. 6b, 6c). However, when the grafts were rejected in group 6, Foxp3$^+$ Tregs observed in either the peripheral blood or spleen, and Foxp3 mRNA expressions in the allografts were not significantly different from the background level. These increased levels of Foxp3$^+$ Tregs in group 5 were further found to be donor-specific (Fig. 6a).

Donor-specific Foxp3$^+$ Tregs were required for donor hyporeactivity by one-way mixed lymphocyte proliferation assays

In an effort to elucidate the role of donor-specific FoxP3$^+$ Tregs in the maintenance of tolerance, we performed *in vitro* one-way MLR assays at the end of the observation period. None of the splenic cells from recipient rats in group 5 showed any reactivity to donor antigen stimulation (S.I = 1.4±0.35), but they remained far more reactive to third-party antigen stimulation (S.I = 6.3±1.3) than baseline levels when naïve Lewis splenic cells were used as responders (S.I = 8.5±1.5 and 7.1±1.5 to donor and third-party antigens, respectively). However, when donor-specific FoxP3$^+$ Tregs

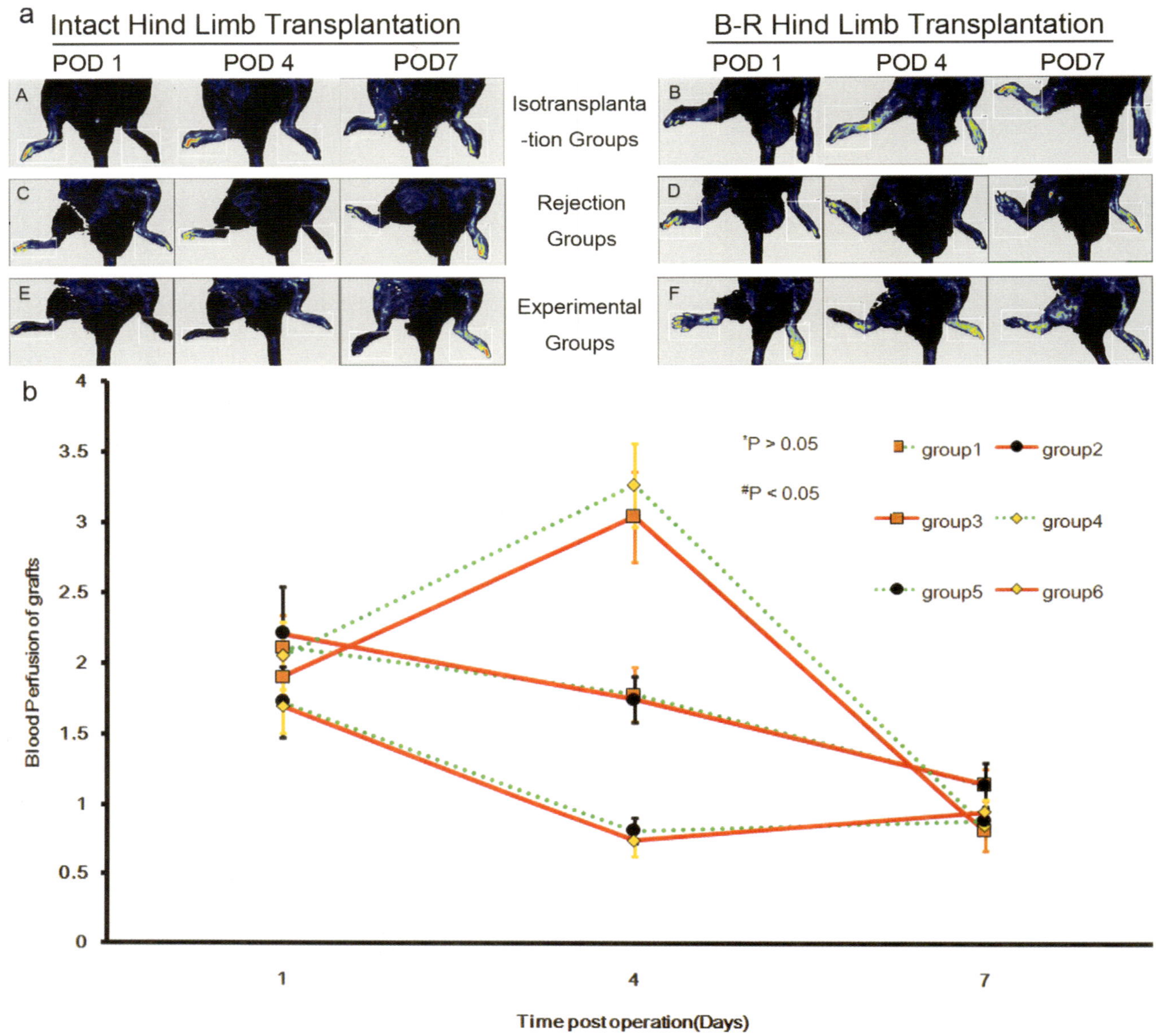

Figure 2. Dynamic changes of blood perfusion in grafts of the recipients. (a) All transplantations were successful, as confirmed by the considerable blood supply of the transplanted grafts according indicated by LDF. (b) The perfusion ratio between intact hind limbs and B–R hind limbs in each group was analyzed. Blood perfusion in isograft controls showed a smooth course of recovery during the observation period. In rejection groups, it peaked at POD 4 and then decreased sharply to a level below that of the contralateral limb. Blood perfusion became undetectable when they were rejected at POD 11. The blood perfusion of transplanted grafts in experimental groups remained low at all times, and ebbed at POD 4. Then it increased to a level below that of the contralateral limb at POD 7. Mean blood perfusion of grafts did not show any significant differences between any two groups given the same treatment at any point in time point ($^{*}P>0.05$). In contrast, all pairs of rejection and experimental groups showed statistical differences at POD 4 ($^{\#}P<0.05$).

were removed from the responder populations, robust antidonor alloreactivity reappeared (S.I 8.8±1.4, roughly equal to the baseline level). Reactivity to the third-party antigens remained generally strong in these assays (Fig. 7). These *in vitro* data confirmed the donor-specific tolerance of recipients in group 5, which was consistent with the long-term graft survival observed in this group.

Discussion

Conventional bone marrow cell transplantation has been found to be effective in inducing chimerism and tolerance, which eliminates the need for lifelong immunosuppression [19,20]. However, this involves significant risk and a time-consuming process including recipient conditioning, donor bone marrow cell isolation, and the administration of substantial amounts of immunosuppressants for achieving transplanted cell engraftment and the repetitive detection for the presence of stable chimerism. In this way, it is not feasible for composite tissue allotransplantation, in which cadaveric donors are always used and recipients are not under the threat of death. Recently, it has been proposed that VBMT may be superior to bone marrow cell transplantation

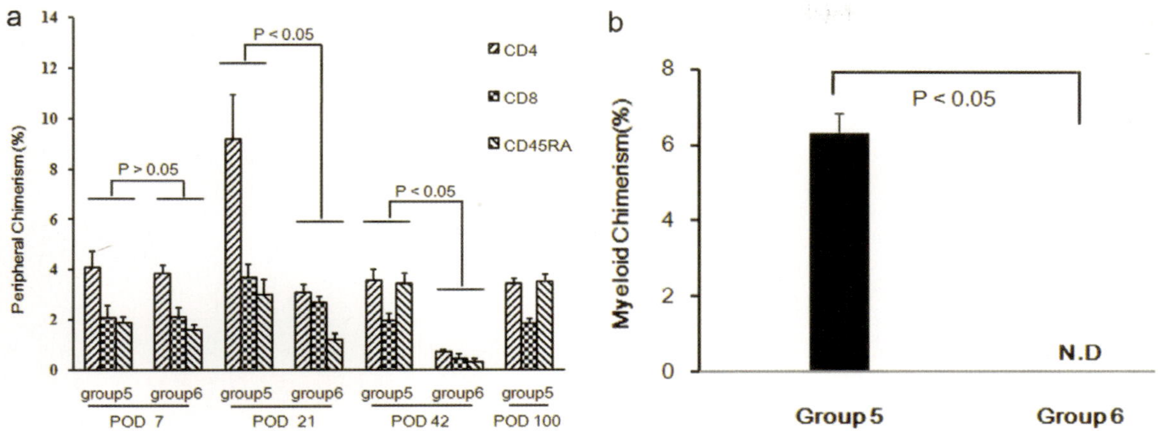

Figure 3. Dynamic changes of peripheral chimerism. Flow cytometry analysis for the presence of donor-specific CD4+/CD8+ T lymphocytes and CD45RA+ B lymphocytes at POD 7, POD 21, and POD 42 of one representative intact allogeneic hind limb recipient with CsA treatment. Levels of donor-specific chimerism were 3.3% in CD4/RT1^n cells, 1.2% in CD8/RT1^n cells, and 1.6% in CD45RA/RT1^n cells at POD 7. They rose to the highest level for donor-origin CD4/RT1^n 13.2%, CD8/RT1^n 2.9%, and CD45RA/RT1^n 2.1% at POD 21, remained at 3.6% CD4/RT1^n, 2.0% CD8/RT1^n, and 3.0% CD45RA/RT1^n. The background levels observed in isograft controls were assessed at 0.3%, 0.2%, and 0.3%, respectively.

for the establishment of chimerism and the induction of tolerance. Several studies have suggested that femoral, sternal, mandibular elements within the allograft may serve as a substantial source of bone marrow cells, resulting in the development of donor-specific chimerism [11,21,22].

Rats make up the most frequent animal model of hind limb allotransplantation with vascularized bone marrow grafts. Previous studies have indicated that transplanted hind limb allografts containing bone marrow cells and stromal microenvironments facilitate allograft tolerance under certain immunosuppressive protocols, but the mechanism underlying this improved tolerance has not been extensively investigated. In this study, with a modified hind limb transplantation model, we observed that, under a minimally toxic recipient immunosuppressive protocol, the intact hind limb survived rejection-free for more than 100 days. However, when the bone components were removed, the allografts tended to be rejected within 2 months. Most importantly, we identified a critical role for donor-specific FoxP3$^+$ Tregs in allografts survival.

Previous studies have shown that transplanted organs and CTAs contain large numbers of immunocompetent cells, including those of myeloid origin. These cells are called passenger leukocytes [23,24]. Once vascular anastomoses are established, these leukocytes may migrate from grafted tissue to peripheral blood and colonize both lymphoid and non-lymphoid organs of the recipient. In this study, we observed that, shortly after operation, donor-origin RT1^n cells were detected in recipients in both the rejection and experimental groups. But due to the lack of immunosuppression, the number of RT1^n cells sharply declined during the course of the rejection process, regardless of whether the bone components had been removed. Likewise, with a tapered CsA protocol, the chimerism in B–R allograft recipients gradually declined and disappeared whenever the graft rejection process took less than 2 months. In contrast, under the same CsA treatment, the intact hind limb survived rejection-free for more than 100 days. Immunocytofluorescence analysis of bone marrow cells from the contralateral recipient innate femur at POD 30 showed the presence of donor-origin cells in intact allograft recipients and an absence of such cells from B–R allograft recipients. This indicated that the passenger leukocytes within the B–R allografts were unable to engraft to the bone marrow compartment of recipients under the tapered CsA protocol. The bone components were required for the induction of myeloid chimerism.

FoxP3$^+$ Tregs have been shown to play a crucial role in maintaining allograft tolerance in experimental models of transplantation recently [25]. In order to disclose the mechanism underlying the long-term survival of transplants to rat recipients with myeloid chimerism, we investigated the contribution of FoxP3$^+$ Tregs to allograft survival in our model. At POD 30, when myeloid chimerism has been successfully achieved in group 5, the frequency of Foxp3$^+$ Tregs in the peripheral blood showed no differences from that of group 6. However, when at POD 100, donor-specific FoxP3$^+$ Tregs were acquired only in intact hind limb recipient rats that had received CsA treatment. This treatment was therefore considered responsible for the donor-specific hyporeactivity by *in vitro* one-way MLR and may be required for the maintenance of tolerance to allografts as supported by the significantly higher FoxP3 mRNA expression in the long-term accepted allografts than in the rejected allografts. Our results are consistent with those of other, supporting the conclusion that Tregs is critical to the maintenance of allograft survival [26,27].

These results conflict with published data, which state that long-term calcineurin inhibitors are associated with a decline of Tregs in patients receiving solid organ transplantation [28]. Considering the complex process of tolerance induction/maintenance to transplanted tissues and the relatively delayed appearance of donor-specific FoxP3$^+$ Tregs in group 5, we deduce that the increased donor-specific FoxP3$^+$ Tregs are likely to be induced by the myeloid chimerism established in intact allogeneic hind limb recipients under the minimally toxic CsA guarantee, which have immunoregulatory effects on the recipients and contribute to long-term allograft survival. However, this has yet to be confirmed. There are also data indicating that the effects of calcineurin inhibition on Treg function may be dose-dependent and that low doses may permit or even support Treg function [29].

We used a noninvasive laser Doppler flowmeter to monitor postoperative blood perfusion status. No significant differences were observed between any 2 groups that received the same treatment, indicating that the B–R procedure did not affect blood perfusion. Isotransplantation and rejection groups showed the same survival period, confirming that this procedure does not

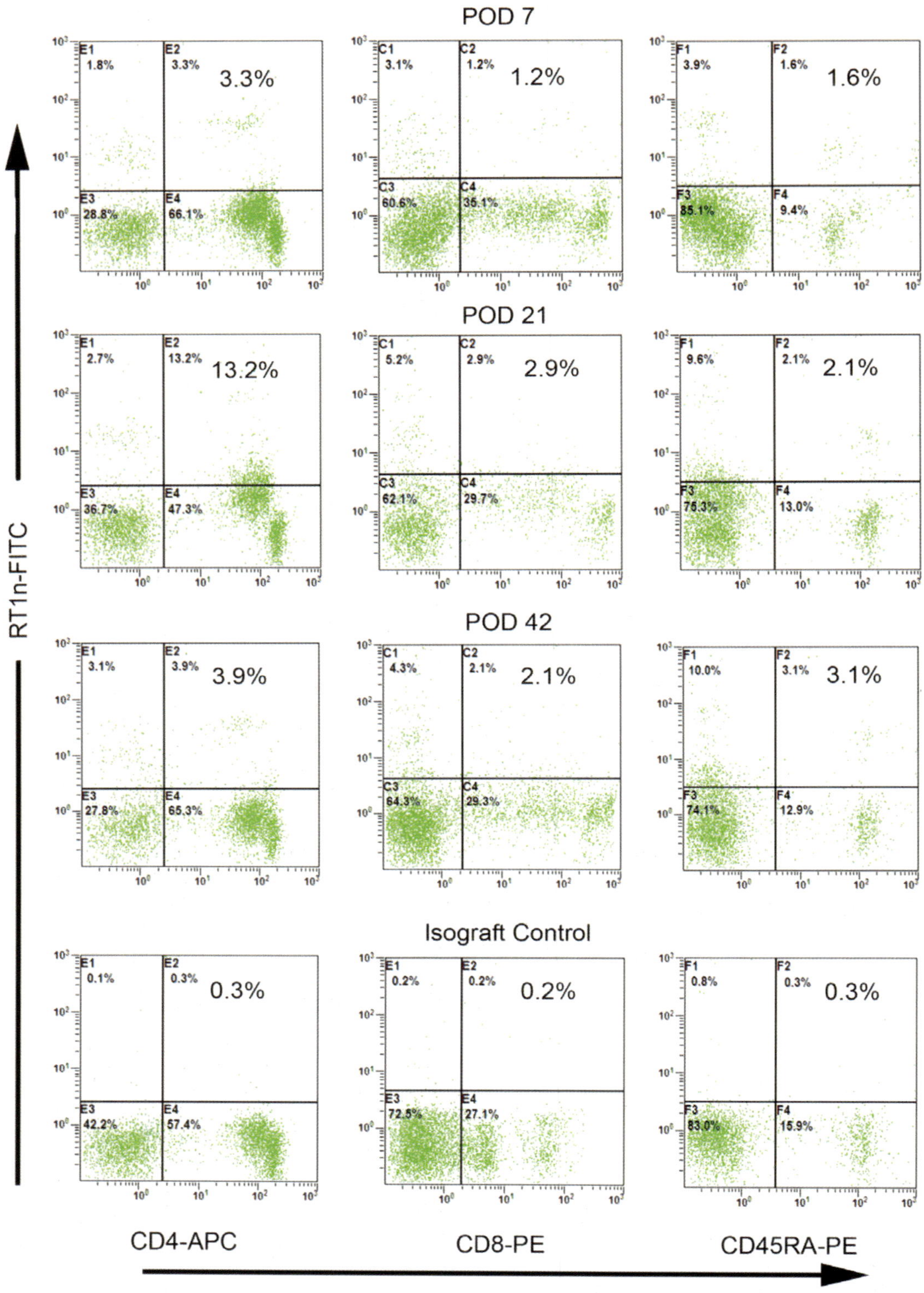

Figure 4. Dynamic changes in peripheral and myeloid chimerism. (a) Time kinetics of chimerism in groups 5 and 6. At POD 7, they showed almost the same chimerism level ($P>0.05$). At POD 21, the level of chimerism in group 6 was mildly decreased, but it increased sharply in group 5 ($P<0.05$). At POD 42, chimerism in group 5 returned to a total level 8.7%±0.6% but it decreased to background level in group 6 ($P<0.05$). In addition, donor-origin CD45RA+ B cells in group 5 prevailed beginning at POD 21 and maintained thereafter. (b) Myeloid chimerism was detectable at 6.3±0.5% at POD 100 in group 5 and it never appeared in group 6 when allografts were rejected (n=6, $P<0.05$).

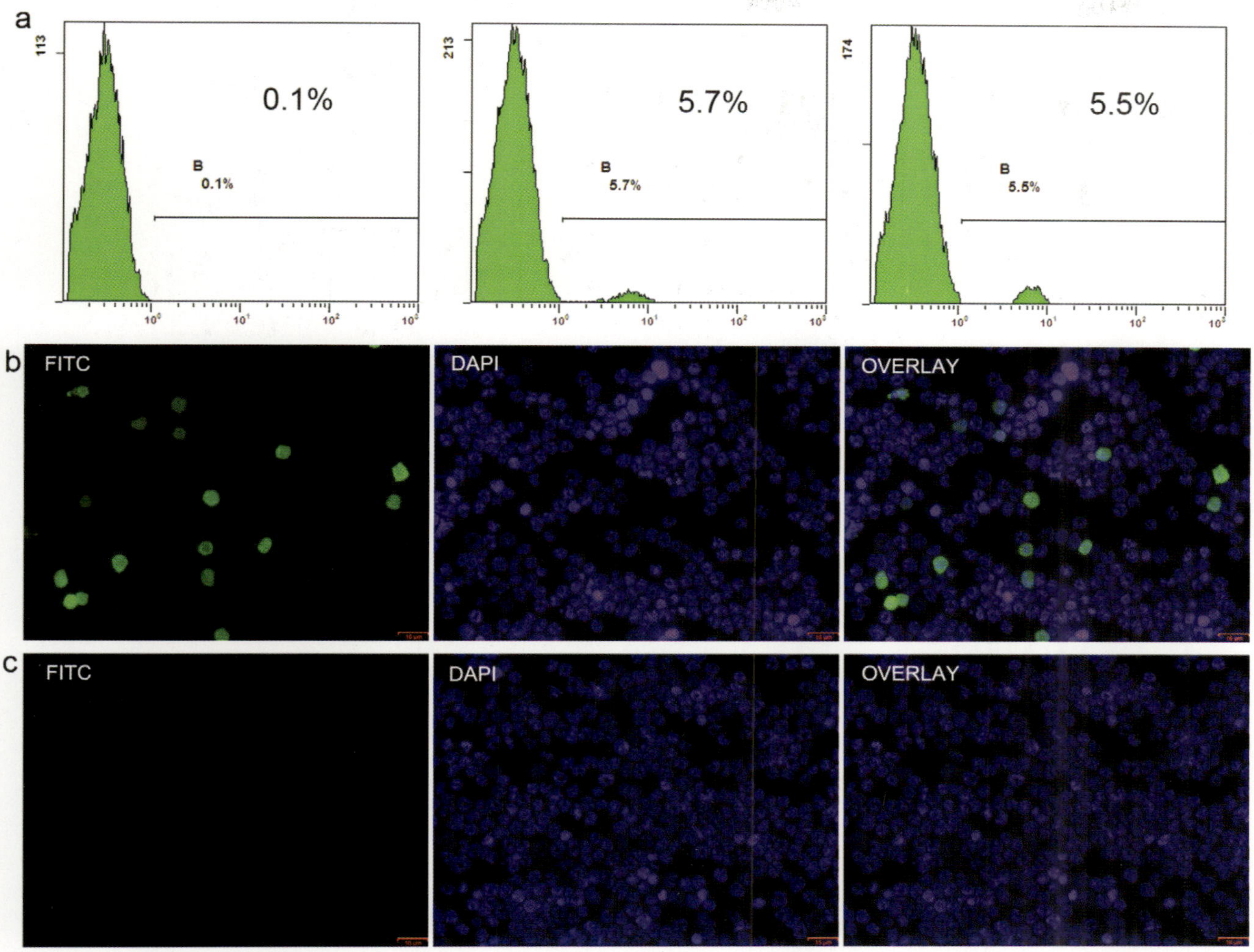

Figure 5. Flow cytometry analysis for myeloid chimerism and immunocytofluorescence staining for the presence of donor-origin cells in recipients' innate femurs. (a)The proportion of donor-origin cells observed from 2 representative recipients at POD 30 were at 5.7% and 5.5%, respectively, with the background level assessed at 0.1%. (b, c) The presence of RT1n cells in the contralateral femurs of recipients in group 5 and their absence in other groups was confirmed by immunocytofluorescence (×20).

cause the final rejection of B–R allografts observed in the experimental groups.

In conclusion, using B–R hind limbs with all the same elements as the intact hind limbs except for its lack of bone components, we observed that, under a minimally toxic recipient immunosuppressive protocol, intact allogeneic hind limbs were able to survive rejection-free for more than 100 days. When the bone components were removed, early rejection episodes and graft loss were observed. Further investigation indicated that donor-specific FoxP3^{+} Tregs are required for donor hyporeactivity in *in vitro* one-way MLR and that they may be responsible for long-term allograft survival. The means by which these cells are generated merits further investigation. The B–R hind limb model might serve as a counterpart to tolerance induction studies of hind limb allotransplantation and so advance realization of the allotransplantation in clinical settings.

Materials and Methods

Animals

Inbred Brown-Norway [BN (RT1^{n})] rats and Lewis [LEW (RT1^{l})] rats with disparate major histocompatibility complexes (MHC) and minor histocompatibility antigens were purchased from Vital River, Inc. (Beijing, China). Eight-to-ten-week-old BN rats weighing 175–200 g were used as donors, LEW rats equal in age and body weight were used as recipients. The research protocol was approved by the Experimental Animal Committee of the Fourth Military Medical University. All rats received humane care in compliance with the *Guide for the Care and Use of Laboratory Animals* published by the National Institutes of Health.

The experimental design is described in Table 1. Forty-eight hind limb transplants were performed. Isograft transplantations were performed in groups 1 and 2 between genetically identical LEW rats (Isotransplantation Groups). Allograft transplantations were performed between BN rats and LEW rats in groups 3 through 6. The rats in groups 3 and 4 (Rejection Groups) were given 1 mL. In groups 5 and 6 (Experimental Groups), all recipients were treated with tapered CsA, which was administered on day 0 at a standard dose of 16 mg/kg per day for 1 week, tapered to 2 mg/kg per day over 4 weeks, and maintained at this level thereafter. The femur, tibia, and fibula were kept intact in groups 1, 3, and 5 (intact grafts), but they were removed in groups

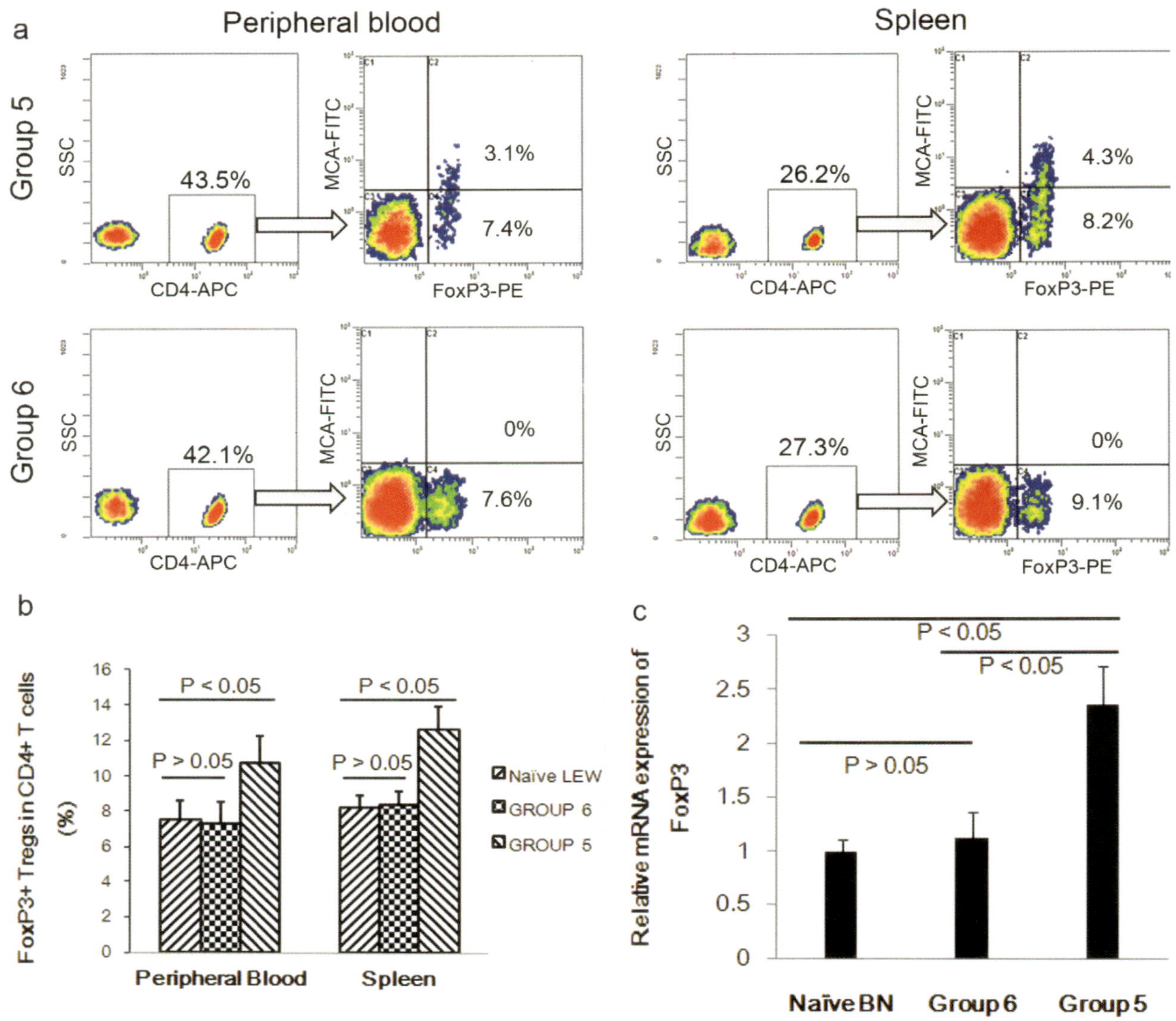

Figure 6. Location of FoxP3⁺ Tregs in rats receiving CsA treatment. (a) Representative dot plots of donor-specific FoxP3⁺ Tregs in peripheral blood and spleen from allograft recipients in groups 5 and 6 at the end of the observation period. Mononuclear cells were obtained by Ficoll solution centrifugation, followed by magnetic isolation of CD4+ T cells. Isolated CD4+ T cells were then co-stained with anti-rat mAb $RT1^n$-FITC and intracellularly stained with anti-mouse/rat Foxp3-PE. All cells were analyzed by flow cytometry. The results demonstrated that donor-specific $FoxP3^+$ Tregs were exclusively obtained in both the peripheral blood and spleens of long-term allograft recipients in group 5. (b) Further analysis indicated an average proportion of 10.7%±1.1% versus 7.6%±1.6% and 12.6%±0.7% versus 8.3%±1.1 $FoxP3^+$ Tregs located in the peripheral blood and spleen in group 5 and 6, respectively, with significant differences (n = 6, $P<0.05$). (c) Expression of FoxP3 mRNA in the allografts was analyzed by real-time PCR normalized to GAPDH. Significantly higher levels of FoxP3 were observed in group 5 (n = 6, $P<0.05$).

2, 4, and 6 (bone-removal grafts, B–R grafts) before transplantation.

Surgical procedure

Bone-removal hind limb preparation. After general anesthesia with sodium pentobarbital (50 mg/kg), the donor BN rats were shaved and below the inguinal level and their skin was sterilized with 75% ethanol solution. A longitudinal incision was made from the sacroiliac joint through the anterior aspect of the ankle joint and the knee joint along the lateral femoral intermuscular septum of the recipient's right hind limb. The femur, tibia, and fibula were removed after the dissection of all adherent tissues and ligation of the vascular branches supplying the femur and tibia. Then a 1.5 mm Kirschner wire was put in place of the femur and tibia. The incisions were then closed with 3/0 sutures. After preparation, B–R hind limbs were immediately transplanted to recipient rats.

Transplantation. Hind limb transplantation was performed according to the technique described by Doi [30]. Briefly, a circumferential skin incision was made in the recipients rear middle thighs. Then the femoral artery, vein, and nerve were dissected, clamped, and transected proximal to the superficial epigastric artery. The limb was amputated at the mid-femoral level. The donor limb was prepared in the same way. Donor limbs were then attached to the recipient's femoral stump with 1.5 mm Kirschner wire. After femoral vessels of the donor and recipient were anastomosed and ascertained to be patent, the incision was

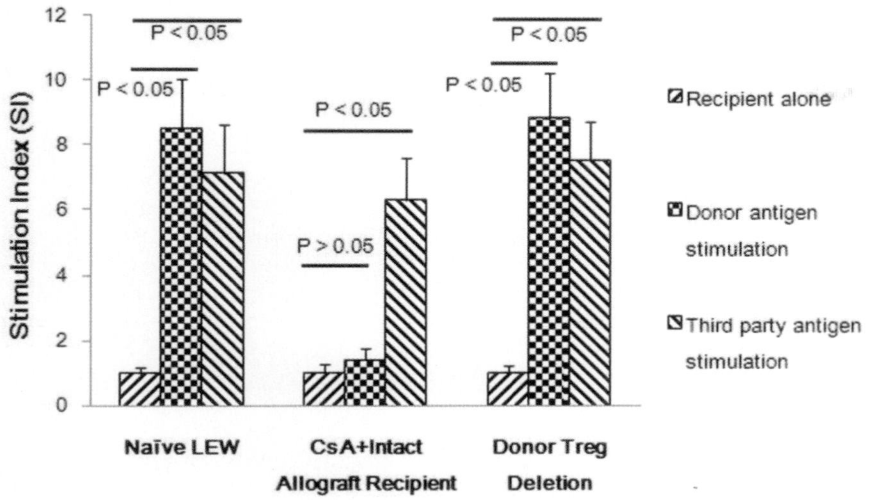

Figure 7. One-way MLR revealed a critical role of donor-specific FoxP3$^+$ Tregs for the maintenance of tolerance. Baseline levels were assessed when naïve Lewis splenic cells were used as responders. Hyporeactivity to donor antigen stimulation and immunocompetence for third-party antigens stimulation (ACI rats) in recipients of group 5 at POD 100 was demonstrated. When donor-specific FoxP3$^+$ Tregs were depleted from the responder populations, robust antidonor alloreactivity reappeared.

closed. Three milliliters of N.S. was injected intraperitoneally to compensate for perioperative fluid loss.

Evaluation of graft survival and assessment of graft-versus-host disease

After the operation, clinical manifestations of rejection, such as changes in color and temperature, progressive edema, loss of hair, desquamation, ulceration, epidermolysis, exudation, stiffness, and progressive shrinkage were recorded and evaluated daily. Clinical criteria for the appearance of graft-versus-host disease (GVHD) included diffuse erythema, hyperkeratosis of the foot pads, dermatitis, weight loss, and diarrhea.

Quantitation of blood perfusion

All recipients were anesthetized under 1% isoflurane in 100% oxygen flow at 1 L/min on postoperative days (POD) 1, 4, and 7. The blood perfusion of both hind limbs was determined by Laser Doppler Flowmeter (PeriFlux System 5000, Perimed, Stockholm, Sweden) scanning, which generated computerized pseudo-color images. To minimize variation, all animals were placed in a supine position on a 37°C heating pad during scanning. After the images were recorded, the perfusion value, indicated by color, was defined within a range of 0 to 1000. Blood perfusion of the hind limb grafts was expressed as the ratio of perfusion value of the transplanted hind limb to that of the contralateral innate hind limb.

Histopathology

Tissue sections were cut from 6 μg skin samples of the grafts for hematoxylin/eosin staining. Each tissue section was evaluated by a pathologist and the histopathological grade of each tissue sample was determined according to previously published criteria [31].

Chimerism evaluation by flow cytometry analysis

One hundred microliters of peripheral blood was collected from recipients in all groups. Bone marrow was harvested from the contralateral innate femurs of 2 representative recipients at POD 30 and from the other 6 animals either at POD 100 or when the allografts in all allotransplantation groups were rejected. Peripheral blood samples were incubated with the combination of mouse anti-rat mAb RT1^n-FITC (BN MHC Class I, clone MCA 156/OX-27, Serotec, U.K.) and either mouse anti-rat mAb of T-cell CD4-APC (clone W3/25), CD8a-PE (clone OX-8), and B-cell CD45RA-PE (clone OX-33; Biolegend, San Diego, CA, U.S.) for 30 minutes at 37°C away from light. Then red cells were lysed by the addition of lysing buffer (FACS lysing solution; Bio Legend

Table 1. Experimental design and survival time of the transplanted grafts.

Groups	Surgical procedure	Treatment	Survival time(d)
Group1(n = 8)	Isotransplantation	No	>100
Group2(n = 8)	Isotransplantation(b–r)	No	>100
Group3(n = 8)	Allotransplantation	N.S	8,9,8,11,10,9,10,12
Group4(n = 8)	Allotransplantation(b–r)	N.S	9,8,11,12,11,10,8,12
Group5(n = 8)	Allotransplantation	CsA	30#,30#, 100*,100*,100*,100*,100*,100*
Group6(n = 8)	Allotransplantation(b–r)	CsA	30#,30#,46,49,47,49,48,51

#At POD 30, 2 recipients in groups 5 and 6 were killed for myeloid chimerism evaluation.
*At POD 100, the other 6 recipients in group 5 were killed for evaluation of myeloid chimerism and determination of underlying mechanisms.

Co.) Cells were incubated for 10 min at room temperature. Cells were finally suspended in 1% paraformadehyde for 30 min and subjected to an EPICS XL flow cytometry (Beckman-Coulter, Fullerton, CA, U.S.). Bone marrow cells from the contralateral innate femurs were loaded on the 1.077 g/mL Ficoll density gradient solution and centrifuged at 316 g for 20 min. The white membrane layer was resuspended in PBS. One million cells stained with mouse anti-rat mAb $RT1^n$-FITC were quantified by flow cytometry and analyzed with Expo 32 ADC analysis software (Beckman-Coulter, Fullerton, CA, U.S.).

Immunocytochemical staining

Bone marrow cells from the contralateral innate femurs stained with mouse anti-rat mAb $RT1^n$-FITC were further stained with DAPI for 5 min. They were then washed with PBS and smeared on the microscope slide, and examined for the presence of donor cells by the Olympus FSX100 Bio Imaging Navigator (OLYMPUS, Japan).

Detection of donor-specific $FoxP3^+$ Tregs by flow cytometry analysis

One and a half milliliters of peripheral blood and 1/3 single spleen cell suspensions from recipients in the experimental groups were isolated at the end of the observation period through 1.077 g/mL Ficoll density gradient. Then >95% pure $CD4^+$ T cells were magnetically isolated using a $CD4^+$ T cell isolation kit in accordance with the manufacturer's protocol (Miltenyi Biotec, Bergisch Gladbach, Germany). Isolated $CD4^+$ T cells were then stained with mouse anti-rat mAb $RT1^n$-FITC for 30 min at 4°C. The stained cells were washed, fixed, and permeabilized with saponin 20% (Sigma-Aldrich) for 30 min at 37°C. Permeabilized cells were stained with Anti-Mouse/Rat Foxp3 PE (Cat. 12577382; eBioscience). All cells were quantified by flow cytometry and analyzed with Expo 32 ADC analysis software.

RNA isolation and real-time PCR

Total RNA from allografts of groups 5 and 6 were isolated with Trizol Reagent (Invitrogen, San Diego, CA, U.S.) according to the manufacturer's instruction. Five hundred ng of RNA was reverse-transcribed using PrimeScript RT Kit (TaKaRa, Dalian, China) in a final volume of 10 µL. Real-time PCR was performed in the Bio-Rad IQ^5 Real-Time System (Bio-Rad, Hercules, CA, U.S.) by using a SYBR® Premix Ex Taq™ II kit (TaKaRa, Dalian, China) in a 20 µL volume of the PCR reaction solution. Primer sequences were as follows: FoxP3: forward 5′-CTTCAGACAGCTTGTT-TGCTGTG-3′, reverse 5′-GGGCCGCATATTATGGTAC-T-TG-3′; GAPDH: forward 5′-GGCACAGTCAAGGCTGAGAA-TG-3′, reverse 5′- ATGGTGGTGAAGACGCCAGTA-3′ The cycling conditions used were as follows: initial denaturation at 95°C for 30 s, followed by 40 cycles with denaturation at 95°C for 10 s, annealing at 60°C for 10 s, and elongation at 72°C for 15 s. The expression level of GAPDH was used for internal control.

In vitro one-way mixed lymphocyte reaction assay

One-way mixed lymphocyte reaction (MLR) assay was used to determine donor-specific tolerance. Spleens were harvested and mashed to yield single cell suspensions. After red cell clearance, they were adjusted to 2×10^6/mL in RPMI 1640 medium (Gibco, U.S.) containing 10% FBS. Responder cells were isolated from naïve Lewis rats or recipients in group 5 at POD 100, when they were killed. In order to determine the role of $FoxP3^+$ Tregs, parts of the responder cells from recipient rats in group 5 were donor-specific $FoxP3^+$ Tregs magnetically depleted. Stimulator cells were isolated from the spleens of BN and third-party August-Copenhagen-Irish (ACI) rats and inactivated by Mitomycin C (Sigma, St. Louis, MO, U.S.) at 50 µg/mL, 37°C for 30 min preincubation. Two-hundred thousand responder cells and equal numbers of stimulator cells were then cocultured in 200 µL of RPMI 1640 medium containing 10% FBS in 96-well plates in a humidified 37°C, 5% CO2 incubator. After 3 days of incubation, cultures were pulsed with 1 µCi [^{3}H] Thymidine for 18 h and assessed by a β-scintillation counter. The stimulation index (SI) was determined by assessing the ratio of the counts per minute (c.p.m.) generated in response to each stimulator to that of the culture medium alone (in the absence of stimulators).

Statistical analysis

All data were expressed as mean ± SEM. To compare average perfusion between B–R hind limbs and intact hind limbs subjected to the same treatment or when average chimerism and $FoxP3^+$ Tregs as well as FoxP3 mRNA expression between groups 5 and 6 were compared, an independent sample T-test was performed. All statistical analyses were performed using SPSS 13.0. Statistical differences were considered significant at $P<0.05$.

Acknowledgments

The authors gratefully acknowledge the assistance of Yingjun Su during the writing of this article.

Author Contributions

Conceived and designed the experiments: YW ZZ DH. Performed the experiments: YW JL FH YL. Analyzed the data: NL XH. Contributed reagents/materials/analysis tools: ZZ. Wrote the paper: YW.

References

1. Ziegler-Graham K, MacKenzie EJ, Ephraim PL, Travison TG, Brookmeyer R (2008) Estimating the prevalence of limb loss in the United States: 2005 to 2050. Arch Phys Med Rehabil 89: 422–429.
2. Robinson E, Rumsey N, Partridge J (1996) An evaluation of the impact of social interaction skills training for facially disfigured people. Br J Plast Surg 49: 281–289.
3. Levine E, Degutis L, Pruzinsky T, Shin J, Persing JA (2005) Quality of life and facial trauma: psychological and body image effects. Ann Plast Surg 54: 502–510.
4. Ye EM (1998) Psychological morbidity in patients with facial and neck burns. Burns 24: 646–648.
5. Ravindra KV, Wu S, Bozulic L, Xu H, Breidenbach WC, et al. (2008) Composite tissue transplantation: a rapidly advancing field. Transplant Proc 40: 1237–1248.
6. Rossini AA, Dale GL, Mordes JP (1999) Induction of immunologic tolerance for transplantation. Physiol Rev 79: 99–141.
7. Rifle G, Mousson C (2003) Donor-derived hematopoietic cells in organ transplantation: a major step toward allograft tolerance?. Transplantation 75 (9Suppl): 3S–7S.
8. Foster RD, Pham S, Li S, Aitouche A (2003) Long-term acceptance of composite tissue allografts through mixed chimerism and CD28 blockade. Transplantation 76: 988–994.
9. Hettiaratchy S, Randolph MA, Petit F, Lee WP, Butler PE (2004) Composite tissue allotransplantation–a new era in plastic surgery?. Br J Plast Surg 57: 381–391.
10. Arsian E, Klimczak A, Siemionow M (2007) Chimerism induction in vascularized bone marrow transplants augmented with bone marrow cells. Microsurgery 27: 190–199.
11. Kulahci Y, Klimczak A, Madajka M, Altuntas S, Siemionow M (2010) Long-term survival of composite hemiface/mandible/tongue allografts correlates with multilineage chimerism development in the lymphoid and myeloid compartments of recipients. Transplantation 90: 843–852.
12. Hori S, Nomura T, Sakaguchi S (2003) Control of regulatory T cell development by the transcription factor Foxp3. Science 299: 1057–1061.

13. Tang Q, Bluestone JA, Kang SM (2012) CD4+ FoxP3+ regulatory T cell therapy in transplantation. Journal of Molecular Cell Biology 4: 11–21.
14. Bonde S, Chan KM, Zavazava N (2008) ES-Cell Derived Hematopoietic Cells Induce Transplantation Tolerance. PLoS ONE 3(9): e3212.
15. Stevens HP, Hovius SE, Heeney JL, van Nierop PW, Jonker M (1991) Immunologic aspects and complications of composite tissue allografting for upper extremity reconstruction: a study in the rhesus monkey. Transplant Proc 23: 623–625.
16. Lanzetta M, Petruzzo P, Margreiter R, Dubernard JM, Schuind F, et al. (2005) The International Registry on Hand and Composite Tissue Transplantation. Transplantation 79: 1210–1214.
17. Piza-Katzer H, Ninkovic M, Pechlaner S, Gabl M, Ninkovic M, et al. (2002) Double hand transplantation: functional outcome after 18 months. J Hand Surg Br 27: 385–390.
18. Dubernard JM, Petruzzo P, Lanzetta M, Parmentier H, Martin X, et al (2003) Functional results of the first human double-hand transplantation. Ann Surg 238: 128–136.
19. Brouha PC, Iidstad ST (2001) Mixed allogeneic chimerism. Past, present, and prospects for the future. Transplantation 72(Suppl 8): S36–S42.
20. Siemionow M, Oke R, Ozer K, Izycki D, Prajapati R (2002) Induction of donor-specific tolerance in rat hind-limb allografts under antilymphocyte serum and cyclosporine A protocol. J Hand Surg Am 27: 1095–1103.
21. Tai CY, France MA, Strande LF, Eydelman R, Sheng X, et al. (2003) An extraperitoneal isolated vascularized bone marrow transplant model in the rat. Transplantation 75: 1591–1593.
22. Santiago SF, de Faria W, Khan TF, Gandia CE, Misiakos EP, et al. (1999) Heterotopic sternum transplant in rats: A new model of a vascularized bone marrow transplantation. Microsurgery 19: 330–334.
23. Kreisel D, Petrowsky H, Krasinskas AM, Krupnick AS, Szeto WY, et al. (2002) The role of passenger leukocyte genotype in rejection and acceptance of rat liver allografts. Transplantation 73:1501–1507.
24. Starzl TE, Zinkernagel RM (1998) Antigen localization and migration in immunity and tolerance. N Engl J Med 339: 1905–1913.
25. Denecke C, Bedi DS, Ge X, Kim IK, Jurisch A, et al. (2010) Prolonged Graft Survival in Older Recipient Mice Is Determined by Impaired Effector T-Cell but Intact Regulatory T-Cell Responses. PLoS ONE 5(2): e9232.
26. Eljaafari A, Badet L, Kanitakis J, Ferrand C, Farre A, et al. (2006) Isolation of regulatory T cells in the skin of a human hand-allograft, up to six years posttransplantation. Transplantation 82: 1764.
27. Bozulic LD, Wen Y, Xu H, Ildstad ST (2011) Evidence that FoxP3+ regulatory T cells may play a role in promoting long-term acceptance of composite tissue allotransplants. Transplantation 91: 908–915.
28. Demirkiran A, Hendrikx TK, Baan CC, van der Laan LJ (2008). Impact of immunosuppressive drugs on CD4+CD25+FOXP3+ regulatory T cells: does in vitro evidence translate to the clinical setting?. Transplantation 85: 783–789.
29. Brandt C, Pavlovic V, Radbruch A, Worm M, Baumgrass R (2009) Low-dose cyclosporine A therapy increases the regulatory T cell population in patients with atopic dermatitis. Allergy 64: 1588–1596.
30. Doi K (1979) Homotransplantation of limbs in rats. Plast Reconstr Surg 64: 613–621.
31. Cendales LC, Kirk AD, Moresi JM, Ruiz P, Kleiner DE (2006) Composite tissue allotransplantation: classification of clinical acute skin rejection. Transplantation 81: 418–422.

8

Rapamycin Combined with Anti-CD45RB mAb and IL-10 or with G-CSF Induces Tolerance in a Stringent Mouse Model of Islet Transplantation

Nicola Gagliani[1,2,3], Silvia Gregori[2], Tatiana Jofra[1], Andrea Valle[1,3], Angela Stabilini[1], David M. Rothstein[4], Mark Atkinson[5], Maria Grazia Roncarolo[2,3], Manuela Battaglia[1]*

1 San Raffaele Diabetes Research Institute, San Raffaele Scientific Institute, Milan, Italy, **2** San Raffaele Telethon Institute for Gene Therapy, San Raffaele Scientific Institute, Milan, Italy, **3** Vita-Salute San Raffaele University, Milan, Italy, **4** Starzl Transplantation Institute, University of Pittsburgh Medical Center, Pittsburgh, Pennsylvania, United States of America, **5** Department of Pathology, The University of Florida, Gainesville, Florida, United States of America

Abstract

Background: A large pool of preexisting alloreactive effector T cells can cause allogeneic graft rejection following transplantation. However, it is possible to induce transplant tolerance by altering the balance between effector and regulatory T (Treg) cells. Among the various Treg-cell types, Foxp3$^+$Treg and IL-10–producing T regulatory type 1 (Tr1) cells have frequently been associated with tolerance following transplantation in both mice and humans. Previously, we demonstrated that rapamycin+IL-10 promotes Tr1-cell–associated tolerance in Balb/c mice transplanted with C57BL/6 pancreatic islets. However, this same treatment was unsuccessful in C57BL/6 mice transplanted with Balb/c islets (classified as a stringent transplant model). We accordingly designed a protocol that would be effective in the latter transplant model by simultaneously depleting effector T cells and fostering production of Treg cells. We additionally developed and tested a clinically translatable protocol that used no depleting agent.

Methodology/Principal Findings: Diabetic C57BL/6 mice were transplanted with Balb/c pancreatic islets. Recipient mice transiently treated with anti-CD45RB mAb+rapamycin+IL-10 developed antigen-specific tolerance. During treatment, Foxp3$^+$Treg cells were momentarily enriched in the blood, followed by accumulation in the graft and draining lymph node, whereas CD4$^+$IL-10$^+$IL-4$^-$ T (i.e., Tr1) cells localized in the spleen. In long-term tolerant mice, only CD4$^+$IL-10$^+$IL-4$^-$ T cells remained enriched in the spleen and IL-10 was key in the maintenance of tolerance. Alternatively, recipient mice were treated with two compounds routinely used in the clinic (namely, rapamycin and G-CSF); this drug combination promoted tolerance associated with CD4$^+$IL-10$^+$IL-4$^-$ T cells.

Conclusions/Significance: The anti-CD45RB mAb+rapamycin+IL-10 combined protocol promotes a state of tolerance that is IL-10 dependent. Moreover, the combination of rapamycin+G-CSF induces tolerance and such treatment could be readily translatable into the clinic.

Editor: Holger K. Eltzschig, University of Colorado Denver, United States of America

Funding: This work has been supported by the Juvenile Diabetes Research Foundation Grant 7-2006-328. The funders had no role in study design, data collection and analysis, decision to publish, or preparation of the manuscript.

Competing Interests: The authors have declared that no competing interests exist.

* E-mail: manuela.battaglia@hsr.it

Introduction

T regulatory (Treg) cells typically control immune responses, and they are also capable of establishing tolerance to non-self molecules that are deliberatively introduced into the host, as occurs in allogeneic transplantation settings [1,2]. However, endogenous Treg cells do not usually occur in sufficient numbers to control the large population of pre-existing alloreactive T effector cells in recipients, and this imbalance increases the potential for graft rejection [3]. Immunosuppressive drugs block/deplete alloreactive T effector cells, and are currently used in the clinic to prevent graft rejection [4]. However, most of these drugs necessitate life-long administration and thus increase the risk of undesirable side effects (*e.g.*, infections and lymphomas). In addition, some immunosuppressive drugs, such as cyclosporine A and FK506, are known to interfere not only with the function of allogeneic T cells but also with that of Treg cells [5]. The twin priorities of overcoming interference with Treg cells and of inducing long-term transplant tolerance argue strongly for a therapeutic approach that simultaneously enables the depletion of pre-existing alloantigen specific T cells and the fostering of Treg cells [1,6].

The CD4$^+$ Treg cells that have most often been associated with tolerance to allogeneic transplantation in mice and humans are CD4$^+$CD25$^+$Foxp3$^+$ (Foxp3$^+$) Treg cells and T regulatory type 1 (Tr1) cells. The expression of CD25 is considered essential for the complete fitness of Foxp3$^+$ Treg cells [7]. In contrast, Tr1 cells do not constitutively express CD25 and Foxp3, and are defined by the production of high levels of IL-10 and the absence of IL-4, as well as by the predominant occurrence of control immune responses via IL-10 and TGF-β release [8,9]. On these bases, Foxp3$^+$-Treg and Tr1 cells are considered to be two distinct types of Treg cells [10,11].

We previously established two distinct models of islet transplantation on the basis of the mean rejection time of untreated transplanted mice, whereby one model could be considered as more stringent than the other [12]. Thus differentiated, these two models were used to test different compounds, either alone or in combination, in order to define the optimal protocol for inducing stable long-term tolerance. Moreover, we attempted to design a clinically relevant protocol by restricting our testing to compounds that were already in use within current clinical settings.

Rapamycin is a non-calcineurin-based inhibitor that is currently used in a variety of immunosuppressive strategies, in combination with other compounds, to block solid organ graft rejection [13]. Of note, this drug not only blocks T cell activation, but also selectively allows for proliferation as well as fostering the suppressive function of Foxp3$^+$ Treg cells [14,15]. IL-10 is a cytokine with potent anti-inflammatory properties that can induce Tr1 cells *in vitro* [12,16]. We previously showed that rapamycin+IL-10 treatment leads to long-term tolerance associated with the induction of Tr1 cells in the non-stringent model of islet transplant [17]. Therefore, a primary goal of this current effort is to test rapamycin+IL-10 therapy in the more stringent mouse model of islet transplantation. Considering the high frequency of alloreactive T cells in the recipient mice of this model, we hypothesized that a depleting agent could improve the efficacy of rapamycin+IL-10 treatment. Therefore, from the several depleting agents available today, we chose to test anti-CD45RB mAb, which transiently depletes alloreactive T cells from the blood [18,19] and, more importantly, has the capacity to increase the Treg-cell suppressive function [20].

Another promising tolerogenic molecule is the granulocyte-colony stimulating factor (G-CSF), which is currently used in clinical practice for the mobilization of bone marrow hematopoietic stem cells. *In vivo* administration of G-CSF blocks graft versus host disease (GvHD) [21], and prevents type 1 diabetes development [22,23]. The effect of this molecule in a setting of islet transplantation has never been investigated, and the issue of whether its tolerogenic effect is associated with increases in IL-10 release or with Foxp3$^+$ Treg-cell expansion is controversial [21,22].

The current study demonstrates that, in a stringent model of islet transplantation, the combination of anti-CD45RB mAb with rapamycin+IL-10 promotes a unique state of tolerance IL-10 dependent and associated with two types of Treg cells. Moreover, the combination of rapamycin+G-CSF induces Tr1 cell-associated tolerance. Considering that both rapamycin and G-CSF are currently in clinical use, we believe these data have powerful clinical implications.

Results

The combined protocol (anti-CD45RB mAb+rapamycin+IL-10) promotes tolerance in a stringent mouse model of islet transplant

Rapamycin+IL-10 treatment promotes transplantation tolerance in chemically-induced diabetic BALB/c (BALB) mice transplanted with C57BL/6 (B6) islets (B6→BALB) [17]. In a more stringent model of islet transplantation (BALB→B6) rapamycin+IL-10, administered in accordance with a previously used schedule and dose regimen [17], did not promote tolerance (Figure 1A). We hypothesized that a therapy capable of combining deletion with immunomodulant effects would promote long-term tolerance in this more stringent model [1,6]. Anti-CD45RB mAb transiently depletes circulating T cells [18], which are responsible for allograft rejection [19,24]; at the same time, it fits the regulatory action of Treg cells [20,25]. Accordingly, three peri-transplant injections of anti-CD45RB mAb duly promoted long-term acceptance of the graft in 75% of BALB mice transplanted with B6 islets (B6→BALB model) (Figure 1B). This treatment transiently reduced the number of circulating lymphocytes and significantly increased the expression of CTLA-4 on Treg cells in the spleen and in graft-draining lymph nodes (dLN) (data not shown), as previously demonstrated [20].

We then tested the efficacy of anti-CD45RB mAb treatment in the stringent mouse transplantation model (BALB→B6). Although the mAb was highly efficient in blocking early graft rejection (*i.e.*, at 15–30 days following islet transplant), it subsequently lost efficacy (*i.e.*, at 60 days or more following islet transplant) (Figure 1C). On the basis of these data, we designed a combined protocol; to a peri-transplant treatment comprising of anti-CD45RB mAb, we added a 30-day therapy with rapamycin+IL-10. When tested separately, neither rapamycin+IL-10 nor anti-CD45RB mAb attained long-term graft survival in the stringent model of islet transplant (Figure 1A and 1C). Nonetheless, the combined protocol (anti-CD45RB mAb+rapamycin+IL-10) prolonged graft survival in 73% of the mice to 100 days following transplantation (Figure 1D). Significantly, upon injection of donor-derived splenocytes (*i.e.*, a donor-derived antigen boost) 100 days after transplant, only 4 out of 21 mice with a long-term functioning graft rejected the allogeneic islets. Overall, the proportion of mice treated with the combined protocol that achieved long-term tolerance (*i.e.*, acceptance of the graft and maintenance of graft survival upon donor-derived Ag re-challenge in the absence of any active immunosuppressive treatment), was 58% (Figure 1D). We accordingly conclude that the combination of rapamycin+IL-10 treatment with anti-CD45RB mAb promotes long-term tolerance in a stringent mouse model of islet transplant.

Engraftment of allogeneic islets endorsed by the combined protocol is associated with CD4$^+$CD25$^+$Foxp3$^+$ and CD4$^+$IL-10$^+$IL-4$^-$ cells, which localize in different tissues

Our next step was to investigate the immunological outcome of the joint administration of anti-CD45RB mAb and rapamycin+IL-10. Kinetic analysis of the peripheral blood of transplanted and treated mice revealed that the number (data not shown) and the frequency of circulating CD4$^+$ and CD8$^+$ T cells was reduced (Figure 2A) as a result of specific CD45RB^{high} T-cell targeting by the anti-CD45RB mAb (Figure 2B), both in mice treated with the combined protocol and in those treated with anti-CD45RB mAb alone. In addition, the selective depletion of CD45RB^{high} cells led to an enrichment of circulating CD4$^+$CD25$^+$Foxp3$^+$ Treg cells (Figure 2B). All these immunological phenomena were transient, since CD4$^+$, CD8$^+$, and CD4$^+$CD25$^+$Foxp3$^+$ Treg cells returned to their physiological basal levels 30 days from the beginning of the treatment (Figure 2).

Given the known activity of rapamycin on Foxp3$^+$ Treg cells, and of IL-10 on Tr1 cells [26], we analyzed these two Treg-cell types in the spleen, in the lymph-node that drain the graft (dLN), and in the graft of treated mice at the end of the treatment (*i.e.*, 30 days following transplantation). These analyses showed that the frequency of Foxp3$^+$ Treg cells increased both in dLN and in the graft, but not in the spleen of mice treated with the combined protocol (Figure 3). In contrast, CD4$^+$IL-10$^+$IL4$^-$ (*i.e.*, Tr1 cells) cells were enriched in the spleen, but not in the dLN nor in the

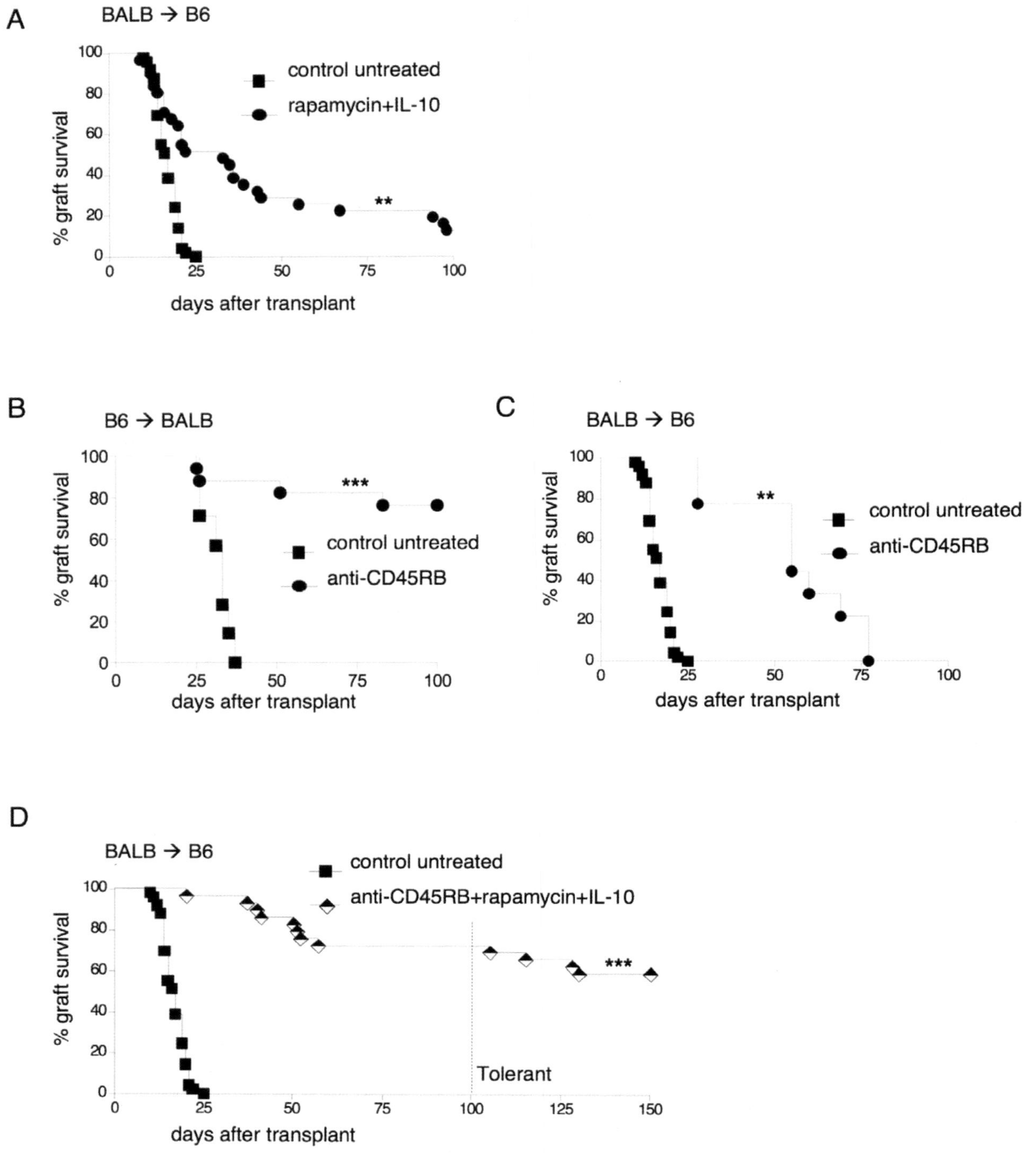

Figure 1. Anti-CD45RB mAb+rapamycin+IL-10 induce long-term tolerance in a stringent model of islet transplantation. (**A**) Diabetic C57BL/6 (B6) mice were transplanted with BALB/c (BALB) islets (BALB→B6). The transplanted mice were either left untreated (n = 49) or treated with rapamycin+IL-10 (n = 30). The treatment was withdrawn 30 days from transplantation. Overall graft survival is shown. (**B**) Diabetic BALB mice were transplanted with B6 islets (B6→BALB). The transplanted mice were either left untreated (n = 17) or treated with anti-CD45RB mAb (n = 17) at days 0, 3 and 5 from transplantation. Overall graft survival is shown. (**C**) Diabetic B6 mice were transplanted with BALB islets (BALB→B6). The transplanted mice were either left untreated (n = 49) or treated with the anti-CD45RB mAb (n = 8) at days 0, 3 and 5 from transplantation. Overall graft survival is shown. (**D**) Diabetic B6 mice were transplanted with BALB islets (BALB→B6). The transplanted mice were either left untreated (n = 49) or treated with anti-CD45RB mAb (at days 0, 3 and 5 from transplantation)+rapamycin+IL-10 (n = 29) for 30 days. One hundred days from transplantation, 30×10^6 splenocytes isolated from BALB mice were injected in tolerant mice to boost their immune system. Mice that were normoglycemic 40–50 days after the boost were considered tolerant. Overall graft survival is shown. These results are cumulative of 5–10 independent experiments performed in parallel. Log-rank (Mantel-Cox) test has been used (*p<0.01;**p<0.001; ***p<0.0001).

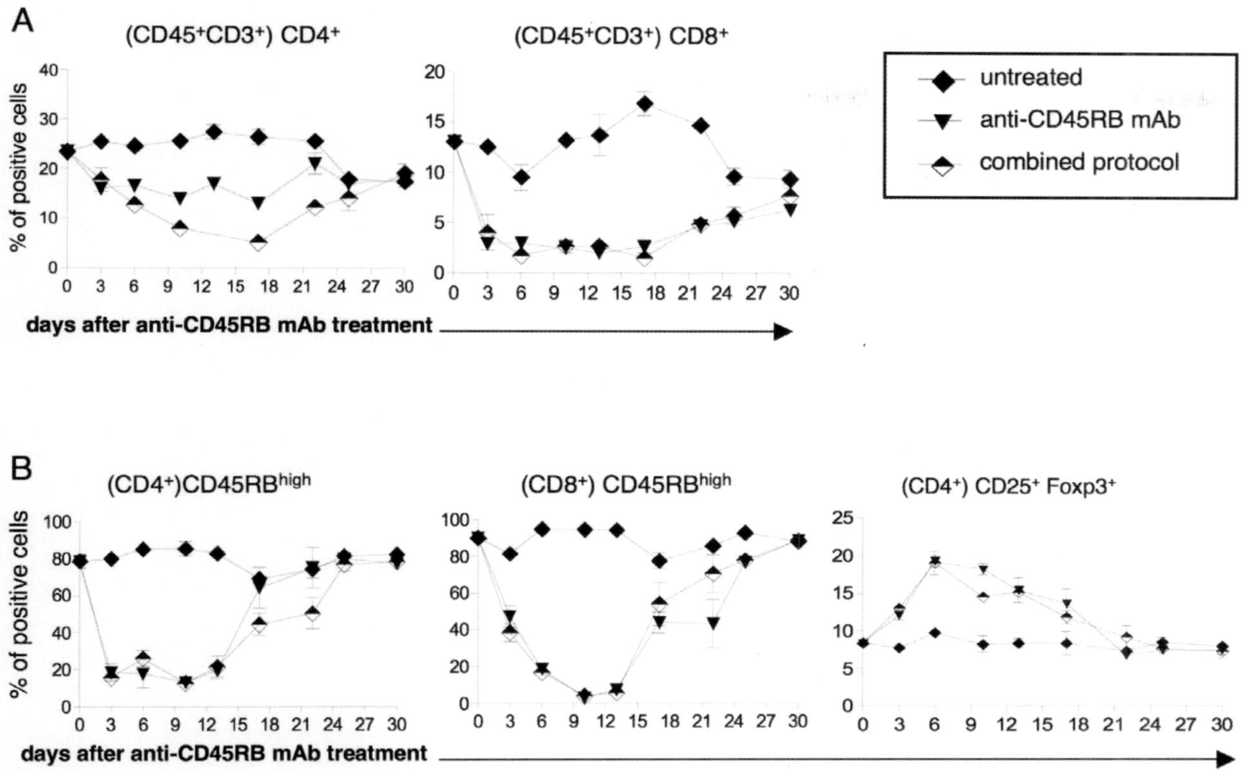

Figure 2. Anti-CD45RB mAb+rapamycin+IL-10 reduce CD45RB^{high} T cells and enrich CD4$^+$CD25$^+$Foxp3$^+$ T cells. Diabetic B6 mice were transplanted with BALB islets and were either left untreated (n = 3), or treated with anti-CD45RB mAb (n = 4), or with the combined protocol (n = 5). (**A**) The frequencies of peripheral-blood CD4$^+$ (left) and CD8$^+$ (right) T cells within CD45$^+$CD3$^+$ cells are shown at different time points after the first injection of the anti-CD45RB mAb. (**B**) The frequencies of peripheral-blood CD45RB^{high} effector T cells within CD45$^+$CD3$^+$CD4$^+$ cells (left) and within CD45$^+$CD3$^+$CD8$^+$ cells (middle), and the frequencies of peripheral-blood CD25$^+$Foxp3$^+$ T cells within CD4$^+$ cells (right), are shown at different time points after the first injection of anti-CD45RB mAb. One representative experiment out of 2 is shown. Means ± SEM are shown.

graft (Figure 4A and data not shown). Accordingly, splenic CD4$^+$ T cells isolated from mice treated with the combined protocol produced more IL-10 than did those isolated from control mice (Figure 4B), where the former also exert a powerful *in vivo* Ag-specific suppressive function, as we previously showed [12]. Interestingly, although treatment with anti-CD45RB mAb alone was not efficient in controlling graft rejection, it led to increased frequency of splenic CD4$^+$IL-10$^+$IL4$^-$ T cells (Figure 4A). Consequently, the CD4$^+$ T cells isolated from the spleen of the same treated mice produced more IL-10 than did those isolated from the spleen of control mice (Figure 4B).

Notably, no differences in the total number of CD4$^+$ T cells were observed among untreated and treated (*i.e.*, anti-CD45RB mAb and combined) mice in the spleen, dLN and graft 30 days (Figure S1) and 150 days (data not show) following islet transplant. On the base of this, the frequencies of Foxp3$^+$ Treg and Tr1 cells mirrored the differences in absolute number. Overall, these data show that the combined treatment promotes both the expansion of Foxp3$^+$ Treg cells in the graft and dLN, and the induction of CD4$^+$IL-10$^+$IL4$^-$ T cells that accumulate in the spleen.

Long-term tolerance to allogeneic transplanted islets endorsed by the combined protocol is associated with splenic CD4$^+$IL-10$^+$IL-4$^-$ cells

To determine whether long-term tolerance (*i.e.*, >150 days following transplantation) observed in mice treated with the combined protocol was still associated with the presence of Treg cells, we analyzed the frequency of Foxp3$^+$ and CD4$^+$IL-10$^+$IL4$^-$ T cells in mice 50 days from donor-derived Ag re-challenge (*i.e.*, 150 days from transplantation). The Foxp3$^+$ Treg cells in the dLN had expanded to levels similar to those in the dLN of mice analyzed 30 days from transplantation, although said levels were not statistically significant in comparison to levels identified in untreated mice (Figure 5A). In the graft, the frequency of Foxp3$^+$ Treg cells did not differ statistically from that found in untreated mice and was lower than that found 30 days following transplantation (Figure 5A). The lack of splenic accumulation of Foxp3$^+$ Treg cell was also confirmed at this later time point (Figure 5A). The CD4$^+$IL-10$^+$IL4$^-$ T cells remained enriched in the spleens of long-term tolerant mice (Figure 5B), and splenic CD4$^+$ T cells produced high levels of IL-10 upon *in vitro* polyclonal stimulation (Figure 5C). In a demonstration of their donor-specificity, CD4$^+$ T cells isolated from the spleen of tolerant mice produced IL-10 exclusively upon stimulation with original Ag (*i.e.*, BALB-derived splenocytes) and not with third party Ag (*i.e.*, C3H-derived splenocytes) (Figure 5D).

We then tested whether the presence of Ag-specific CD4$^+$IL-10$^+$IL4$^-$ T cells was associated with Ag-specific long-term tolerance. The original graft was removed from long-term tolerant mice, in which diabetes promptly resumed, and a second transplant with islets isolated from the original donors or third-party donors was performed. Only mice receiving third party islets rejected the graft (Figure 5E), a finding that proved the establishment of Ag-specific long-term tolerance in mice trans-

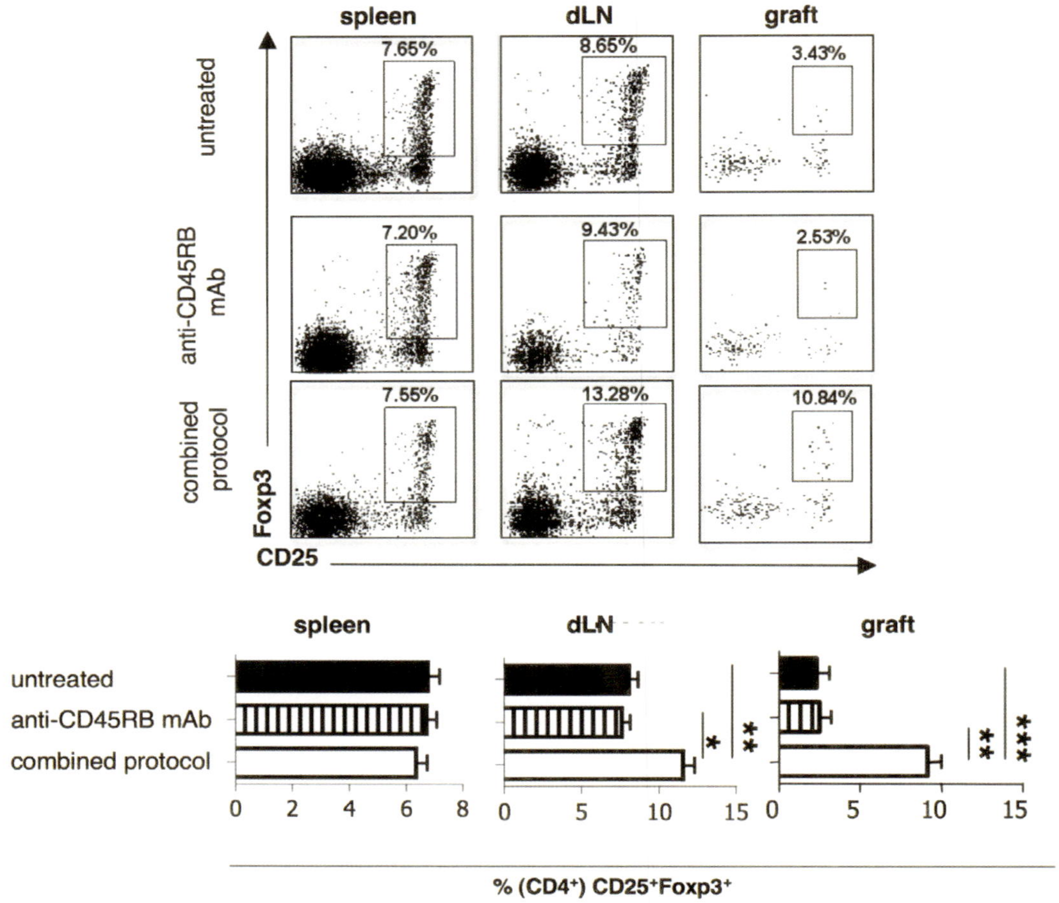

Figure 3. Localization of CD4$^+$Foxp3$^+$CD25$^+$ Treg cells in engrafted mice after the combined protocol. Diabetic B6 mice were transplanted with BALB islets and were either left untreated (n = 13), or treated with anti-CD45RB mAb (n = 7), or with the combined protocol (n = 7). Thirty days after transplantation, treated mice were analyzed. Untreated control mice were analyzed once the graft was rejected. The frequencies of CD25$^+$Foxp3$^+$ cells within CD4$^+$ cells in the spleen, in dLN, and in the graft are shown. Representative dot plots of the stainings are shown in the upper panel, while the results collected from all mice analyzed are shown in the lower panel. Means ± SEM are shown (*$p<0.05$;**$p<0.005$; ***$p<0.0005$).

planted with allogeneic islets and treated with the combined protocol.

IL-10 is required for the maintenance of long-term tolerance

The combined protocol promotes a state of long term-tolerance associated with the accumulation IL-10-producing splenic CD4$^+$ T cells. However, the role of IL-10 in this state of tolerance remains unknown. In order to address this point, tolerant mice were injected with anti-IL-10R mAb. Interestingly all the mice promptly rejected the graft upon mAb injection (Figure 6A).

Although the number and the frequencies of Foxp3$^+$ T cells in tolerant mice were not significantly higher as compared to those in control mice, the combined treatment could have boost the regulatory activity of Foxp3$^+$ T cells, for instance by increasing the expression of CTLA-4 [20]. Therefore, one could still hypothesize a role of these type of Treg cells in the maintenance of tolerance. Interestingly, the depletion of Foxp3$^+$ T cells mediated by the injection of anti-CD25 mAb (Figure S2) did not alter the state of tolerance induced by the combined treatment (Figure 6B). These data show the key role of IL-10 in the maintenance of tolerance and suggest that Foxp3$^+$ T cells are not the IL-10-producers.

A clinically translatable protocol (G-CSF+rapamycin) induces long-term tolerance

One important goal in the field of experimental (*i.e.*, preclinical) transplantation is to develop an immunomodulatory protocol that is readily translatable to the clinic setting. Since recombinant IL-10 is not available for clinical use, we chose to replace it with G-CSF. G-CSF is a growth factor currently used for the clinical mobilization of hematopoietic stem cells [27]. Importantly, both in mice [21] and in humans [28], G-CSF has tolerogenic properties that resemble those of IL-10. The combination of G-CSF+rapamycin, in the absence of any depleting agents, led to long-term graft survival in 80% of B6 mice transplanted with BALB islets (*i.e.*, stringent model) (Figure 7A). Upon injection of donor-derived splenocytes (*i.e.*, donor-derived antigen boost) 100 days from transplant, only 7 out of 25 mice with a long-term functioning graft rejected the allogeneic islets. Overall, 58% of mice treated with G-CSF+rapamycin achieved long-term tolerance (Figure 7A). Finally, graft removal from all tolerant mice promptly induced a return to hyperglycemia in each animal, and thus confirmed the lack of any endogenous islet regeneration (Figure 7B).

Treated mice were analyzed, and increased percentages of CD4$^+$IL-10$^+$IL4$^-$ T cells were found in the spleen 30 and 150

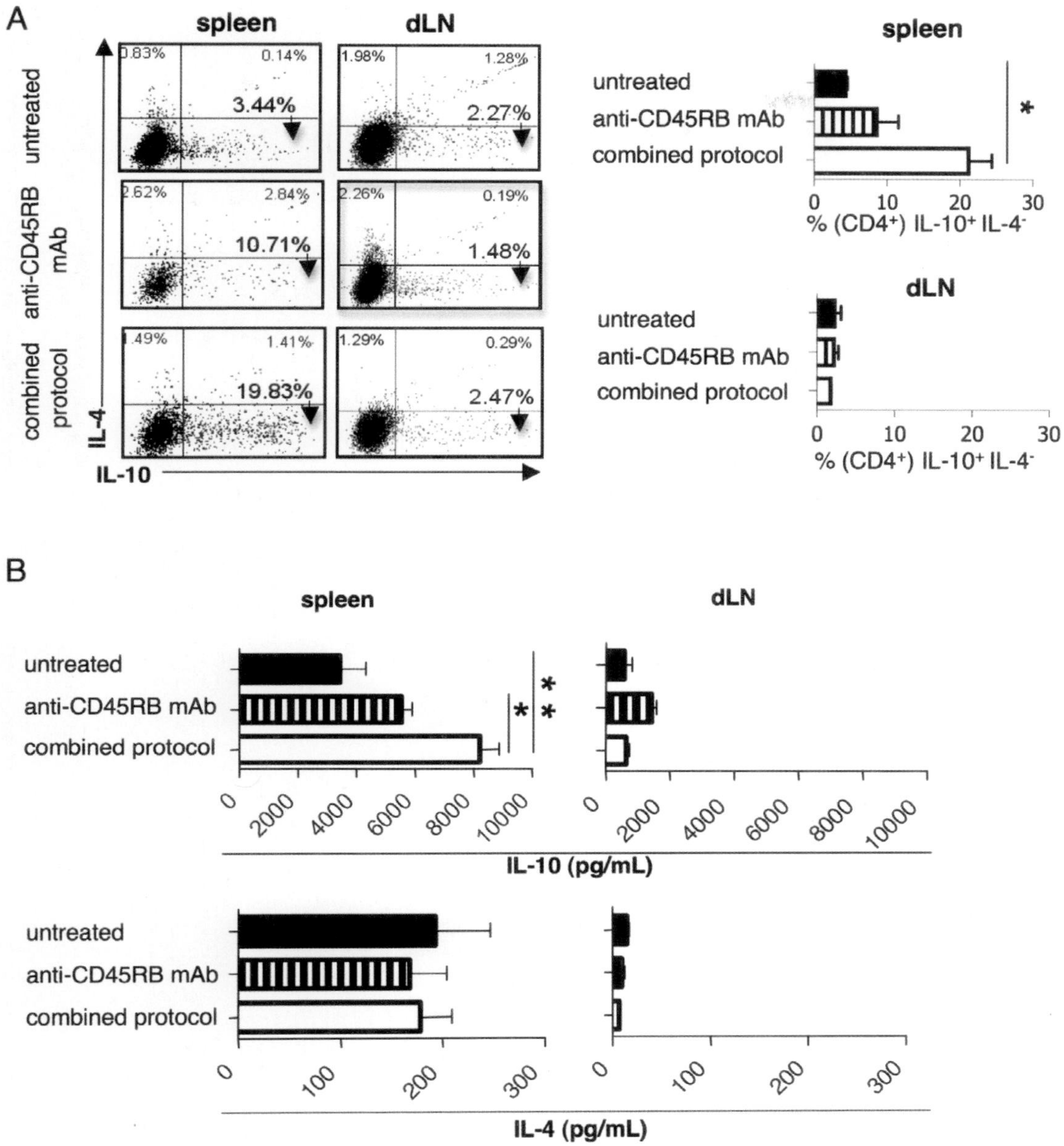

Figure 4. Localization of CD4$^+$Foxp3$^+$CD25$^+$ Treg cells and ag-specific CD4$^+$IL-4$^-$IL-10$^+$ T cells in engrafted mice after the combined protocol. Diabetic B6 mice were transplanted with BALB islets and were either left untreated (n = 13), or treated with anti-CD45RB mAb (n = 7), or with the combined protocol (n = 7). Thirty days after transplantation, treated mice were analyzed. Untreated control mice were analyzed once the graft was rejected. (**A**) Representative dot plots of the intracellular stainings for the detection of IL-10 and IL-4 production by CD4$^+$ T cells from the spleens and the dLN are shown in the left panel, while the results collected from all mice analyzed are shown in the right panel. (**B**) The amounts of IL-10 (upper) and IL-4 (lower) released *in vitro* after polyclonal stimulation of CD4$^+$ T cells isolated from the spleen (left) or the dLN (right) are shown. Cells isolated from spleen and dLN were cultured for 5 days in the presence of αCD3 (10 ug/ml) and αCD28 (1 ug/ml) mAbs. At the end of the culture the cells were finally re-stimulated for 5 h in the presence of TPA/ionomycin to test the ability to produce IL-10 and IL-4 was tested by intracellular staining. Means ± SEM are shown (*$p<0.05$;**$p<0.005$).

days from transplantation (Figure 7C). In contrast, Foxp3$^+$ Treg cells were not found expanded in the spleen, dLN, or in the cells infiltrating the graft; these findings were confirmed both at the end of the treatment and in long-term tolerant mice (Figure 7D).

These data demonstrate that treatment with G-CSF+rapamycin endorses long-term tolerance in a stringent mouse model of islet transplantation, without any need for a deletion compound. Such transplant tolerance is associated with the induction of splenic CD4$^+$ with a Tr1-cell phenotype. However, further studies are required to demonstrate the role of Tr1 cells for the maintenance of tolerance upon G-CSF+rapamycin treatment.

Discussion

Firstly, we have proved that the combination of rapamycin, IL-10 and anti-CD45RRB mAb is an efficient protocol to induce Ag-specific tolerance as associated with two different types of Treg cells localized in different tissues. Interestingly, the engraftment

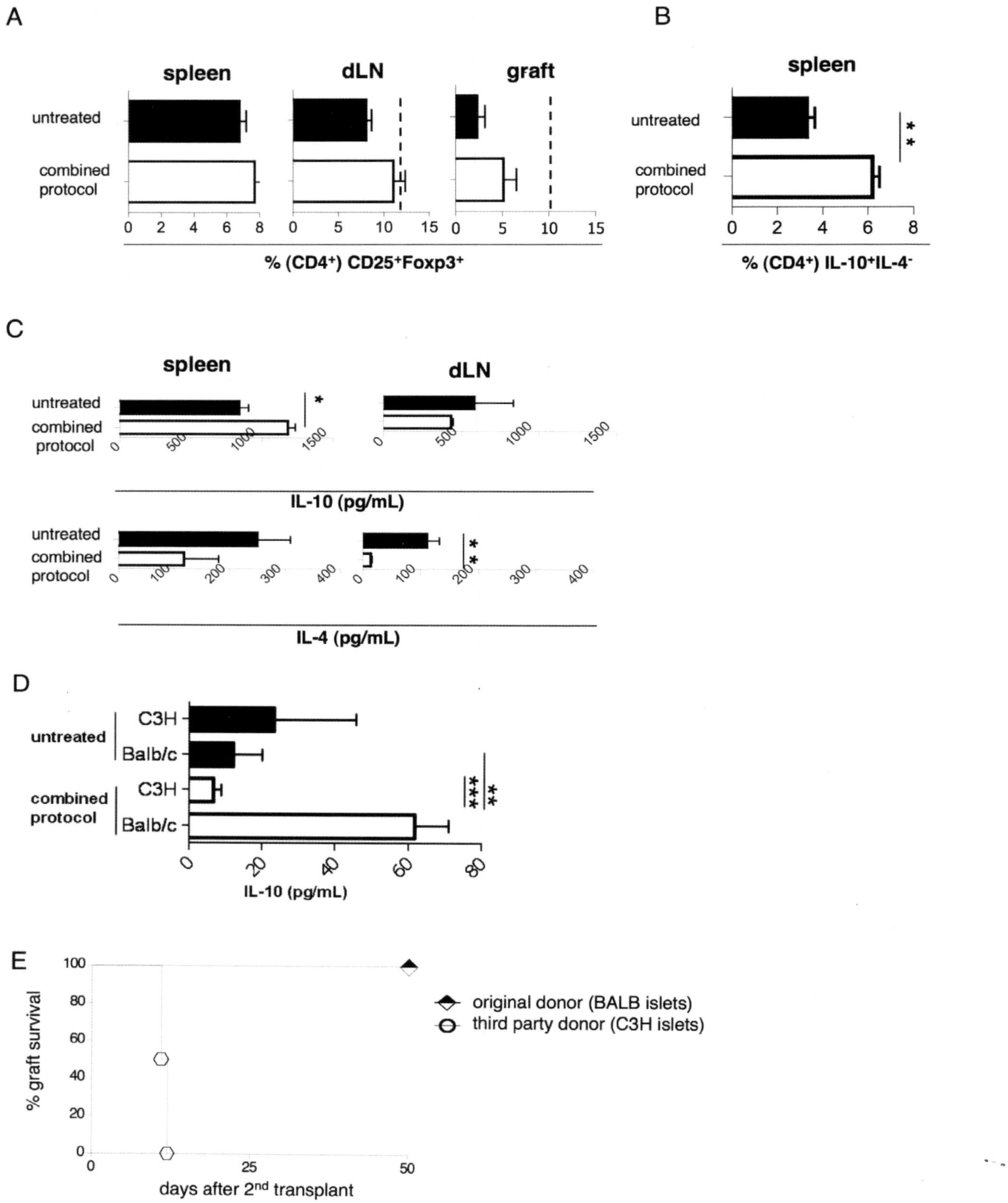

Figure 5. Ag-specific CD4^{+}IL-4^{-}IL-10^{+} T cells remain expanded in the spleen of tolerant mice and are associated with Ag-specific tolerance. Diabetic B6 mice were transplanted with BALB islets and were either left untreated (n = 8), or treated with the combined protocol (n = 5). Fifty days after boosting with donor-derived Ag (i.e., 150 days from transplantation), treated mice were analyzed. Untreated control mice were analyzed once the graft was rejected. (**A**) The frequencies of CD25^{+}Foxp3^{+} cells within CD4^{+} cells in the spleen, in dLN, and in the graft are shown.

The dash bars report the frequencies of $CD25^{+}Foxp3^{+}$ cells within $CD4^{+}$ cells of transplanted mice treated with the combined protocol and sacrificed 30 days after transplantation. (**B**) The frequencies of $IL\text{-}10^{+}IL\text{-}4^{-}$ cells within splenic $CD4^{+}$ cells were detected by intracellular staining, and **t**he results collected from all mice analyzed are shown. (**C**) The amounts of IL-10 (upper) and IL-4 (lower) released *in vitro* after polyclonal stimulation of $CD4^{+}$ T cells isolated from the spleen (left) or the dLN (right) are shown. (**D**) The amounts of IL-10 released from the splenic $CD4^{+}$ T cells *in vitro* after stimulation with third party Ag (C3H) or donor-specific Ag (BALB) are shown. Means ± SEM are shown (*$p<0.05$;**$p<0.005$; ***$p<0.0005$). (E) Diabetic B6 mice were transplanted with islets from BALB mice and were treated with the combined protocol. One hundred days after transplantation, the graft was removed and all the mice returned to being hyperglycemic. A second transplant was performed with islets isolated either from the original donor (BALB, n = 5) or from a third party donor (C3H, n = 4). The percentages of graft survival following the second islet transplant are shown.

was accompanied by the accumulation of $Foxp3^{+}$ Treg cells in the target organ (*i.e.*, graft) and of Ag-specific $CD4^{+}IL\text{-}10^{+}IL\text{-}4^{-}$ T cells in the spleen. In contrast, long-term donor-specific transplantation tolerance is characterized by a small collection of $Foxp3^{+}$ Treg cells in dLN and by the maintenance of Ag-specific $CD4^{+}$ $IL\text{-}10^{+}$ $IL\text{-}4^{-}$ T cells in the spleen. Accordingly the tolerance is maintained by IL-10, while $Foxp3^{+}$ Treg cells are dispensable. Secondly, we have shown that the combination of rapamycin with G-CSF, two drugs already in clinical practices, promotes long-term tolerance in the stringent mouse model of islet transplantation. It is interesting to note that this tolerance was again associated with the presence of $CD4^{+}IL\text{-}10^{+}$ $IL\text{-}4^{-}$ T cells in the spleen of treated mice. However, the role of IL-10 and in turn of Tr1 cells remains to be investigated.

Previous studies had already shown the transient deletion of circulating lymphocytes following treatment with anti-CD45RB mAb [18,19]. We have confirmed this phenomenon and demonstrated that $Foxp3^{+}$ Treg cells are spared, while naïve/effector $CD4^{+}$, $CD8^{+}$ T cells and B cells (data not shown) are the main targets. The injection of anti-CD45RB mAb promotes $Foxp3^{+}$ Treg-cell enrichment in the blood since the expression of CD45RB by $Foxp3^{+}$ Treg cells is low [29]. The frequency of $Foxp3^{+}$ Treg cells returns to normal levels upon the repopulation of the blood with naive/effector $CD4^{+}$ and $CD8^{+}$ T cells. This

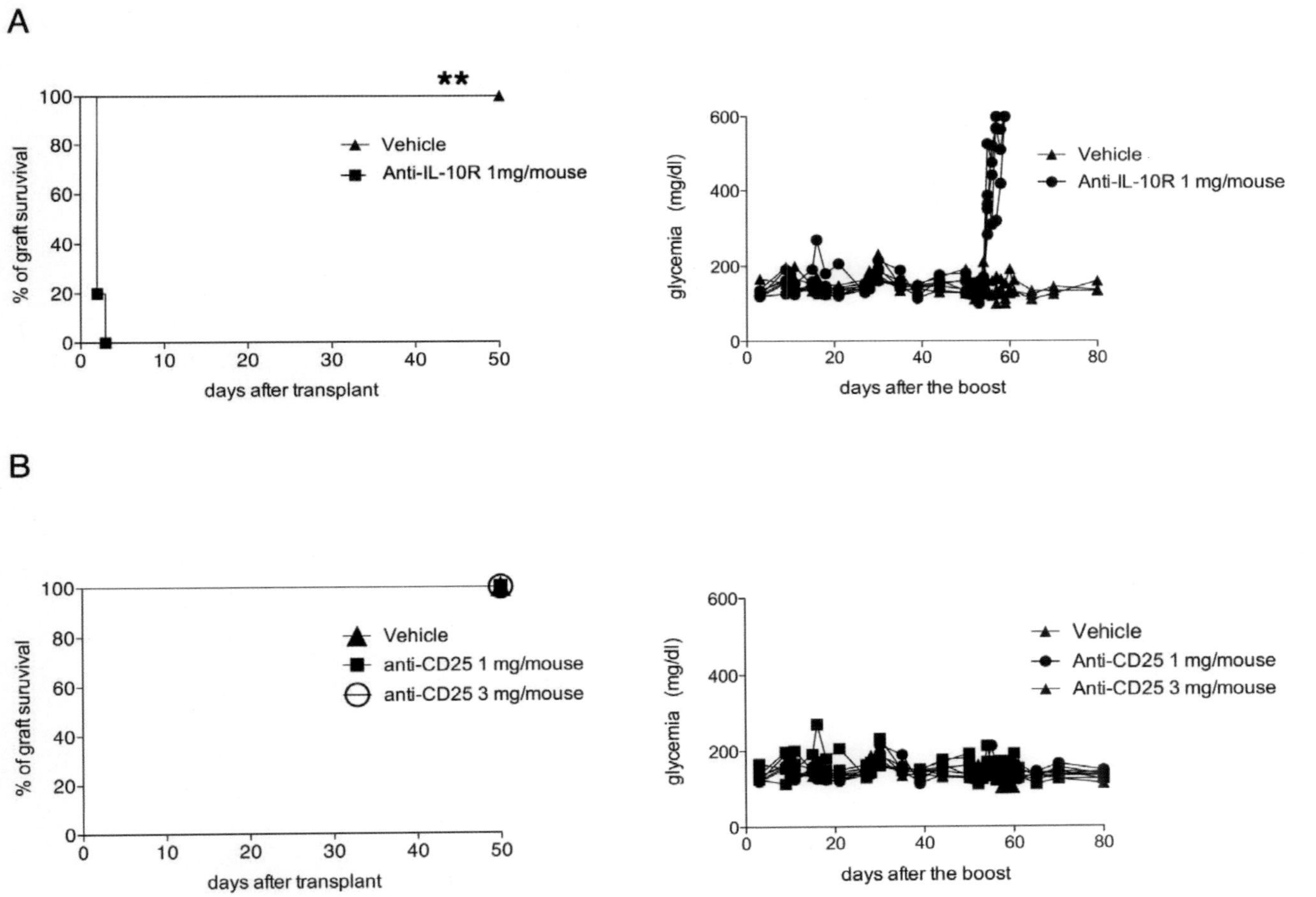

Figure 6. IL-10 and not CD4+ CD25+ Foxp3+ Treg cells is required to maintain long-term tolerance in transplanted mice upon the combined treatment. Diabetic B6 mice were transplanted with BALB islets and were treated with the combined protocol. (**A**) The percentage for graft survival (left) and the concentration of glycemia in the blood (right) of tolerant mice injected with the anti-IL-10R mAb (anti-IL-10R 1 mg/mouse) or with PBS (vehicle) at 150 days transplantation are shown. (**B**) The percentage for graft survival (left) and the concentration of glycemia in the blood (right) of tolerant mice injected with the low doe of anti-CD25 mAb (anti-CD25 mAb 1 mg/mouse), high dose (anti-CD25 mAb 3 mg/mouse) or with PBS (vehicle) at 150 days after transplantation are shown.

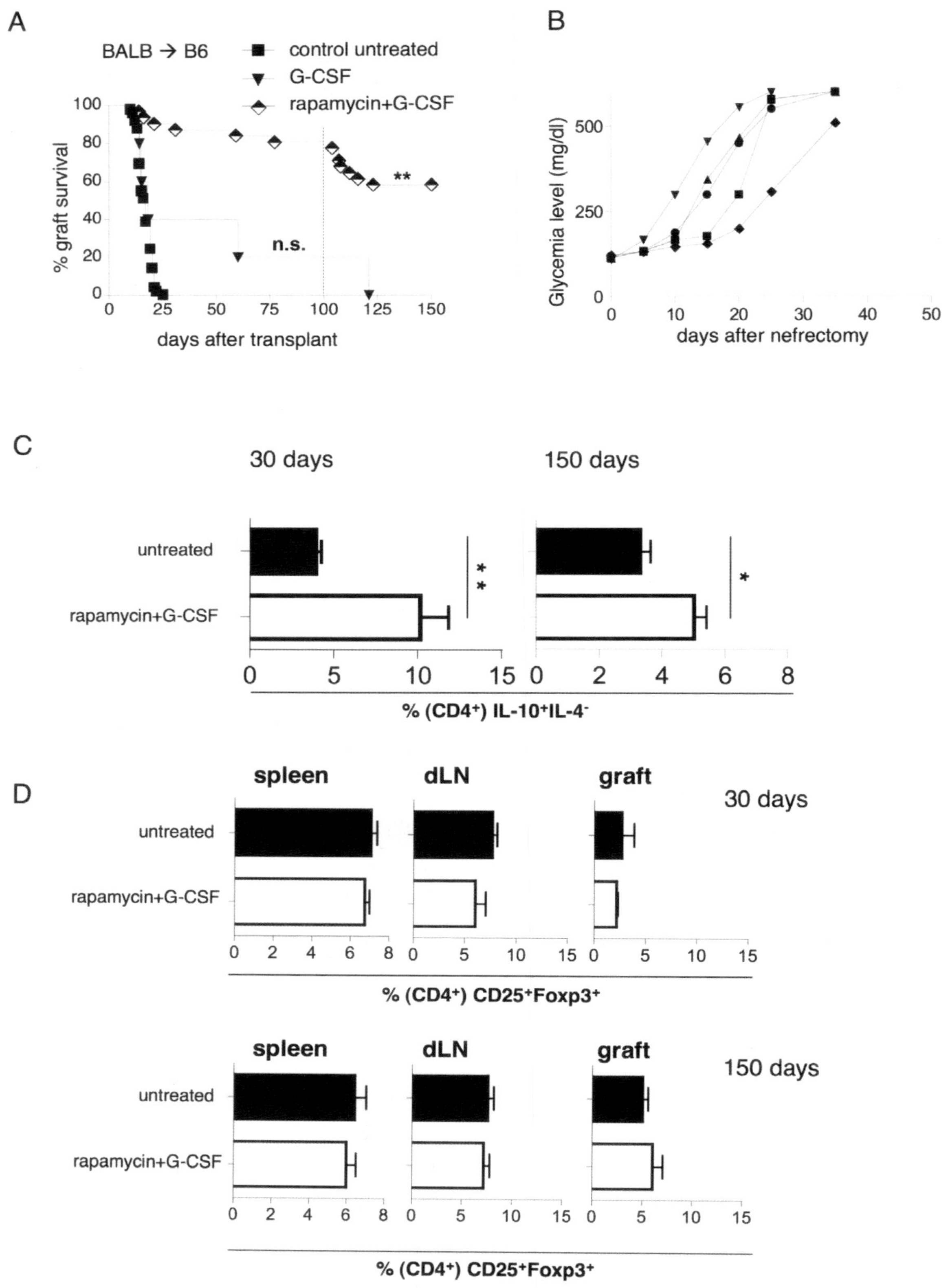

Figure 7. G-CSF+rapamycin induces long-term tolerance associated with splenic CD4^{+}IL-4^{-}IL-10^{+} T cells. Diabetic B6 mice were transplanted with BALB islets. (**A**) The transplanted mice were either left untreated (n = 47) or treated with G-CSF alone (n = 5) or with rapamycin+G-CSF (n = 30). The treatment was withdrawn 30 days after transplantation. One hundred days after transplantation, donor-derived splenocytes were injected into tolerant mice to boost their immune system. Overall graft survival is shown. These results are cumulative of 2 independent experiments performed in parallel. Log-rank (Mantel-Cox) test has been used (*$p<0.01$;**$p<0.001$;) (**B**) The graft was surgically removed from tolerant mice (n = 5)

to verify graft functionality. Glycemia levels in the blood of each mouse tested are shown. (**C**) The frequencies of IL-10$^+$IL-4$^-$ T cells within splenic CD4$^+$ T cells 30 (left) and 150 (right) days after transplantation in control untreated (n = 5) and rapamycin+G-CSF–treated (n = 5) mice are shown. Cells isolated from spleen and dLN were cultured for 5 days in the presence of αCD3 (10 ug/ml) and αCD28 (1 ug/ml) mAbs. At the end of the culture the cells were finally restimulated for 5 h in the presence of TPA/ionomycin to test the ability to produce IL-10 and IL-4 was tested by intracellular staining. (**D**) The frequencies of CD25$^+$Foxp3$^+$ T cells within CD4$^+$ cells in the spleen, in dLN and in graft 30 (upper) and 150 days (lower) after transplantation in control untreated (n = 5) and rapamycin+G-CSF–treated (n = 5) mice are shown. Means ± SEM are shown (*$p<0.05$;**$p<0.005$).

paper shows that these effects are maintained when anti-CD45RB mAb is combined with rapamycin+IL-10 treatment.

It is also known that the anti-CD45RB mAb fits the regulatory properties of Foxp3$^+$ Treg cells by increasing the expression of CTLA-4 and by promoting long-term graft survival [20]. We confirm that increased CTLA-4 expression coincides with high engraftment efficacy in anti-CD45RB mAb-treated mice. However, none of these treated animals reached a state of long-term tolerance. This result partially contrasts with previously published data [30]. We suggest that these varying results could be explained by: (I) differences in administration schedules; (II) differences in gender ratios of the mice used as recipients and donors; and (III) differences in approach used to verify the state of tolerance (*e.g.,* boost with splenocytes versus a second transplantation). Importantly, we have clearly demonstrated that anti-CD45RB mAb radically increases the efficacy of rapamycin+IL-10 treatment in the stringent mouse model of islet transplantation.

Our data demonstrate that after the combined treatment, Foxp3$^+$ Treg cells and CD4$^+$IL-10$^+$IL-4$^-$ T cells localized in different organs. Data from mice and also from humans have already reported that Foxp3$^+$ Treg cells occur in tolerant grafts [31]. Other authors suggest that the presence of Foxp3$^+$ Treg cells in dLN are key for their regulatory action [31]. In our model, we observed Foxp3$^+$-Treg cells in the graft and in dLN 30 days from transplantation, and their subsequent accumulation in the dLN of long-term tolerant mice. This suggests that Foxp3$^+$ Treg cells may migrate from the graft to dLN. In agreement with our hypothesis, this Foxp3$^+$ Treg-cell migration (*i.e.,* from the graft to dLN) has been found to be a requisite for the blocking of islet allograft rejection [32]. Interestingly, our data suggest that at later time points, once immunological tolerance is established, the Foxp3$^+$ Treg cells slightly accumulate in the dLN and they are dispensable for the maintenance of tolerance. Accordingly, studies performed in mouse models of islet transplant have demonstrated that Foxp3$^+$ Treg cells are fundamental only during the early phase after transplantation [33,34,35]. On the basis of this, one could hypothesizes that Foxp3$^+$ Treg cells migrate to the graft at early time points, exert their main role *in situ*, and become dispensable lately once localized in the dLN.

Unlike the localization of Foxp3$^+$ Treg cells, Tr1 cells localize mainly in the spleen, as we previously observed in various animal models of tolerance [17,26] and as we reassert, with increased evidence, in this study. It is especially interesting to note that splenic DCs alone have the capacity, in the presence of TGF-β, to induce Tr1 cells [36]. However, the issue of whether the spleen is the key organ for Tr1-cell regulatory activity is still inadequately addressed.

All in all, the combined treatment promoted a state of tolerance that was associated with two different types of Treg cells, which in turn localized in differing tissues. This model represents a unique opportunity to study some still ill-defined aspects of the biology of Foxp3$^+$ Treg and Tr1 cells: whether, where and how these two different types of Treg cells work together to induce and promote transplantation tolerance.

Exogenous treatment with recombinant IL-10 has not clearly demonstrated beneficial effects in a number of clinical trials [37], and at present is not clinically available. On this basis, we developed a new combined protocol that uses previously approved compounds. G-CSF is used for the mobilization of stem cells, and it shows tolerogenic capacities that are interestingly similar to those of the IL-10 treatment [27]. We accordingly substituted IL-10 with G-CSF; without using any depleting agents, and against all expectation, the combination of rapamycin+G-CSF promoted tolerance in the stringent mouse model of islet transplantation. Although it is known that G-CSF promotes the in vivo expansion of CD4$^+$CD25$^+$ T cells [22,23], we could not find any enrichment of these cells in any target organs of treated mice. Differences in G-CSF administration schedules and/or the combination with rapamycin could explain why our data vary from previous findings.

It is also known that G-CSF promotes the release of IL-10 from human and mouse CD4$^+$ T cells [21,28]. In turn, we find a strong in vivo expansion of splenic CD4$^+$ IL-10$^+$ IL-4$^-$ T cells, both under the umbrella of the treatment and in tolerant mice. Although the cytokine profile of CD4$^+$ IL-10$^+$ IL-4$^-$ T cells found in the spleen of treated mice reflects that of Tr1 cells, future efforts must verify their regulatory capacity. We are currently developing new tools that will selectively isolate or delete Tr1 cells as a way to understand their specific role in the induction of tolerance. Finally, it is interesting to note that two different treatments induce CD4$^+$ IL-10$^+$ IL-4$^-$ T cells, which in both cases localize in the spleen and occur in tolerant mice.

Materials and Methods

Mice and islet transplant

BALB/c (BALB) and C57BL/6 (B6) female mice were purchased from Charles River (Calco, Italy). All mice were maintained under specific pathogen-free conditions. Diabetes was induced by intravenous (*i.v.*) injection of 170 mg/kg streptozotocin (Sigma-Aldrich, St. Louis, MO). Glucose levels in tail venous blood were quantified with the Glucometer Elite system (Bayer, Wuppertal, Germany), and measurements invariably took place in the morning. Pancreatic islet transplant was performed as previously described [17]. Graft rejection was diagnosed on the basis of two sequential glucose measurements >300 mg/dl.

The transplanted mice that did not reject the graft 100 days after transplantation were boosted *in vivo* with donor-origin splenocytes. A total of 30×10^6 splenocytes isolated from the original islet donors were injected intraperitoneally (*i.p.*), and blood glucose levels were monitored daily thereafter. Mice still normoglycemic 30–50 days from boosting were considered long-term tolerant. The study was approved by the San Raffaele Hospital Institutional Animal Care and Use Committee (permit no IACUC 350).

Treatment of transplanted mice

Transplanted mice were treated with anti-CD45RB mAb (MB23G2 clone from ATCC) alone or with the addition of rapamycin (Rapamune; Wyeth Europe, Taplow, U.K.)+r-hu-IL-10 (BD Pharmingen, San Diego, CA). Anti-CD45RB mAb was injected *i.v.* at days 0, 1, and 5 following transplantation at 100 μg per dose. Rapamycin was diluted in water and administered by gavage for 30 consecutive days once a day at 1 mg/kg. Recombinant hu-IL-10 was diluted in PBS and administered *i.p.* twice a day for 30 consecutive days at 0.05 μg/kg. G-CSF (Myelostim, rHuG-CSF, Italfarmaco) was diluted in PBS and injected *s.c.* for 30 consecutive days at 200 μg/kg. Neither treatments with the vehicles (water, PBS), nor with the isotype control for anti-CD45RB mAb (Rat IgG2a), following the same administration and schedule of the original treatments, show any delay in the survival of the graft respect to untreated mice (data not shown).

Some tolerant mice (combined treatment) were injected either with the anti-IL-10 receptor (anti-IL-10R) (1B1.2 clone from ATCC, Manassas, VA) or with the anti-CD25Rα (PC61 clone from ATCC) monoclonal antibody (mAb). The anti-IL-10R mAb diluted in PBS (vehicle) was administered *i.p.* for three consecutive days to reach a dose of 1 mg/mouse. The PC61 mouse (500 mg/mouse/dose) was diluted in PBS (vehicle) and administered *i.p.* for two consecutive days every week for either 1 or 3 weeks to reach the dose of 1 mg/mouse and 3 mg/mouse respectively. The doses of anti-IL-10R and PC61 mAbs were chosen in accordance with the literature [17,33,34].

Cell isolation

Spleen, dLN and graft were isolated from transplanted mice and mashed to yield single cell suspensions. Splenic $CD4^+$ T cells were magnetically isolated in accordance with the protocol of the "$CD4^+$ T cell isolation kit" (Miltenyi Biotec, Bergisch Gladbach, German; purity 90–95%).

Cell staining and enzyme-linked immunosorbent assay

Surface cell staining was performed with anti-CD45 PercP, anti-CD3 APC, anti-CD4 Pacific Blue, anti-CD25 APC or PeCy7, and anti-CD8 PE mAbs (all from BD Pharmingen). The CD45RB expression was tested with the anti-CD45RB PE mAb (clone 16A from BD Pharmingen), which had previously been demonstrated to bind to an epitope different than that bound by MB23G2 mAb [20]. Foxp3 expression was tested with the Foxp3 staining kit (eBioscience, San Diego, California; clone FjK-16s). Intracellular staining and ELISA were performed as previously described [12]. Cells were acquired on a FACSCanto (BD Bioscience) and analyzed with FCS express V3 (De Novo Software, Los Angeles, CA).

Statistical analysis

Differences between groups were assessed with the Student t test. P values were two-tailed with a confidence of 95%. Islet allograft survivals were determined with Kaplan-Meier survival curves, and were compared by means of the log-rank test. Statistical analysis was performed with the Prism V4.03 software (Graph-Pad, San Diego, California USA).

Supporting Information

Figure S1 Diabetic B6 mice were transplanted with BALB islets and were either left untreated (Untreated), or treated with anti-CD45RB mAb (aCD45RB), combined protocol (Combine), G-CSF (C-CSF) and rapamycin plus G-CSF (rapamycin+G-CSF). Thirty days after transplantation, treated mice were analyzed. Untreated control mice were analyzed once the graft was rejected. The total number of CD4+ T cells within CD45+ cells in the spleen, in dLN, and in the graft is shown. Results are cumulative from three independent experiments. The study was approved by the San Raffaele Hospital Institutional Animal Care and Use Committee (permit no IACUC 350).

Figure S2 B6 mice were injected i.v. with 1 mg (2 injections) or with 3 mg (6 injections) of anti-CD25 mAb (clone PC61) and 7 days after the last injection the % of CD25+ Foxp3+ within CD4+ T cells in the blood, spleen and mLN were analyzed. The clone 7D4 for mAb anti-CD25 has been used for the FACS staining. The study was approved by the San Raffaele Hospital Institutional Animal Care and Use Committee (permit no IACUC 350).

Acknowledgments

We would like to acknowledge all members of the Battaglia's and Roncarolo's laboratories for helpful and continuous discussion. Especially we are grateful to Andrea Annoni and Laura Passerini.

Author Contributions

Conceived and designed the experiments: NG MB. Performed the experiments: NG SG TJ AS AV. Analyzed the data: NG SG TJ AV MB. Contributed reagents/materials/analysis tools: DR. Wrote the paper: NG SG MA MB. Discussed the data and corrected the manuscript: MGR.

References

1. Walsh PT, Taylor DK, Turka LA (2004) Tregs and transplantation tolerance. J Clin Invest 114: 1398–1403.
2. Li XC, Turka LA (2010) An update on regulatory T cells in transplant tolerance and rejection. Nat Rev Nephrol 6: 577–583.
3. Sanchez-Fueyo A, Strom TB (2011) Immunologic basis of graft rejection and tolerance following transplantation of liver or other solid organs. Gastroenterology 140: 51–64.
4. Grinyo JM, Cruzado JM (2009) Mycophenolate mofetil and calcineurin-inhibitor reduction: recent progress. Am J Transplant 9: 2447–2452.
5. Battaglia M (2011) Potential T regulatory cell therapy in transplantation: how far have we come and how far can we go? Transpl Int 23: 761–770.
6. Turka LA, Lechler RI (2009) Towards the identification of biomarkers of transplantation tolerance. Nat Rev Immunol 9: 521–526.
7. Fontenot JD, Rasmussen JP, Gavin MA, Rudensky AY (2005) A function for interleukin 2 in Foxp3-expressing regulatory T cells. Nat Immunol 6: 1142–1151.
8. Pot C, Apetoh L, Awasthi A, Kuchroo VK (2010) Molecular pathways in the induction of interleukin-27-driven regulatory type 1 cells. J Interferon Cytokine Res 30: 381–388.
9. Roncarolo MG, Battaglia M (2007) Regulatory T-cell immunotherapy for tolerance to self antigens and alloantigens in humans. Nat Rev Immunol 7: 585–598.
10. Maynard CL, Harrington LE, Janowski KM, Oliver JR, Zindl CL, et al. (2007) Regulatory T cells expressing interleukin 10 develop from Foxp3+ and Foxp3- precursor cells in the absence of interleukin 10. Nat Immunol 8: 931–941.
11. Vieira PL, Christensen JR, Minaee S, O'Neill EJ, Barrat FJ, et al. (2004) IL-10-secreting regulatory T cells do not express Foxp3 but have comparable regulatory function to naturally occurring CD4+CD25+ regulatory T cells. J Immunol 172: 5986–5993.
12. Gagliani N, Jofra T, Stabilini A, Valle A, Atkinson M, et al. (2010) Antigen-specific dependence of Tr1-cell therapy in preclinical models of islet transplant. Diabetes 59: 433–439.
13. Ponticelli C (2004) The pleiotropic effects of mTor inhibitors. J Nephrol 17: 762–768.
14. Battaglia M, Stabilini A, Roncarolo MG (2005) Rapamycin selectively expands CD4+CD25+FoxP3+ regulatory T cells. Blood 105: 4743–4748.
15. Monti P, Scirpoli M, Maffi P, Piemonti L, Secchi A, et al. (2008) Rapamycin monotherapy in patients with type 1 diabetes modifies CD4+CD25+FOXP3+ regulatory T-cells. Diabetes 57: 2341–2347.
16. Groux H, O'Garra A, Bigler M, Rouleau M, Antonenko S, et al. (1997) A CD4+ T-cell subset inhibits antigen-specific T-cell responses and prevents colitis. Nature 389: 737–742.
17. Battaglia M, Stabilini A, Draghici E, Gregori S, Mocchetti C, et al. (2006) Rapamycin and interleukin-10 treatment induces T regulatory type 1 cells that mediate antigen-specific transplantation tolerance. Diabetes 55: 40–49.

18. Lazarovits AI, Poppema S, Zhang Z, Khandaker M, Le Feuvre CE, et al. (1996) Prevention and reversal of renal allograft rejection by antibody against CD45RB. Nature 380: 717–720.
19. Luke PP, Deng JP, Lian D, O'Connell PJ, Garcia B, et al. (2006) Prolongation of allograft survival by administration of anti-CD45RB monoclonal antibody is due to alteration of CD45RBhi: CD45RBlo T-cell proportions. Am J Transplant 6: 2023–2034.
20. Fecteau S, Basadonna GP, Freitas A, Ariyan C, Sayegh MH, et al. (2001) CTLA-4 up-regulation plays a role in tolerance mediated by CD45. Nat Immunol 2: 58–63.
21. Morris ES, MacDonald KP, Rowe V, Johnson DH, Banovic T, et al. (2004) Donor treatment with pegylated G-CSF augments the generation of IL-10-producing regulatory T cells and promotes transplantation tolerance. Blood 103: 3573–3581.
22. Kared H, Masson A, Adle-Biassette H, Bach JF, Chatenoud L, et al. (2005) Treatment with granulocyte colony-stimulating factor prevents diabetes in NOD mice by recruiting plasmacytoid dendritic cells and functional CD4(+)CD25(+) regulatory T-cells. Diabetes 54: 78–84.
23. Hadaya K, Kared H, Masson A, Chatenoud L, Zavala F (2005) G-CSF treatment prevents cyclophosphamide acceleration of autoimmune diabetes in the NOD mouse. J Autoimmun 24: 125–134.
24. Davies JD, O'Connor E, Hall D, Krahl T, Trotter J, et al. (1999) CD4+ CD45RB low-density cells from untreated mice prevent acute allograft rejection. J Immunol 163: 5353–5357.
25. Ariyan C, Salvalaggio P, Fecteau S, Deng S, Rogozinski L, et al. (2003) Cutting edge: transplantation tolerance through enhanced CTLA-4 expression. J Immunol 171: 5673–5677.
26. Battaglia M, Stabilini A, Draghici E, Migliavacca B, Gregori S, et al. (2006) Induction of tolerance in type 1 diabetes via both CD4+CD25+ T regulatory cells and T regulatory type 1 cells. Diabetes 55: 1571–1580.
27. Rutella S (2007) Granulocyte colony-stimulating factor for the induction of T-cell tolerance. Transplantation 84: S26–30.
28. Rutella S, Pierelli L, Bonanno G, Sica S, Ameglio F, et al. (2002) Role for granulocyte colony-stimulating factor in the generation of human T regulatory type 1 cells. Blood 100: 2562–2571.
29. Sakaguchi S, Miyara M, Costantino CM, Hafler DA (2010) FOXP3+ regulatory T cells in the human immune system. Nat Rev Immunol 10: 490–500.
30. Basadonna GP, Auersvald L, Khuong CQ, Zheng XX, Kashio N, et al. (1998) Antibody-mediated targeting of CD45 isoforms: a novel immunotherapeutic strategy. Proc Natl Acad Sci U S A 95: 3821–3826.
31. Dijke IE, Weimar W, Baan CC (2008) Regulatory T cells after organ transplantation: where does their action take place? Hum Immunol 69: 389–398.
32. Zhang N, Schroppel B, Lal G, Jakubzick C, Mao X, et al. (2009) Regulatory T cells sequentially migrate from inflamed tissues to draining lymph nodes to suppress the alloimmune response. Immunity 30: 458–469.
33. Webster KE, Walters S, Kohler RE, Mrkvan T, Boyman O, et al. (2009) In vivo expansion of T reg cells with IL-2-mAb complexes: induction of resistance to EAE and long-term acceptance of islet allografts without immunosuppression. J Exp Med 206: 751–760.
34. Muller YD, Mai G, Morel P, Serre-Beinier V, Gonelle-Gispert C, et al. (2010) Anti-CD154 mAb and rapamycin induce T regulatory cell mediated tolerance in rat-to-mouse islet transplantation. PLoS One 5: e10352.
35. Luo X, Pothoven KL, McCarthy D, DeGutes M, Martin A, et al. (2008) ECDI-fixed allogeneic splenocytes induce donor-specific tolerance for long-term survival of islet transplants via two distinct mechanisms. Proc Natl Acad Sci U S A 105: 14527–14532.
36. Maynard CL, Hatton RD, Helms WS, Oliver JR, Stephensen CB, et al. (2009) Contrasting roles for all-trans retinoic acid in TGF-beta-mediated induction of Foxp3 and Il10 genes in developing regulatory T cells. J Exp Med 206: 343–357.
37. Asadullah K, Sterry W, Volk HD (2003) Interleukin-10 therapy–review of a new approach. Pharmacol Rev 55: 241–269.

9

Insights from Computational Modeling in Inflammation and Acute Rejection in Limb Transplantation

Dolores Wolfram[1]*, Ravi Starzl[2], Hubert Hackl[3], Derek Barclay[4], Theresa Hautz[5], Bettina Zelger[6], Gerald Brandacher[7], W. P. Andrew Lee[7], Nadine Eberhart[1], Yoram Vodovotz[4], Johann Pratschke[5], Gerhard Pierer[1], Stefan Schneeberger[5,7]

1 Department of Plastic, Reconstructive and Aesthetic Surgery, Innsbruck Medical University, Innsbruck, Austria, **2** Language Technologies Institute, Carnegie Mellon University, Pittsburgh, Pennsylvania, United States of America, **3** Division of Bioinformatics, Biocenter, Innsbruck Medical University, Innsbruck, Austria, **4** Department of Immunology, University of Pittsburgh, Pittsburgh, Pennsylvania, United States of America, **5** Department of Visceral, Transplant and Thoracic Surgery, Innsbruck Medical University, Innsbruck, Austria, **6** Department of Pathology, Innsbruck Medical University, Innsbruck, Austria, **7** Department of Plastic and Reconstructive Surgery, Johns Hopkins University School of Medicine, Baltimore, Maryland, United States of America

Abstract

Acute skin rejection in vascularized composite allotransplantation (VCA) is the major obstacle for wider adoption in clinical practice. This study utilized computational modeling to identify biomarkers for diagnosis and targets for treatment of skin rejection. Protein levels of 14 inflammatory mediators in skin and muscle biopsies from syngeneic grafts [n = 10], allogeneic transplants without immunosuppression [n = 10] and allografts treated with tacrolimus [n = 10] were assessed by multiplexed analysis technology. Hierarchical Clustering Analysis, Principal Component Analysis, Random Forest Classification and Multinomial Logistic Regression models were used to segregate experimental groups. Based on Random Forest Classification, Multinomial Logistic Regression and Hierarchical Clustering Analysis models, IL-4, TNF-α and IL-12p70 were the best predictors of skin rejection and identified rejection well in advance of histopathological alterations. TNF-α and IL-12p70 were the best predictors of muscle rejection and also preceded histopathological alterations. Principal Component Analysis identified IL-1α, IL-18, IL-1β, and IL-4 as principal drivers of transplant rejection. Thus, inflammatory patterns associated with rejection are specific for the individual tissue and may be superior for early detection and targeted treatment of rejection.

Editor: Valquiria Bueno, UNIFESP Federal University of São Paulo, Brazil

Funding: Funding for this work was provided by the Armed Forces Institute for Advanced Regenerative Medicine Program (TATRC, DOD) Program, Department of Defense grant WX81XWH-07-1-0415, the Austrian Research Fund (Erwin Schrödinger Stipendium), the Austrian Society of Plastic and Reconstructive Surgery and the and the Pennsylvania Department of Health Commonwealth Universal Research Enhancement (CURE) program. The funders had no role in study design, data collection and analysis, decision to publish, or preparation of the manuscript.

Competing Interests: The authors have declared that no competing interests exist.

* E-mail: dolores.wolfram@i-med.ac.at

Introduction

Rejection in Vascular Composite Allotransplantation (VCA) is characterized by an inflammatory cell-mediated cytotoxic process, which progressively harms the epidermis and the junction between dermis and epidermis, unless reversed or prevented by immunosuppression. Understanding the immune signaling patterns of skin rejection would enable the development of targeted and local therapy with fewer side effects.

The current gold standard for the diagnosis of rejection is histological evaluation of tissue biopsies according to the BANFF 2007 working classification [1]. Assessing rejection by histology suffers from latency between initiation of tissue damage and diagnosis. Often, histological signs of skin rejection have been found in protocol biopsies despite absence of clinical signs of rejection. As stated previously by our group and others, the histopathological alterations associated with rejection are not specific, but rather similar to several common inflammatory dermatoses [2,3] or the result of an inflammatory trigger [4]. The differential diagnosis between skin rejection, infection and unspecific inflammation can be challenging in hand- and especially face transplantation. The conditions are similar in their appearance and may interfere with or trigger each other [5].

Traditional methods are of limited value for elucidation of how the immune/inflammatory response in the skin affects VCA through intricate signaling patterns and context-dependent behaviors. Advanced computational methods such as language technologies and machine learning offer significant advances in deciphering complex processes from other areas of science [6,7].

We hypothesized that mechanisms of rejection in VCA are tissue specific and can be detected in advance of gross histological damage by assessing leukocyte expression patterns with advanced computational tools. Based on our findings, promising diagnostic markers for skin and muscle rejection as well as possible targets for new therapeutic interventions in VCA have been identified.

Methods

Experimental design

All animal procedures, care, and housing were reviewed and approved by the Institutional Animal Care and Use Committee

(IACUC) of the University of Pittsburgh (protocol number: 0808858B-2), and followed the National Institutes of Health guidelines for the care and use of laboratory animals. A summary of the cohorts and the conditions they represent are presented in Table 1. Limb transplantations including skin, muscle, bone and vessels, were performed as per a standardized technique between eight- to ten-week-old male Brown-Norway (BN) and Lewis rats (LEW) weighing 200–250 g with (group 3) or without (group 1) immunosuppression and compared with untreated isografts (group 2) [8]. Animals were anesthetized with a combination of xylazine (Xylasol, 5 mg/kg) and ketamine (Ketavet, 100 mg/kg), injected intramuscularly.

Assessment of rejection

Animals were inspected daily for signs of rejection. Skin rejection was classified per appearance: Grade 0 – no signs of rejection; Grade I – erythema of the transplanted leg, Grade II – erythema and edema, Grade III – epidermolysis of the transplanted skin, Grade IV – mummification of the leg (limb necrosis). In untreated animals (allografts, ATC), rejection occurs after 3-4 days (Grade I rejection) and progresses to Grade IV rejection between day 9 and 11. Samples from allograft skin and muscle were collected at postoperative days (POD) 3, 5, 7, 9 and 11 in all three groups in a staggered fashion. To out rule an impact of the trauma an the readout of subsequent tissue samples, biopsies were taken from sites distant to another on days 3, 5, 7 and 11, or days 5, 9 and 11 (see Table 2). Since all animals showed mummification of the graft on POD 11 with super infection in some, samples from this time point were excluded from the study.

The size of each tissue biopsy per chosen time point was approximately 25×10 mm. This tissue sample was divided into 3 identical parts for further analyses. One biopsy part (piece) was fixed in 10% buffered formalin and processed routinely for hematoxilyn and eosin (H&E) staining. Sections were evaluated for lymphocytic infiltration, dermal/epidermal interphase reaction, dermal-epidermal separation and necrosis by a pathologist in a blinded fashion. The other biopsy parts were preserved in RNALater for protein analysis and RNA isolation.

Protein isolation and protein expression analysis

Proteins from skin and muscle samples were isolated using a disperser (T10, basic ULTRA-TURRAX, IKA, Germany) with 1 ml 1 x Cell Lysis Buffer (Cell Signaling, Danvers, USA) per sample on ice. Proteins were quantified after homogenizing using the BCA Protein Assay Kit according to the manufacturer's protocol.

Inflammatory mediator expression at the protein levels was measured using the Luminex inflammatory mediator bead set (RCYTO-80K-PMX-14-plex Milliplex Map Kit from Millipore, Billerica, MA) that included interferon (IFN)-γ, IL-1α, IL-1β, IL-2, IL-4, IL-5, IL-6, IL-10, IL-12p70, IL-18, monocyte chemotactic protein (MCP-1), GRO/KC, TNF-α, and granulocyte-macrophage colony stimulating factor (GM-CSF) in a Luminex 100 IS (Luminex Corporation, USA) and analyzed by xPonent 3.1 Rev.2 Software (Luminex Corporation, USA). Results for each of the 14 analytes were read in pg/ml and subsequently normalized to total mass of sample protein (pg inflammatory mediator/mg protein) by multiplying with 0.025 ml standard sample volume and dividing with 0.1 mg added total protein for each sample. Any analytes indicating a concentration above 20,000 pg/μl were excluded from analysis (NA) as being outside the linear range of the Luminex assay.

Table 1. Study groups and design.

Group (Name)	Animals per group	Donor	Recipient	Treatment	Samples per time point (POD 3,5,7,9)	Samples per animal	Tissue
1 (ATC)	10	BN	LEW	none	5	3	Skin & Muscle
2 (ISO)	10	LEW	LEW	none	5	3	Skin & Muscle
3 (TAC)	10	BN	LEW	Tacrolimus*	5	3	Skin & Muscle

* 1 mg/kg/day (for 11 days).

Table 2. Appearance (Grading for skin rejection: I–IV) of each allograft on POD 1–11.

Animals ID	POD (Postoperative Day)										
	1	**2**	**3**	**4**	**5**	**6**	**7**	**8**	**9**	**10**	**11**
ATC 1	0	0	0	I	**I**	II	II	III	**III**	IV	**IV**
ATC 2	0	0	0	I	**II**	II	III	III	**IV**	IV	**IV**
ATC 3	0	0	**0**	0	**I**	II	**III**	III	IV	IV	**IV**
ATC 4	0	0	**0**	0	**I**	II	**II**	III	IV	IV	**IV**
ATC 5*	0	0	**0**								
ATC 6	0	0	**0**	0	I	II	**II**	III	**III**	IV	**IV**
ATC 7	0	0	**0**	I	II	II	**III**	III	**IV**	IV	**IV**
ATC 8	0	0	0	I	**II**	II	**II**	III	IV	IV	**IV**
ATC 9	0	0	0	I	**II**	II	II	III	**IV**	IV	IV
ATC 10	0	0	**0**	I	I	II	**II**	III	III	IV	IV
ATC 11	0	0	0	I	**II**	II	II	III	**III**	IV	**IV**

*This animal died on POD 3 during the anesthesia. Bold numbers mark biopsy timepoints (skin and muscle) for each animal.

Statistical and computational analysis

Analyses were performed with the statistical framework R 2.13.1 using packages including *stats, nnet, multtest, MASS, beeswarm, randomForest.* The non-parametric Kruskal-Wallis test was used to compare mediator abundance among groups 1-3 (ATC, ISO, TAC) at POD 3/POD 5. The Wilcoxon rank-sum test was used to identify the tissue levels of those mediators whose levels varied significantly between animals exhibiting rejection (ATC) and animals treated with tacrolimus to prevent rejection (TAC) in the early postoperative phase (POD 3/POD 5), as well for selected inflammatory mediators at POD 3. All p-values were adjusted for multiple hypothesis testing based on the false discovery rate (FDR) [9].

The multivariate extension of the one-way analysis of variance (MANOVA) or the discriminant function analysis (based on the same formulation as MANOVA with inflammatory mediators as independent variables and the rejection group as dependent variable in the latter case) are used to determine the coefficients of the two orthogonal discriminant vectors (DV), which enable maximal separation of the groups. As a measure of contribution to these vectors for each mediator, the sum of the absolute values of the respective coefficients (loadings) were used and related to the overall sum. Pillai's trace statistic was used to test for the differences in the vectors of means. The mediators showing significant differences among the 3 groups and with >2.5% contribution to the DVs in both skin and muscle were subjected to multinomial (logistic) regression analyses. A model for skin and one model for muscle were selected based on minimal Akaike information criterion [AIC]. Classifier performance was assessed using a 8-fold cross validation procedure and visualized using confusion tables. Accuracy was defined as 1- misclassification rate and Welch's test was used to test the differences between the mean of the number of true predicted and the mean of the sum of the respective number of false predicted.

To assess similarity of inflammatory mediator levels among different time points and tissue types, complete-linkage hierarchical clustering was performed and visualized as heat map using Genesis [10] based on mean-centered log2-transformed profiles. For this analysis, the mean value for each group and mediator was used.

A Random Forest (RF) [11] approach was used for classification of the rejection group (ATC, ISO, TAC) including all time points. This method was also used to identify those mediators most important for classification or diagnosis. Classifier performances were assessed by confusion tables and the out-of-bag (OOB) error rate. Principal Component Analysis (PCA) was used to rank most variable (important) mediators and potential therapeutic target candidates [12]. PCA reduces a multidimensional dataset to a few principal components, which account for the most variability in the dataset. The underlying hypothesis is that a mediator which changes during a process is important to that process [12,13]. In this analysis, the data were combined from skin and muscle, mean centered, and variance scaled. Components sufficient to capture at least 70% of total data variance observed were included.

Results

Progression of rejection

Appearance. On postoperative day (POD) 3, none of the allografts (n = 10) showed signs of rejection, on POD 5, 50% of the allografts displayed Grade I rejection and 5 animals (50%) II rejection. On postoperative day 7, rejection Grade II was present in 7 animals (70%) and rejection Grade III in 3 animals (30%). On day 9, 4 animals displayed Grade III rejection and 6 animals

Grade IV. None of the syngeneic controls or tacrolimus treated animals showed any signs of skin rejection/inflammation (Table 2).

Histological evaluation of skin biopsies. Histological evaluation of allograft skin biopsies on day 3 showed no or minimal inflammatory infiltrates (Grade 0) in six animals and a mild perivascular infiltrate (Grade I) in one biopsy. No tacrolimus-treated animals showed any signs of rejection while a mild perivascular infiltration was seen in one of the syngeneic control animal. On POD 5, biopsies from allogeneic transplants displayed Grade I rejection in three animals, as well as a moderate to severe perivascular inflammation with or without mild epidermal and/or adnexal epidermal dyskeratosis or apoptosis (Grade II) in three animals. One biopsy taken from the allogeneic group showed a severe skin rejection (Grade III), with dense inflammation and epidermal involvement with epithelial apoptosis, dyskeratosis and keratinolysis on POD 5. No inflammatory response was observed in isografts on POD 5, but two out of five biopsies in the tacrolimus treated animals did show an inflammatory infiltrate. On POD 7, allogeneic animals showed Grade III rejection and, one skin biopsy taken from the isograft group and one from the tacrolimus group displayed a moderate inflammation corresponding with Grade I/II rejection. At the endpoint, all samples from allografts showed rejection Grade III and one biopsy (n = 5) taken from the isografts displayed the characteristics of Grade I rejection. Two out of five biopsies in the tacrolimus group showed a mild rejection (Grade I) and one biopsy was classified as Grade II rejection (Table 3 and Figure 1).

Histological evaluation of muscle biopsies. H&E stains from allograft muscle samples showed no or rare inflammatory cells on POD 3 in four biopsies and Grade I rejection in two biopsies. Muscle biopsies from syngeneic controls showed a mild infiltration in two biopsies, severe inflammation similar to rejection Grade II in one graft, and no inflammatory response at this time point in two animals. On POD 5, two biopsies from the allogeneic transplants were classified as Grade 0 rejection, three samples as Grade I and one muscle biopsy as Grade II rejection, four biopsies from the isografts showed no or rare inflammation and only one sample a mild inflammation.

On POD 7, all biopsies (n = 5) from allografts displayed Grade I rejection and only one biopsy from an isografts showed a mild muscle inflammation on both day 7 and 9. Allograft muscle biopsies on day 9 showed rejection Grade I (n = 1, Grade II (n = 2) or Grade III (n = 2). Tacrolimus treated animals did not show any signs of rejection except for one animal displaying mild inflammation in the muscle on POD 9 (Table 4 and Figure 1).

Significant differences of inflammatory mediator levels at early postoperative time points among the different transplant models

We examined the levels of 14 inflammatory analytes in skin and muscle biopsies of allogeneic, syngeneic and immunosuppressed hind limb transplants at different postoperative days (POD 3, 5, 7, and 9) with a focus on the early postoperative phase where no histological alterations were observed (POD 3 and 5, Figure 2 and Figure S2). Non-parametric univariate analysis of the inflammatory mediators from skin and muscle were performed. Five inflammatory mediators (GM-CSF, IL1-α, IL-4, IL-12p70, IL-5, TNF-α) were significantly different at least in one group (adjusted $p<0.05$; Kruskal-Wallis test [KW]) in both skin and muscle. IL-12p70 and TNF-α were highly significantly different in the allograft versus the tacrolimus-treated animals (adjusted $p<0.005$; Wilcoxon-rank sum test [WR]; Table 5).

In Figure 2, the levels of the concentrations of these inflammatory mediators at POD 3 of all three groups within skin

Table 3. Histological evaluation of skin biopsies from postoperative (POD) 3 to 9.

SKIN	POD 3				POD 5				POD 7				POD 9			
GRADE	0	I	II	III	0	I	II	III	0	I	II	III	0	I	II	III
ATC	6	1				3	3	1				6				5
ISO	3	1			4				4		1		4	1		
TAC	5				3	2			4	1			2	2	1	

Number of biopsies taken on each postoperative day (POD 3,5,7,9) in skin according to their histological grading (Grad 0-III) based on H&E staining.

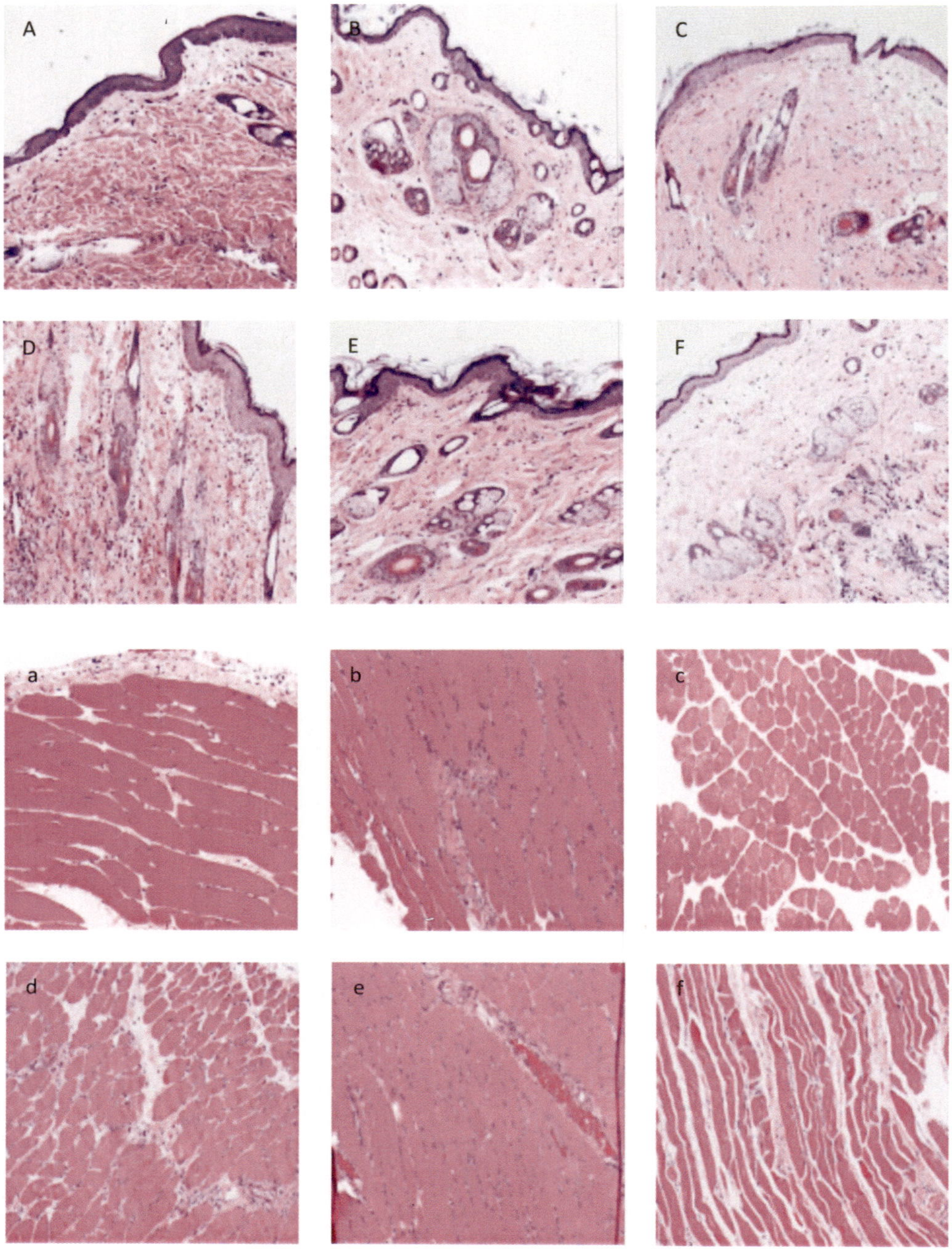

Figure 1. Histological evaluation of skin and muscle rejection in the early postoperative phase (POD 3 and 5). (A–C) Skin sample taken on POD 3 from an allograft without immunosuppression (A), from an isograft (B) and an allograft under TAC (C) showing no/rare inflammatory response (Grade 0 rejection). (D–F) Skin biopsies taken on POD 5 from a rejecting animal (D) displaying Grade 1 rejection, from an isograft (E) showing no/rare inflammatory response and a TAC treated allograft (F) characterized by a mild inflammatory response (Grade 0-I) in the deep dermis. (a–c) Muscle sample taken on POD 3 from an allograft without immunosuppression (a), from an isograft (b) and an allograft under TAC (c) showing no/rare inflammatory response (Grade 0 rejection). (d–f) Skin biopsies taken on POD 5 from a rejecting animal (d) displaying a mild inflammatory response (Grad 0-I rejection), from an isograft (E) and a TAC treated allograft (f) showing no/rare inflammatory response.

and muscle are depicted. Significantly higher concentrations of IL-12p70 in the skin from the allograft animals compared to the tacrolimus-treated animals (adjusted $p = 0.026$) as well as lower abundance of TNF-α in the allogeneic compared to the immunosuppressed transplants (adjusted $p = 0.026$) were detected. In muscle, numerical differences did not reach statistical significance (adjusted $p = 0.056$ in both cases).

For identification of inflammatory mediators with the highest predicting value, at early time points, multivariate analyses were performed. We fitted multivariate analysis of variance (MANOVA) models which resulted in $p = 8.9 \times 10^{-10}$ for skin and $p = 3.4 \times 10^{-5}$ for muscle from Pillai's trace statistic. Using these models, a functional discriminant analysis was performed. Mediators with the greatest absolute coefficients in the two resulting discriminant vectors might contribute most to the separation of groups (Table 5). The partition to the discrimination vectors for GM-CSF, IL-4, IL-12p70, IL-5, and TNF-α were > 2.5% in both tissues. We selected these inflammatory mediators as promising biomarkers candidates for further analyses.

Inflammatory mediators at early time points discern the procedure to which animals were subjected

A major goal of this study was to determine markers for early and accurate diagnosis of skin rejection in advance of major histological alterations. We applied several multivariate multinomial logistic regression models in skin and muscle samples for the classification of the three study groups at early postoperative time points (POD 3 and POD 5) using a combination of the selected inflammatory mediators (GM-CSF, IL-4, IL-12p70, IL-5, and TNF-α) as independent variables and study group as outcome. Based on the Akaike information criterion (AIC), which is a measure of the trade-off between the complexity of the model, i.e. number of variables, and the goodness of fit, optimal models for differentiation of the study groups could be found in skin rejection (based on IL-4, IL-12p70, and TNF-α: AIC = 16.0; residual deviance = 1.7×10^{-4}) and in muscle (based on IL-12p70 and TNF-α: AIC = 12.0; residual variance = 1.6×10^{-4}). The coefficients of the inflammatory mediators in the logistic regression models and classifier performance as assessed by 8-fold cross validation are detailed in Table 5. The prediction accuracy within skin was 87.1% and in muscle 100%, as derived from classification tables. A pairwise multivariate logistic regression analysis between the study groups (ATC vs. TAC, TAC vs. ISO, ISO vs. ATC) and applying a leave-one-out cross validation strategy resulted in an area under curve (AUC) from receiver operating characteristics (ROC) for skin of 0.5, 0.69, and 0.86 and for muscle of 1.0, 1.0, and 1.0, indicating a substantially better discrimination than by chance (AUC = 0.5) (Table 6).

Inflammatory mediator profiles are similar within each group

Hierarchical clustering was performed for all inflammatory mediators in the three experimental groups. Each row of the data matrix corresponds with one of the 14 inflammatory mediators, and each column corresponds with a group. The $\log_2$-transformed and mean-centered values (mean concentrations from each condition) are visualized as a heat map, with color codes shown in the color bar (Figure 3). The dendrogram on the x-axis shows the similarities among the samples. As expected, the rejection group (ATC skin and muscle samples), especially samples from later time points with pronounced histological changes, exhibit a completely different mediator clustering pattern vs. the control groups, with high abundance of IL-5, IL-18, IL-1β, MCP-1, IL-6, GRO-KC, and TNF-α. In TAC-treated animals, only IL-1α and TNF-α were highly abundant, whereas the expression of all other mediators assessed appeared suppressed.

The separation of the tacrolimus-treated group was also evident from the cluster analysis. Within sample cluster A (17 samples), 5.9% were from the tacrolimus and 94.1% were from study group ISO/ATC. In contrast, in cluster B (7 samples), 100% were from tacrolimus and 0% from the ISO/ATC groups. A Fisher's exact test ($p = 2.3\times10^{-5}$) suggested that the distribution between clusters A and B was not random. Profiles of MCP-1, IL-4, IL-1β, and IL-6 characterize rejecting grafts, whereas GM-CSF and IL-4 characterize isografts. This was also indicated by an absolute value of point-biserial correlation coefficient >0.6 comparing each group with the other groups. Interestingly, there appeared to be an

Table 4. Histological evaluation of muscle biopsies from postoperative (POD) 3 to 9.

MUSCLE	POD 3				POD 5				POD 7				POD 9			
GRADE	**0**	**I**	**II**	**III**	**0**	**I**	**II**	**III**	**0**	**I**	**II**	**III**	**0**	**I**	**II**	**III**
ATC	4	2			2	3	1			5				1	2	2
ISO	2	2	1		4	1			4	1			4	1		
TAC	5				5				5				4	1		

Number of biopsies taken on each postoperative day (POD 3,5,7,9) in muscle according to their histological grading (Grad 0-III) based on H&E grading. The first biopsy was taken from the lateral proximal part of the thigh, the second one from the lateral distal thigh, the third one from the ventral thigh and the last one from the medial part of the thigh.

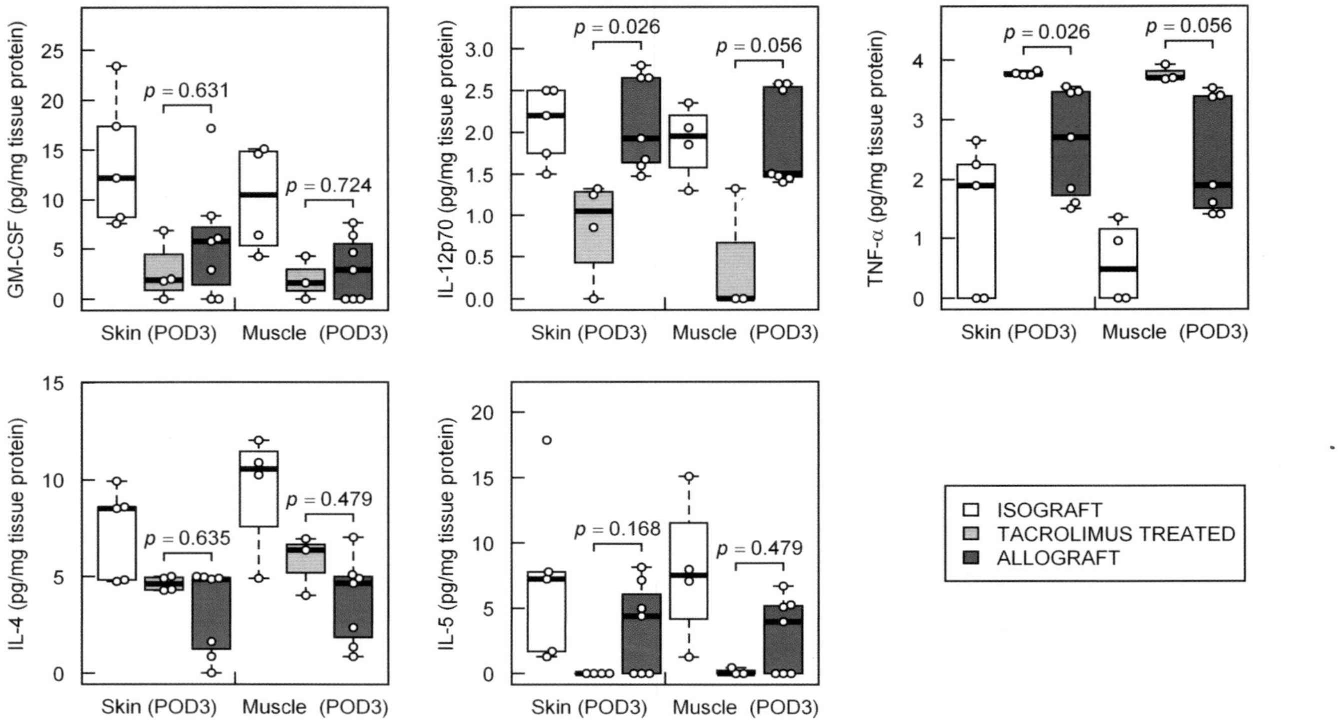

Figure 2. Distribution of inflammatory mediator levels at the earliest postoperative measurements (POD 3) in rat limb transplantation models. Adjusted p-values from Wilcoxon rank-sum test between the rejection group (ATC) vs. Tacrolimus treated group (TAC) for selected inflammatory mediators, which were tested to be included in a prediction model by multinomial logistic regression analysis, are presented.

Table 5. Statistical analysis for all 14 inflammatory mediator levels in skin and in muscle at early postoperative time points (combined group of POD 3 and POD 5).

	Skin POD 3/5			Muscle POD 3/5		
	p_{KW}	p_{WR}	Partition on DVs [%]	p_{KW}	p_{WR}	Partition on DVs [%]
GM-CSF	**0.0018**	0.3260	**4.26**	**0.0083**	0.6178	**2.60**
IL-1α	**0.0244**	1.0000	0.01	**0.0105**	0.0773	0.01
MCP-1	**0.0011**	**0.0026**	0.72	**0.0466**	0.3673	0.79
IL-4	**0.0040**	0.3421	**24.21**	**0.0194**	0.5312	**18.68**
IL-1β	0.2042	0.1577	0.10	0.8251	0.7577	0.09
IL-2	0.2042	0.2868	0.83	0.1779	0.5312	0.29
IL-6	0.1322	0.2824	0.27	0.5127	0.6178	0.29
IL-10	0.2777	0.2805	0.55	0.8251	0.8657	0.39
IL-12p70	**0.0019**	**0.0013**	**15.65**	**0.0030**	**0.0025**	**31.59**
IL-5	**0.0022**	**0.0123**	**4.85**	**0.0010**	0.2112	**5.03**
IFN-γ	0.2956	0.3729	**5.67**	0.2562	0.3619	1.90
IL-18	0.3462	0.2868	0.03	**0.0425**	0.7498	0.03
GRO-KC	**0.0040**	**0.0021**	0.27	0.5127	0.5312	0.11
TNF-α	**1.7×10^{-4}**	**0.0013**	**42.59**	**0.0001**	**0.0025**	**38.21**

Most promising inflammatory mediators for classification of rejection, based on early identification before histological manifestation of rejection is evident, are selected (p_{KW}<0.05 and *Partition on DVs* >1%, symbols in bold) and subjected to multinomial logistic regression analyses. For all measured inflammatory mediators adjusted p-values from Kruskal-Wallis test (KW) of overall equality between all 3 cohorts (ISO, TAC, ATC) and Wilcoxon rank-sum test (WR) for comparison between the rejection group (ATC) and the Tacrolimus treated group (TAC) as well as partition of each inflammatory mediator on the two discriminant vectors (DVs), which maximizes the separation between the 3 rejection groups, resulting from discriminant function analysis, are given.

Table 6. Results for multinomial logistic regression models in skin and muscle for classification of the rejection groups based inflammatory mediator/chemokine levels at early postoperative time points (POD 3/5) in rat transplantation models.

	Skin POD3/5			Muscle POD3/5		
ln(p(*TAC*)/p(*ATC*))	**-6.7-2.6**IL4*-61.3**IL12p70*+25.6**TNFa***			**-6.9-18.8**IL12p70*+11.3**TNFa***		
ln(p(*ISO*)/p(*ATC*))	**-1094.8+112.6**IL4*+250.4**IL12p70*-28.6**TNFa***			**-10.0+25.1**IL12p70*-27.0**TNFa***		
	ATC^{pred}	**TAC^{pred}**	**ISO^{pred}**	**ATC^{pred}**	**TAC^{pred}**	**ISO^{pred}**
ATC	12	0	1	13	0	0
TAC	0	8	0	0	7	0
ISO	3	0	7	0	0	9
	Accuracy = 87.1% $p = 0.020$			Accuracy = 100% $p = 0.031$		

Best prediction models for skin and muscle and their respective logistic prediction functions and classifier performance including confusion table (assessed by an 8-fold cross validation procedure) are summarized.

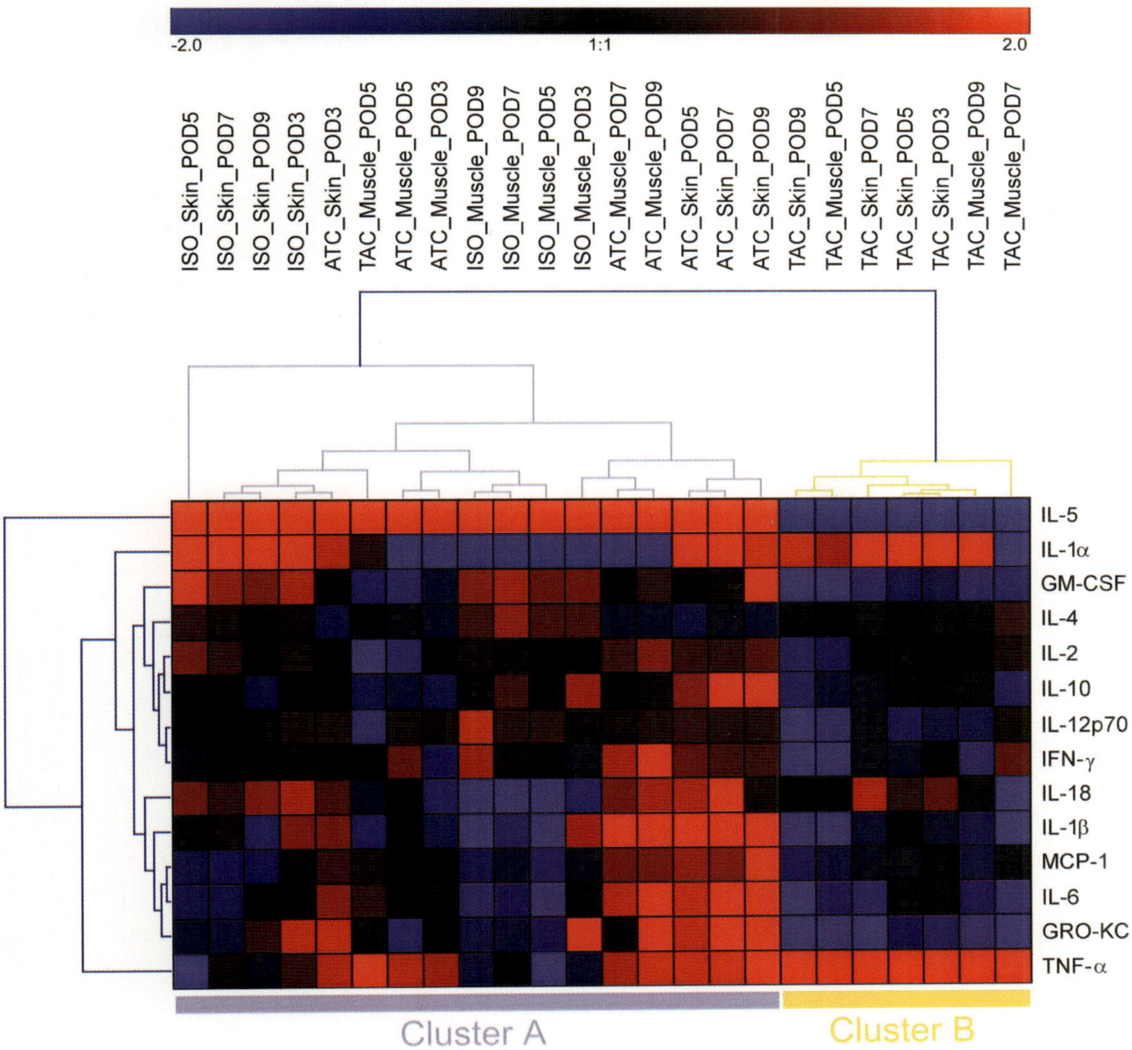

Figure 3. Similarity of sample groups and association between inflammatory mediators in rat limb transplantation models based on their profiles of mean levels in each condition. Heatmap as a result of complete linkage hierarchical clustering on log2-transformed and mean centered data. Log2-fold differences against the respective mean levels of each inflammatory mediator are color coded (red means higher inflammatory mediator levels and blue means lower inflammatory mediator levels than the mean levels of the respective inflammatory mediator according to the color scheme at the top). Dendrograms (trees) show similarity between different conditions and different inflammatory mediator profiles, respectively.

overlap in the expression pattern of the isografts and the rejecting animals for IL-5, IL-1α, IL-18, and GRO-KC.

Mediators relevant for classifications and progression of rejection

Random forest (RF) classification was performed for skin and muscle samples in all three cohorts at POD 3–9. The overall out-of-bag error rate was 6.7% for skin and 7.0% for muscle. The classification tables are shown in Figure 4. The importance of a variable in discriminating among study groups was demonstrated by ranked mean decrease accuracy as depicted in Figure 4. The mediator best capable of differentiating among experimental groups samples was MCP-1 in skin and TNF-α in muscle. Discriminant analysis suggested that the mediators best capable of discriminating among experimental groups in the early postoperative time points were GM-CSF, IL-4, IL-12p70, IL-5, and TNF-α; these mediators also appear within the seven top-ranked mediators in the RF analysis.

To identify inflammatory cytokines with high dynamic variability, we performed principal component analysis (PCA) on the combined mean-centered dataset including the whole postoperative time series over all study groups and tissues. The PCA scores of the first four principle components (explaining >70% of the variance) of all 14 cytokines were ranked based on the sum of the absolute PCA scores (loadings) of all 4 PCs (Figure 5). The top prioritized cytokines IL-1α, IL-18, IL-1β, and IL-4 might be promising candidates for new therapeutic regimens.

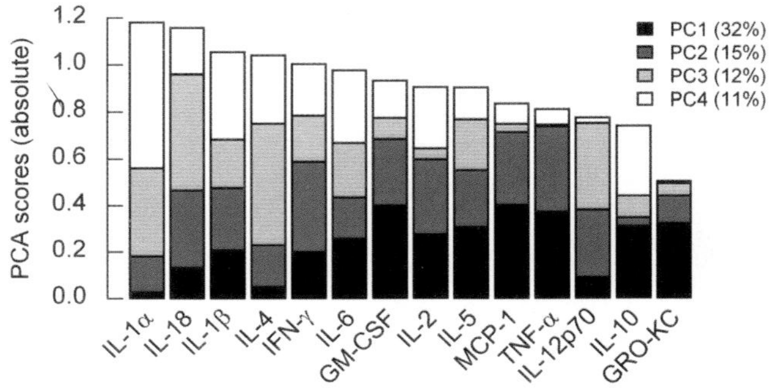

Figure 5. Most variable mediators identified by principal component analysis (PCA) suggesting new potential targets for therapeutic interventions to suppress limb transplant rejection. PCA scores (loadings) for the first four principal components (PCs), which represent more than 70% of information within the data, are displayed in a stacked bar plot for all inflammatory mediators (ranked by the overall PCA score of the 4 PCs).

Discussion

Experimental transplant rejection can be detected reliably in advance of the current clinical gold standard of histologic evaluation, using computational modeling that involves 14 inflammatory mediators in this model. These findings support the hypothesis that the immune signaling associated with rejection follows specific patterns of expression and is driven by different principal components than those associated with inflammation following syngeneic transplantation.

Detailed cellular and molecular assessment provides valuable insights into the role of the immune/inflammatory response in post-transplant pathophysiology [14,15]. Translation of these findings into biomarkers applied clinically, however, has been very limited. It remains a major challenge to reduce the complexity of dynamic biological systems to elements with diagnostic or therapeutic clinical value [16,17]. Data-driven investigations of genomic and proteomic studies in combination with mechanistic computational modeling based on measurements of circulating inflammatory mediators have given insight into the

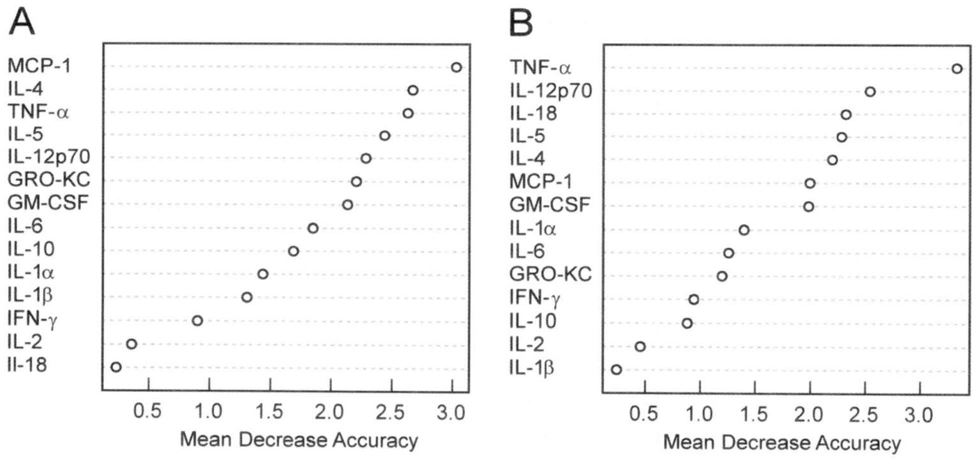

Skin	ATC^{pred}	TAC^{pred}	ISO^{pred}	class error
ATC	22	0	2	8.3 %
TAC	0	16	0	0.0 %
ISO	2	0	18	10.0 %
error rate (OOB)				6.67 %

Muscle	ATC^{pred}	TAC^{pred}	ISO^{pred}	class error
ATC	23	0	1	4.2 %
TAC	1	14	0	6.7 %
ISO	2	0	16	11.1 %
error rate (OOB)				7.02 %

Figure 4. Results from Random Forest classification of the different rejection groups (ISO, TAC, ATC) using over the whole time course (POD 3, POD 5, POD 7, POD 9) measured inflammatory mediators in skin (A) and muscle (B) samples of rat limb transplantation models. Most important mediators for the decision trees based classification approach are evident by ranked mean decrease accuracy. Performances of the classifiers are indicated by the confusion table and the out-of-bag (OOB) error rate.

pathophysiology of trauma, shock as well as organ transplantation [18–22].

Herein, we demonstrate that data-driven and expression pattern-oriented analyses of a high-content dataset can help to decipher the complexity of acute inflammation in VCA. In the present study, these advanced computational algorithms allowed to diagnose rejection in advance of gross histological damage. We suggest that measuring inflammatory mediators expressed in skin and muscle is clinically feasible in the setting of VCA since skin and muscle are more accessible as compared to solid organs. Isografts were compared to allografts and tacrolimus treated allografts in order to delineate between surgery/trauma/ischemia induced inflammation and allograft rejection. Tacrolimus treatment was sufficient to diminish rejection (but not completely eliminate the immune response).

In the samples analyzed in the present study, skin rejection was detected in advance of histological alterations based on the inflammatory mediators IL-4, IL-12p70 and TNF-α, with a prediction accuracy of >87%. In muscle rejection, IL-12p70 and TNF-α were identified as best and accurate classifiers. TNF-α, a canonical inflammatory mediator, is mainly produced by activated monocytes, macrophages, and T-cells, and exerts a direct effect on the proliferation, apoptosis, necrosis, differentiation, and function of virtually every cell type [23]. In the skin, mast cells appear to be the predominant source of preformed TNF-α, which can be released upon inflammatory stimuli [24]. TNF-α activates T-cells; increases the release of other inflammatory mediators; and induces neutrophil adherence, infiltration and the production of enzymes and reactive oxygen. These mechanisms are harmful to the allograft, and subsequently cause tissue injury as well as organ dysfunction [23]. Several studies have demonstrated increased TNF-α levels in the serum during episodes of rejection in liver, kidney and pancreas transplant recipients [25–27]. Interestingly, the increase in TNF-α levels occurred two days before clinical manifestation of rejection.

The production of IL-12 strongly promotes the development of IFN-γ producing helper T (TH)-cells. IL-12 may not only be essential for macrophage-mediated allograft rejection via induction of TH1 responses, but IL-12 may be involved in delaying rejection via induction of inducible nitric oxide synthase (iNOS) and indolamine 2,3 dioxygenase (IDO) [28]. This positive effect was shown in several skin or heart allograft models, as well as in the course of graft-versus-host disease (GVHD) [29–31].

Good performance of the multinomial logistic regression model, which models linear decision boundaries effectively, indicates that the patterns of inflammatory mediator expression in skin are fundamentally different in isograft and allograft skin tissue, and that this difference can be captured with reasonable performance by computationally efficient algorithms. Multinomial logistic regression performance for discrimination of rejection is even stronger and the consistency with which this distinction is made across a rather complex set of features implies a high level of biological significance. In other words, not only is the specific inflammatory mediator, but also the particular combination of mediators in the local inflammatory milieu seems to play a determinative role in the nature and progression of inflammation expressed.

The RF classification approach including more time points (POD 3-POD 9) achieves high levels of accuracy and continues to improve with the addition of variables. This finding implies that there are specific inflammatory mediator interactions that are relevant only under certain contexts [32], and that these interactions can be leveraged to identify potential targets for therapeutic intervention.

We hypothesized that mediators with time-dependent changes might be important in the different dynamic processes and describe principal drivers (principal components, PC), which could turn out as therapeutic targets. We were focusing on the first four PCs since they comprise more than 70% of the total variance. The four top-ranked mediators were IL-1α, IL-18, IL-1β, and IL-4 (Figure 5).

To discern the effect of the inflammatory mediators within each group, we performed the same PCA procedure for each group individually (Figure S1). The impact of IL12p70 already shown as potential early diagnostic marker for rejection was not as pronounced in the tacrolimus-treated animals as in the isograft and allograft study group. Interferon-γ and IL-4 had a high ranking in all groups (ISO, TAC, ATC) indicating a more unspecific effect in inflammation; In contrast, IL-1α and IL-18 exhibited an expression profile which indicates a possible key role in VCA rejection and makes these cytokines interesting candidates for therapeutic interventions.

Our studies identified IL-1α and IL-18 as possible candidates for the treatment of skin rejection. These inflammatory mediators share similarities regarding structure, receptor family, signal transduction pathways, and biological effects. Both inflammatory mediators are produced by monocytes/macrophages but also constitutively expressed by keratinocytes [33]. IL-1α plays an important role in sterile inflammation. During necrotic cell death, the IL-1α precursor is released [34] and binds to its receptor expressed on adjacent macrophages and epithelial cells, which in turn triggers a pro-inflammatory response characterized by an influx of neutrophils followed by macrophages [35,36]. IL-18, together with IL-2, IL-12, and IL-15, is a dominant IFN-γ inducing factor. Several human diseases, such as systemic lupus erythematosus, rheumatoid arthritis, Crohn's disease, psoriasis and graft-versus-host-disease are thought to be mediated in part by IL-18 [37]. Moreover, IL-18 stimulates ICAM-1 expression on monocytic cell lines, which is important for the recruitment of T-cells and other immune cells to the skin. Lymphocyte recruitment is known as a key mechanism in inflammatory skin disorders and [38,39]. Hautz et al. showed, that expression of ICAM-1 correlated closely with severity of skin rejection [8].

Based on our findings, IL-1α and IL-18 appear as interesting potential targets for intervention. Yuan J et al. already showed the efficacy of IL-1 receptor antagonist (IL-1ra) gene transfer treatment for acute corneal graft rejection in a rat model [40] The group demonstrated during acute rejection, that TGF-β1, RANTES and IL-1 levels were lower in the IL-1ra treatment group. Thus antagonizing the biological activitiy of IL-1 could effectively prolong graft survival. IL-ra, a specific inhibitor of both IL-1α and IL-β generically known as anakinra is clinically applied for the treatment of rheumatoid arthritis. IL-18-binding protein (IL-18BP), a specific inhibitor or IL-18 which neutralizes IL-18 bioactivity, was discovered during the search for soluble IL-18 receptors in humane urine [41]. A clinical preparation of human IL-18BP has been shown to be safe and effective in patients with RA or plaque psoriasis [42]. A soluble form of the IL-18 receptor accessory protein (sIL-18Rβ) has recently been identified as novel IL-18 inhibitor in collagen-induced arthritis in mice [43].

In summary, we herein provide information, which could help identifying a diagnostic profile and novel targets for treatment of skin rejection in VCA. The present study demonstrates that the application of advanced computational methods can be successfully applied in molecular assessment of skin rejection and provides novel insights into the inflammatory mediator communication patterns. The study remains observational in its nature and investigational trials are warranted in order to address the true functional value of the postulated treatment targets.

Supporting Information

Figure S1 Most variable (influential) mediators identified by principal component analysis (PCA) for each of the three study groups (ISO/TAC/ATC). PCA scores (loadings) for the first four principal components (PCs), which represent more than 75% of information, are displayed in a stacked bar plot for all inflammatory mediators (ranked by the overall PCA score of the 4 PCs) and a scatter plot of the first two PCs.

Figure S2 Distribution of inflammatory mediator levels (boxplots) at postoperative day 5 in rat limb transplantation models for selected inflammatory mediators. Adjusted p-values from Wilcoxon rank-sum test between the rejection group (ATC) versus Tacrolimus treated group (TAC) are provided.

Acknowledgments

We gratefully acknowledge the effort of Dr. Mario Cherubino and Dr. Yong Wang for performing a major part of hindlimb transplants. The help of Prof. Bernhard Zelger in preparing and evaluating histological sections and the editorial work by Mary Margreiter are also gratefully acknowledged.

Author Contributions

Conceived and designed the experiments: DW SS GB RS WAL YV. Performed the experiments: DW DB TH NE HH. Analyzed the data: DW HH RS TH NE BZ. Contributed reagents/materials/analysis tools: YV JP GP. Wrote the paper: DW HH SS.

References

1. Cendales LC, Kanitakis J, Schneeberger S, Burns C, Ruiz P, et al. (2008) The Banff 2007 working classification of skin-containing composite tissue allograft pathology. Am J Transplant 8: 1396–1400.
2. Kanitakis J, Jullien D, Nicolas JF, Frances C, Claudy A, et al. (2000) Sequential histological and immunohistochemical study of the skin of the first human hand allograft. Transplantation 69: 1380–1385.
3. Kanitakis J (2008) The challenge of dermatopathological diagnosis of composite tissue allograft rejection: a review. J Cutan Pathol 35: 738–744.
4. Schneeberger S, Gorantla VS, van Riet RP, Lanzetta M, Vereecken P, et al. (2008) Atypical acute rejection after hand transplantation. Am J Transplant 8: 688–696.
5. Hautz T, Wolfram D, Grahammer J, Starzl R, Krapf C, et al. (2012) Mechanisms and mediators of inflammation: potential models for skin rejection and targeted therapy in vascularized composite allotransplantation. Clin Dev Immunol: 1–9.
6. Tarca AL, Carey VJ, Chen XW, Romero R, Draghici S (2007) Machine learning and its applications to biology. PLoS Comput Biol 3: e116.
7. Coin L, Bateman A, Durbin R (2003) Enhanced protein domain discovery by using language modeling techniques from speech recognition. Proc Natl Acad Sci U S A 100: 4516–4520.
8. Hautz T, Zelger B, Grahammer J, Krapf C, Amberger A, et al. (2010) Molecular markers and targeted therapy of skin rejection in composite tissue allotransplantation. Am J Transplant 10: 1200–1209.
9. Benjamini Y, Hochberg Y (1995) Controlling the false discovery rate: A practical and powerful approach to multiple testing. J R Statist Soc B 57: 289–300.
10. Sturn A, Quackenbush J, Trajanoski Z (2002) Genesis: cluster analysis of microarray data. Bioinformatics 18: 207–208.
11. Breiman L (2001) Random Forests. Machine Learning 45: 5–32.
12. Mi Q, Constantine G, Ziraldo C, Solovyev A, Torres A, et al. (2011) A dynamic view of trauma/hemorrhage-induced inflammation in mice: principal drivers and networks. PLoS One 6: e19424.
13. Namas RA, Namas R, Lagoa C, Barclay D, Mi Q, et al. (2012) Hemoadsorption reprograms inflammation in experimental gram-negative septic peritonitis: insights from in vivo and in silico studies. Mol Med 18: 1366–1374.
14. Page EK, Dar WA, Knechtle SJ (2012) Biologics in organ transplantation. Transpl Int 25: 707–719.
15. Sarwal MM (2006) Chipping into the human genome: novel insights for transplantation. Immunol Rev 210: 138–155.
16. Vodovotz Y (2006) Deciphering the complexity of acute inflammation using mathematical models. Immunol Res 36: 237–245.
17. Mesarovic MD, Sreenath SN, Keene JD (2004) Search for organising principles: understanding in systems biology. Syst Biol (Stevenage) 1: 19–27.
18. Calvano SE, Xiao W, Richards DR, Felciano RM, Baker HV, et al. (2005) A network-based analysis of systemic inflammation in humans. Nature 437: 1032–1037.
19. Warren HS, Elson CM, Hayden DL, Schoenfeld DA, Cobb JP, et al. (2009) A genomic score prognostic of outcome in trauma patients. Mol Med 15: 220–227.
20. Chow CC, Clermont G, Kumar R, Lagoa C, Tawadrous Z, et al. (2005) The acute inflammatory response in diverse shock states. Shock 24: 74–84.
21. Bohra R, Klepacki J, Klawitter J, Thurman JM, Christians U (2013) Proteomics and metabolomics in renal transplantation-quo vadis? Transpl Int 26: 225–241.
22. Azhar N (2013) Analysis of serum inflammatory mediators identifies unique dynamic networks associated with death and spontaneous survival in pediatric acute liver failure.
23. Grenz A, Schenk M, Zipfel A, Viebahn R (2000) TNF-alpha and its receptors mediate graft rejection and loss after liver transplantation. Clin Chem Lab Med 38: 1183–1185.
24. Walsh LJ, Trinchieri G, Waldorf HA, Whitaker D, Murphy GF (1991) Human dermal mast cells contain and release tumor necrosis factor alpha, which induces endothelial leukocyte adhesion molecule 1. Proc Natl Acad Sci U S A 88: 4220–4224.
25. Imagawa DK, Millis JM, Olthoff KM, Derus LJ, Chia D, et al. (1990) The role of tumor necrosis factor in allograft rejection. I. Evidence that elevated levels of tumor necrosis factor-alpha predict rejection following orthotopic liver transplantation. Transplantation 50: 219–225.
26. Bubnova LN, Kabakov A, Serebrianaya N, Ketlinky S (1992) Interleukin-1 beta and tumor necrosis factor-alpha serum levels in renal allograft recipients. Transplant Proc 24: 2545.
27. Grewal HP, Kotb M, Salem A, el Din AB, Novak K, et al. (1993) Elevated tumor necrosis factor levels are predictive for pancreas allograft transplant rejection. Transplant Proc 25: 132–135.
28. Goriely S, Goldman M (2008) Interleukin-12 family members and the balance between rejection and tolerance. Curr Opin Organ Transplant 13: 4–9.
29. Piccotti JR, Chan SY, Goodman RE, Magram J, Eichwald EJ, et al. (1996) IL-12 antagonism induces T helper 2 responses, yet exacerbates cardiac allograft rejection. Evidence against a dominant protective role for T helper 2 cytokines in alloimmunity. J Immunol 157: 1951–1957.
30. Verma ND, Boyd R, Robinson C, Plain KM, Tran GT, et al. (2006) Interleukin-12p70 prolongs allograft survival by induction of interferon gamma and nitric oxide production. Transplantation 82: 1324–1333.
31. Dey BR, Yang YG, Szot GL, Pearson DA, Sykes M (1998) Interleukin-12 inhibits graft-versus-host disease through an Fas-mediated mechanism associated with alterations in donor T-cell activation and expansion. Blood 91: 3315–3322.
32. Nathan C, Sporn M (1991) Cytokines in context. J Cell Biol 113: 981–986.
33. Dinarello CA (1999) IL-18: A TH1-inducing, proinflammatory cytokine and new member of the IL-1 family. J Allergy Clin Immunol 103: 11–24.
34. Carmi Y, Voronov E, Dotan S, Lahat N, Rahat MA, et al. (2009) The role of macrophage-derived IL-1 in induction and maintenance of angiogenesis. J Immunol 183: 4705–4714.
35. Rider P, Carmi Y, Guttman O, Braiman A, Cohen I, et al. (2011) IL-1alpha and IL-1beta recruit different myeloid cells and promote different stages of sterile inflammation. J Immunol 187: 4835–4843.
36. van de Veerdonk FL, Netea MG (2013) New Insights in the Immunobiology of IL-1 Family Members. Front Immunol 4: 167.
37. Dinarello CA (2009) Immunological and inflammatory functions of the interleukin-1 family. Annu Rev Immunol 27: 519–550.
38. Robert C, Kupper TS (1999) Inflammatory skin diseases, T cells, and immune surveillance. N Engl J Med 341: 1817–1828.
39. Schon MP, Ludwig RJ (2005) Lymphocyte trafficking to inflamed skin—molecular mechanisms and implications for therapeutic target molecules. Expert Opin Ther Targets 9: 225–243.
40. Yuan J, Liu Y, Huang W, Zhou S, Ling S, et al. (2013) The experimental treatment of corneal graft rejection with the interleukin-1 receptor antagonist (IL-1ra) gene. PLoS One 8: e60714.
41. Novick D, Kim SH, Fantuzzi G, Reznikov LL, Dinarello CA, et al. (1999) Interleukin-18 binding protein: a novel modulator of the Th1 cytokine response. Immunity 10: 127–136.
42. Tak PP, Bacchi M, Bertolino M (2006) Pharmacokinetics of IL-18 binding protein in healthy volunteers and subjects with rheumatoid arthritis or plaque psoriasis. Eur J Drug Metab Pharmacokinet 31: 109–116.
43. Veenbergen S, Smeets R, Bennink M, Arntz O, Joosten L, et al. (2010) The natural soluble form of IL-18 receptor beta exacerbates collagen-induced arthritis via modulation of T-cell immune responses. Ann Rheum Dis 69: 276–283.

10

Flt3L Combined with Rapamycin Promotes Cardiac Allograft Tolerance by Inducing Regulatory Dendritic Cells and Allograft Autophagy in Mice

Ali Xiong[1], Lihua Duan[1], Jie Chen[1], Zhigang Fan[1], Fang Zheng[1], Zheng Tan[1], Feili Gong[1,2,3]*, Min Fang[1,2,3]*

1 Department of Immunology, Tongji Medical College, Huazhong University of Science and Technology, Wuhan, Hubei, China, **2** Key Laboratory of Organ Transplantation, Ministry of Education, Wuhan, Hubei, China, **3** Key Laboratory of Organ Transplantation, Ministry of Health, Wuhan, Hubei, China

Abstract

The induction of immune tolerance is still a formidable challenge in organ transplantation. Dendritic cells (DCs) play an important role in orchestrating immune responses by either mediating protective immune responses or inducing antigen specific tolerance. Previous studies demonstrated that the fms-like tyrosine kinase 3 receptor (Flt3) and its ligand (Flt3L) play an essential role in the regulation of DC commitment and development. Here, we report a synergic effect between Flt3L and low-dose rapamycin (Rapa) in the protection of allograft rejction. It was found that Flt3L combined with Rapa significantly prolonged murine cardiac allograft survival time as compared with that of untreated recipients or recipients treated with Rapa or Flt3L alone. Mechanistic studies revealed that Flt3L combined with low-dose of Rapa induced the generation of tolerogenic DCs along with the production of $CD25^{+}$ $Foxp3^{+}$ regulatory T cells and IL-10 secretion. We also observed enhanced autophagy in the cardiac allograft, which could be another asset contributing to the enhanced allograft survival. All together, these data suggest that Flt3L combined with low-dose of Rapa could be an effective therapeutic approach to induce tolerance in clinical setting of transplantation.

Editor: Maria G. Castro, University of Michigan School of Medicine, United States of America

Funding: This work was supported by the National Natural Science Foundation of China (Grant No. 81072440), NSFC-Guangdong Union Grant (Grant No. U0832003). The funders had no role in study design, data collection and analysis, decision to publish, or preparation of the manuscript.

Competing Interests: The authors have declared that no competing interests exist.

* E-mail: minfang89@mail.hust.edu.cn (MF); flgong@163.com (FG)

Introduction

Organ transplantation has become the primary treatment for patients with end-stage organ failure [1]. Although the application of immunosuppressive drugs has contributed significantly to the success of allograft survival, side effects resulted from immunosuppression or drug toxicity also markedly impact the quality of life of recipients [2,3]. Therefore, establishment of strategies aimed at inducing allograft tolerance is wanting.

In the setting of transplantation, DCs actively mediate graft rejection by presenting donor-derived alloantigens to naïve T cells. However, there is emerging evidence indicating that other than mediation of allograft rejection, DCs also possess the capability to induce allograft tolerance [4]. Therefore, DCs are capable of inducing either immune response or tolerance depending on their activation and maturation status [5,6].

Flt3, a member of the tyrosine-kinase receptor family, was initially cloned from fetal liver of cells with hematopoietic stem cell activity [7]. Flt3L is the ligand for Flt3, which is a key regulator for DC commitment and development. Mice administered with Flt3L displayed the expansion of certain subtypes of DCs such as the plasmacytoid DCs (pDCs) and conventional DCs (cDCs) in the spleen [8]. Studies have shown that pDCs play an important role in the induction of Tregs in vivo manifested by that their precursors are able to prolong graft survival [9]. Studies in hematopoietic cell transplantation also revealed that Flt3L is a potent mobilizer to induce murine hematopoietic chimerism, while long-term persistence of donor hematopoietic cells in peripheral lymphoid and non-lymphoid tissues of organ allograft recipients is postulated to be an essential prerequisite for the induction of donor-specific tolerance [10,11].

Autophagy in eukaryotic cells is a cellular quality control process to deliver cytoplasmic constituents for lysosomal degradation, which enables cells to recycle nutrients for survival during nutrient starvation [12]. Rapamycin, an inhibitor of the mammalian target of rapamycin (mTOR) has been used to stimulate autophagy. In the steady state, autophagy-mediated antigen processing in thymic epithelial cells could have a crucial role in the induction and maintenance of $CD4^{+}$ T-cell tolerance [12,13].

In this study, we examined the effects of Flt3L in combination with Rapamycin in a BALB/c-to-C57BL/6 cardiac allograft model. Our results demonstrate that Flt3L combined with low-dose of Rapamycin prevented acute allograft rejection and prolonged allograft survival time. The enhanced allograft survival is associated with the induction of tolerogenic DCs along with the production of $CD25^{+}$ $Foxp3^{+}$ regulatory T cells and increased allograft autophagy. Our data suggest that Flt3L combined with low-dose of Rapa could be a promising therapeutic strategy in clinical transplantation.

Results

Flt3L Combined with Low-dose of Rapa Prolongs Cardiac Allograft Survival

We first sought to investigate the regulatory effect of Flt3L combined with a short-term of low-dose Rapa treatment on allograft acute rejection. A murine cardiac allograft transplantation model was employed to address this question. As shown in Figure 1A, untreated recipients rapidly rejected their grafts (7.6±0.516 days) along with typical pathological features of acute rejection (Fig. 1B). Similar pathological features were observed in recipients treated with either PBS or rGST (controls, Figure 1B). As expected, administration of Rapa significantly increased graft mean survival time (MST) (16.9±2.767 days, Fig. 1A). Similarly, recipients treated with Flt3L doubled allograft MST (13.1±1.287 days, Fig. 1A). In sharp contrast, a significant enhanced graft survival was observed in mice treated with Flt3L and low-dose of Rapa (36.4±18.704 days, Fig. 1A). Remarkably, about 20% of recipients showed long-term graft survival (MST>100 days, Fig. 1A). In consistent with these results, a significant reduction for inflammatory infiltration was observed in the allograft sections (Fig. 1B).

Flt3L Combined with Rapa Induces Tolerogenic DCs in the Recipient Mice

We next examined DC phenotypes in the recipient mice. It was noted that a significant increase in the number of pDCs in mice treated with Flt3L or Flt3L with low-dose of Rapa as compared with that of control mice (Fig. 2A). Similarly, we also detected a significantly higher proportion of splenic $CD8a^+$ DCs in Flt3L or Flt3L/Rapa treated mice (Fig. 2A). Since both $CD8a^+$ DCs and pDCs have regulatory functions [14], Our data suggest that Flt3Lcombined with Rapa could induce the expansion of regulatory DCs in the recipient mice.

Rapamycin has been shown to inhibit the up-regulation of maturation markers expressed by DCs [15], while immature DCs have been demonstrated with capability to prolong allograft survival [16,17]. In line with this notion, Flt3L combined with Rapa significantly blocked $CD11c^+$ DC maturation as manifested by the decreased CD40, CD80 expression (Fig. 2B). Since $CCR9^+$ pDCs had previously been reported to be potent inducers for Tregs [18], we then investigated whether $CCR9^+$ pDCs are implicated in the induction of allograft tolerance. Indeed, recipients treated with Flt3L and low-dose of Rapa displayed a significant increase for $CCR9^+$ pDCs as compared with those recipients treated with Flt3L or Rapa alone or other groups (Fig. 2C).

Flt3L Combined with Rapa Promotes the Production of $CD4^+$ $CD25^+$ $Foxp3^+$ and $CD8^+$ $CD25^+$ $Foxp3^+$ T Cells

The above results prompted us to examine the proportion of $CD4^+CD25^+Foxp3^+$ and $CD8^+CD25^+Foxp3^+$ Tregs. To this end, splenic T cells isolated from each group of recipient mice were stained for intracellular Foxp3 after co-staining with anti-CD4/CD25 antibodies or anti-CD3/CD8/CD25 antibodies, and the cells were next analyzed by flow cytometry. A significant increase of $CD4^+$ $CD25^+$ $Foxp3^+$ and $CD8^+CD25^+Foxp3^+$ Tregs was observed in recipients treated with Flt3L and Rapa as compared with recipients in other groups (Fig. 3).

Flt3L/Rapa Therapy Favors Anergic Induction in Alloreactive T Cells

We then tested the reactivity of bulk T cells isolated from the spleens of the recipients against donor-derived DCs. As shown in Figure 4A, T cells derived from Flt3L/Rapa treated mice exhibited a significantly lower proliferative response against donor BALB/c DCs in MLR when compared with that of T cells derived from untreated, rGST-treated and PBS-treated recipients. Unexpectedly, a similar proliferation rate was noted in recipients treated with either Flt3L or Rapa alone as compared with that of recipients treated with Flt3L/Rapa. This result promoted us to further examine cytokine production in the culture supernatants by ELISA. Of Interestingly note, the production of IL-10 was significantly higher in the Flt3L/Rapa treated mice. More importantly, although T cells derived from Flt3L or Rapa treated mice showed similar potency for proliferation (Fig. 4A), but their capacity for secretion of IL-10 was similar to those T cells from control mice (Fig. 4B). Collectively, our data suggest that Flt3L/Rapa treatment enhances IL-10 secretion which could favor the induction of T anergy.

$CD8^+$ T Cells and pDCs Play a Dominant Role to Promote Allograft Long-term Survival

Given that Flt3L/Rapa therapy resulted in reproducible long-term allograft survival in about 20% of recipients without immunosuppression (Fig. 1A), we thus employed adoptive transfer studies to characterize the cell subpopulations for sustained allograft survival. For this purpose, $CD4^+$ T cells, $CD8^+$ T cells, pDCs and total splenocytes were first isolated from long-term survival recipients, and then adoptively transferred into naive recipients. The mice were next transplanted with cardiac allografts as described. As shown in Figure 5, transferred $CD8^+$ T cells and pDCs exhibited the ability to prolong allograft survival. Unexpectedly, compared with $CD8^+$ T cells and pDCs, adoptive transfer of $CD4^+$ T cells failed to provide protection against allograft rejection.

Flt3L/Rapa Therapy Enhances Autophagy in the Grafts

To determine whether the prolonged allograft survival was associated with enhanced autophagy, we examined the levels of autophagy-related protein beclin-1, microtubule associated protein1 light chain 3 (LC3) I and II by Western blot analysis. As shown in Fig. 6A, only low levels of Beclin-1 and LC3 II were detected in control mice (rGST, untreated and PBS groups), but higher levels of Beclin-1 and LC3 II were observed in mice treated with Flt3L or Rapa alone. Importantly, the highest Beclin-1 and LC3 II expressions were noted in Flt3L/Rapa treated mice. To further confirm these results, we did immunohistochemical analysis, and similar results were obtained (Fig. 6A). To examine the functional relevance for the enhanced autophagy in allograft survival, we performed similar transplantation along with the administration of 3-MA, an autophagy inhibitor [19,20]. As expected, administration of 3-MA significantly repressed autophagy as determined by Western blot and immunohitochemical analysis (Fig. 6B). Remarkably, repression of autophagy significantly attenuated Flt3L/Rapa therapy mediated protection against allograft rejection (Fig. 6C). In consistent with this result, we also observed a decrease for the number of regulatory T cells and regulatory DCs (Fig. 6D). Taken together, these data indicate that autophagy plays an essential role in Flt3L/Rapa therapy mediated protection against allograft rejection.

Discussion

Despite the benefit of Flt3L and Rapa for anti-rejection in setting of transplantation, the effect for Flt3L or Rapa based mono-therapy on allograft survival remains poor [21,22,23,24]. In the present study, we have demonstrated that Flt3Lcombined with low-dose of Rapa could markedly increase graft survival time as

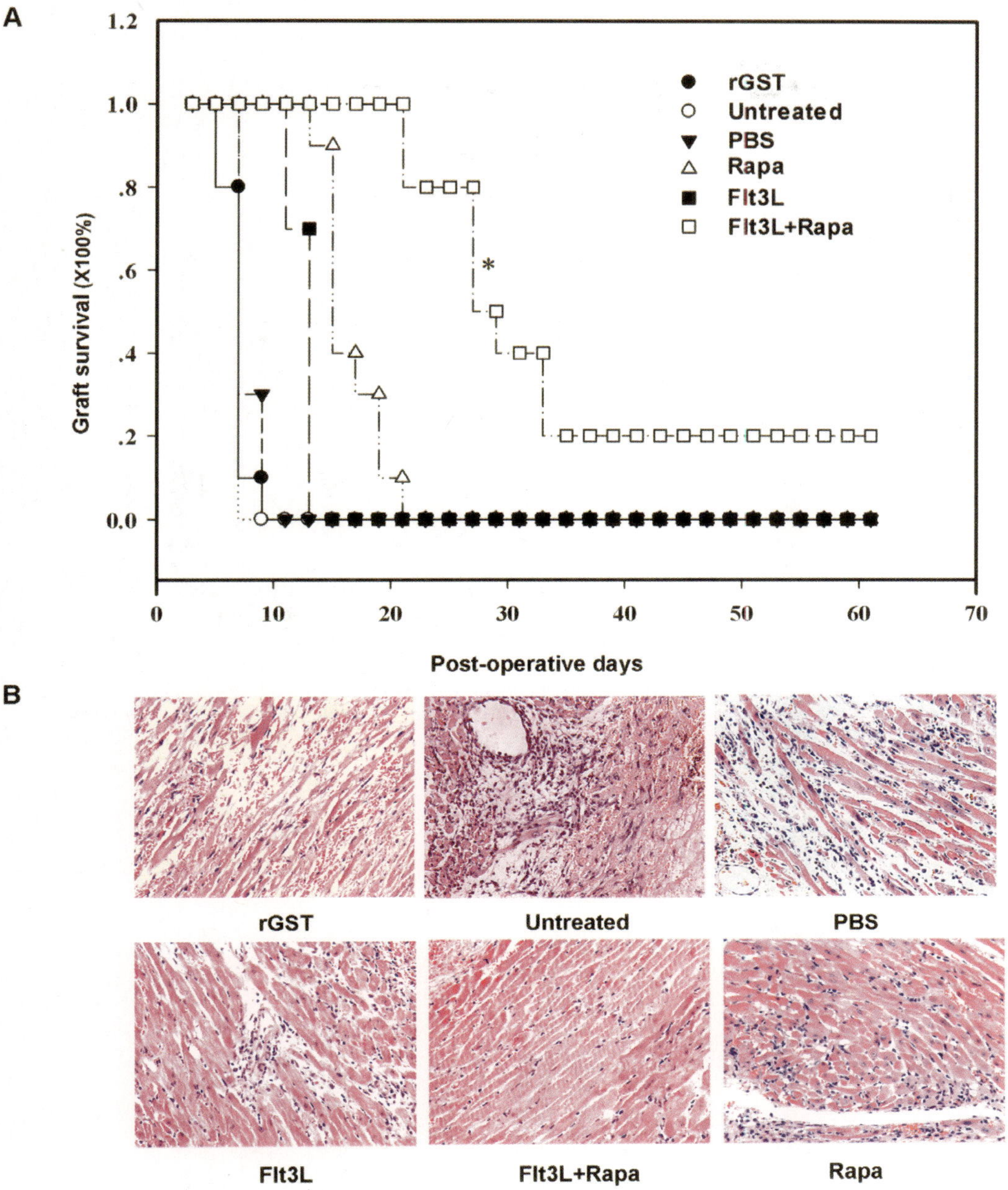

Figure 1. Flt3L combined with low-dose of Rapa prolongs cardiac allograft survival and attenuates infiltrates in the graft. (A) Heart allograft survival. The cardiac allograft survival time in recipients treated with Flt3L (10 μg/day, i.v.) and low-dose of Rapa (2 mg/kg/day; p.o, POD0-15) was significant longer than those of the untreated and monotherapy groups (n = 10) (* $P<0.05$, combination therapy group vs. other groups). (B) Histology of cardiac allografts. Grafts were harvested at the time of rejection or at study endpoint (POD 100) and evaluated by H&E staining of paraffin sections (original magnification, ×200). The results are representative of three independently performed experiments.

compared with that of Flt3L or Rapa alone. The enhanced protective effect was achieved by promoting the generation of tolerogenic DCs and Tregs along with increased autophagy in the allograft.

It has been reported that DCs expanded by Flt3L only express low levels of costimulatory molecules, and therefore, they are able to delay allograft rejection in transplantation settings [25,26]. In contrast to Flt3L or Rapa alone, our data show that Flt3L combined with low-dose of Rapa are more potent to expand DCs with tolerogenic characteristics. Moreover, short-term of low-dose Rapa exerts the effect to expand Tregs while to avoid side effect due to high-dose of Rapa.

Several DC subsets have been reported to promote tolerance induction [4,27]. The $CD11c^+$ $CD8a^+$ DC subset could promote peripheral self-tolerance and prolong the survival of cardiac allografts in rodents [28,29]. More recently, pDC precursors have been identified and are implicated in the induction of allogeneic T-cell hyporesponsiveness [9,30]. In line with these findings, our phenotypic analysis of splenic DCs in the recipient mice revealed that Flt3L/Rapa treatment increased the proportion of DC subsets with regulatory effect such as $CD11c^+$ $CD8a^+$ DCs and pDCs. It is

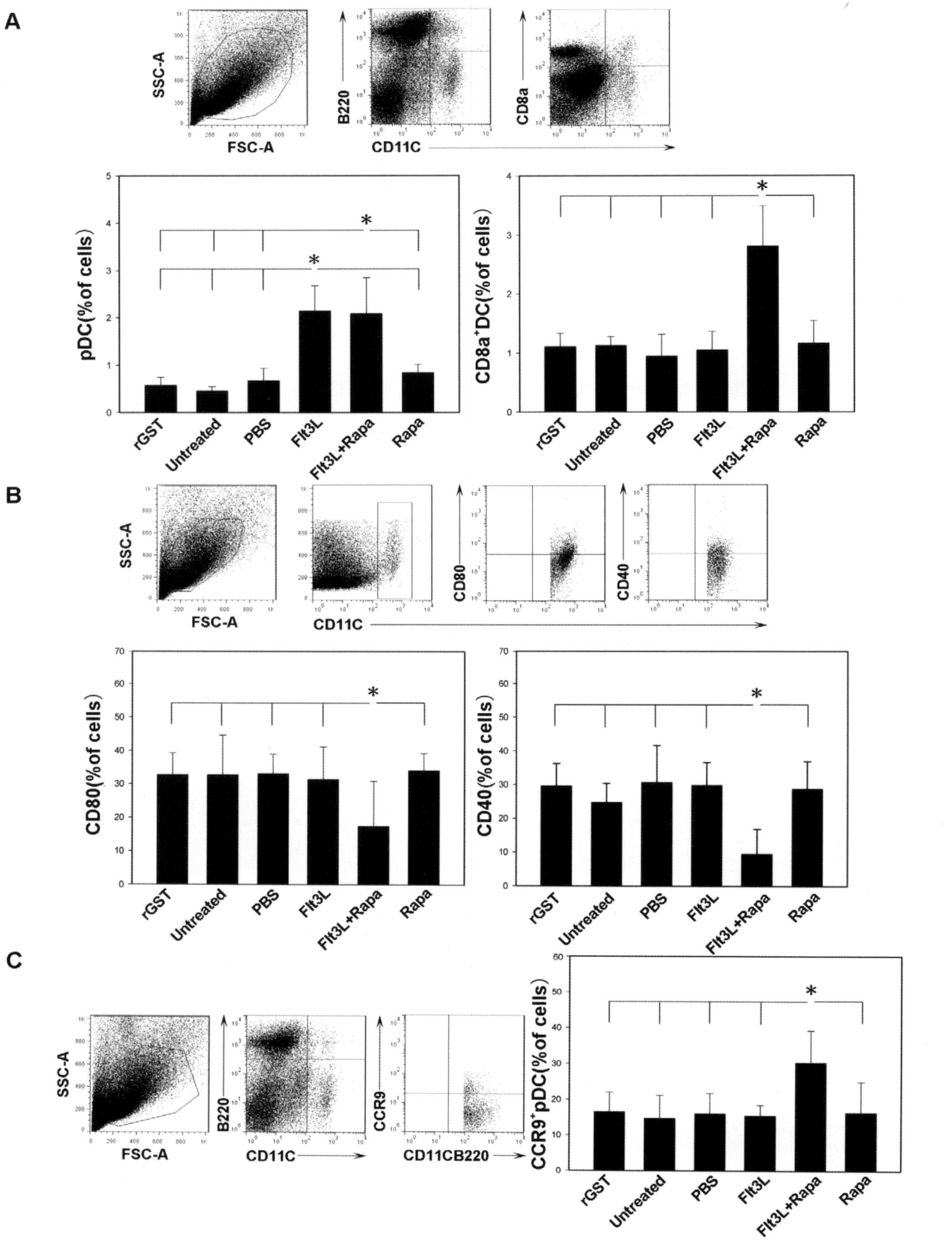
A
SSC-A
FSC-A
B220
CD11C
CD8a
pDC(%of cells)
CD8a⁺DC(%of cells)
*
rGST
Untreated
PBS
Flt3L
Flt3L+Rapa
Rapa
B
SSC-A
FSC-A
CD11C
CD80
CD40
CD80(%of cells)
CD40(%of cells)
C
SSC-A
FSC-A
B220
CD11C
CCR9
CD11CB220
CCR9⁺pDC(%of cells)

Figure 2. DCs from recipients treated with Flt3L/Rapa display a tolerogenic phenotype. Spleen cells isolated from mice treated with Flt3L/Rapa and other control mice at the time of rejection or at study endpoint (POD 100) were stained with PE-cy7-labeled anti-mouse CD11c mAb, Per-cy5.5-labeled anti-mouse B220 mAb, APC-cy7-labeled anti-mouse CD8a mAb, FITC-labeled anti-mouse CCR9 mAb, APC-labeled anti-mouse CD80 mAb and APC-labeled anti-mouse CD40 mAb. $CD11c^+$ and $CD11c^+$ $B220^+$ gated DCs were analyzed by flow cytometry for expression of the various DC markers. (A) The bar graph was a summary of percentages of pDC and $CD8a^+$ DC in the recipients. (B) $CD11c^+$-gated DCs were analyzed for expression of costimulatory markers CD80 and CD40 to assess their maturation state. (C) The percentage of $CCR9^+$ cell of gated pDC subsets was assessed by FACS analysis. The results are representative of three independently performed experiments (* $P<0.05$).

known that immature DCs not only fail to prime T cells effectively, but also serve to promote tolerance induction [31]. Our studies show that Flt3L combined with Rapa could block DC maturation and increase the ratio of $CCR9^+$ pDCs, while $CCR9^+$ pDCs are immature pDCs with potency to suppress antigen-specific immune responses both in vitro and in vivo [18].

Regulatory T cells are a subpopulation of T cells that have the ability to suppress immune reactions and maintain tolerance. They were believed to play a key role in transplant tolerance induction. The most important representative of regulatory T cells is the naturally occurring regulatory T cells (Tregs), with a $CD4^+$ $CD25^+$ $Foxp3^+$ phenotype. They were found to mediate donor-specific

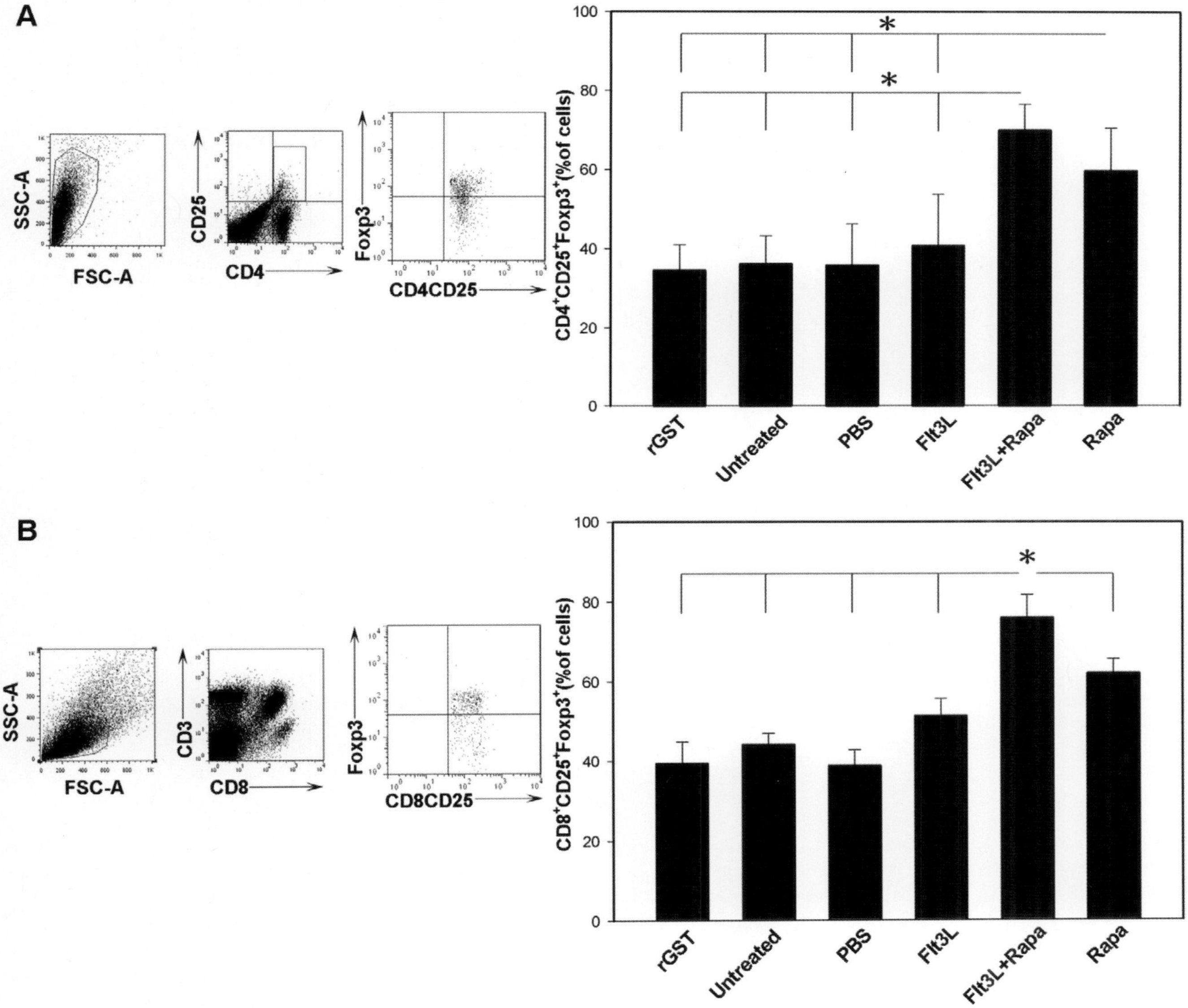

Figure 3. Flt3L combined with Rapa promotes the production of $CD4^+CD25^+Foxp3^+$ and $CD8^+CD25^+Foxp3^+$ T cells. Spleen cells isolated from mice treated with Flt3L/Rapa and other control mice at the time of rejection or at study endpoint (POD 100) were analyzed to determine the proportion of $CD4^+$ $CD25^+$ $Foxp3^+$ and $CD8^+$ $CD25^+$ $Foxp3^+$ T cells. (A, B) The expression of Foxp3 by $CD4^+$ $CD25^+$ and $CD8^+$ $CD25^+$ T cells was analyzed by flow cytometry after intracellular staining. The bar graph was a summary of percentages of $CD4^+$ $CD25^+$ $Foxp3^+$ T cells and $CD8^+$ $CD25^+$ $Foxp3^+$ T cells in the recipients. The data shown are representative of three independent experiments that yielded comparable results (* $P<0.05$).

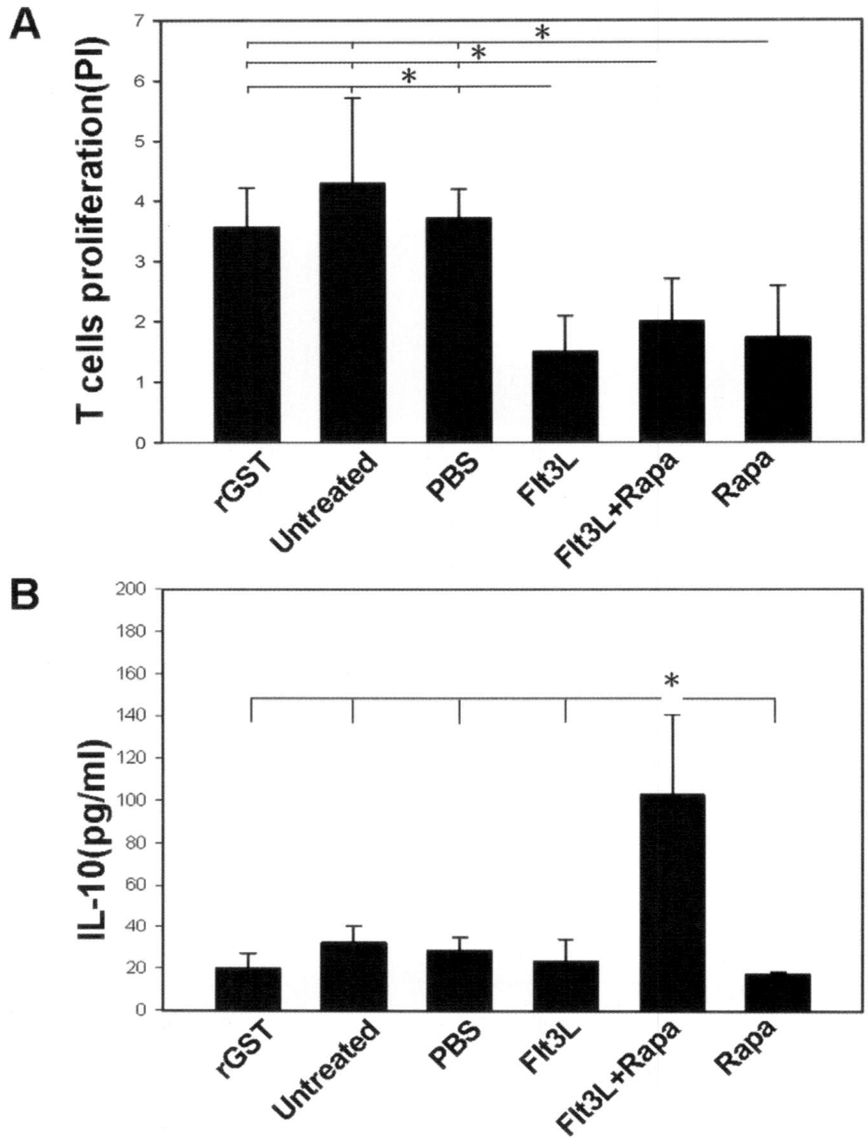

Figure 4. Flt3L/Rapa therapy favors anergic induction in alloreactive T cells. (A) Splenic T cells originated from cardiac allograft recipient mice at the time of rejection or at study endpoint (POD 100) were used as responder cells for MLR assay with donor-derived DCs (DC: T ratio of 1:5). Bar graph was the summary of proliferation index (PI) of T cells isolated from different recipients. (B) The culture supernatants were harvested and cytokine IL-10 levels were quantification by ELISA. The data shown are representative of three independent experiments ($^{*}P<0.05$).

unresponsiveness in some stable renal [32,33,34,35,36] and liver [37] transplant patients. In addition, adoptive transfers of Tregs could prevent allograft rejection and prolong graft survival in the mouse models [38]. Previously, addition of rapamycin to human and murine T cell cultures preferentially expanded regulatory T cells [39,40]. Our data indicated that infusion of Flt3L with Rapa and Rapa alone enhances the production of $CD4^{+}$ $CD25^{+}$ $Foxp3^{+}$ Tregs. In addition, we found a significant increase of splenic $CD8^{+}CD25^{+}Foxp3^{+}$ T cell populations in the recipient mice treated with Flt3L/Rapa, while $CD8^{+}CD25^{+}Foxp3^{+}$ T cell have been found being able to inhibit antigen-specific $CD4^{+}$ and $CD8^{+}$ T cell responses by cell contact inhibition, secretion of cytokines and other ways [41].

Our adoptive transfer studies showed that $CD8^{+}$ T cells are responsible for induction of long-lasting tolerance toward donor alloantigen. We therefore proposed that Flt3L-mobilized recipient DCs might process indirect antigen presentation of allopeptides to induce tolerance for host $CD8^{+}$ alloreactive T cells, which are the main effector mechanism of cellular rejection across an MHC class I barrier. This notion is well supported by a recent study, in which Rapa-conditioned, alloAg-pulsed DC can present acquired MHC-peptide complexes from donor cells and modulate directly-reactive $CD8^{+}$ T cell function, and through which, these DCs enhance Ag-specific $CD8^{+}$ T cell undergoing apoptosis [42]. Furthermore, $CD8^{+}CD28$ T cells may also play an important role in tolerance induction. These T cells represent a transient state of effector $CD8^{+}$ T cells, which promotes the production of the immuno-suppressive cytokine IL-10 [43,44]. Emerging data suggest that the appearance of these T cells in transplant recipients is associated with better graft acceptance along with stable function [45,46,47].

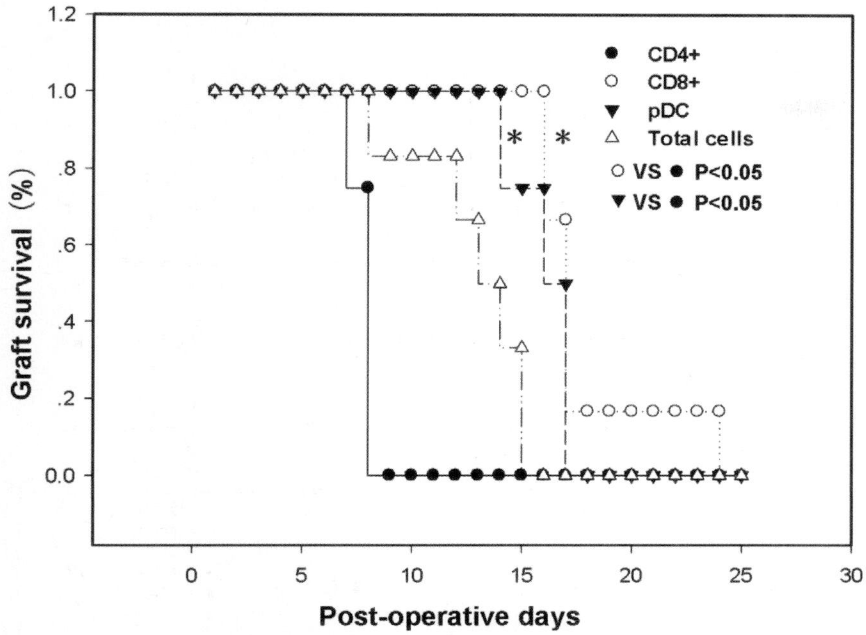

Figure 5. CD8$^+$ T cells and pDCs play a dominant role to promote allograft long-term survival. The purified CD4$^+$ T cells (5×10^6), CD8$^+$ T cells (5×10^6), pDCs (5×10^5) and total splenotytes (5×10^6) originated from recipients with long-term allograft survival were then adoptively transferred into naive recipients respectively. One day after the adoptive transfer, the mice were transplanted with cardiac allograft. The survival time of cardiac allografts was monitored. The data shown are representative of three independent experiments (*$P<0.05$).

Finally, our data indicate that autophagy plays an important role in the protective effect of Flt3L in combination with Rapa on cardiac allograft survival. The possible mechanisms is that autophagy delivers self-proteins for MHC class II loading, and their peptidic fragments are essential for the deletion of self-reactive T cells in the thymus. Recent studies have also suggested that the possible link between autophagy and tolerance is that autophagy plays a role in the removal of apoptotic cell corpses [48]. Regarding to the effect of autophagy on allograft survival seems controversial. In a rat liver transplantation study, it has been shown that autophagy-associated hepatocyte death triggers liver graft dysfunction, and suppression of autophagy prevent cold ischemia-warm reperfusion injury associated with liver transplantation [49]. Thus, further relevant investigations are needed.

Conclusion

In summary, Flt3L combined with Rapamycin is able to promote the prolongation of allograft survival. This protective effect is associated with the generation of tolerogenic DC subsets, CD25$^+$ Foxp3$^+$ regulatory T cells (Tregs), and enhanced allograft autophagy.

Materials and Methods

Mice

Six to eight week-old female C57BL/6 (H-2^b), BALB/c (H-2^d) mice were obtained from the animal facilities at Tongji Medical College. All mice were maintained under specific pathogen-free conditions and the studies were carried out in compliance with the institutional animal care and use guidelines.

Reagents and Antibodies

CFSE was purchased from Invitrogen (Eugene, OR, USA). All kits were obtained as follows: Mouse IL-10 ELISA MAX^{TM} Deluxe was derived from Biolegend. Mouse CD4 (L3T4) MicroBeads (Miltenyi Biotec, CA), Mouse Plasmacytoid Dendritic Cell Isolation Kit II (Miltenyi Biotec, CA), Mouse CD8a (Ly-2) MicroBeads were derived from Miltenyi Biotec, CA. Rapamycin was purchased from Wyeth, USA. 3-Methyladenine was purchased from Sigma. Antibodies for Beclin-1,and LC3B were purchased from cell signaling. PE-cy7-labeled anti-Mouse CD11c (clone N418), Per-cy5.5-labeled anti-Mouse B220 (clone RA3-6B2), FITC-labeled anti-Mouse CCR9 (clone CW-1.2), PE-labeled anti-rat CD3 (clone G4.18), PE-cy7-labeled anti-Mouse CD3 (clone 145-2C11), APC-labeled anti-Mouse CD80 (clone 16-10A1), APC-labeled anti-Mouse CD40 (clone 1C10), anti-Mouse CD16/32 (clone 93), FITC-labeled anti-Mouse CD4 (clone GK1.5), PE-labeled anti-Mouse CD25 (clone PC61.5), APC-cy7-labeled anti-Mouse CD8a (clone 53-6.7), APC-labeled anti-Mouse/Rat Foxp3 (clone FJK-16s) were obtained from eBioscience (San Diego, CA, USA).

Expression and Purification of Recombinant Flt3L

DNA sequence encoding Flt3L (696 bp) was amplified from the C57BL/6 mouse spleen cDNA using the following oligonucleotides: 5′-CGG GAT CCA TGA CAG TGC TGG CGC C-3′ and 5′-CGG AAT TCA TCC TAG GGA TGG GAG-3′. The resulting products were subsequently cloned into a pGEX-4T3 vector with a glutathione S-transferase tag. The plasmid was transformed into Escherichia coli strain BL21. Recombinant Flt3L expression was induced by addition of 1 mM IPTG and then purified using the glutathione sepharose 4B resin columns as instructed by the manufacturer. A GST vector protein was also expressed and purified to homogeneity. The proteins were passed over polymyxin B columns (PIERCE) to remove any contaminated LPS and further concentrated by 3KD Micropore Filters. The purified recombinant Flt3L and rGST were stored in aliquots at −80°C until use.

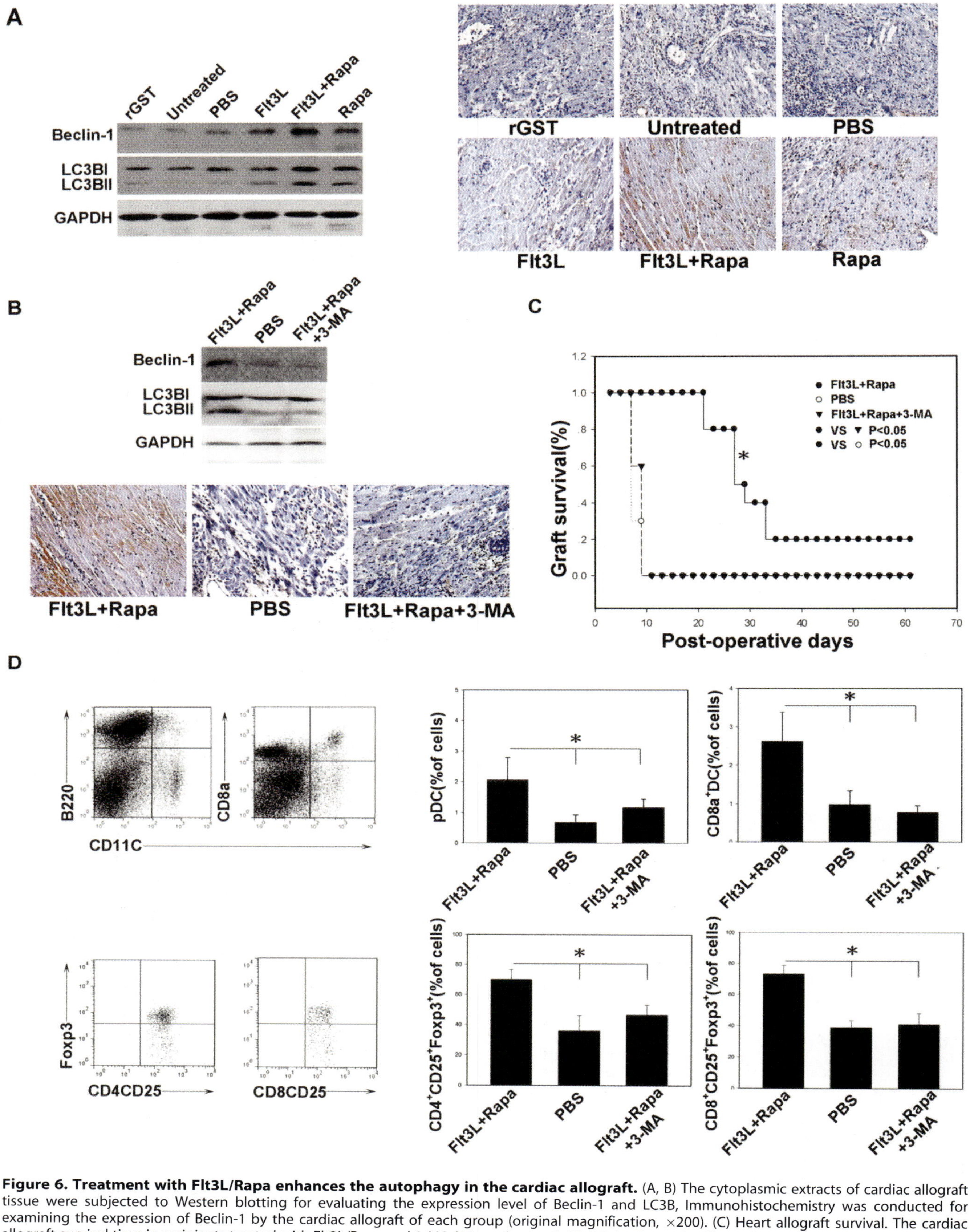

Figure 6. Treatment with Flt3L/Rapa enhances the autophagy in the cardiac allograft. (A, B) The cytoplasmic extracts of cardiac allograft tissue were subjected to Western blotting for evaluating the expression level of Beclin-1 and LC3B, Immunohistochemistry was conducted for examining the expression of Beclin-1 by the cardiac allograft of each group (original magnification, ×200). (C) Heart allograft survival. The cardiac allograft survival time in recipients treated with Flt3L/Rapa and 3-MA (24 mg/kg, i.p, 5, 10, 15 days) was significant shorter than that of the recipients treated with Flt3L/Rapa (* $P<0.05$). (D) The percentage of pDC, $CD8a^+$ DC, $CD4^+$ $CD25^+$ $Foxp3^+$ and $CD8^+$ $CD25^+$ $Foxp3^+$ T cells was assessed by FACS

analysis (* $P<0.05$, combination therapy group vs. other groups at endpoint). All data presented here are representative of three separate experiments with consistent results.

Heart Transplantation Model

Heterotopic cardiac transplantation was performed as previously described [50]. In this study, transplant surgery involved the transfer of fully MHC-mismatched hearts from BALB/c (H-2^d) donors to C57BL/6 (H-2^b) recipients. Heart beat of the grafts was monitored and evaluated daily by direct abdominal palpation to detect the state of cardiac health/rejection.

Experimental Groups

Heart transplant recipients were randomly assigned to six groups (n = 10): Group 1, rGST alone; Group 2, untreated control; Group 3, PBS alone; Group 4, Flt3L alone (10 μg/day, i.v) for 10 consecutive days before heart transplantation; Group 5, Rapa alone (2 mg/kg/day; p.o, POD0-15); Group 6, combination treatment of Flt3L and Rapa.

Graft Histology

Allograft samples were fixed in 4% paraformaldehyde. Serial sections (5 μm in thickness) were prepared using a microtome and stained with hematoxylin/eosin for the analysis of pathological changes.

Flow Cytometric Analysis

Spleen cells isolated from mice treated with Flt3L/Rapa and other control mice were incubated with anti-CD16/CD32 monoclonal antibody to block FcR, and then stained with PE-cy7-labeled anti-mouse CD11c mAb, Per-cy5.5-labeled anti-mouse B220 mAb, APC-cy7-labeled anti-CD8a mAb, FITC-labeled anti-mouse CCR9 mAb, APC-labeled anti-mouse CD80 mAb and APC-labeled anti-mouse CD40 mAb. CD11c$^+$ and CD11c$^+$ B220$^+$ gated DCs were analyzed by flow cytometry for expression of the various DC markers. For analysis of regulatory T cells, splenocytes were isolated from the recipient mice and subsequently co-stained with CD4, CD25 or CD3, CD8a CD25 antibodies. The cells were further stained with Foxp3 using established techniques [51]. Cells were then analyzed using FACS flow cytometer as previously reported [52].

Mixed Lymphocyte Reaction, Cell Proliferation and Cytokine Quantification

Splenic T cells (purified using nylon wool columns) isolated from naive or grafted C57BL/6 mice serving as responders (2×10^6/well) were incubated for 7 days in the presence of Mitomycin C-treated (50 μg/ml, Sigma-Aldrich) DCs used as stimulators derived from naive BALB/c mice (4×10^5/well, DC: T ratio of 1:5) in 12-well flat bottom plates (Nunc, Roskilde, Denmark). Cultures were kept at 37°C in 5% CO_2 atmosphere. Supernatants were recovered after 7 days for determination of IL-10 production. Cytokine level was quantified using Mouse IL-10 ELISA MAX^{TM} Deluxe. T-cell proliferation was assessed by serial dilution of the intracellular CFSE dye as described previously [53].

Western Blot Analysis

Proteins (50 μg) extracted from cardiac allograft were subjected to electrophoresis on a 12% SDS–PAGE and then transferred onto PVDF membranes. The membranes were then incubated with primary antibodies for Beclin-1, LC3B and GAPDH at 37°C for 2 h, respectively. The blots were visualized using enhanced chemiluminescence (Amersham).

Immunohistochemistry

After deparaffin and rehydration, the paraffin-embedded heart sections (5 μm) were treated with 3% H_2O_2 for 5 min. The non-specific proteins were blocked with 5–10% goat serum for 10 min. For Beclin-1 staining, specimens were incubated with a rabbit anti-mouse Bcelin-1 Monoclonal antibody (1:200) at 4°C overnight, followed by incubation with a HRP conjugated goat anti-rabbit secondary antibody. The sections were finally incubated with DAB chromogenic substrate and counterstained with hematoxylin.

Adoptive Transfer Experiments

Total T cells were first enriched with T cells using nylon wool columns, and then subjected to isolation of mouse CD4$^+$ T cells using the (L3T4) MicroBeads, and CD8$^+$ T cells using the mouse CD8a (Ly-2) MicroBeads as instructed (Miltenyi Biotec, CA)., pDCs were isolated using a mouse Plasmacytoid Dendritic Cell Isolation Kit II as instructed (Miltenyi Biotec, CA). The purified CD4$^+$ T cells (5×10^6), CD8$^+$ T cells (5×10^6), pDCs (5×10^5) and total splenocytes (5×10^6) originated from recipients with long-term survival allograft were then adoptively transferred into naive recipients, respectively. One day after the adoptive transfer, the mice were transplanted with cardiac allografts and monitored for allograft survival as described above.

Statistical Analysis

The data are presented as means ± SD. Statistical differences were determined by one-way ANOVA. Allograft survival differences between groups were determined using the log-rank test. P values less than 0.05 were considered with statistical significant.

Author Contributions

Conceived and designed the experiments: AX MF FG. Performed the experiments: AX LD JC. Analyzed the data: AX MF ZF. Contributed reagents/materials/analysis tools: FZ ZT. Wrote the paper: AX MF FG.

References

1. Sayegh MH, Carpenter CB (2004) Transplantation 50 years later–progress, challenges, and promises. N Engl J Med. 2004/12/24 ed. 2761–2766.
2. Fishman JA (2007) Medical progress: Infection in solid-organ transplant recipients. New England Journal of Medicine 357: 2601–2614.
3. Tantravahi J, Womer KL, Kaplan B (2007) Why hasn't eliminating acute rejection improved graft survival? Annu Rev Med 58: 369–385.
4. Morelli AE, Thomson AW (2007) Tolerogenic dendritic cells and the quest for transplant tolerance. Nat Rev Immunol 7: 610–621.
5. Banchereau J, Briere F, Caux C, Davoust J, Lebecque S, et al. (2000) Immunobiology of dendritic cells. Annu Rev Immunol 18: 767–811.
6. Steinman RM, Hawiger D, Nussenzweig MC (2003) Tolerogenic dendritic cells. Annu Rev Immunol 21: 685–711.
7. Matthews W, Jordan CT, Wiegand GW, Pardoll D, Lemischka IR (1991) A receptor tyrosine kinase specific to hematopoietic stem and progenitor cell-enriched populations. Cell 65: 1143–1152.
8. Schmid MA, Kingston D, Boddupalli S, Manz MG (2010) Instructive cytokine signals in dendritic cell lineage commitment. Immunol Rev 234: 32–44.
9. Abe M, Wang Z, de Creus A, Thomson AW (2005) Plasmacytoid dendritic cell precursors induce allogeneic T-cell hyporesponsiveness and prolong heart graft survival. Am J Transplant 5: 1808–1819.
10. Starzl TE, Demetris AJ, Trucco M, Murase N, Ricordi C, et al. (1993) Cell migration and chimerism after whole-organ transplantation: the basis of graft acceptance. Hepatology 17: 1127–1152.

11. Starzl TE, Demetris AJ, Murase N, Trucco M, Thomson AW, et al. (1996) The lost chord: microchimerism and allograft survival. Immunol Today 17: 577–584; discussion 588.
12. Lunemann JD, Munz C (2009) Autophagy in CD4+ T-cell immunity and tolerance. Cell Death Differ 16: 79–86.
13. Schmid D, Pypaert M, Munz C (2007) Antigen-loading compartments for major histocompatibility complex class II molecules continuously receive input from autophagosomes. Immunity 26: 79–92.
14. Steinman RM, Banchereau J (2007) Taking dendritic cells into medicine. Nature 449: 419–426.
15. Hackstein H, Taner T, Zahorchak AF, Morelli AE, Logar AJ, et al. (2003) Rapamycin inhibits IL-4-induced dendritic cell maturation in vitro and dendritic cell mobilization and function in vivo. Blood 101: 4457–4463.
16. Fu F, Li Y, Qian S, Lu L, Chambers F, et al. (1996) Costimulatory molecule-deficient dendritic cell progenitors (MHC class II+, CD80dim, CD86-) prolong cardiac allograft survival in nonimmunosuppressed recipients. Transplantation 62: 659–665.
17. Rastellini C, Lu L, Ricordi C, Starzl TE, Rao AS, et al. (1995) Granulocyte/macrophage colony-stimulating factor-stimulated hepatic dendritic cell progenitors prolong pancreatic islet allograft survival. Transplantation 60: 1366–1370.
18. Hadeiba H, Sato T, Habtezion A, Oderup C, Pan J, et al. (2008) CCR9 expression defines tolerogenic plasmacytoid dendritic cells able to suppress acute graft-versus-host disease. Nat Immunol 9: 1253–1260.
19. Blommaart EF, Krause U, Schellens JP, Vreeling-Sindelarova H, Meijer AJ (1997) The phosphatidylinositol 3-kinase inhibitors wortmannin and LY294002 inhibit autophagy in isolated rat hepatocytes. Eur J Biochem 243: 240–246.
20. Petiot A, Ogier-Denis E, Blommaart EF, Meijer AJ, Codogno P (2000) Distinct classes of phosphatidylinositol 3′-kinases are involved in signaling pathways that control macroautophagy in HT-29 cells. J Biol Chem 275: 992–998.
21. Saunders RN, Metcalfe MS, Nicholson ML (2001) Rapamycin in transplantation: a review of the evidence. Kidney Int 59: 3–16.
22. Kahan BD, Camardo JS (2001) Rapamycin: clinical results and future opportunities. Transplantation 72: 1181–1193.
23. Steptoe RJ, Fu F, Li W, Drakes ML, Lu L, et al. (1997) Augmentation of dendritic cells in murine organ donors by Flt3 ligand alters the balance between transplant tolerance and immunity. J Immunol 159: 5483–5491.
24. Ge W, Jiang J, Baroja ML, Arp J, Zassoko R, et al. (2009) Infusion of mesenchymal stem cells and rapamycin synergize to attenuate alloimmune responses and promote cardiac allograft tolerance. Am J Transplant 9: 1760–1772.
25. Coates PT, Duncan FJ, Colvin BL, Wang Z, Zahorchak AF, et al. (2004) In vivo-mobilized kidney dendritic cells are functionally immature, subvert alloreactive T-cell responses, and prolong organ allograft survival. Transplantation 77: 1080–1089.
26. Emmanouilidis N, Guo Z, Dong Y, Newton-West M, Adams AB, et al. (2006) Immunosuppressive and trafficking properties of donor splenic and bone marrow dendritic cells. Transplantation 81: 455–462.
27. Munn DH, Sharma MD, Hou D, Baban B, Lee JR, et al. (2004) Expression of indoleamine 2,3-dioxygenase by plasmacytoid dendritic cells in tumor-draining lymph nodes. J Clin Invest 114: 280–290.
28. Belz GT, Behrens GM, Smith CM, Miller JF, Jones C, et al. (2002) The CD8alpha(+) dendritic cell is responsible for inducing peripheral self-tolerance to tissue-associated antigens. J Exp Med 196: 1099–1104.
29. O'Connell PJ, Li W, Wang Z, Specht SM, Logar AJ, et al. (2002) Immature and mature CD8alpha+ dendritic cells prolong the survival of vascularized heart allografts. J Immunol 168: 143–154.
30. Liu YJ (2005) IPC: professional type 1 interferon-producing cells and plasmacytoid dendritic cell precursors. Annu Rev Immunol 23: 275–306.
31. Dhodapkar MV, Steinman RM, Krasovsky J, Munz C, Bhardwaj N (2001) Antigen-specific inhibition of effector T cell function in humans after injection of immature dendritic cells. J Exp Med 193: 233–238.
32. Velthuis JH, Mol WM, Weimar W, Baan CC (2006) CD4+CD25bright+ regulatory T cells can mediate donor nonreactivity in long-term immunosuppressed kidney allograft patients. Am J Transplant 6: 2955–2964.
33. Baan CC, Velthuis JH, van Gurp EA, Mol WM, Klepper M, et al. (2007) Functional CD25(bright+) alloresponsive T cells in fully immunosuppressed renal allograft recipients. Clin Transplant 21: 63–71.
34. Velthuis JH, Hesselink DA, Hendrikx TK, van der Mast BJ, Klepper M, et al. (2007) Kinetic analysis reveals potency of CD4+ CD25bright+ regulatory T-cells in kidney transplant patients. Transpl Immunol 18: 159–165.
35. Hendrikx TK, van Gurp EA, Sewgobind VD, Mol WM, Schoordijk W, et al. (2009) Generation of donor-specific regulatory T-cell function in kidney transplant patients. Transplantation 87: 376–383.
36. Wang Z, Fu XY, Shi BY, Qian YY, Xiao L, et al. (2009) Antigen-specific suppression by induced CD4+CD25high regulatory T cells in kidney recipients. Transplant Proc 41: 1574–1576.
37. Yoshizawa A, Ito A, Li Y, Koshiba T, Sakaguchi S, et al. (2005) The roles of CD25+CD4+ regulatory T cells in operational tolerance after living donor liver transplantation. Transplant Proc 37: 37–39.
38. Lee MKt, Moore DJ, Jarrett BP, Lian MM, Deng S, et al. (2004) Promotion of allograft survival by CD4+CD25+ regulatory T cells: evidence for in vivo inhibition of effector cell proliferation. J Immunol 172: 6539–6544.
39. Battaglia M, Stabilini A, Migliavacca B, Horejs-Hoeck J, Kaupper T, et al. (2006) Rapamycin promotes expansion of functional CD4+CD25+FOXP3+ regulatory T cells of both healthy subjects and type 1 diabetic patients. J Immunol 177: 8338–8347.
40. Battaglia M, Stabilini A, Roncarolo MG (2005) Rapamycin selectively expands CD4+CD25+FoxP3+ regulatory T cells. Blood 105: 4743–4748.
41. Lee HK, Mattei LM, Steinberg BE, Alberts P, Lee YH, et al. (2010) In vivo requirement for Atg5 in antigen presentation by dendritic cells. Immunity 32: 227–239.
42. Fischer RT, Turnquist HR, Wang Z, Beer-Stolz D, Thomson AW (2011) Rapamycin-conditioned, alloantigen-pulsed myeloid dendritic cells present donor MHC class I/peptide via the semi-direct pathway and inhibit survival of antigen-specific CD8(+) T cells in vitro and in vivo. Transpl Immunol 25: 20–26.
43. Trandem K, Zhao J, Fleming E, Perlman S (2011) Highly activated cytotoxic CD8 T cells express protective IL-10 at the peak of coronavirus-induced encephalitis. J Immunol 186: 3642–3652.
44. Zhang N, Bevan MJ (2011) CD8(+) T cells: foot soldiers of the immune system. Immunity 35: 161–168.
45. Suciu-Foca N, Manavalan JS, Scotto L, Kim-Schulze S, Galluzzo S, et al. (2005) Molecular characterization of allospecific T suppressor and tolerogenic dendritic cells: review. Int Immunopharmacol 5: 7–11.
46. Lin YX, Wang LL, Yan LN, Cai P, Li B, et al. (2009) Analysis of CD8+CD28− T-suppressor cells in living donor liver transplant recipients. Hepatobiliary Pancreat Dis Int 8: 241–246.
47. Strioga M, Pasukoniene V, Characiejus D (2011) CD8+ CD28− and CD8+ CD57+ T cells and their role in health and disease. Immunology 134: 17–32.
48. Qu X, Zou Z, Sun Q, Luby-Phelps K, Cheng P, et al. (2007) Autophagy gene-dependent clearance of apoptotic cells during embryonic development. Cell 128: 931–946.
49. Gotoh K, Lu Z, Morita M, Shibata M, Koike M, et al. (2009) Participation of autophagy in the initiation of graft dysfunction after rat liver transplantation. Autophagy 5: 351–360.
50. Corry RJ, Winn HJ, Russell PS (1973) Heart transplantation in congenic strains of mice. Transplant Proc 5: 733–735.
51. Huang Y, Yin H, Han J, Huang B, Xu J, et al. (2007) Extracellular hmgb1 functions as an innate immune-mediator implicated in murine cardiac allograft acute rejection. Am J Transplant 7: 799–808.
52. Yu G, Fang M, Gong M, Liu L, Zhong J, et al. (2008) Steady state dendritic cells with forced IDO expression induce skin allograft tolerance by upregulation of regulatory T cells. Transpl Immunol 18: 208–219.
53. Lyons AB (2000) Analysing cell division in vivo and in vitro using flow cytometric measurement of CFSE dye dilution. J Immunol Methods 243: 147–154.

11

Common Gamma Chain Cytokines Promote Rapid *In Vitro* Expansion of Allo-Specific Human CD8$^+$ Suppressor T Cells

Yuming Yu[1,2], Jennifer R. Zitzner[1], Josetta Houlihan[1], Nancy Herrera[1], Luting Xu[1], Joshua Miller[1], James M. Mathew[1], Anat R. Tambur[1], Xunrong Luo[1,3]*

1 Comprehensive Transplant Center, Northwestern University Feinberg School of Medicine, Chicago, Illinois, United States of America, **2** Department of Organ Transplantation, Nanfang Hospital, Southern Medical University, Guangzhou, Guangdong, China, **3** Department of Medicine, Northwestern University Feinberg School of Medicine, Chicago, Illinois, United States of America

Abstract

Human CD8$^+$ regulatory T cells, particularly the CD8$^+$CD28$^-$ T suppressor cells, have emerged as an important modulator of alloimmunity. Understanding the conditions under which these cells are induced and/or expanded would greatly facilitate their application in future clinical trials. In the current study, we develop a novel strategy that combines common gamma chain (γc) cytokines IL-2, IL-7 and IL-15 and donor antigen presenting cells (APCs) to stimulate full HLA-mismatched allogeneic human CD8$^+$ T cells which results in significant expansions of donor-specific CD8$^+$CD28$^-$ T suppressor cells *in vitro*. The expanded CD8$^+$CD28$^-$ T cells exhibit increased expressions of CTLA-4, FoxP3, and CD25, while down-regulate expressions of CD56, CD57, CD127, and perforin. Furthermore, these cells suppress proliferation of CD4$^+$ T cells in a contact-dependent and cytokine-independent manner. Interestingly, the specificity of suppression is restricted by the donor HLA class I antigens but promiscuous to HLA class II antigens, providing a potential mechanism for linked suppression. Taken together, our results demonstrate a novel role for common γc cytokines in combination with donor APCs in the expansion of donor-specific CD8$^+$CD28$^-$ T suppressor cells, and represent a robust strategy for *in vitro* generation of such cells for adoptive cellular immunotherapy in transplantation.

Editor: Gernot Zissel, University Medical Center Freiburg, Germany

Funding: This work was supported by grants from the National Institutes of Health Training Grant T32 DK077662 (JH), NIH K08 DK070029 (XL) and NIH Directors New Innovator Award DP2 DK083099 (XL). The funders had no role in study design, data collection and analysis, decision to publish, or preparation of the manuscript.

Competing Interests: The authors have declared that no competing interests exist.

* E-mail: xunrongluo@northwestern.edu

Introduction

Allogeneic organ transplantation has emerged as the current best therapeutic option for selected patients with end stage organ failure. Tolerance induction is highly desirable in this population, because long-term immunosuppressive therapy is associated with significant risks for opportunistic infections, degenerative and metabolic diseases, as well as malignancies. Regulatory T cell (Treg) based therapy has emerged as a promising means for immunomodulation to achieve transplant tolerance. Great interest has been focused on CD4$^+$ Tregs [1], and cell therapies using adoptive transfer of *in vitro* generated CD4$^+$ Treg cells have demonstrated promising efficacy for immunomodulation in animal models of allogeneic transplantation as well as in clinical trials of human allogeneic bone marrow transplantation for the control of graft versus host disease [2,3,4]. However, evidence also suggests that CD8$^+$ Tregs may play an important regulatory role in transplant tolerance [5,6,7,8], in addition to possible immunomodulatory roles in autoimmune disorders [9,10], cancers [11] and aging [12]. Several subsets of CD8$^+$ Tregs have been observed. Natural CD8$^+$ Tregs have been reported to be CD8$^+$CD25$^+$, CD8$^+$CD122$^+$, or CD8$^+$CXCR3$^+$ in different systems [13,14,15]. Induced CD8$^+$ Tregs have also been reported to bear various phenotypic characteristics, such as CD28$^-$, CD56$^+$, CD57$^+$, CTLA4$^+$, CD103$^+$, CD25$^+$Foxp3$^+$ or LAG3$^+$CCL4$^+$ [5,16,17,18,19]. These natural or induced CD8$^+$ Tregs exert their suppressive function by cell-cell contact [5] or by producing soluble cytokines [15,17], and in some circumstances by inducing tolerogenicity in antigen presenting cells (APCs) [20].

Among the various CD8$^+$ Tregs, CD8$^+$CD28$^-$ T suppressor cells have emerged as an important modulator of alloimmunity. Human *allo-specific* CD8$^+$CD28$^-$ cells have been shown to emerge after repeated stimulation with allogeneic APCs with supplemental recombinant human IL-2 *in vitro* [5]. These cells have subsequently been termed "Ts cells". Similarly, *autoantigen-specific* CD8$^+$ Tregs including CD8$^+$CD28$^-$ cells have been reported to be induced *in vitro* via stimulation of peripheral T cells obtained from patients with systemic lupus erythematosus (SLE) in the presence of a combination of common gamma chain (γc) cytokines IL-2, IL-7 and IL-15 [21]. These conditions under which CD8$^+$CD28$^-$ cells are induced are distinct from those in which CD4$^+$ Tregs are induced, in that the latter frequently require the presence of tolerance promoting agents such as TGF-β, IL-10, or rapamycin in the culture [22,23,24,25]. While the mechanisms by which

CD8$^+$CD28$^-$ cells are induced under such apparently non-tolerance promoting conditions remain unclear, the induced CD8$^+$CD28$^-$ cells nevertheless exhibit potent antigen-specific suppressive capacities [5,21]. The γc cytokines have also been reported to induce stable loss of CD28 expression in actively dividing CD8$^+$CD28$^+$ T cells [26,27], thereby promoting the generation of a preponderance of CD8$^+$CD28$^-$ T cells. We therefore questioned if γc cytokines in combination with donor APCs may be used to expand *donor-specific* CD8$^+$CD28$^-$ T suppressor cells in large numbers *in vitro*, and if so, what the mechanisms of donor-specific suppression are.

In this report, we utilized APCs and T cells variably matched for human leukocyte antigen (HLA) class I or class II to study the ability and mechanisms of suppression of the CD8$^+$CD28$^-$ T cells generated *in vitro* by this novel approach of combining allogeneic APCs plus γc cytokines. Our findings indicate that large numbers of CD8$^+$CD28$^-$ T cells with potent donor-specific suppressive capacity can be effectively generated *in vitro* using this approach. Furthermore, their suppressive capacity is contact-dependent and is restricted only by the donor HLA class I antigens but promiscuous to HLA class II antigens. To our knowledge, this is the first report demonstrating a role of combination γc cytokines in the *in vitro* generation of large numbers of human donor-specific CD8$^+$CD28$^-$ suppressor cells. Findings from this study may have important implications for designing future Treg based therapies for prevention of rejection in human organ or tissue transplantation.

Results

Donor APCs plus γc cytokines induce rapid expansion of CD8$^+$CD28$^-$ T cells in culture

The CD28$^-$ cell population accounts for a small fraction of freshly isolated human CD8$^+$ T cells from PBMCs (5.5%, Figure 1A, top panel, Day 0). Fresh CD8$^+$ T cells were stimulated with HLA-A, -B and -DR complete-mismatched APCs in the presence of IL-2 alone or a combination of γc cytokines IL-2, IL-7 and IL-15 as described in *Materials and Methods* [21]. As shown in Figure 1A bottom panels (Day 6, Day 9), culture in the presence of IL-2 alone allowed only minimal increase of the CD28$^-$ population over time. In contrast, culture in the presence of a combination of γc cytokines IL-2, IL-7 and IL-15 significantly increased this population from 5.5% of all CD8$^+$ cells on day 0 to 45.7% (51.5+/−8.5%) on day 6, and 55.5% (58.5+/−7.2%) on day 9 (Figure 1*A*), likely representing down-regulation of cell surface CD28 during the *in vitro* cell activation as previously described [26,27]. The total number of CD8$^+$CD28$^-$ recovered at the end of the 9 day culture increased by ~26.7+/−7.5 fold (Figure 1*B*). The most dramatic increase of this population was observed when IL-15 was added to the culture, with moderate effect observed with IL-7 on the expansion of this population (data not shown).

In vitro expanded CD8$^+$CD28$^-$ T cells suppress CD4$^+$ T cells proliferation in a donor-specific manner

CD8$^+$CD28$^-$ T cells were generated from individual A by culturing with allogeneic APCs from individual B (designated as B-$_{APC}$) in the presence of the γc cytokine combination as described above. After 9 days of culture, the resulting CD8$^+$CD28$^-$ T cells were isolated (purity>95%) and used as suppressors (S) to test for their suppressive capacity in mixed lymphocyte reactions (MLRs) using CD4$^+$ T cells from individual A (designated as A-T4) as responders (R). Suppressor to responder ratios (S:R) of 0.5:1, 0.1:1 and 0.02:1 were tested (with the cell number of "R" kept constant). As shown in Figure 2*A*, when APCs from the original priming stimulator (B-$_{APC}$) were used as stimulators of the MLRs, proliferation of A-T4 (measured by CFSE dilution) was markedly suppressed in a dose-dependent manner by the *in vitro* expanded CD8$^+$CD28$^-$ T cells. Suppression was also confirmed by using ^{3}H-thymidine incorporation as a read-out (Figure 2*B*). In contrast, when APCs from an HLA-A, -B and -DR mismatched indifferent stimulator (I-$_{APC}$) were used as stimulators of the MLRs, CD8$^+$CD28$^-$ cells exhibited only marginal suppression at the highest S:R ratio tested (0.5:1, shown in Fig. 2*A*, middle panels). No suppression could be demonstrated when anti-CD3/CD28 coated Dynabeads were used for stimulating the CD4$^+$ T cells (Figure 2*A*, bottom panels). Taken together, our results indicate that the CD8$^+$CD28$^-$ T cell generated from donor APCs plus γc cytokine-driven *in vitro* expansion suppress CD4$^+$ T cells proliferation *only* in a donor-specific manner.

Suppression by the *in vitro* expanded CD8$^+$CD28$^-$ T cells is restricted by donor HLA class I antigens but promiscuous to HLA class II antigens

To determine whether the donor specificity observed in the above suppression of proliferation was restricted via recognition of HLA class I antigens only, we examined the ability of the CD8$^+$CD28$^-$ T cells generated from culturing with B-$_{APC}$ to suppress proliferation stimulated by APCs from a third-party donor (C-$_{APC}$) who shared identical HLA class I but not class II antigens with individual B. The ability of suppressing C-$_{APC}$ driven proliferation was compared with that of suppressing I-$_{APC}$ driven proliferation (I-$_{APC}$ were from an indifferent individual who was mismatched with individual A for *both* HLA class I and class II antigens). Table 1 provides one example of the HLA class I and class II antigen typing of individuals A, B, C, and I used for one of three such experiments. As shown representatively in Figure 3, proliferation of A-T4 was profoundly suppressed when B-$_{APC}$ was used as the stimulator as expected. Interestingly, a significant suppression was also observed, albeit at a slightly reduced level, when C-$_{APC}$ was used as the stimulator. In contrast, suppression was almost completely lost when I-$_{APC}$ was used as the stimulator. These data support the hypothesis that suppression by the *in vitro* expanded CD8$^+$CD28$^-$ T cells is mediated via specific interactions between the T cell receptor (TCR) on the CD8$^+$ cells and donor HLA class I molecules on the APCs, and such interactions can lead to suppression of CD4$^+$ cells with TCRs specific for HLA class II molecules co-expressed on the same interacting APCs (the C-$_{APC}$ in this case) but different from those expressed on the original priming APCs (the B-$_{APC}$ in this case). This finding corroborates with the previous observation that CD8 suppressor cells are capable of exerting linked suppression via interactions with APCs [28].

Suppression by the *in vitro* expanded CD8$^+$CD28$^-$ T cells is contact dependent but IFN-γ or TGF-β independent

The role of cell-cell contact in suppression was examined using transwell assays as shown in Figure 4*A*. The lower chamber was plated with CFSE-labeled responder cells (R) and stimulator cells (B-$_{APC}$), and the *in vitro* expanded CD8$^+$CD28$^-$ T cells (S) were added either in the lower chamber to allow cell-cell contact or in the upper chamber to prevent cell-cell contact. As shown in Figure 4*A*, suppression of proliferation by CD8$^+$CD28$^-$ T cells was abolished when these cells were plated in the upper chamber of the transwells, indicating that suppression by these cells requires cell-cell contact between the CD8$^+$CD28$^-$ T cells, stimulator APCs and/or the responder CD4$^+$ T cells. This finding is

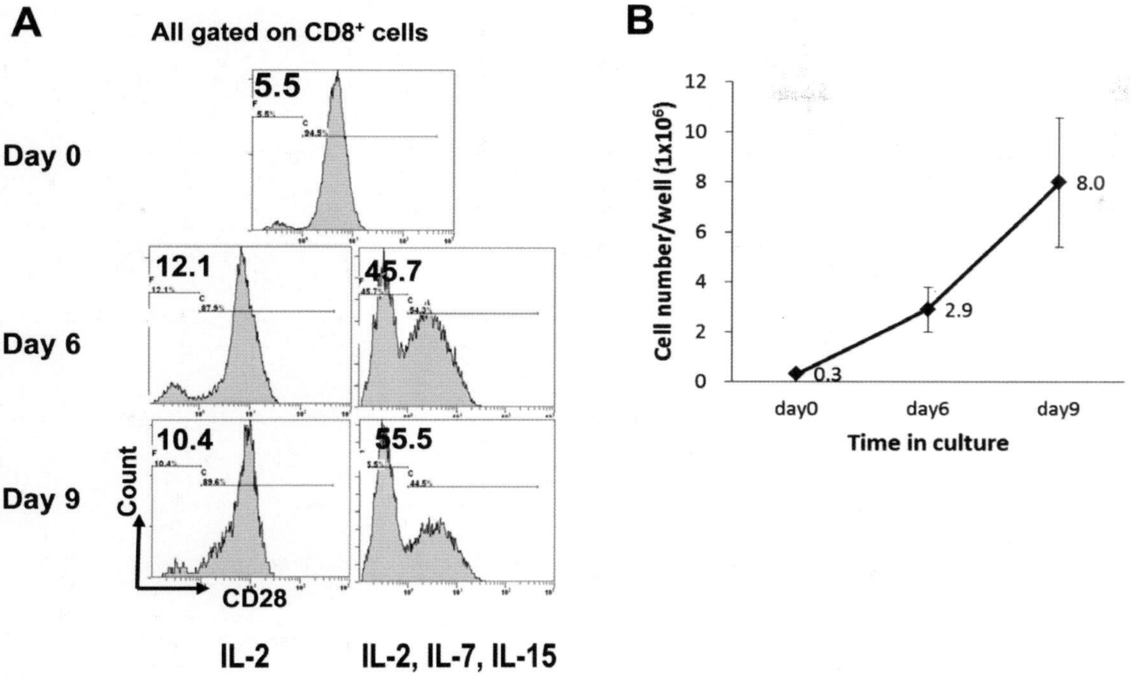

Figure 1. Donor APCs plus γc cytokines induce rapid expansion of CD8$^+$CD28$^-$ T cells in culture. Freshly purified CD8$^+$ T cells (2×10^6 per well) from healthy volunteers were stimulated by HLA-A, B and DR mismatched allogeneic APCs (1×10^6 per well) for 9 days in 24-well plates supplemented with IL-2 alone or a combination of IL-2, IL-7 and IL-15. *A*, Expression of CD28 on CD8$^+$ cells over time. Histograms were gated on the CD8$^+$ population. *B*, Expansion of cell numbers of the CD8$^+$CD28$^-$ population over time by donor APC plus γc cytokines stimulation. The numbers of the CD8$^+$CD28$^-$ cells per well of 24-well culture plates were calculated for day 0, 6 and 9. Data shown in *A* are representative of three independent experiments. Data shown in *B* is the average of three independent experiments.

consistent with the characteristic donor HLA class I restriction of the suppressive activity of the *in vitro* expanded CD8$^+$CD28$^-$ T cells observed in Figure 3.

Several reports have implicated TGF-β [13,29,30] and IFN-γ [8,31,32] in the mechanisms of regulation by CD8$^+$ suppressor cells. To test for a potential role of TGF-β or IFN-γ in the

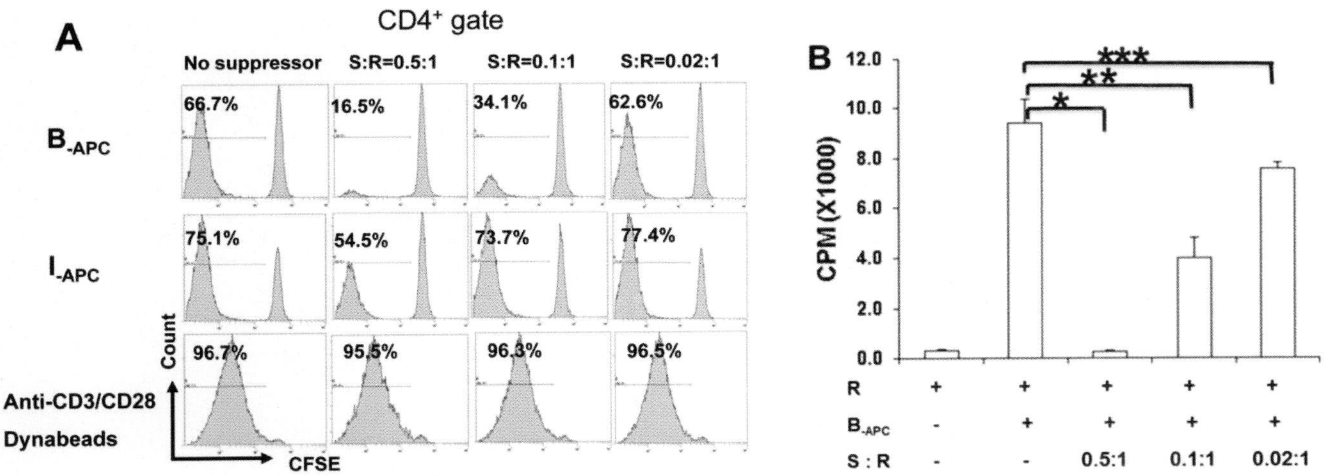

Figure 2. *In vitro* expanded CD8$^+$CD28$^-$ T cells suppress CD4$^+$ T cells proliferation in a donor-specific manner. CD8$^+$ T cells from donor A were stimulated with APCs from donor B plus γc cytokines for 9 days, followed by enrichment of the CD8$^+$CD28$^-$ population as described in *Materials and Methods.* 5×10^4 CFSE labeled purified responder CD4$^+$ T cells (R) from donor A were stimulated with 5×10^4 APCs from donor B (B-$_{APC}$) or from an indifferent donor (I-$_{APC}$, HLA-A, B and DR fully mismatched with donor B), or 1×10^4 anti-CD3/CD28 coated Dynabeads in triplicates in 96-well plates. The *in vitro* expanded CD8$^+$CD28$^-$ T cells were added as putative suppressors (S) at S:R ratios of 0.5:1, 0.1:1 and 0.02:1 (with the cell number of "R" kept constant). Proliferation of the CD4$^+$ cells was measured by CFSE dilution (*A*) or by ^{3}H thymidine uptake (*B*). Data shown are representative of three independent experiments. * $P=0.002$; ** $P=0.009$; *** $P=0.008$.

Table 1. Representative HLA typing of donors used for experiments demonstrating HLA class I antigen specificity shown in Figure 3.

Cell type	HLA-A		HLA-B		HLA-DR	
A ($CD8^+CD28^-$ cells or A-T4	11	-	18	35	1	7
B_{-APC}	1	2	8	44	4	15(2)
C_{-APC}	1	2	8	44	3	12(5)
I_{-APC}	24	26	7	61	9	10

The HLA typing of donors for $CD8^+$ T cells for generation of $CD8^+CD28^-$ suppressor cells, the priming B_{-APC} cells, the partially matched C_{-APC} cells (which shared identical HLA-A, -B, but not HLA-DR, with B_{-APC}), or the fully mismatched I_{-APC} cells (HLA-A, B and DR fully mismatched with B_{-APC}) are shown. Two additional sets of donors A, B, C, and I were used for repeating this experiment for a total of three independent times.

suppressive capacity of the *in vitro* expanded $CD8^+CD28^-$ T cells in our system, anti-human IFN-γ or anti-human TGF-β antibody was added to the suppression assays described above (baseline suppression without the blocking antibodies is shown in Figure 4*B*). As shown in Figure 4*C* and Figure 4*D*, neither anti-IFN-γ nor anti-TGF-β antibodies at increasing concentrations affected suppression by $CD8^+CD28^-$ T cells.

In vitro expanded $CD8^+CD28^-$ T cells do not exhibit cytotoxicity

To test whether cytotoxicity towards the stimulating APCs contributes to the suppression of donor-specific proliferation observed above, we assessed the cytotoxicity of $CD8^+CD28^-$ T cells using a CFSE-based assay [33]. We designed this assay to specifically determine the ability of the $CD8^+CD28^-$ T cells to lyse allogeneic donor APCs used as stimulators in the above MLRs. In this assay, "effector cells" were the $CD8^+CD28^-$ T cells generated by the donor APC plus γc cytokine-driven *in vitro* cultures as above. The $CD8^+CD28^+$ T cells generated by the same cultures were used as control effector cells because of their known cytotoxicity [5,34,35]. Target cells were either the original priming APCs which were labeled with a high concentration of CFSE (B_{-APC}-$CFSE^{high}$), or control APCs from an HLA-A, -B, and -DR mismatched indifferent individual which were labeled with a low concentration of CFSE (I_{-APC}-$CFSE^{low}$). A 1:1 mixture of I_{-APC}-$CFSE^{low}$ and B_{-APC}-$CFSE^{high}$ cells were plated either by themselves or with the same number of the putative ($CD8^+CD28^-$) or control ($CD8^+CD28^+$) effector cells. At 24, 72, and 120 hr of culture, cells were collected and analyzed by FACS to enumerate $CFSE^{low}$ and $CFSE^{high}$ cells. The ratio of cell numbers of I_{-APC}-$CFSE^{low}$ over B_{-APC}-$CFSE^{high}$ (shown as "R" in Figure 5) over time provided a measure of specific cytolytic effect of the putative effector cells on these two target populations. As shown in Figure 5 left panels, minimal spontaneous lysis was observed as the ratio R remained stable over time in the absence of any effector cells. When the $CD8^+CD28^+$ T cells were added as effector cells (Figure 5, middle panels), R increased to 1.5 at 72 hrs and 2.9 at 120 hrs, demonstrating that B_{-APC}-$CFSE^{high}$ cells were specifically killed by the $CD8^+CD28^+$ T cells. In contrast, when the $CD8^+CD28^-$ T cells were added as effector cells, R remained unchanged over time, indicating that the $CD8^+CD28^-$ T cells exhibit no specific cytolysis towards the B_{-APC} cells (Figure 5, right panels).

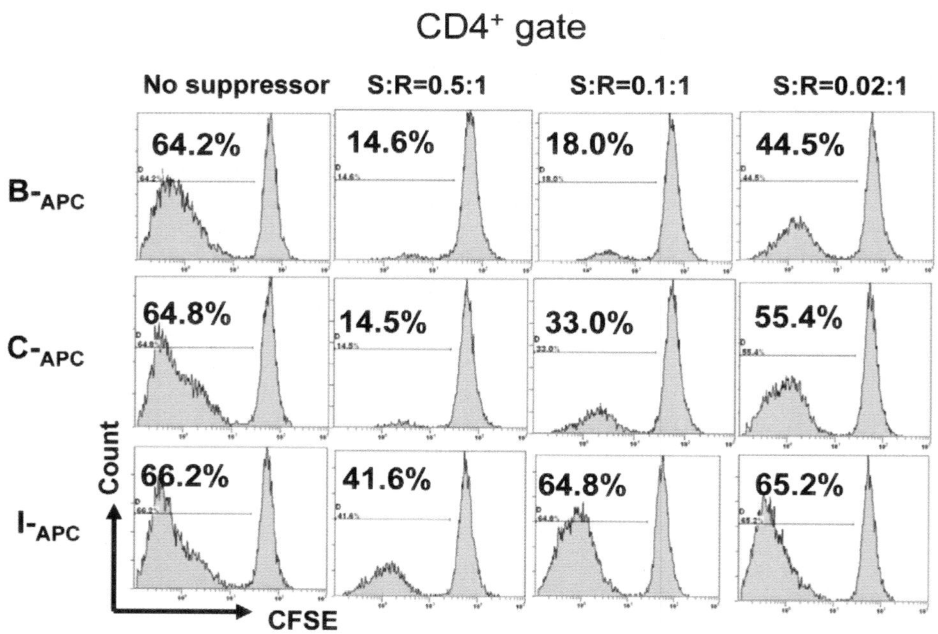

Figure 3. Suppression by the *in vitro* expanded $CD8^+CD28^-$ T cells is restricted by donor HLA class I antigens. Suppression assays were set up as described in Figure 2, with the exception that the stimulator APCs for $CD4^+$ proliferation were from either the priming donor (B_{-APC}), an indifferent donor (I_{-APC}, HLA-A, B and DR fully mismatched with donor B), or a partially matched donor (C_{-APC}, who shared identical HLA class I, but not class II antigens, with donor B). Proliferation of the $CD4^+$ cells was measured by CFSE dilution. Data shown are representative of three independent experiments using three pairs of donors B, C and I. Table 1 provides one example of the HLA class I and class II antigen typing of individuals B, C, and I used for one of three such experiments.

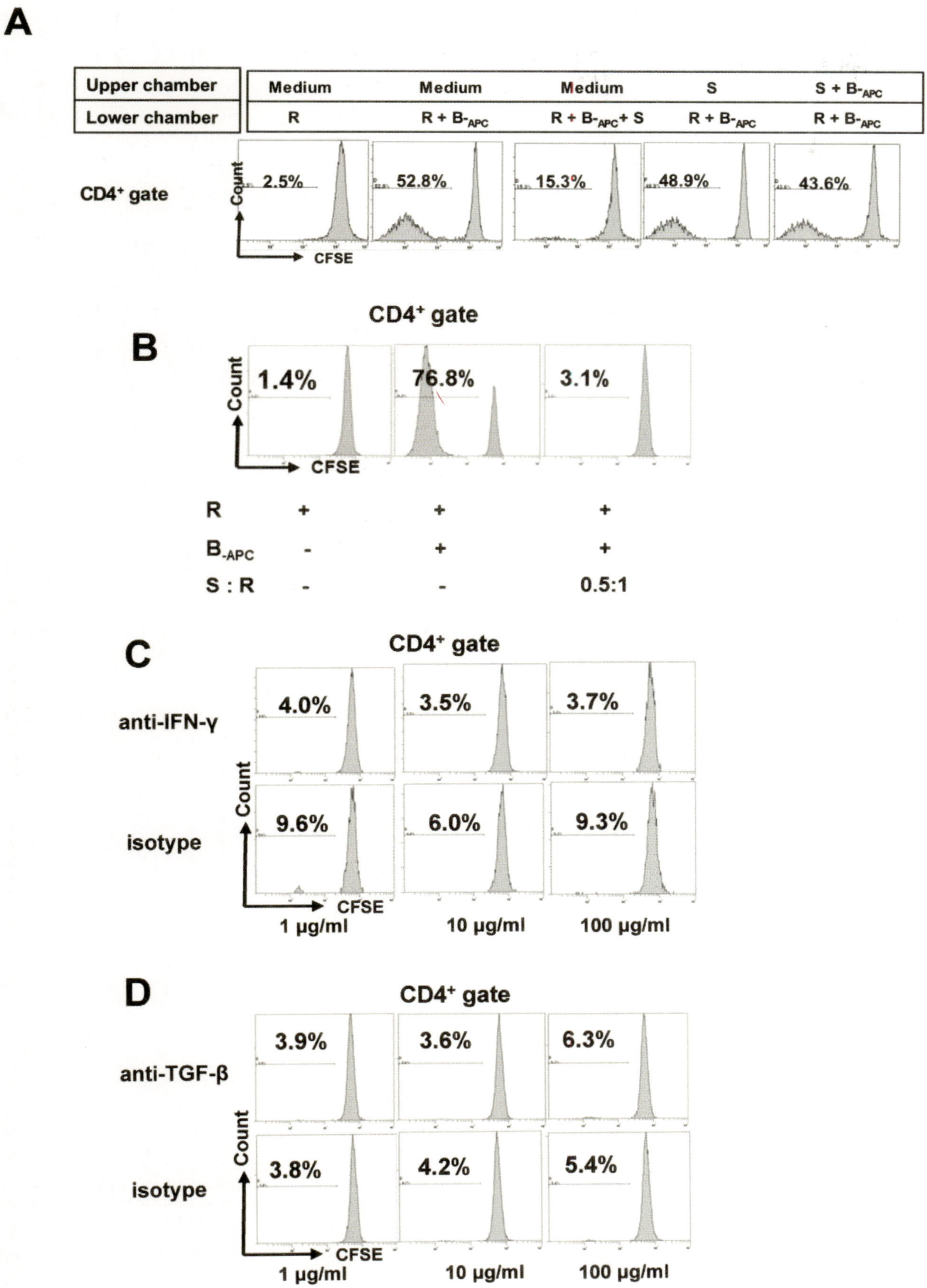
A
Upper chamber
Lower chamber
Medium
R
Medium
R + B-APC
Medium
R + B-APC + S
S
R + B-APC
S + B-APC
R + B-APC
CD4+ gate
Count
CFSE
2.5%
52.8%
15.3%
48.9%
43.6%
B
CD4+ gate
1.4%
76.8%
3.1%
R + + +
B-APC - + +
S : R - - 0.5:1
C
CD4+ gate
anti-IFN-γ
4.0%
3.5%
3.7%
isotype
9.6%
6.0%
9.3%
1 μg/ml
10 μg/ml
100 μg/ml
D
CD4+ gate
anti-TGF-β
3.9%
3.6%
6.3%
isotype
3.8%
4.2%
5.4%
1 μg/ml
10 μg/ml
100 μg/ml

Figure 4. Suppression by the *in vitro* expanded $CD8^+CD28^-$ T cells is contact dependent but IFN-γ or TGF-β independent. Suppression assays were set up as described in Figure 2 at an S:R ratio of 0.5:1. Proliferation of the $CD4^+$ cells was measured by CFSE dilution. *A*, Transwell assays: the lower chambers of 24-well transwell plates were plated with CFSE-labeled responder cells (3×10^5 of R) and stimulator cells (3×10^5 of B_{-APC}), and the *in vitro* expanded $CD8^+CD28^-$ T cells were added either in the lower chamber to allow cell-cell contact or in the upper chamber to prevent cell-cell contact. Data shown are representative of three independent experiments. *B*, Control suppression without any blocking antibodies. *C*, Suppression in the presence of anti-human IFN-γ antibody or its isotype control antibody at concentrations of 1 μg/ml, 10 μg/ml and 100 μg/ml. *D*, Suppression in the presence of anti-human TGF-β antibody or its isotype control antibody at concentrations of 1 μg/ml, 10 μg/ml and 100 μg/ml. Data shown for *B* and *C* are representative of three independent experiments. Abbreviations used for *A–D*: "R": $CD4^+$ responder cells from donor A; "B_{-APC}": APC stimulators from donor B; "S": the *in vitro* expanded $CD8^+CD28^-$ T cells.

Phenotypic characteristics of the *in vitro* expanded $CD8^+CD28^-$ T cells

Phenotypic characteristics of $CD8^+CD28^-$ T cells were examined before and after donor APCs plus γc cytokine-driven *in vitro* expansion to determine if reported markers of CD8 Tregs such as CTLA-4, FoxP3, CD25, CD56 and CD57 [5,16,17,18,19] were also expressed by the $CD8^+CD28^-$ T cells generated by our protocol. As shown in Figure 6*A*, among freshly isolated $CD8^+$ T cells prior to *in vitro* stimulation, $CD8^+CD28^-$ T cells comprised a small fraction. At baseline, they expressed CD56 (35.0%), CD57 (76.5%), CD62L (28.0%), CD127 (13.6%), and perforin (36.6%), but exhibited minimal expressions of CTLA-4, FoxP3, CD25 (Figure 6*A*). Following donor APCs plus γc cytokine-driven expansion, $CD28^-$ cells became the predominant population among $CD8^+$ cells, and they significantly up-regulated expressions of CTLA-4 (78.7%), FoxP3 (16.0%), and CD25 (37.5%) compared with basline, while down-regulated expressions of CD56, CD57, CD62L, CD127, and perforin (Figure 6*B*). While the exact percentages of these markers varied between the $CD8^+CD28^-$ cells from different individuals (data not shown), the trend of up- or down-regulations before and after stimulation in cultures remained the same (1 of 3 representative experiments is shown in Figure 6).

Discussion

In this study, we reported the novel finding that large numbers of donor-specific human $CD8^+CD28^-$ T suppressor cells can be

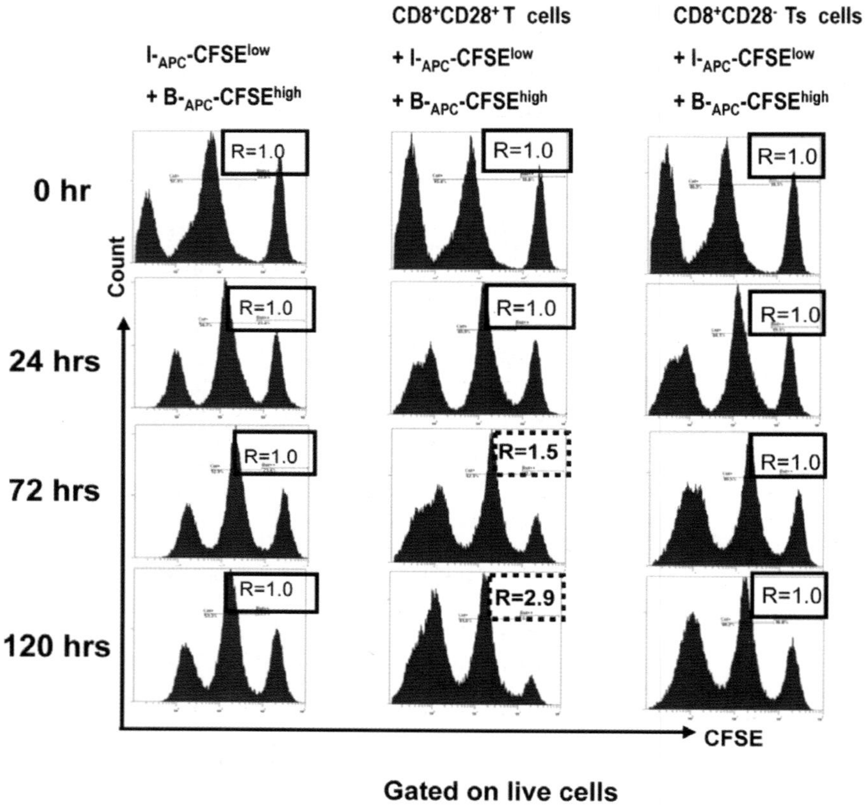

Figure 5. Cytotoxicity does not contribute to the suppression of proliferation by the *in vitro* expanded $CD8^+CD28^-$ T cells. A CFSE based cytotoxicity assay was set up as follows: target cells were the original priming APCs (for generating the $CD8^+CD28^-$ T cells) labeled with a high concentration (2.0 μM) of CFSE (B_{-APC}-$CFSE^{high}$), or APCs from an HLA-A, -B, and -DR mismatched indifferent individual labeled with a low concentration (0.2 μM) of CFSE (I_{-APC}-$CFSE^{low}$). A 1:1 mixture of I_{-APC}-$CFSE^{low}$ and B_{-APC}-$CFSE^{high}$ cells were plated either by themselves (left panels), or with the same number of control ($CD8^+CD28^+$, middle panels) or putative ($CD8^+CD28^-$, right panels) effector cells in 96 U-bottom plates in triplicates. At 24, 72, and 120 hr of culture, cells were collected and analyzed by FACS to enumerate $CFSE^{low}$ and $CFSE^{high}$ cells. The ratio of cell numbers of I_{-APC}-$CFSE^{low}$ over B_{-APC}-$CFSE^{high}$ was calculated as "R" for all time points. An increase in the value of R indicates specific killing of B_{-APC}-$CFSE^{high}$ cells by the effector cells, whereas a stable value of R at 1.0 indicates no specific killing of B_{-APC}-$CFSE^{high}$ cells by the effector cells. Data shown are representative of two independent experiments.

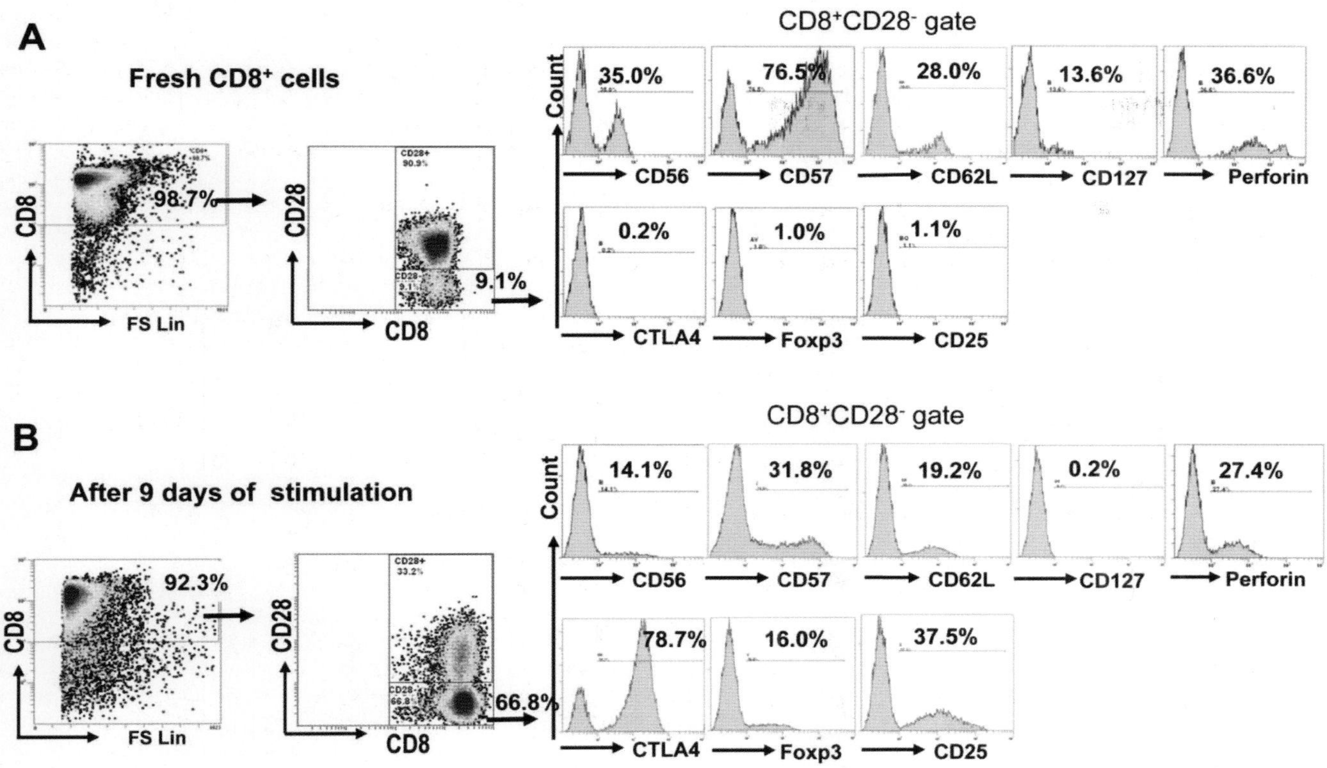

Figure 6. Phenotypic characteristics of the *in vitro* expanded CD8$^+$CD28$^-$ T cells. CD8$^+$ T cells freshly isolated from healthy volunteers (*A*) or after *in vitro* stimulation with donor APCs plus γc cytokines for 9 days (*B*) were analyzed for cell surface or intracellular markers by multichromatic flow cytometry. Date shown are representative of three independent experiments.

generated *in vitro* using a combination of donor APCs and γc cytokines stimulated proliferation. Common γc cytokines IL-2, IL-7 and IL-15 play critical roles in T cell homeostasis [36]. Recent reports have demonstrated that IL-15 can promote the generation and proliferation of CD8$^+$ memory T cells when stimulated by anti-CD3 and anti-CD28 antibodies [12,26]. In contrast, a combination of γc cytokines including IL-2, IL-7 and IL-15 has been used to expand CD8$^+$Foxp3$^+$ Treg *in vitro* from autoimmune patients with SLE who have undergone autologous bone marrow transplant [21]. Human allo-specific CD8$^+$CD28$^-$ suppressor T cells have been reported to be generated by two rounds of stimulation by allogeneic APCs in which IL-2 was the only cytokine added during the last four days of cultures [20]. These cells have been termed as Ts cells. Here, we demonstrated that the combination of IL-2, IL-7 and IL-15, compared with IL-2 alone, was superior in inducing significant expansions of allo-specific CD8$^+$CD28$^-$ cells in cultures activated by donor APC stimulation (Figure 1*A*, 1*B*), and that the expanded CD8$^+$CD28$^-$ cells were highly functionally suppressive. The role of each individual cytokine in the expansion versus inducing the "suppressive" characteristics of this cell population remains to be further elucidated.

The phenotypic and functional characteristics of the CD8$^+$CD28$^-$ T cells generated in our protocol with a combination of γc cytokines closely resemble those of previously described Ts cells [19,20]. They both up-regulate CTLA-4, FoxP3 and CD25, and have variable degrees of down-regulation of CD62L during expansion; possess minimal cytotoxicity; and exhibit suppressive capacity in a contact dependent fashion. We further demonstrated that our *in vitro* expanded CD8$^+$CD28$^-$ T cells exert linked suppression of CD4 T cells of a different HLA class II specificity as long as the HLA class II molecules are co-expressed with the priming HLA class I molecules on the same APCs. This has also been previously indirectly demonstrated as a characteristic of Ts cells [5]. The ability to generate large numbers of functionally suppressive donor-specific CD8$^+$CD28$^-$ T cells that closely mimic Ts cells with this novel approach of using common γc cytokines thus has significant potential for facilitating future clinical use of Treg cell-based immunotherapy for tolerance induction in transplantation.

Several mechanisms of suppression by CD8 suppressor cells have been described. These include direct cytotoxicity [37], secretion of inhibitory cytokines [32,38], down-regulation of co-stimulatory molecules [5,19], and generation of tolerogenic APCs [20]. In our suppression assays, the CD8$^+$CD28$^-$ T cells generated by donor APCs plus γc cytokines suppress proliferation of CD4$^+$ T cells in a donor-specific and dose-dependent manner. Interestingly, distinct from CD4 Treg cells, the CD8$^+$CD28$^-$ T cells do not have the ability to suppress proliferation driven by non-specific stimulation by anti-CD3 and anti-CD28 coated Dynabeads. This finding indicates the importance of the interacting APCs in mediating the suppression by the CD8$^+$CD28$^-$ T cells. Further studies characterizing phenotypic and functional changes of the interacting APCs will provide definitive evidence for this hypothesis. Furthermore, the transwell assay showed that separation of the CD8$^+$CD28$^-$ T cells alone or CD8$^+$CD28$^-$ T cells together with stimulator APCs from the responder CD4$^+$ T cells abolished the ability of the CD8$^+$CD28$^-$ T cells to suppress. These data further indicate that suppression of CD8$^+$CD28$^-$ T cells is mediated through cell-cell contact in a three-cell system, i.e. not only between the $CD8^{+}CD28^{-}$ T cells and the APCs, but also between the APCs (or the $CD8^{+}CD28^{-}$ T cells) and the responding $CD4^{+}$ T cells.

The finding that suppression by the $CD8^{+}CD28^{-}$ T cells is restricted by HLA class I but is promiscuous towards HLA class II specificities with which the responding CD4 TCRs interact suggests a potential mechanism for linked suppression. Linked suppression classically depicts a situation in which co-expression of an indifferent antigen and a tolerant antigen on the same graft allows acceptance of the indifferent antigen in a host previously tolerized to the tolerant antigen [39]. Dendritic cells are thought to play a critical role in the process of linked suppression [39]. In our studies, C-$_{APC}$ cells co-express both matched HLA class I antigens with the priming donor B-$_{APC}$ and mismatched HLA class II antigens with the priming donor B-$_{APC}$. Therefore linked suppression by the $CD8^{+}CD28^{-}$ T cells occurs via C-$_{APC}$ cells, and proliferation of $CD4^{+}$ responder to the mismatched class II antigens is suppressed. These findings have significant implications for designing and understanding the therapeutic value of this $CD8^{+}$ suppressor population.

The role of cytotoxicity in mechanisms of regulation by $CD8^{+}$ suppressor cells has been debated. Suppressive $CD8^{+}CD28^{-}$ Ts cells generated by repeated stimulations with alloantigens have been shown to have no cytotoxicity towards the stimulating allogeneic APCs [5]. In contrast, Zheng et al [37] reported that human $CD8^{high}$ T cells induced by allogeneic CD40-activated B cells have regulatory property that is at least in part mediated through cytotoxicity towards the allogeneic priming PBMC. In our *in vitro* CFSE-based cytotoxicity assay (Figure 5), it appears that the $CD8^{+}CD28^{-}$ T cells generated by our protocol do not possess strong cytotoxicity towards their priming APCs. This is consistent with the down-regulation of perforin in these cells after culturing (Figure 6). It should be noted, however, that cytotoxicity and other possible regulatory mechanisms, such as cytokine production or those mediated through high levels of expression of FoxP3 and CTLA-4, need not be mutually exclusive.

Both cytokine TGF-β [13,29,30] and IFN-γ [8,31,32] have been implicated in the regulatory mechanisms of $CD8^{+}$ suppressor cells in different studies. In our system, neither anti-IFN-γ nor anti-TGF-β antibody reversed the suppressive effect of the expanded $CD8^{+}CD28^{-}$ T cells (Figure 4*C*, *D*). CD56 and CD57 are two markers of natural killer cells previously reported to over-express on $CD8^{+}CD28^{-}$ Ts cells [19]. However, in our culture system the expression of these markers on the $CD8^{+}CD28^{-}$ cells decreased after culture, suggesting that they may not play a major role in the functionality of expanded $CD8^{+}CD28^{-}$ cells in our system.

Two proteins, FoxP3 and CTLA-4, are discernibly up-regulated in the expanded $CD8^{+}CD28^{-}$ T cells. FoxP3 has been described as an important marker for $CD8^{+}$ suppressor cells in humans [18,20,40,41]. However, unlike in mice, in humans non-regulatory T cells including effector cells can also up-regulate FoxP3 expression transiently upon activation [42,43]. Moreover, there are also $CD8^{+}$ suppressor cells that are not characterized with FoxP3 expression [16,32,38]. Whether or not FoxP3 up-regulation in our *in vitro* expanded $CD8^{+}CD28^{-}$ T cells contribute to their suppressive function remains to be elucidated. CTLA-4 is another marker described in $CD8^{+}$ suppressor cells [18,20,40,41]. CTLA-4 is a homologue of CD28, and is known as a negative co-stimulatory receptor which upon signaling from CD80 and CD86 delivers inhibitory signals to T cells to down-regulate T cell activation [44,45]. Recent data also suggest that signaling between CTLA-4 and CD80/CD86 can be bi-directional. CTLA-4 expressed on surface of $CD4^{+}$ Tregs has been shown to interact with CD80/CD86 expressed on APCs and subsequently down-regulate their expression, possibly via a process of trans-endocytosis [46], thereby decreasing the ability of APCs to stimulate T cells through CD28 [47,48]. CTLA-4 has also been reported to up-regulate indolamine 2,3 dioxygenase (IDO) in some subsets of APCs as yet another mechanism for regulating T cell responses [49]. Given the profound up-regulation of this molecule (from 0.2% to 78.7%, Figure 6) and simultaneous down-regulation of CD28 in our $CD8^{+}CD28^{-}$ T cells, CTLA-4 mediated negative signaling to the interacting APCs is a highly attractive potential mechanism of suppression by this cell population.

While robust suppression is observed from our *in vitro* expanded $CD8^{+}CD28^{-}$ T cells, an important issue which remains to be resolved is how these cells would behave *in vivo* upon adoptive transfer. Significant plasticity has been described of $CD4^{+}CD25^{+}FoxP3^{+}$ T cells. Studies of *in vivo* viability, stability and functionality of the expanded human $CD8^{+}CD28^{-}$ T cells in our protocol will necessitate the use of functional humanized mouse models of allogeneic immune responses. Such studies are critical before this approach can be safely translated into clinical applications and are currently being actively pursued in our laboratory.

In conclusion, our findings show that donor APCs plus γc cytokines can be harnessed for efficient *in vitro* expansion of human donor-specific $CD8^{+}CD28^{-}$ T suppressor cells in a simple and robust culture system. This approach may hold promise for clinical application of using regulatory T cell-based immunotherapy for tolerance induction in transplantation in the future.

Materials and Methods

Ethics Statement

This study was approved by the Northwestern Institutional Review Board and written consent was obtained from the participants.

Human subjects and HLA typing

Peripheral blood mononuclear cells (PBMCs) were obtained from healthy volunteers. HLA typing was performed by the Northwestern Histocompatibility Laboratory using molecular methods. Donors for T cells and APCs were selected for their HLA- A, B and DR compatibility or incompatibility based on the specific requirements of individual experiments.

Isolation of PBMCs and cell subsets

PBMCs were isolated from fresh whole blood using Lymphocyte Separation Medium (Mediatech Inc., Manassas, VA) by density gradient centrifugation. $CD8^{+}$ and $CD4^{+}$ T cells were purified from PBMCs using CD8 or CD4 isolation kits (Miltenyi Biotec) through positive selection according to the manufacturer's protocols. Purities for both T cells were confirmed by flow cytometry and were routinely >98%. APCs were isolated from PBMCs by depletion of $CD3^{+}$ cells using CD3 microbeads (Miltenyi Biotech). After culturing of the $CD8^{+}$ cells for indicated number of days, $CD28^{+}$ cells were removed by positive selection using human CD28 MicroBead Kit (Miltenyi Biotech, purity>99%), and the flow-through was collected as $CD28^{-}$ cells (purity>95%). Again, purity of all isolated cells was confirmed by flow cytometry.

In vitro generation and expansion of $CD8^{+}CD28^{-}$ cells with allogeneic APCs and γc cytokines

2×10^{6} purified $CD8^{+}$ T cells from individual A were cultured with 1×10^{6} HLA-A, -B, -DR mismatched APCs from individual B in 2 ml culture medium (RPMI-1640 supplemented with 15% normal human blood group AB serum, 2 mM L-glutamine, 10 mM HEPES and 1×antibiotic-antimycotic solution; all from Gibco-BRL, Gaithersburg, MD) supplemented with IL-2 (20 U/ml), IL-7 (50 ng/ml) and IL-15 (50 ng/ml) (PeproTech Inc., Rocky Hill, NJ) in 24-well plates at 37°C in 5% CO_2. Supplemented culture medium was changed on days 4, 7 and 8 (by replacing 1 ml of the culture medium with fresh medium containing cytokines). Cells in each well were split into two wells on day 6 and harvested on day 9, and the $CD28^-$ population was isolated as described above.

Suppression of donor-specific proliferation by *in vitro* generated $CD8^+CD28^-$ cells

5×10^4 CFSE labeled purified $CD4^+$ T cells from individual A (A-T4) were used as "responders (R)" and stimulated with 5×10^4 APCs from the original priming donor (individual B; $B\text{-}_{APC}$). APCs from an HLA-A,-B,-DR complete-mismatched indifferent donor ($I\text{-}_{APC}$) or 1×10^4 anti-CD3/anti-CD28 Dynabeads (Invitrogen, Carlsbad, CA) were used as third party or non-specific stimulation controls respectively. All cultures were prepared in triplicates and incubated in 96-well U-bottom plates in 37°C 5% CO_2 incubator. The $CD8^+CD28^-$ cells were added as "suppressor (S)" at S:R ratios of 0.5:1, 0.1:1 and 0.02:1 (the cell number of "R" was kept constant). CFSE dilution was assessed on day 7 to determine extent of proliferation. In selected experiments, anti-human IFN-γ (eBioscience Inc.), anti-human TGF-β antibody (BioXcell, West Lebanon, NH), or respective isotype controls were added to cultures at concentrations of 1 µg/ml, 10 µg/ml or 100 µg/ml. Parallel cultures were analyzed using ^{3}H-thymidine incorporation. 1 µCi ^{3}H-thymidine (PerkinElmer, San Jose, CA) was added per well for the last 18 hrs of a 7-day culture, and incorporated radioactivity was measured as counts per minute (CPM) with a Perkin-Elmer scintillation counter.

Transwell experiments

The lower chambers of 24-well transwell plates were plated with either 3×10^5 CFSE labeled naïve $CD4^+$ T cells from individual A (A-T4), or with A-T4 and 3×10^5 priming APCs from individual B ($B\text{-}_{APC}$) in the presence or absence of 3×10^4 $CD8^+CD28^-$ cells (total volume 600 µl). The upper chambers were plated with medium only, $CD8^+CD28^-$ cells only, or $CD8^+CD28^-$ cells plus priming APCs ($B\text{-}_{APC}$). Cells collected from the lower chamber after 7 days of culture were assessed by FACS for CFSE dilution.

Cytotoxicity by $CD8^+CD28^-$ cells

CFSE-based cytotoxic assay was set up according to published methods [33] as follows. APCs serving as target cells were labeled with two concentrations of CFSE: high concentration (2.0 µM) for APCs from the priming donor ($B\text{-}_{APC}\text{-}CFSE^{high}$) and low concentration (0.2 µM) for APCs from an HLA-A,-B,-DR complete-mismatched indifferent donor ($I\text{-}_{APC}\text{-}CFSE^{low}$). The *in vitro* generated $CD8^+CD28^-$ cells or their $CD8^+CD28^+$ counterpart were used as putative or control effector cells respectively. 5×10^4 effector cells were cultured with 5×10^4 each of $B\text{-}_{APC}\text{-}CFSE^{high}$ and $I\text{-}_{APC}\text{-}CFSE^{low}$ together in 96-well U-bottom plates in triplicate wells. Cultured $B\text{-}_{APC}\text{-}CFSE^{high}$ and $I\text{-}_{APC}\text{-}CFSE^{low}$ in the absence of effector cells were used as controls for spontaneous cytolysis. $B\text{-}_{APC}\text{-}CFSE^{high}$ and $I\text{-}_{APC}\text{-}CFSE^{low}$ were enumerated by FACS after 0, 24, 72 and 120 hrs of culture. The ratios of cell numbers of $I\text{-}_{APC}\text{-}CFSE^{low}$ over $B\text{-}_{APC}\text{-}CFSE^{high}$ in the absence or the presence of effector cells were calculated over time to estimate specific killing of $B\text{-}_{APC}\text{-}CFSE^{high}$.

Multi-color flow cytometric analysis

The following anti-human antibodies and their isotype controls were used: FITC conjugated anti-CD3 (OKT3), CD4(OKT4), CD8(SK1), CD56(MEM188), CD57(TBO1), CD62L(DREG56), CD127(RDR5), Perforin(dG9), all from eBioscience; FITC conjugated anti-human CTLA-4(A3.4H2.H12, Cedarlane USA, Burlington, NC), CD25(BC96), Granzyme B(GB11, Biolegend, San Diego, CA); PE conjugated anti-human Foxp3(eBioscience, San Diego, CA); ECD conjugated anti-human CD8(SFCI21Thy2D3), PE-cyanin 5 (PC5) conjugated anti-human CD28(28.2), PE-cyanin 7 (PC7) conjugated anti-human CD8(SFCI21Thy2D3, Beckman Coulter, Miami, FL). Surface and intra-cellular staining was performed following manufacturers' recommended protocols. Data was acquired on a 5-color FC500 flow cytometer and analyzed using the CXP program (Beckman-Coulter).

Statistical analysis

Comparisons were made by paired Student's *t* test. Differences were considered significant if the *P* value was <0.05.

Acknowledgments

We wish to thank Dr. Syamal Datta for helpful discussions and critical reading of this manuscript. We also wish to thank Ms. Sam Malladi for meticulous proof-reading of the manuscript.

Author Contributions

Conceived and designed the experiments: YY ART XL. Performed the experiments: YY JRZ JH NH. Analyzed the data: YY JRZ ART XL. Contributed reagents/materials/analysis tools: LX JM JMM ART. Wrote the paper: YY JRZ ART XL.

References

1. Sakaguchi S (2005) Naturally arising Foxp3-expressing CD25+CD4+ regulatory T cells in immunological tolerance to self and non-self. Nat Immunol 6: 345–352.
2. Tsang JY, Tanriver Y, Jiang S, Leung E, Ratnasothy K, et al. (2009) Indefinite mouse heart allograft survival in recipient treated with CD4(+)CD25(+) regulatory T cells with indirect allospecificity and short term immunosuppression. Transpl Immunol 21: 203–209.
3. Joffre O, Santolaria T, Calise D, Al Saati T, Hudrisier D, et al. (2008) Prevention of acute and chronic allograft rejection with CD4+CD25+Foxp3+ regulatory T lymphocytes. Nat Med 14: 88–92.
4. Trzonkowski P, Bieniaszewska M, Juscinska J, Dobyszuk A, Krzystyniak A, et al. (2009) First-in-man clinical results of the treatment of patients with graft versus host disease with human ex vivo expanded CD4+CD25+CD127− T regulatory cells. Clin Immunol 133: 22–26.
5. Liu Z, Tugulea S, Cortesini R, Suciu-Foca N (1998) Specific suppression of T helper alloreactivity by allo-MHC class I-restricted CD8+CD28− T cells. Int Immunol 10: 775–783.
6. Dijke IE, Caliskan K, Klepper M, de Kuiper R, Balk AH, et al. (2009) Donor-specific immune regulation by CD8 lymphocytes expanded from rejecting human cardiac allografts. Am J Transplant 9: 397–403.
7. Li XL, Menoret S, Bezie S, Caron L, Chabannes D, et al. (2010) Mechanism and localization of CD8 regulatory T cells in a heart transplant model of tolerance. J Immunol 185: 823–833.
8. Guillonneau C, Hill M, Hubert FX, Chiffoleau E, Herve C, et al. (2007) CD40Ig treatment results in allograft acceptance mediated by CD8CD45RC T cells, IFN-gamma, and indoleamine 2,3-dioxygenase. J Clin Invest 117: 1096–1106.
9. Konya C, Goronzy JJ, Weyand CM (2009) Treating autoimmune disease by targeting CD8(+) T suppressor cells. Expert Opin Biol Ther 9: 951–965.
10. Tsai S, Shameli A, Yamanouchi J, Clemente-Casares X, Wang J, et al. (2010) Reversal of autoimmunity by boosting memory-like autoregulatory T cells. Immunity 32: 568–580.
11. Jarnicki AG, Lysaght J, Todryk S, Mills KH (2006) Suppression of antitumor immunity by IL-10 and TGF-beta-producing T cells infiltrating the growing

tumor: influence of tumor environment on the induction of CD4+ and CD8+ regulatory T cells. J Immunol 177: 896–904.
12. Godlove J, Chiu WK, Weng NP (2007) Gene expression and generation of CD28−CD8 T cells mediated by interleukin 15. Exp Gerontol 42: 412–415.
13. Cosmi L, Liotta F, Lazzeri E, Francalanci M, Angeli R, et al. (2003) Human CD8+CD25+ thymocytes share phenotypic and functional features with CD4+CD25+ regulatory thymocytes. Blood 102: 4107–4114.
14. Rifa'i M, Kawamoto Y, Nakashima I, Suzuki H (2004) Essential roles of CD8+CD122+ regulatory T cells in the maintenance of T cell homeostasis. J Exp Med 200: 1123–1134.
15. Shi Z, Okuno Y, Rifa'i M, Endharti AT, Akane K, et al. (2009) Human CD8+CXCR3+ T cells have the same function as murine CD8+CD122+ Treg. Eur J Immunol 39: 2106–2119.
16. Uss E, Rowshani AT, Hooibrink B, Lardy NM, van Lier RA, et al. (2006) CD103 is a marker for alloantigen-induced regulatory CD8+ T cells. J Immunol 177: 2775–2783.
17. Joosten SA, van Meijgaarden KE, Savage ND, de Boer T, Triebel F, et al. (2007) Identification of a human CD8+ regulatory T cell subset that mediates suppression through the chemokine CC chemokine ligand 4. Proc Natl Acad Sci U S A 104: 8029–8034.
18. Mahic M, Henjum K, Yaqub S, Bjornbeth BA, Torgersen KM, et al. (2008) Generation of highly suppressive adaptive CD8(+)CD25(+)FOXP3(+) regulatory T cells by continuous antigen stimulation. Eur J Immunol 38: 640–646.
19. Davila E, Kang YM, Park YW, Sawai H, He X, et al. (2005) Cell-based immunotherapy with suppressor CD8+ T cells in rheumatoid arthritis. J Immunol 174: 7292–7301.
20. Chang CC, Ciubotariu R, Manavalan JS, Yuan J, Colovai AI, et al. (2002) Tolerization of dendritic cells by T(S) cells: the crucial role of inhibitory receptors ILT3 and ILT4. Nat Immunol 3: 237–243.
21. Zhang L, Bertucci AM, Ramsey-Goldman R, Burt RK, Datta SK (2009) Regulatory T cell (Treg) subsets return in patients with refractory lupus following stem cell transplantation, and TGF-beta-producing CD8+ Treg cells are associated with immunological remission of lupus. J Immunol 183: 6346–6358.
22. Luo X, Tarbell KV, Yang H, Pothoven K, Bailey SL, et al. (2007) Dendritic cells with TGF-beta1 differentiate naive CD4+CD25− T cells into islet-protective Foxp3+ regulatory T cells. Proc Natl Acad Sci U S A 104: 2821–2826.
23. Saito M, Nagasawa M, Takada H, Hara T, Tsuchiya S, et al. (2011) Defective IL-10 signaling in hyper-IgE syndrome results in impaired generation of tolerogenic dendritic cells and induced regulatory T cells. J Exp Med 208: 235–249.
24. Bedke T, Pretsch L, Karakhanova S, Enk AH, Mahnke K (2010) Endothelial cells augment the suppressive function of CD4+ CD25+ Foxp3+ regulatory T cells: involvement of programmed death-1 and IL-10. J Immunol 184: 5562–5570.
25. Hippen KL, Merkel SC, Schirm DK, Nelson C, Tennis NC, et al. (2011) Generation and Large-Scale Expansion of Human Inducible Regulatory T Cells That Suppress Graft-Versus-Host Disease. Am J Transplant.
26. Chiu WK, Fann M, Weng NP (2006) Generation and growth of CD28nullCD8+ memory T cells mediated by IL-15 and its induced cytokines. J Immunol 177: 7802–7810.
27. Borthwick NJ, Lowdell M, Salmon M, Akbar AN (2000) Loss of CD28 expression on CD8(+) T cells is induced by IL-2 receptor gamma chain signalling cytokines and type I IFN, and increases susceptibility to activation-induced apoptosis. Int Immunol 12: 1005–1013.
28. Kapp JA, Honjo K, Kapp LM, Xu X, Cozier A, et al. (2006) TCR transgenic CD8+ T cells activated in the presence of TGFbeta express FoxP3 and mediate linked suppression of primary immune responses and cardiac allograft rejection. Int Immunol 18: 1549–1562.
29. He H, Yang P, Jiang L, Zhang J, Zhao C, et al. (2008) Upregulation of CD94 on CD8+T cells in anterior chamber-associated immune deviation. BMC Immunol 9: 53.
30. Hahn BH, Singh RP, La Cava A, Ebling FM (2005) Tolerogenic treatment of lupus mice with consensus peptide induces Foxp3-expressing, apoptosis-resistant, TGFbeta-secreting CD8+ T cell suppressors. J Immunol 175: 7728–7737.
31. Myers L, Croft M, Kwon BS, Mittler RS, Vella AT (2005) Peptide-specific CD8 T regulatory cells use IFN-gamma to elaborate TGF-beta-based suppression. J Immunol 174: 7625–7632.
32. Seo SK, Choi JH, Kim YH, Kang WJ, Park HY, et al. (2004) 4-1BB-mediated immunotherapy of rheumatoid arthritis. Nat Med 10: 1088–1094.
33. Martin AJ, McCarthy D, Waltenbaugh C, Goings G, Luo X, et al. (2010) Ethylenecarbodiimide-treated splenocytes carrying male CD4 epitopes confer histocompatibility Y chromosome antigen transplant protection by inhibiting CD154 upregulation. J Immunol 185: 3326–3336.
34. Koide J, Engleman EG (1990) Differences in surface phenotype and mechanism of action between alloantigen-specific CD8+ cytotoxic and suppressor T cell clones. J Immunol 144: 32–40.
35. Damle NK, Engleman EG (1989) Antigen-specific suppressor T lymphocytes in man. Clin Immunol Immunopathol 53: S17–24.
36. Surh CD, Sprent J (2008) Homeostasis of naive and memory T cells. Immunity 29: 848–862.
37. Zheng J, Liu Y, Qin G, Chan PL, Mao H, et al. (2009) Efficient induction and expansion of human alloantigen-specific CD8 regulatory T cells from naive precursors by CD40-activated B cells. J Immunol 183: 3742–3750.
38. Gilliet M, Liu YJ (2002) Generation of human CD8 T regulatory cells by CD40 ligand-activated plasmacytoid dendritic cells. J Exp Med 195: 695–704.
39. Cobbold SP, Adams E, Nolan KF, Regateiro FS, Waldmann H (2010) Connecting the mechanisms of T-cell regulation: dendritic cells as the missing link. Immunol Rev 236: 203–218.
40. Bisikirska B, Colgan J, Luban J, Bluestone JA, Herold KC (2005) TCR stimulation with modified anti-CD3 mAb expands CD8+ T cell population and induces CD8+CD25+ Tregs. J Clin Invest 115: 2904–2913.
41. Herold KC, Gitelman SE, Masharani U, Hagopian W, Bisikirska B, et al. (2005) A single course of anti-CD3 monoclonal antibody hOKT3gamma1(Ala-Ala) results in improvement in C-peptide responses and clinical parameters for at least 2 years after onset of type 1 diabetes. Diabetes 54: 1763–1769.
42. Allan SE, Crome SQ, Crellin NK, Passerini L, Steiner TS, et al. (2007) Activation-induced FOXP3 in human T effector cells does not suppress proliferation or cytokine production. Int Immunol 19: 345–354.
43. Morgan ME, van Bilsen JH, Bakker AM, Heemskerk B, Schilham MW, et al. (2005) Expression of FOXP3 mRNA is not confined to CD4+CD25+ T regulatory cells in humans. Hum Immunol 66: 13–20.
44. Sansom DM, Walker LS (2006) The role of CD28 and cytotoxic T-lymphocyte antigen-4 (CTLA-4) in regulatory T-cell biology. Immunol Rev 212: 131–148.
45. Fife BT, Griffin MD, Abbas AK, Locksley RM, Bluestone JA (2006) Inhibition of T cell activation and autoimmune diabetes using a B cell surface-linked CTLA-4 agonist. J Clin Invest 116: 2252–2261.
46. Qureshi OS, Zheng Y, Nakamura K, Attridge K, Manzotti C, et al. (2011) Trans-endocytosis of CD80 and CD86: a molecular basis for the cell-extrinsic function of CTLA-4. Science 332: 600–603.
47. Wing K, Onishi Y, Prieto-Martin P, Yamaguchi T, Miyara M, et al. (2008) CTLA-4 control over Foxp3+ regulatory T cell function. Science 322: 271–275.
48. Onishi Y, Fehervari Z, Yamaguchi T, Sakaguchi S (2008) Foxp3+ natural regulatory T cells preferentially form aggregates on dendritic cells in vitro and actively inhibit their maturation. Proc Natl Acad Sci U S A 105: 10113–10118.
49. Huang L, Baban B, Johnson BA, 3rd, Mellor AL (2010) Dendritic cells, indoleamine 2,3 dioxygenase and acquired immune privilege. Int Rev Immunol 29: 133–155.

12

Host-Based Th2 Cell Therapy for Prolongation of Cardiac Allograft Viability

Shoba Amarnath[1*], Hao Chen[2,3], Jason E. Foley[1], Carliann M. Costanzo[1], Joel D. Sennesh[4], Michael A. Solomon[2,5], Daniel H. Fowler[1]

1 Experimental Transplantation and Immunology Branch, National Cancer Institute, National Institutes of Health, Bethesda, Maryland, United States of America, **2** Critical Care Medicine, Clinical Center, National Institutes of Health, Bethesda, Maryland, United States of America, **3** Department of Cardiac Surgery, Huadong Hospital, Fudan University, Shanghai, China, **4** Department of Pathology, Inova Fairfax Hospital, Fairfax, Virginia, United States of America, **5** Cardiovascular and Pulmonary Branch, National Heart, Lung and Blood Institute, National Institutes of Health, Bethesda, Maryland, United States of America

Abstract

Donor T cell transfusion, which is a long-standing approach to prevent allograft rejection, operates indirectly by alteration of host T cell immunity. We therefore hypothesized that adoptive transfer of immune regulatory host Th2 cells would represent a novel intervention to enhance cardiac allograft survival. Using a well-described rat cardiac transplant model, we first developed a method for ex vivo manufacture of rat host-type Th2 cells in rapamycin, with subsequent injection of such Th2.R cells prior to class I and class II disparate cardiac allografting. Second, we determined whether Th2.R cell transfer polarized host immunity towards a Th2 phenotype. And third, we evaluated whether Th2.R cell therapy prolonged allograft viability when used alone or in combination with a short-course of cyclosporine (CSA) therapy. We found that host-type Th2.R cell therapy prior to cardiac allografting: (1) reduced the frequency of activated T cells in secondary lymphoid organs; (2) shifted post-transplant cytokines towards a Th2 phenotype; and (3) prolonged allograft viability when used in combination with short-course CSA therapy. These results provide further support for the rationale to use "direct" host T cell therapy for prolongation of allograft viability as an alternative to "indirect" therapy mediated by donor T cell infusion.

Editor: Aric Gregson, University of California Los Angeles, United States of America

Funding: This work was supported by the Center for Cancer Research, National Cancer Institute, and Critical Care Medicine Department, Clinical Center Intramural Research Program. The funders had no role in study design, data collection and analysis, decision to publish, or preparation of the manuscript.

Competing Interests: The authors have declared that no competing interests exist.

* E-mail: samarnath@mail.nih.gov

These authors contributed equally to this work.

Introduction

Clinical interventions to prolong cardiac allograft survival have relied primarily on long-term post-transplant administration of calcineurin inhibitors such as cyclosporine A (CSA) for suppression of host T cells that mediate rejection [1] [reviewed in [2]]. However, long-term calcineurin inhibitor therapy is typically only partially effective and the T cell immune deficiency predisposes to life threatening infection and malignancy [reviewed in [3]]. As such, new approaches in transplantation seek to limit patient exposure to calcineurin inhibitors and to promote immune tolerance through either pharmacologic or cellular interventions [reviewed in [4,5]].

"Donor specific tolerance" was observed when recipients of T cell-containing, third-party blood transfusion prior to clinical organ transplantation were found to have a reduced incidence of graft rejection [6,7,8]. Recent animal model experiments have demonstrated that the reduction in graft rejection through donor T cell infusion occurs "indirectly" through modulation of host T cells [9,10]. Most recently, in a murine model of transplantation tolerance, donor regulatory T (Treg) cells contained within transferred blood products were found to induce naive host T cells to adopt a Treg phenotype [11].

As such, various T cell transfer methods that result in the modulation of host T cell populations represent a general approach to prolong allograft survival. Recently, we have shown that donor T cells polarized into a Th2 phenotype modulate host T cells towards a Th2 phenotype, thereby preventing graft rejection in a murine model of hematopoietic stem cell transplantation [12,13]. Based on this background, we now project that host Th2 cell adoptive transfer may represent a "direct" pathway to prolong solid organ allograft viability. Host T cell therapy would be particularly useful for cardiac allograft recipients due to the lack of cadaveric donor T cells. In addition, rat cardiac allograft rejection has been characterized as a Th1-type process [14], and therefore predictably amenable to Th2 cell therapy, which we have shown to be capable of modulating Th1-type transplantation responses [12]. Towards this aim, we tested our hypothesis in a well-characterized rat cardiac allograft transplantation model.

In murine models of graft rejection [12] and graft-versus-host disease [15], we found that adoptive transfer of Th2 cells that were manufactured ex vivo in rapamycin ("Th2.R cells") were more effective than control Th2 cells; the increased in vivo efficacy of Th2.R cells is likely due to their rapamycin-induced anti-apoptotic phenotype, which permits prolonged in vivo T cell persistence [13]. In light of these data, we hypothesized that adoptive cell therapy using host-type Th2.R cells may represent a novel approach to modulate host immunity towards a Th2 phenotype for prolongation of solid organ transplant survival.

Results

Ex vivo manufacture of rat CD4$^+$ Th2 cells with or without rapamycin

There are no reports in the literature pertaining to the ex vivo manufacture of rat Th2 cells in the presence of rapamycin; as such, we first evaluated if rat CD4$^+$ T cells could be polarized to a Th2 phenotype during rapamycin exposure. In previous experiments evaluating Th2 cell therapy in the context of murine allogeneic bone marrow transplantation, we identified an effective strategy whereby cytokine polarization occurred ex vivo in a polyclonal manner, with subsequent acquisition of allosensitization in vivo [16]; as such, for these studies, we performed cytokine polarization in the context of polyclonal co-stimulation. Co-stimulation and IL-4 priming in the presence or absence of rapamycin resulted in T cells expressing a Th2 phenotype, as defined by minimal IFN-γ secretion (Fig. 1a, panel i; Fig. 1b, panels i, ii, iii) and high levels of IL-4 secretion (Fig. 1a, panel ii; Fig. 1b, panel iv, v, vi). Relative to control Th2 cells ("Th2"), rapamycin treated Th2 cells ("Th2.R") secreted higher amounts of IL-4 ($P<0.05$ for supernatant assay in Fig. 1a; $p = 0.03$ for i.c. flow cytometry assay in Fig. 1b). Control Th2 cells and Th2.R cells each had minimal expression of the Treg transcription factor, Foxp3 (Fig. 1c; percent CD4$^+$Foxp3$^+$ expression, mean ± SEM, Th2 vs. Th2.R: 2.0±0.5 vs. 0.5±0.6). As such, ex vivo rapamycin enhanced host T cell Th2 polarity without promoting a Treg phenotype.

Th2.R cell therapy combined with CSA therapy reduces T cell activation during allograft challenge and augments post-transplant Th2 polarity

Expanded host-type Th2.R cells were infused intravenously into recipient (host-type) rats following cardiac transplantation surgery at day 0. Cohorts received the allograft either alone ("allograft") or in combination with: CSA for 28 days (CSA 28); CSA for 18 days (CSA 18); Th2.R cells; or Th2.R cells plus (CSA 18). At the final day 28 post-transplant endpoint, recipients in the rejection control cohort that did not receive CSA or Th2.R cells had low frequencies of CD4$^+$CD25$^+$Foxp3$^+$ T cells (Fig. 2a top panels) and had high frequencies of CD4$^+$CD25$^+$Foxp3$^-$ activated effector T cells (Fig. 2a, bottom left panel) and CD8$^+$CD25$^+$ Foxp3$^-$ activated effector T cells (Fig. 2a, bottom right panel) in the spleen, inguinal lymph nodes, and mesenteric lymph nodes. By comparison, recipients of daily subcutaneous CSA therapy had undetectable levels of activated effector CD4$^+$ and CD8$^+$ T cells. Statistical analyses were performed, with comparison of each experimental cohort to the rejection control cohort. Relative to rejection controls, recipients of a short-course of CSA alone, Th2.R cells alone, or the combination of short-course CSA plus Th2.R cells had decreased frequencies of effector CD4$^+$ and CD8$^+$ T cells; as such, both CSA and Th2.R cell infusion reduced in vivo host T cell activation during allograft challenge.

Next, we evaluated the cytokine profile of the various cohorts at day 28 post-transplant; post-transplant T cell cytokine production was induced after polyclonal stimulation using co-stimulation (Fig. 2b) and by syngeneic and allogeneic antigen-presenting-cell (APC) stimulation to determine allospecific cytokine secretion (Fig. 2c). Upon co-stimulation and allogeneic APC activation, spleen and lymphoid cells isolated from recipients of short-course CSA or the combination of short-course CSA plus Th2.R cells had increased secretion of IL-4 relative to spleen and lymphoid cells isolated from recipients of either continuous daily CSA therapy or Th2.R cell therapy alone (Fig. 2b and 2c, respectively); the mechanism(s) whereby short-course CSA consistently increased post-transplant IL-4 secretion capacity is not clear and was not addressed in our experiments. The rejection control cohort secreted low levels of IL-4. As such, whereas daily CSA therapy suppressed the host Th2 response, short-course CSA and Th2 cell transfer promoted Th2 immunity. Furthermore, infusion of Th2.R cells in the context of short-course CSA therapy reduced post-transplant T cell capacity to secrete IFN-γ in both a polyclonal and an allospecific manner (Fig. 2b and 2c, respectively).

Evaluation of Th2.R cell therapy timing and rapamycin co-administration

Further experiments were performed in host-type BN rats to optimize Th2.R cell therapy. We hypothesized that infusion of host Th2.R cells one or two weeks prior to the allogeneic transplant might induce more marked host skewing towards a Th2 state, thereby enhancing a Th2.R cell protection against graft rejection. In lieu with our prior finding that murine Th2.R cells were relatively resistant to in vivo rapamycin drug therapy [17], we also hypothesized that pre-transplant co-administration of rapamycin might further augment the host Th2 state. Indeed, at day 7 after host Th2.R cell infusion, there was a dramatic increase in host capacity to secrete IL-4 (Fig. 3a); however, co-administration of rapamycin actually abrogated this host Th2 shift. Of note, host immunity was not significantly polarized at day 14 after Th2.R cell infusion; as such, further experiments focused on an anti-rejection strategy incorporating Th2.R cell infusion at day −7 pre-transplant. Seven days after treatment with CD4$^+$ Th2.R cells, no significant increase in Foxp3$^+$ T cells was observed (Fig. 3b). Both host CD4$^+$ and CD8$^+$ T cells were enriched for IL-4 secretion capacity (Fig. 3c; Representative flow plot panel i gated on CD8$^+$ T cells and ii gated on CD4$^+$ T cells; summary iii and iv); as such, similar to our previous work in murine models, the adoptive transfer of highly purified rat CD4$^+$ Th2.R cells resulted in the transfer of Th2 immunity to other host T cell populations. Of note, Th2.R cell induction of host CD4$^+$ and CD8$^+$ T cell IL-4 secretion was inhibited by rapamycin co-administration. Th2 skewing was confirmed by the ability of the host CD8+ T cells to secrete IL4. Furthermore, seven days after host Th2.R cell infusion, we observed a marked decrease in host CD4$^+$ T cell capacity for IFN-γ secretion (Fig. 3c; v). Interestingly, rapamycin drug therapy did not reduce CD4$^+$ T cell IFN-γ secretion in a statistically significant manner. In addition, Th2.R cells or rapamycin did not significantly alter IFN-γ secretion capacity within host CD8$^+$ T cells (Fig. 3c; vi). Since rapamycin was not permissive for Th2 polarization in our system, further experiments tested Th2.R cell therapy in the setting of CSA rather than rapamycin drug therapy.

Th2.R cell therapy combined with short-course CSA therapy prolongs cardiac allograft viability

We next evaluated host-based Th2.R cell therapy in a stringent, 28-day model of allograft rejection that utilized CSA for only the initial 10 days post-transplant. At day 28 post-transplant, as anticipated, recipients of daily CSA (through day 28 post-transplant) had reduced CD8$^+$ T cell activation in the spleen, inguinal lymph nodes, and mesenteric lymph nodes relative to recipients of short-course CSA (Fig. 4a; top panels). Remarkably, host Th2.R cell infusion plus short-course CSA also reduced CD8$^+$ T cell activation at these tissue sites to levels comparable with daily CSA therapy; in general, this CD8$^+$ T cell inhibition occurred whether Th2.R cells were administered at day −7, day 0, or day −7 plus day 0. However, Th2.R cell infusion without short-course CSA did not inhibit CD8$^+$ T cell activation. In marked contrast to

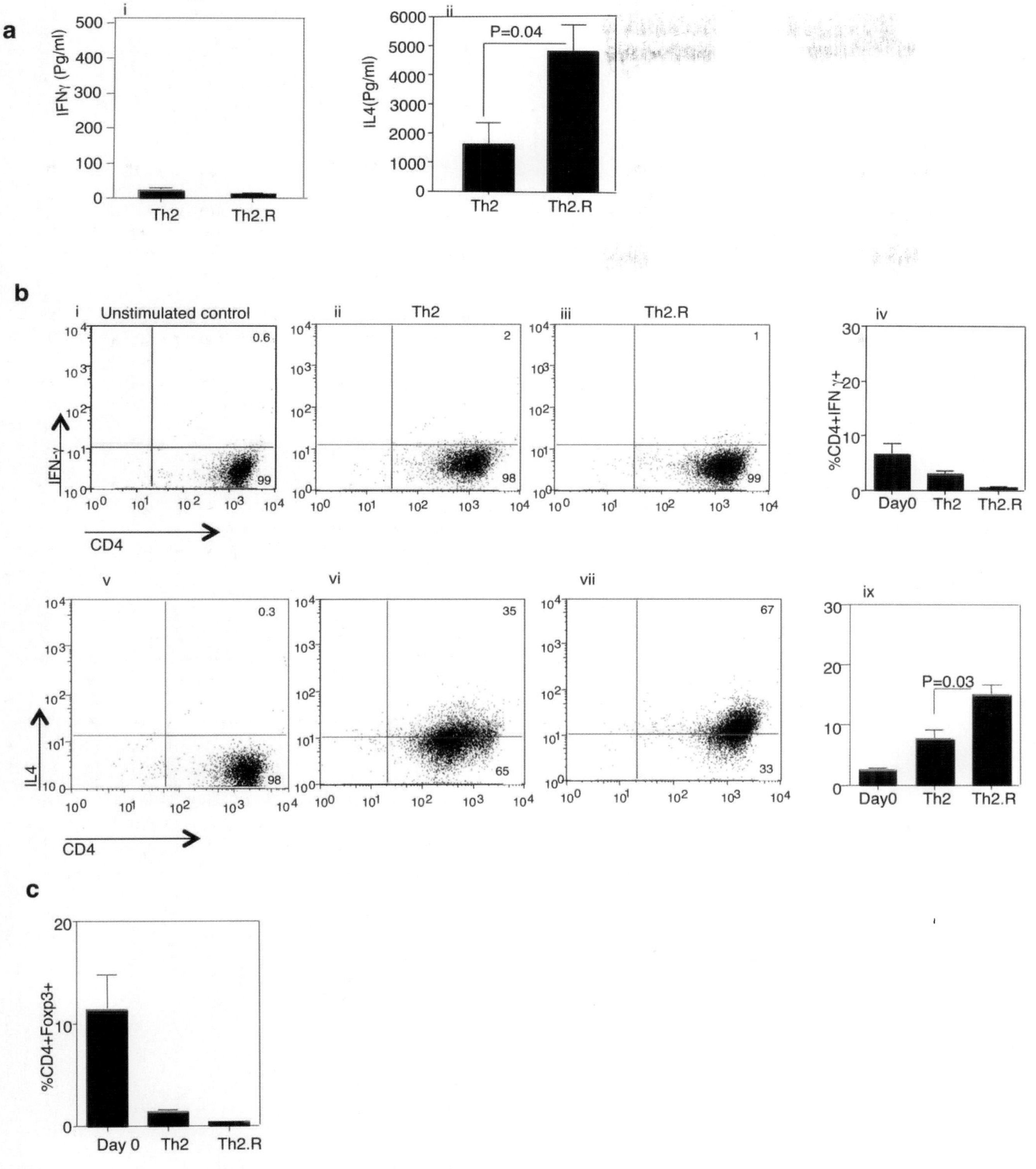

Figure 1. Characterization of rat Th2 cells. CD4^{+} T cells were isolated and expanded using anti-CD3 and anti-CD28 co-stimulation in the presence of rhIL-2, rrIL-4, and rhIL-7 either with rapamycin ("Th2.R") or without rapamycin ("Th2") for 3 days. (a) Expanded Th2 and Th2.R cells were subjected to repeat co-stimulation, and the 24 h supernatant was tested for cytokine content using multiplex bead array. (b) After repeat co-stimulation, Th2 and Th2.R cells were evaluated for intra-cellular expression of IFN-γ and IL-4 by flow cytometry. (c) On day 3, cells were harvested and intra-cellular flow cytometry was performed to evaluate Foxp3 transcription factor expression. Results are a summary of n = 10 cultures.

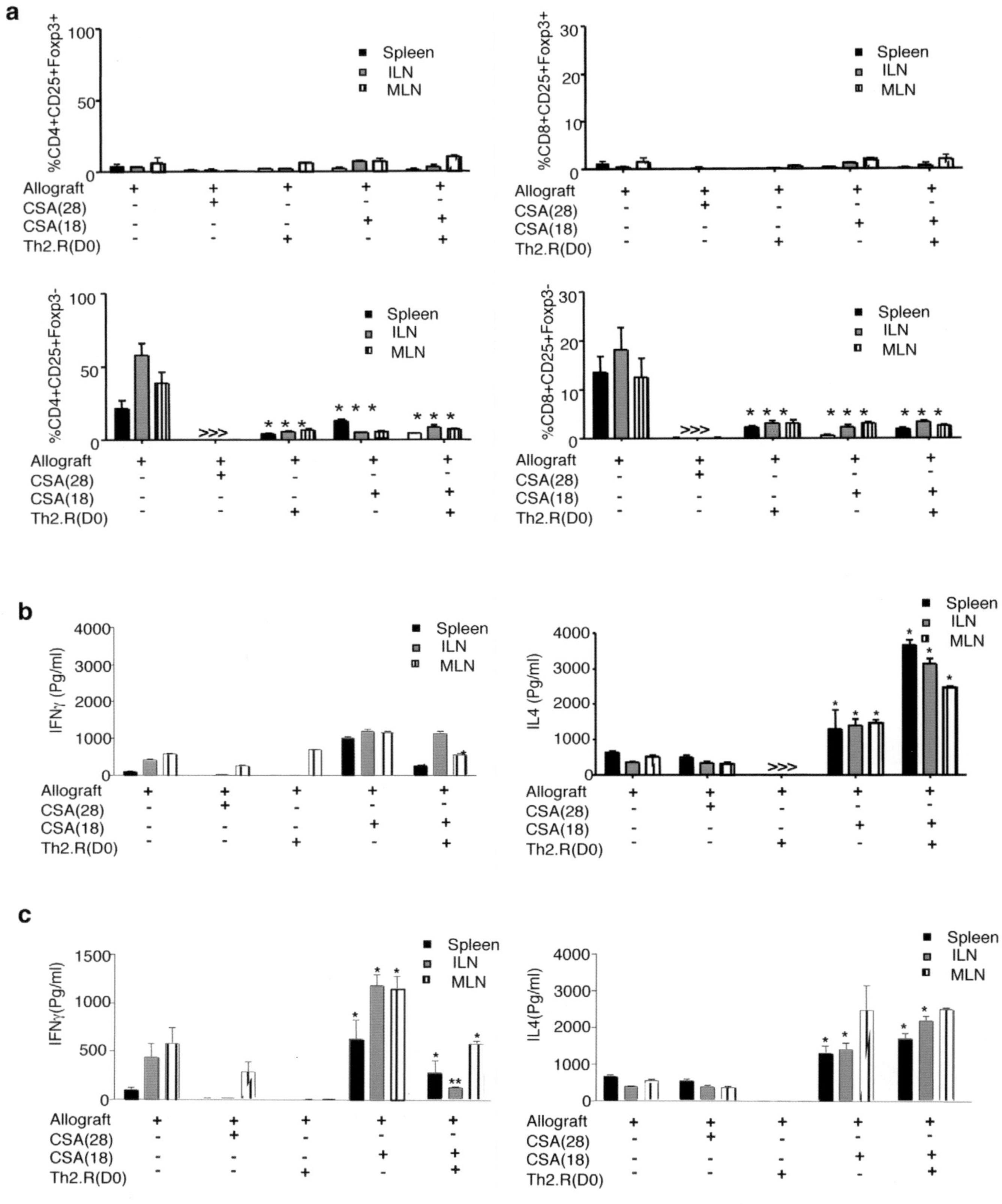

Figure 2. Host Th2.R cell infusion prolongs cardiac allograft survival. Rat allogeneic cardiac transplants was performed and assigned to one of five treatment cohorts, including: no drug and no cell therapy ("rejection control"); 28-day daily cyclosporine A therapy ["CSA(28);" engraftment control]; Th2.R adoptive cell therapy alone on the day of transplant ["Th2.R(d0)"]; 18-day, short-course CSA therapy alone ["CSA(18)"; experimental control]; or a combination of short-course CSA plus Th2.R cell therapy ["CSA(18)+Th2.R(d0)"]. (a) At day 28 post-transplant, recipients were euthanized and spleen, inguinal lymph nodes, and mesenteric lymph nodes were harvested. The frequency of activated $CD4^+$ and $CD8^+$ T cells in each cohort at

each organ site was then determined by flow cytometry (percent of $CD4^+$ or $CD8^+$ T cells that co-expressed CD25 in the absence of Foxp3 expression; results are mean ± SEM of 3 evaluated per cohort; *, indicates p≤0.05; **, indicates p≤0.005). Cells harvested at day 28 post-transplant were co-stimulated (b) or allo-stimulated (c & d), and the 24 h supernatants were tested for cytokine content by multiplex assay.

these $CD8^+$ T cell results, CSA therapy and/or Th2.R cell therapy did not significantly alter $CD4^+$ T cell activation (Fig. 4a; bottom panels); it is possible that the substantial $CD4^+$ T cell activation in Th2.R cell recipients reflects activation of the adoptively transferred Th2.R cells.

Next, we evaluated the in vivo cytokine profile at day 28 post-transplant. Spleen cells from recipients of daily CSA therapy secreted very low levels of IFN-γ in a polyclonal manner (Fig. 4b) or in an allospecific manner (Fig. 4d). In contrast, spleen cells from recipients of either short-course CSA alone or Th2.R cells alone had increased polyclonal and allospecific secretion of IFN-γ. Of note, multiple infusions of Th2.R cells (both day −7 and day 0) prior to transplantation resulted in a decrease in IFN-γ secretion relative to recipients of a single dose Th2.R cells. Recipients of short-course CSA plus Th2.R cells (independent to Th2.R cell timing) had decreased polyclonal and allospecific IFN-γ secretion relative to recipients of short-course CSA alone. Relative to recipient of short-course CSA alone, recipients of short-course CSA plus Th2.R cell infusion had an increase in allospecific IL-4 secretion (Fig. 4e); this increase in allospecific IL-4 secretion was observed in each of the three cohorts to receive Th2.R cells. Interestingly, limited differences was noted in IL-4 secretion between cohorts on polyclonal stimulation (Fig. 4c).

Furthermore, at day 28 post-transplant, we tested for the presence of activated T cells within the cardiac allografts. As anticipated, recipients of short-course CSA alone had a high frequency of activated $CD4^+$ and $CD8^+$ T cells infiltrating the graft (Fig. 4f); by comparison, recipients of daily CSA had minimal evidence of intra-cardiac activated T cells. Relative to recipients of short-course CSA alone, recipients of Th2.R cell therapy in combination with short-course CSA therapy had reduced frequencies of intra-cardiac activated $CD8^+$ T cells. Interestingly, Th2.R cell therapy reduction in the frequency of intra-graft activated $CD4^+$ T cells was modest relative to $CD8^+$ T cells; however, marked reductions of intra-graft activated $CD4^+$ T cells were observed in recipients of Th2.R cells on day 0 of transplant. Most importantly, intra-cardiac T cells from Th2.R cell recipients had greatly reduced capacity to secrete IFN-γ in an allospecific manner relative to recipients of short-course CSA (Fig. 4g).

As anticipated, the control group that received short-course CSA universally had non-viable cardiac allografts by day 28 post-transplant (Fig. 4h); recipients of Th2.R cells alone also universally had nonviable allografts. Administration of daily CSA predictably increased the incidence of clinical graft viability (graft viability frequency, 85%). Remarkably, recipients of short-course CSA combined with Th2.R cells at day 0, day −7, or day −7 plus day 0 were also generally protected from graft failure (graft viability frequencies: 86%, 100%, 100%, respectively; Table 1). Haematoxylin and eosin staining obtained at day 28 post-transplant demonstrated that recipients of short-course CSA, who had poor allograft viability, had severe myocardial necrosis and a dense mononuclear cell infiltration (Fig. 5a). In contrast, recipients of short-course CSA combined with host Th2.R cell therapy had minimal myocardial necrosis in the setting of substantial mononuclear cell infiltration; importantly, recipients of short-course CSA plus Th2 cells on day 0 of transplant had a statistically significant reduction in rejection by standard histology criteria (Fig. 5b). Of note, recipients of Th2 cells at day −7 plus day 0 of transplant or day −7 of transplant, who had 100% graft viability, did not have reduced histology scores.

Discussion

Utilizing a well-characterized experimental rat cardiac transplantation model, we have shown that allograft viability can be prolonged by direct modulation of host immunity via adoptive T cell therapy using rapamycin-generated Th2-type cells. These data add to the growing body of information relating to cellular approaches to rejection prevention, and squarely places an emphasis upon use of host T cell populations as an alternative to indirect modulation of host immunity via third-party donor cell infusions. Importantly, as a step towards potential clinical translation, we have determined that host Th2-type cell adoptive transfer is efficacious when used in combination with calcineurin inhibitor therapy, which remains the standard of care therapy.

Reports more than 30 years ago determined that donor-specific [18] or third-party [19] transfusions reduced solid organ transplantation rejection through a phenomenon termed donor-specific-tolerance. However, further clinical advances with respect to use of adoptive cell therapy for rejection abrogation did not ensue, in part because the mechanism(s) underlying transfusion-induced tolerance have not been fully characterized and in part because adoptive cell therapy is only now becoming a burgeoning translational medical approach [20]. It has long been proposed that modulation of host T cell immunity might be harnessed to promote graft tolerance, including an early study of "host T cell vaccination" prior to experimental transplantation [21]; however, further investigations into host derived T cell based engraftment strategies have been limited. Extensive mechanistic data exists on donor specific tolerance [11], [14] where adoptive transfer of ex vivo generated host Treg cells prevents allograft rejection [22,23]. Although focus has been placed upon host Tregs for cellular induction of transplantation tolerance [reviewed in [24,25]], other host T cell populations such as $CD4^-CD8^-$ "double-negative" T cells have been shown to facilitate engraftment [26]. In this context, our current results using host-type, rapamycin-generated Th2 cells indicate that a diversity of functionally-defined host T cell subsets represent candidate populations to prevent solid organ graft rejection.

The current study is the first to demonstrate that the adoptive transfer of Th2 polarized host T cells represents a candidate approach to prolong cardiac allograft viability. Although enthusiasm for the potential role of Th2 responses for the regulation of Th1-mediated solid organ rejection has waned with the resurgence of Treg cell research [reviewed in [27]], several previous studies have supported a beneficial role of Th2 cells in cardiac transplantation models, including: evidence that type II cytokines help promote 'infectious tolerance' [28]; modulation of the Th1/Th2 balance via ICAM/LFA blockade [14]; and Treg cell up-regulation of IL-4 and Th2 responses during infectious tolerance [29]. In our studies, the phenotype of the ex vivo, rapamycin-generated host T cell population was consistent with an effector Th2 phenotype, as indicated by prolific secretion of IL-4, a high precursor frequency of cells capable of IL-4 secretion, and minimal expression of the Treg cell transcription factor, FoxP3. These results stand somewhat in contrast to other ex vivo results that described rapamycin to promote Treg cell differentiation [30], but

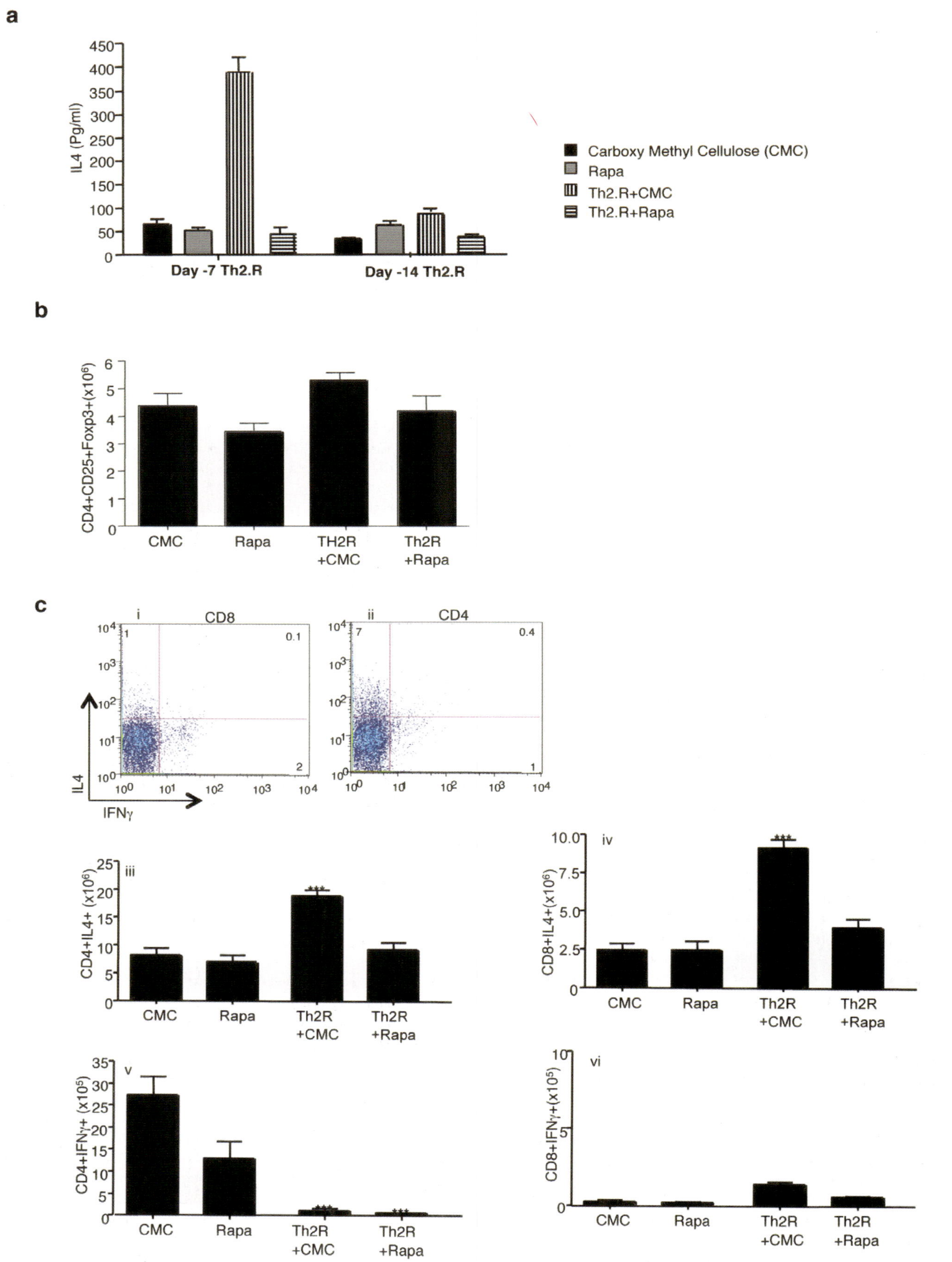
a
IL4 (Pg/ml)
Day -7 Th2.R
Day -14 Th2.R
Carboxy Methyl Cellulose (CMC)
Rapa
Th2.R+CMC
Th2.R+Rapa
b
CD4+CD25+Foxp3+(x10^6)
CMC
Rapa
TH2R +CMC
Th2R +Rapa
c
i CD8
ii CD4
IL4
IFNγ
iii CD4+IL4+ (x10^6)
iv CD8+IL4+(x10^6)
v CD4+IFNγ+ (x10^5)
vi CD8+IFNγ+(x10^5)
CMC
Rapa
Th2R +CMC
Th2R +Rapa

Figure 3. Evaluation of Th2.R cell timing and rapamycin co-administration. Host-type BN rats received an intravenous infusion of isogeneic Th2.R cells either at day −7 or day −14 prior to host euthanasia at "day 0", with subsequent immune evaluation; Th2 cell therapy was administered either alone or in combination with in vivo rapamycin therapy. (a) Harvested spleen, inguinal lymph node, and mesenteric lymph node cells were harvested and subjected to co-stimulation; resultant 24 h supernatants were then tested for cytokine content by Multiplex assay. (b) % Foxp3 expression was measured using IC flow on splenocytes at day7 (c) After co-stimulation, $CD4^+$ and $CD8^+$ T cells from recipients in each cohort were evaluated by intra-cellular flow cytometry for IFN-γ and IL-4 production. * indicates $P<0.05$; $n=5$ per cohort.

are consistent with our murine results that have identified a capacity to generate either effector Th1 and Th2 populations in rapamycin depending upon polarizing cytokine exposure [17,31].

Most importantly, the adoptively transferred T cells mediated a Th2-type response in vivo, as evidenced by: increased post-transfer IL-4 secretion; reduced post-transfer IFN-γ secretion; and minimal induction of Foxp3-expressing T cells. We also observed that recipients of the $CD4^+$ Th2.R cells were enriched for post-transplant $CD8^+$ T cell capacity for IL-4 secretion capacity; this result indicates that the post-transplant Th2 polarization induced through Th2.R cell infusion could be attributable not only to the infused Th2 cell product but also to the transfer of Th2 polarity to endogenous T cells. Similar to our previous observations in murine bone marrow transplant models that utilizing donor-derived Th2.R cells [15,32], we also observed that host adoptive Th2 cell therapy significantly reduced the number of post-transplant $CD8^+$ T cells in secondary lymphoid organs; given the major role for host $CD8^+$ T cells in mediating cardiac allograft rejection [33,34], we speculate that Th2-mediated control of $CD8^+$ T cell immunity may account in part for allograft survival effect we observed in this model. It is interesting to note that Th2.R cell infusion alone did not achieve post-transplant skewing towards a Th2 phenotype, whereas Th2.R cell infusion plus short-course CSA consistently yielded increased post-transplant IL-4 and reduced post-transplant IFN-γ. We speculate that CSA therapy is limiting the expansion of the host Th1-type rejection response, thereby allowing expansion of the infused Th2 cells; in the absence of CSA, the Th2 cells may be inhibited by a predominant Th1 response.

Our results stand somewhat in contrast to previous studies that found Tc2 cells [35] or IL-4 [36] to be detrimental to graft survival. We speculate that our use of purified $CD4^+$ T cells that secreted high levels of IL-4 may help account for the positive results we achieved with a type II cytokine strategy; further experiments will be required to clarify specific molecular mechanisms that account for the Th2.R cell therapeutic effect. It should be mentioned that our model utilizes a relatively short recipient follow-up for assessment of allograft viability, and as such, the effect of the Th2 cell strategy on long term allograft viability would require further study [37]. We observed that both the long-term immune suppression cohort and the short-course suppression plus Th2.R cohort each had prolonged allograft viability; therefore, from these experiments, we can not conclude that one strategy is advantageous relative to the other. Rather, we conclude that short-course suppression plus infusion of a T cell modulation population such as the host Th2.R cells may represent an alternative to long-term immune suppression. Determination of the relative risks and benefits of each approach would require further comparative studies in additional models.

It is important to point out that, in spite of the increase in cardiac viability in Th2.R cell recipients, such recipients did not have a reduction in the rejection score by standard histology criteria. It should be noted that the rejection score is based heavily on mononuclear cell infiltration; because we found that Th2.R cell recipients had relatively dense intra-cardiac T cell infiltration by cells that did not secrete allospecific IFN-γ, it is possible that in the context of interventions such as host-type Th2.R cell transfer, cardiac infiltration by mononuclear cells alone may not accurately predict rejection. Finally, it should also be noted that we did not assess the impact of Th2.R cell infusion on alloantibody formation, which can play an important role as a mediator of kidney allograft rejection [reviewed in [38]].

Infusion of host-type Th2.R cells one week pre-transplant optimally promoted host Th2-type immunity at the time of transplant and preserved allograft viability in 100% of recipients. Since the Th2.R cell product was generated in high-dose rapamycin, we predicted that the Th2.R cells may be relatively resistant to the effects of in vivo rapamycin, thereby further promoting an in vivo Th2 shift; however, to the contrary, co-administration of rapamycin drug therapy abrogated the ability of Th2.R cells to polarize host immunity towards a Th2 phenotype. In our previous murine studies, we did observe that ex vivo rapamycin resistance does not necessarily confer resistance to rapamycin in vivo [17]; such observations may be due to rapamycin blockade of non-T cell pathways in vivo, such as antigen-presenting-cell populations [39] that may help drive T cell expansion in vivo. Furthermore, we also determined that administration of rapamycin did not increase $Foxp3^+$ regulatory T cells in vivo. In contrast to these results using in vivo rapamycin, we found that cyclosporine therapy was permissive for the immune modulatory effect generated through Th2 cell therapy. As such, although experimental models indicate that rapamycin has more tolerance-induction properties relative to cyclosporine therapy [40,41,42], our data indicate that calcineurin inhibitor therapy may be preferentially utilized in the setting of polarized Th2.R cell therapy for solid organ allografting. It is also important to note that infusion of Th2.R cells on the same day as cardiac allografting was sufficient to prolong allograft survival; this lack of requirement for pre-infusion of Th2 cells would be advantageous for clinical translation because of the unpredictability of cardiac allograft availability.

In conclusion, the adoptive transfer of ex vivo generated, rapamycin-resistant host Th2-type cells represents an effective new approach to the prolongation of cardiac allograft viability. These data support the current momentum in the field to develop adoptive cell therapies for tolerance induction in a calcineurin-inhibitor sparing manner, and suggests that functionally-defined and cytokine-polarized effector T cells, as well as Treg cells, may contribute to the future armamentarium to protect against solid organ allograft rejection.

Materials and Methods

Animal care

The experiments were performed as part of a protocol approved by the Animal Care and Use Committee (ACUC) of the Clinical Center of the National Institutes of Health (NIH; Animal study protocol approval number CCM 06-02). Inbred male brown Norway (BN) and dark agouti (DA) rats, weighing 200–250 g, were purchased from Charles River Laboratories (Wilmington, MA) and maintained under pathogen free conditions.

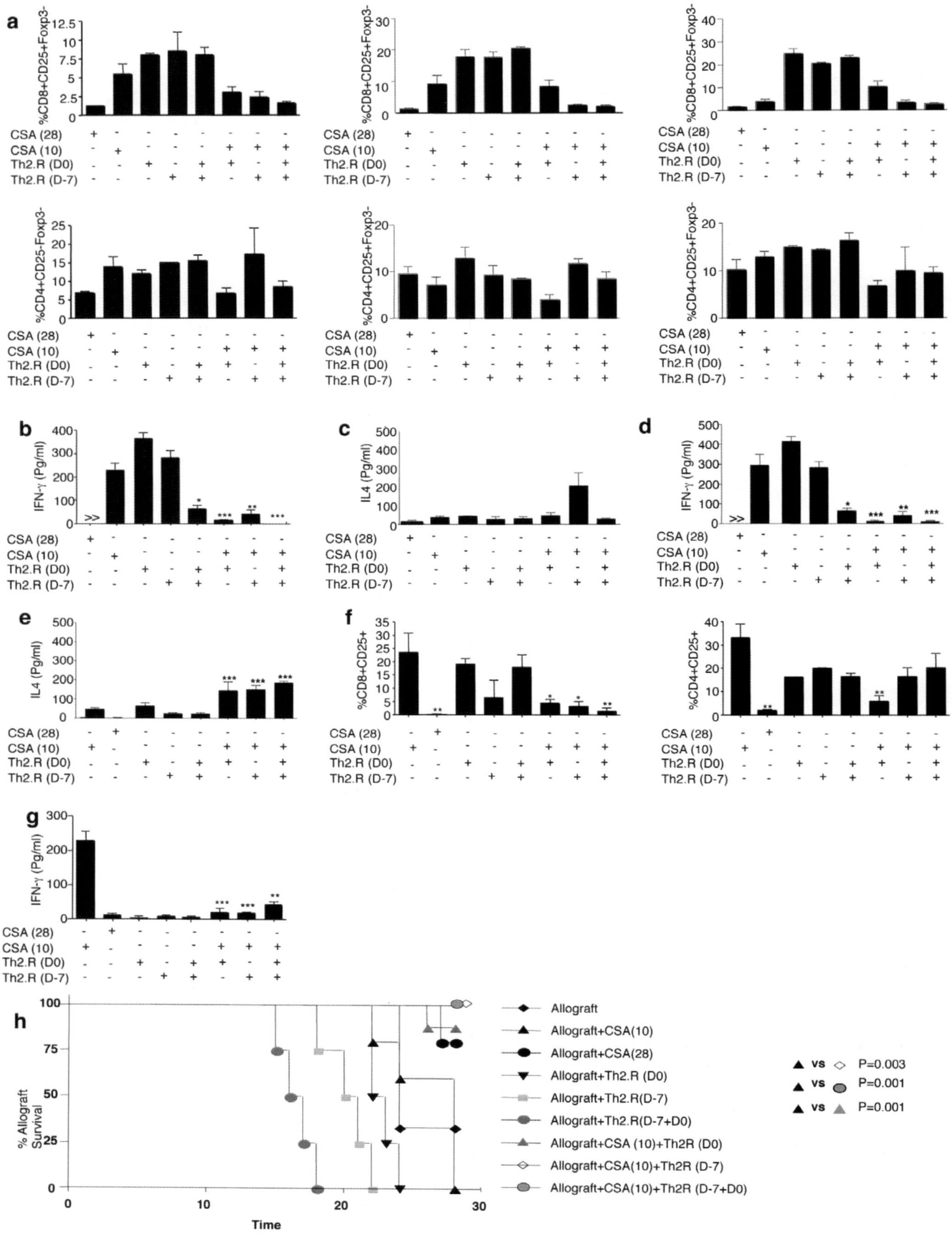
a
%CD8+CD25+Foxp3-
%CD4+CD25-Foxp3-
%CD4+CD25+Foxp3-
CSA (28)
CSA (10)
Th2.R (D0)
Th2.R (D-7)
b
IFN-γ (Pg/ml)
c
IL4 (Pg/ml)
d
e
f
%CD8+CD25+
%CD4+CD25+
g
h
% Allograft Survival
Time
Allograft
Allograft+CSA(10)
Allograft+CSA(28)
Allograft+Th2.R (D0)
Allograft+Th2.R(D-7)
Allograft+Th2.R(D-7+D0)
Allograft+CSA (10)+Th2R (D0)
Allograft+CSA(10)+Th2R (D-7)
Allograft+CSA(10)+Th2R (D-7+D0)
vs P=0.003
vs P=0.001
vs P=0.001

Figure 4. Th2.R cell therapy plus cyclosporine reduces host T cell activation, induces a host Th2 phenotype, and reduces intracardiac allospecific T cells. Rat allogeneic cardiac transplants were performed and assigned to one of eight treatment cohorts, including; 28-day daily cyclosporine A therapy ["CSA(28)"; engraftment control]; Th2.R adoptive cell therapy alone ("Th2.R") at day 0 (D0), day-7 (D-7) or both (D-7+D0); 10-day, short-course CSA therapy alone ["CSA(10);" experimental control]; or a combination of short-course CSA plus Th2.R cell therapy ["CSA(10)+Th2.R"] at day 0 (D0), day-7 (D-7) or both (D-7+D0). (a) At day 28 post-transplant, transplant recipients were euthanized and splenocytes were harvested. The frequency of activated $CD4^+$ and $CD8^+$ T cells in each cohort at each organ site was then determined by flow cytometry (percent of $CD4^+$ or $CD8^+$ T cells that co-expressed CD25 in the absence of Foxp3 expression; results are mean ± SEM of 5 or 7 evaluated per cohort; *, indicates $p<0.05$). Splenocytes were harvested and subjected to either co-stimulation (b & c) or syngeneic and allogeneic APC stimulation (d & e; allospecific cytokine secretion is shown); resultant 24 h supernatants were then tested for cytokine content by Multiplex assay. (f) The frequency of activated $CD4^+$ and $CD8^+$ T cells in harvested cardiac tissue was determined by flow cytometry (percent of $CD4^+$ or $CD8^+$ T cells that co-expressed CD25 in the absence of Foxp3 expression; results are mean ± SEM of 7 evaluated per cohort; *, indicates $p<0.05$). (g) Intracardiac T cells were subjected to stimulation with allogeneic dendritic cells; resultant 24 h supernatants were then tested for cytokine content by Multiplex assay. (h) Survival of cardiac allografts between various cohorts is shown.

Antibodies and reagents

RPMI media, rapamycin, and sodium pyruvate was obtained from Sigma (St.Louis, MO) and FCS was from Gem Cell (West Sacramento, CA). CD4 microbeads were from Miltenyi Biotec (Auburn, CA). Goat anti-rat Ig G was from Qiagen (Valencia, CA). Anti-CD3, anti-CD28 coated tosyl-activated magnetic beads were manufactured as previously described [43]. Recombinant human (rh) IL-2, (rh) IL-7 and (rr) IL-4 were from PeproTech (Rocky Hill, NJ). Penicillin-streptomycin-glutamine, nonessential amino acid and N-acetyl-L-cysteine was obtained from Invitrogen

Table 1. Summary of experimental design.

Experimental Design for data in Figure #2			
Treatment Cohorts (n)	**Cardiac Allograft[1]**	**CSA Drug Therapy (Total Days)[2]**	**Immunotherapy Th2.R (Day administered)[3]**
1. n = 3 (Rejection Control)	Y	N	N
2. n = 3 (Treatment Control)	Y	Y (28)	N
3. n = 3 (Sub-optimal Drug Therapy)	Y	Y (18)	N
4. n = 3 (Immunotherapy)	Y	N	Y (0)
5. n = 3 (Immunotherapy)	Y	Y (18)	Y (0)
Experimental Design for data in Figure #3			
Treatment Cohorts (n)	**Cardiac Allograft**	**Rapamycin Drug Therapy (Total Days prior to transplant)[4]**	**Immunotherapy Th2.R (Day administered)**
1(Experimental Control), n = 5	N	CMC (7)	N
2(Experimental Control), n = 5	N	RAPA (7)	N
3(Immunotherapy), n = 5	N	CMC (7)	Y (−7)
4(Immunotherapy), n = 5	N	RAPA (7)	Y (−7)
5(Experimental Control), n = 5	N	CMC (14)	N
6(Experimental Control), n = 5	N	RAPA (14)	N
7(Immunotherapy), n = 5	N	CMC (14)	Y (−14)
8(Immunotherapy), n = 5	N	RAPA (14)	Y (−14)
Experimental Design for data in Figure #4&5			
Treatment Cohorts	**Cardiac Allograft**	**CSA Drug Therapy (Total Days)**	**Immunotherapy Th2.R (Day administered)**
1(Rejection Control), n = 7	Y	Y (10)	N
2(Treatment Control), n = 7	Y	Y (28)	N
3(Immunotherapy), n = 7	Y	N	Y (0)
4(Immunotherapy), n = 5	Y	N	Y (−7)
5(Immunotherapy), n = 4	Y	N	Y (0 & −7)
6(Immunotherapy), n = 5	Y	Y (10)	Y (0)
7(Immunotherapy), n = 7	Y	Y (10)	Y (−7)
8(Immunotherapy), n = 7	Y	Y (10)	Y (0 & −7)

[1]Y = yes, N = no; DA donor hearts transplanted into BN recipient rats.
[2]Cyclosporine (CSA) administered subcutaneously (10 mg/kg/day).
[3]Th2.R = Th2 cells were generated from host BN CD4+ T cells.
[4]Rapamycin (Rapa) administered i.p (1.5 mg/kg/day); CMC = carboxymethylcellulose.

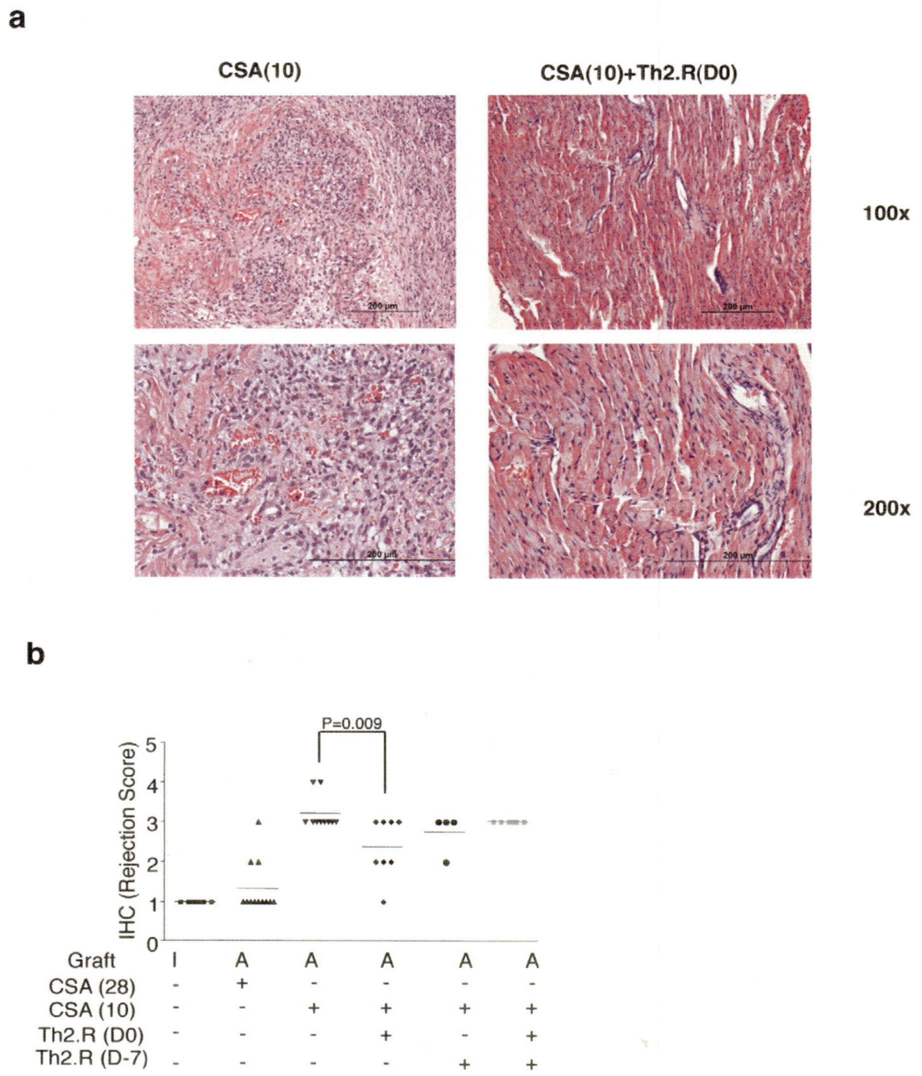

Figure 5. Th2.R cell therapy plus cyclosporine prolongs cardiac allograft survival. Allograft recipients were monitored for cardiac viability through the 28-day post-transplant period of observation. Rejection and engraftment control cohorts received a 10-day short-course of cyclosporine A ["CSA(10]" or a daily 28-day course of "CSA [CSA(28)"]. Other cohorts received either no cyclosporine A or short-course CSA(10) in combination with Th2.R cell therapy at day −7 ["Th2.R(D-7)" or "CSA(10)+Th2.R(D-7)"], day 0 ["Th2.R(D0)" or "CSA(10)+Th2.R(D0)"], or day −7 plus day 0 ["Th2.R(D-7+D0)" or "CSA(10)+Th2.R(D-7+DO)"]. (a) Hematoxylin and eosin staining was performed at day 28 post-transplant. Left panels show a representative example of severe allograft rejection in recipients of short-course CSA(10) alone (characterized by diffuse inflammation and necrosis); right panels show a representative example of relatively preserved myocardial cell structure and reduced mononuclear cell infiltration in recipients of short-course CSA(10) therapy plus Th2.R cell therapy. (b) Cumulative histology score between various cohorts is shown. I = isograft, A = Allograft; IHC score = Immunohistochemistry score.

Life Technologies (Carlsbad, CA). All antibodies (unless otherwise stated) were purchased from BD Biosciences (BD; San Diego, CA); anti-rat Foxp3 APC was from eBioscience (San Diego, CA). Luminex kits for detection of rat IL-2, IL-4, IFN-γ and IL-10 were from Bio-Rad (Hercules, CA). Cyclosporine A (CSA or Sandimmune®) was from Novartis (Hanover, NJ).

T cell subset isolation and ex vivo culture of Th2.R cells

Spleens were harvested from host type BN rats, RBC lysed and B cells were depleted (goat anti-rat IgG beads); CD4 T cells were enriched using Miltenyi CD4 microbeads as per manufacturer's instructions. Total $CD4^+$ T cells were cultured in polystyrene tissue culture flasks (Corning; Lowell, MA). Cells were activated by anti-CD3 (clone:G4.18), anti-CD28 (clone: JJ316) co-stimulation (bead:cell ratio, 3:1) and cultured in RPMI media containing 10% FCS, 1× Sodium pyruvate, 1× non-essential amino acids, β-ME (5×10^{-5} M), 1× streptomycin-penicillin and glutamine. Cytokines (rh) IL-2 (100 IU/ml), (rh) IL-7 (20 ng/ml), (rr) IL-4 (10000 IU/ml) and rapamycin (10 μM) were added to the culture at day 0. Cultures were started at 1.5×10^6 cells/ml, and (rh) IL-2 was again added at day 2. Cultures were harvested on day 3 for phenotyping and adoptive transfer experiments.

Heterotropic cardiac transplantation

Brown-Norway (BN) rats served as recipient and Dark Agouti (DA) rats served as allograft cardiac donor. Allogeneic cardiac

Table 2. Summary of cardiac viability by palpation (day 28 post-transplant).

Treatment Cohort	Frequency of Isograft/Allograft Viability	Percent Allograft Viability	Median Graft Survival (Days)
1	10/10	100%	N/A
2	1/3	33%	24
3	0/7	0%	22
4	6/7	83%	N/A
5	0/7	0%	22.5
6	0/5	0%	20.5
7	0/4	0%	16.5
8	4/5	80%	N/A
9	7/7	100%	N/A
10	7/7	100%	N/A

1 = Isograft alone.
2 = Allograft alone.
3 = Allograft+CSA (10 days of therapy).
4 = Allograft+CSA (28 days of therapy).
5 = Allograft+Th2.R (Day 0 infusion).
6 = Allograft+Th2.R (Day −7 infusion).
7 = Allograft+Th2.R (Day −7+Day 0 infusion).
8 = Allograft+CSA (10 days)+Th2.R (Day 0 infusion).
9 = Allograft+CSA (10 days)+Th2.R (Day −7 infusion).
10 = Allograft+CSA (10 days)+Th2.R (Day −7+Day 0 infusion).

transplantations were performed using a modified version of the heterotopic cardiac transplantation model reported by Yokoyama *et al* [44]. As previously described [45], preparation of the donor heart for transplantation entailed ligation of pulmonary vessels, superior vena cava and inferior vena cava (IVC), creation of an atrial septal defect, and disruption of the tricuspid valve leaflets. The donor ascending aorta was anastamosed to the recipient abdominal aorta and the donor right atrium was anastamosed to the recipient IVC. Upon re-establishment of blood flow, all transplanted hearts resumed spontaneous contractions, had coordinated atrioventricular activity, and were free of gross surgical injury at the time of closure. The transplanted animals were subjected to various treatments with CSA (0, 10, 18, or 28 day regimen), rapamycin, and adoptive transfer of 1×10^7 Th2.R cells per injection (at day 0 of transplant and/or day −7 pre-transplant), as summarized in Table 2. Survival of cardiac grafts was evaluated by daily palpation; cessation of heartbeat was interpreted as lack of viability. Specimens were processed for histopathology using hematoxylin and eosin staining [46].

Flow cytometry

T cells were washed with PBS supplemented with 0.1% BSA and 0.01% azide, and stained using anti-: CD4 PE-cy5 (clone ox-35), CD8 APC (clone ox-8), CD3 biotin (clone g.18), Streptavidin PE-cy7 and CD25 PE (clone ox-39). For intra-cellular (IC) flow cytometry, fixation and permeabilization buffer was utilized (eBioscience); Intracellular flow cytometry was performed with combinations of anti-: IFN-γ FITC (clone DB-1; Biolegend, San Diego, CA), IL-4 PE (clone ox-81), CD4 PE-Cy7 and Foxp3 Pacific Blue (clone FJK-16s; eBioscience). Cells were analyzed using a BD Biosciences LSR II (San Jose, CA) equipped with 488, 633, 405 and 355 nm lasers and thirteen detectors. Data was acquire using DiVa ver. 5.1 (BD Biosciences), and analyzed using FlowJo ver. 8.8 (Treestar Software, Ashland, WA).

Allogeneic mixed lymphocyte reaction (MLR)

Bone marrow DC were generated from DA and BN rats, RBC lysed and cultured in RPMI media with 5% FCS, (rr) GM-CSF (50 ng/ml), and (rr) IL-4 (20 ng/ml) for 5 days. Bacterial LPS (1 μg/ml; Sigma) was added to the culture for 24 hrs and DC were harvested. The DC from syngeneic and allogeneic hosts were utilized to stimulate spleen cells for measuring allo-specific responses.

Cytokine analysis using multibead array

The expanded Th2 cells were harvested at day 3 and extensively washed with media prior to restimulation with anti-CD3 and anti-CD28. Supernatants were collected 24 hr post-stimulation and analyzed for cytokines using the Biorad Multiplex bead array. Single cell suspensions of spleen (1×10^6/ml), inguinal lymph nodes (1×10^6/ml), and mesenteric lymph nodes (1×10^6/ml) were obtained from rats post-transplant and stimulated with anti-CD3, anti-CD28 coated beads followed by incubation at 37°C for 24 hrs. The supernatants were harvested and Th1/Th2 cytokine profile was measured using a Biorad multiplex bead array. In some experiments, T cells were stimulated with BN or DA dendritic cells (DC) (spleen cell to DC ratio, 10:1) for 24 h. Allogeneic cytokine secretion was subtracted out of syngeneic cytokine secretion and is presented as allo-specific responses.

Statistical analysis

Flow cytometry and cytokine data were analyzed using student's 2-tailed *t* tests. Comparison values of $p<0.05$ were considered statistically significant. Survival was determined using Kaplan Meier test.

Acknowledgments

The authors would like to thank Joanna M Swerczek for her invaluable technical Support. The authors would also like to thank Dr. William Telford for flow cytometry advice.

Author Contributions

Conceived and designed the experiments: SA HC MAS DHF. Performed the experiments: SA HC JEF CMC. Analyzed the data: SA HC JDS. Wrote the paper: SA HC MAS DHF.

References

1. Cooley D FO, Panvini G (1983) Cardiac and cardiopulmonary transplantation using cyclosporine for immunosuppresion:recent texas Heart Institute experience. Transplant Proc 15.
2. Patel JK, Kobashigawa JA (2004) Cardiac transplant experience with cyclosporine. Transplant Proc 36: 323S–330S.
3. Maes BD, Vanrenterghem YF (2004) Cyclosporine: advantages versus disadvantages vis-a-vis tacrolimus. Transplant Proc 36: 40S–49S.
4. Khush KK, Valantine HA (2009) New developments in immunosuppressive therapy for heart transplantation. Expert Opin Emerg Drugs 14: 1–21.
5. Egidi MF, Gaber AO (2003) Outcomes of African-American kidney-transplant recipients treated with sirolimus, tacrolimus, and corticosteroids. Transplantation 75: 572; author reply 573.
6. Woodruff MF, van Rood JJ (1983) Possible implications of the effect of blood transfusion on allograft survival. Lancet 1: 1201–1203.
7. Kitade H, Kawai M, Koshiba T, Giulietti A, Overbergh L, et al. (2004) Early accumulation of interferon-gamma in grafts tolerized by donor-specific blood transfusion: friend or enemy? Transplantation 78: 1747–1755.
8. Levy AE, Alexander JW, Babcock GF (1997) A strategy for generating consistent long-term donor-specific tolerance to solid organ allografts. Transpl Immunol 5: 83–88.

9. Kataoka M, Shimizu Y, Margenthaler JA, Landeros K, Otomo N, et al. (2002) Transfer of "infectious" cardiac allograft tolerance induced by donor-specific transfusion. Surgery 132: 167–172.
10. Kataoka M, Margenthaler JA, Ku G, Eilers M, Flye MW (2003) "Infectious tolerance" develops after the spontaneous acceptance of Lewis-to-Dark Agouti rat liver transplants. Surgery 134: 227–234.
11. Abe Y, Urakami H, Ostanin D, Zibari G, Hayashida T, et al. (2009) Induction of Foxp3-expressing regulatory T-cells by donor blood transfusion is required for tolerance to rat liver allografts. PLoS One 4: e7840.
12. Mariotti J, Foley J, Ryan K, Buxhoeveden N, Kapoor V, et al. (2008) Graft rejection as a Th1-type process amenable to regulation by donor Th2-type cells through an interleukin-4/STAT6 pathway. Blood 112: 4765–4775.
13. Mariotti J, Foley J, Jung U, Borenstein T, Kantardzic N, et al. (2008) Ex vivo rapamycin generates apoptosis-resistant donor Th2 cells that persist in vivo and prevent hemopoietic stem cell graft rejection. J Immunol 180: 89–105.
14. Isobe M, Suzuki J, Yamazaki S, Yazaki Y, Horie S, et al. (1997) Regulation by differential development of Th1 and Th2 cells in peripheral tolerance to cardiac allograft induced by blocking ICAM-1/LFA-1 adhesion. Circulation 96: 2247–2253.
15. Foley JE, Jung U, Miera A, Borenstein T, Mariotti J, et al. (2005) Ex vivo rapamycin generates donor Th2 cells that potently inhibit graft-versus-host disease and graft-versus-tumor effects via an IL-4-dependent mechanism. J Immunol 175: 5732–5743.
16. Jung U, Foley JE, Erdmann AA, Eckhaus MA, Fowler DH (2003) CD3/CD28-costimulated T1 and T2 subsets: differential in vivo allosensitization generates distinct GVT and GVHD effects. Blood 102: 3439–3446.
17. Jung U, Foley JE, Erdmann AA, Toda Y, Borenstein T, et al. (2006) Ex vivo rapamycin generates Th1/Tc1 or Th2/Tc2 Effector T cells with enhanced in vivo function and differential sensitivity to post-transplant rapamycin therapy. Biol Blood Marrow Transplant 12: 905–918.
18. Opelz G, Terasaki PI, Graver B, Sasaki N, Langston M, et al. (1979) Correlation between number of pretransplant blood transfusions and kidney graft survival. Transplant Proc 11: 145–147.
19. Cochrum K, Hanes D, Potter D, Perkins H, Amend W, et al. (1981) Improved graft survival following donor-specific blood transfusions. Transplant Proc 13: 1657–1661.
20. Paulos CM, Suhoski MM, Plesa G, Jiang T, Basu S, et al. (2008) Adoptive immunotherapy: good habits instilled at youth have long-term benefits. Immunol Res 42: 182–196.
21. Shapira OM, Mor E, Reshef T, Pfeffermann RA, Cohen IR (1993) Prolongation of survival of rat cardiac allografts by T cell vaccination. J Clin Invest 91: 388–390.
22. Golshayan D, Jiang S, Tsang J, Garin MI, Mottet C, et al. (2007) In vitro-expanded donor alloantigen-specific CD4+CD25+ regulatory T cells promote experimental transplantation tolerance. Blood 109: 827–835.
23. Joffre O, Santolaria T, Calise D, Al Saati T, Hudrisier D, et al. (2008) Prevention of acute and chronic allograft rejection with CD4+CD25+Foxp3+ regulatory T lymphocytes. Nat Med 14: 88–92.
24. Cobbold SP, Adams E, Graca L, Daley S, Yates S, et al. (2006) Immune privilege induced by regulatory T cells in transplantation tolerance. Immunol Rev 213: 239–255.
25. Kang SM, Tang Q, Bluestone JA (2007) CD4+CD25+ regulatory T cells in transplantation: progress, challenges and prospects. Am J Transplant 7: 1457–1463.
26. Young KJ, Yang L, Phillips MJ, Zhang L (2002) Donor-lymphocyte infusion induces transplantation tolerance by activating systemic and graft-infiltrating double-negative regulatory T cells. Blood 100: 3408–3414.
27. Zhai Y, Ghobrial RM, Busuttil RW, Kupiec-Weglinski JW (1999) Th1 and Th2 cytokines in organ transplantation: paradigm lost? Crit Rev Immunol 19: 155–172.
28. Onodera K, Hancock WW, Graser E, Lehmann M, Sayegh MH, et al. (1997) Type 2 helper T cell-type cytokines and the development of "infectious" tolerance in rat cardiac allograft recipients. J Immunol 158: 1572–1581.
29. Ke B, Ritter T, Kato H, Zhai Y, Li J, et al. (2000) Regulatory cells potentiate the efficacy of IL-4 gene transfer by up-regulating Th2-dependent expression of protective molecules in the infectious tolerance pathway in transplant recipients. J Immunol 164: 5739–5745.
30. Battaglia M, Stabilini A, Roncarolo MG (2005) Rapamycin selectively expands CD4+CD25+FoxP3+ regulatory T cells. Blood 105: 4743–4748.
31. Amarnath S, Flomerfelt FA, Costanzo CM, Foley JE, Mariotti J, et al. Rapamycin generates anti-apoptotic human Th1/Tc1 cells via autophagy for induction of xenogeneic GVHD. Autophagy 6.
32. Fowler DH, Kurasawa K, Husebekk A, Cohen PA, Gress RE (1994) Cells of Th2 cytokine phenotype prevent LPS-induced lethality during murine graft-versus-host reaction. Regulation of cytokines and CD8+ lymphoid engraftment. J Immunol 152: 1004–1013.
33. Yamada A, Laufer TM, Gerth AJ, Chase CM, Colvin RB, et al. (2003) Further analysis of the T-cell subsets and pathways of murine cardiac allograft rejection. Am J Transplant 3: 23–27.
34. Schenk AD, Nozaki T, Rabant M, Valujskikh A, Fairchild RL (2008) Donor-reactive CD8 memory T cells infiltrate cardiac allografts within 24-h posttransplant in naive recipients. Am J Transplant 8: 1652–1661.
35. Hall BM, Plain KM, Verma ND, Tran GT, Boyd R, et al. (2007) Transfer of allograft specific tolerance requires CD4+CD25+T cells but not interleukin-4 or transforming growth factor-beta and cannot induce tolerance to linked antigens. Transplantation 83: 1075–1084.
36. Delfs MW, Furukawa Y, Mitchell RN, Lichtman AH (2001) CD8+ T cell subsets TC1 and TC2 cause different histopathologic forms of murine cardiac allograft rejection. Transplantation 71: 606–610.
37. Illigens BM, Yamada A, Anosova N, Dong VM, Sayegh MH, et al. (2009) Dual effects of the alloresponse by Th1 and Th2 cells on acute and chronic rejection of allotransplants. Eur J Immunol 39: 3000–3009.
38. Lucas JG, Co JP, Nwaogwugwu UT, Dosani I, Sureshkumar KK (2011) Antibody-mediated rejection in kidney transplantation: an update. Expert Opin Pharmacother 12(4): 579–592.
39. Hackstein H, Taner T, Zahorchak AF, Morelli AE, Logar AJ, et al. (2003) Rapamycin inhibits IL-4–induced dendritic cell maturation in vitro and dendritic cell mobilization and function in vivo. Blood 101: 4457–4463.
40. Li Y, Zheng XX, Li XC, Zand MS, Strom TB (1998) Combined costimulation blockade plus rapamycin but not cyclosporine produces permanent engraftment. Transplantation 66: 1387–1388.
41. Gao W, Lu Y, El Essawy B, Oukka M, Kuchroo VK, et al. (2007) Contrasting effects of cyclosporine and rapamycin in de novo generation of alloantigen-specific regulatory T cells. Am J Transplant 7: 1722–1732.
42. Raimondi G, Sumpter TL, Matta BM, Pillai M, Corbitt N, et al. Mammalian target of rapamycin inhibition and alloantigen-specific regulatory T cells synergize to promote long-term graft survival in immunocompetent recipients. J Immunol 184: 624–636.
43. Levine BL, Bernstein WB, Connors M, Craighead N, Lindsten T, et al. (1997) Effects of CD28 costimulation on long-term proliferation of CD4+ T cells in the absence of exogenous feeder cells. J Immunol 159: 5921–5930.
44. Yokoyama H, Ohmi M, Murata S, Nakame T, Tabayashi K, et al. (1995) Proposal of a working left heart model with a heterotopic transplantation technique in rats. J Heart Lung Transplant 14: 706–712.
45. Deans KJ, Minneci PC, Chen H, Kern SJ, Logun C, et al. (2009) Impact of animal strain on gene expression in a rat model of acute cardiac rejection. BMC Genomics 10: 280.
46. Stewart S, Winters GL, Fishbein MC, Tazelaar HD, Kobashigawa J, et al. (2005) Revision of the 1990 working formulation for the standardization of nomenclature in the diagnosis of heart rejection. J Heart Lung Transplant 24: 1710–1720.

Adiponectin Mediated MHC Class II Mismatched Cardiac Graft Rejection in Mice Is IL-4 Dependent

Daxu Li[1¤], Julia Y. S. Tsang[1], Jiao Peng[1], Derek H. H. Ho[2], Yee Kwan Chan[3], Jiang Zhu[1], Vincent C. H. Lui[1], Aimin Xu[4], Jonathan R. Lamb[5], Paul K. H. Tam[1*], Yan Chen[1,2*]

1 Paediatric Surgery Division, Department of Surgery, The University of Hong Kong, Hong Kong SAR, China, **2** Department of Chemistry, The University of Hong Kong, Hong Kong SAR, China, **3** School of Biological Science, The University of Hong Kong, Hong Kong SAR, China, **4** Department of Medicine, The University of Hong Kong, Hong Kong SAR, China, **5** Division of Cell and Molecular Biology, Faculty of Natural Sciences, Imperial College London, London, United Kingdom

Abstract

Background: Adiponectin regulates glucose and fatty-acid metabolism but its role in chronic graft rejection mediated by Th2 cytokines remains ill-defined.

Methodology/Principal Findings: Wild type and adiponectin-null mice were used as graft recipients in mouse MHC class II disparate cardiac transplantation (bm12 toB6) and the graft rejection was monitored. In adiponectin-null mice we observed that the cellular infiltrate of eosinophils, $CD4^+$ and $CD8^+$ T cells was reduced in grafts compared to the controls as was collagen deposition and vessel occlusion. A similar outcome was observed for skin transplants except that neutrophil infiltration was increased. Low levels of IL-4 were detected in the grafts and serum. The effect of adiponectin signaling on IL-4 expression was further investigated. Treatment with AMPK and p38 MAPK inhibitors blocked adiponectin enhanced T cell proliferation in mixed lymphocyte reactions. Inhibition of AMPK reduced eosinophil infiltration in skin grafts in wild type recipients and in contrast AMPK activation increased eosinophils in adiponectin-null recipients. The addition of adiponectin increased IL-4 production by the T cell line EL4 with augmented nuclear GATA-3 and phospho-STAT6 expression which were suppressed by knockdown of adiponectin receptor 1 and 2.

Conclusions: Our results demonstrate a direct effect of adiponectin on IL-4 expression which contributes to Th2 cytokine mediated rejection in mouse MHC class II histoincompatible transplants. These results add to our understanding of the interrelationship of metabolism and immune regulation and raise the possibility that AMPK inhibitors may be beneficial in selected types of rejection.

Editor: Francesco Annunziato, University of Florence, Italy

Funding: This work was supported by Seed Funding Programme for Basic Research from the University of Hong Kong (200811159035) and the General Research Fund (HKU 762108M). The funders had no role in study design, data collection and analysis, decision to publish, or preparation of the manuscript.

Competing Interests: The authors have declared that no competing interests exist.

* E-mail: ychenc@hku.hk (YC); paultam@hku.hk (PT)

¤ Current address: Bureau of Health of Ordos Municipality, Inner Mongolia, China

Introduction

In mammals body metabolism and immune function are tightly linked. Adiponectin (APN) is an adipokine mainly produced by adipocytes and functions in glucose and fatty-acid metabolism but it has also been shown to have anti-inflammatory activities [1]. The mechanism was initially attributed to up-regulated IL-10 [2]. Later, work on human macrophages suggested many other factors are involved including A20 and SOCS-3 but not IL-10 [3]. This difference may be due to the various isoforms of APN in that globular adiponectin functions via IL-10 and HO-1 pathways while full length APN uses the IL-4/STAT6 pathway to polarize macrophages to an M2 phenotype [4]. APN can also modulate adaptive immunity. Two adiponectin receptors AdipoR1 and AdipoR2 are present in both human and mouse derived T cells and ligation of these receptors has inhibitory effects on activated T cells [5,6]. Bone marrow derived dendritic cells (DC) treated with APN showed only moderate differences in differentiation but their function was altered such that they reduced the proliferative capacity of allogeneic T cells and enhanced regulatory T cell production [7]. In animal models of fully mismatched MHC class II heart transplantation in which the Th1 cytokines play dominant role increasing APN expression with a PPAR-γ agonist reduced graft rejection and prolonged survival [8,9]. However, the role of APN in regulating Th2 dominant rejection remains to be clarified.

Mouse MHC class II mismatched cardiac transplantation with bm12 to B6 as donor and recipient is a model often used to study chronic rejection. The absence of alloreactive $CD8^+$ T cells biases immune rejection to a Th2 phenotype [10]. IL-4 is central in initiation of the response since IL-4 deficient mice or the administration of an IL-4 neutralizing antibody reduces graft rejection and promotes long-term survival [11,12]. Using this model we have reported that the PPAR-γ agonist rosiglitazone increased eosinophil infiltration in heart transplants [5] suggesting that in this type of graft rejection APN plays a different role.

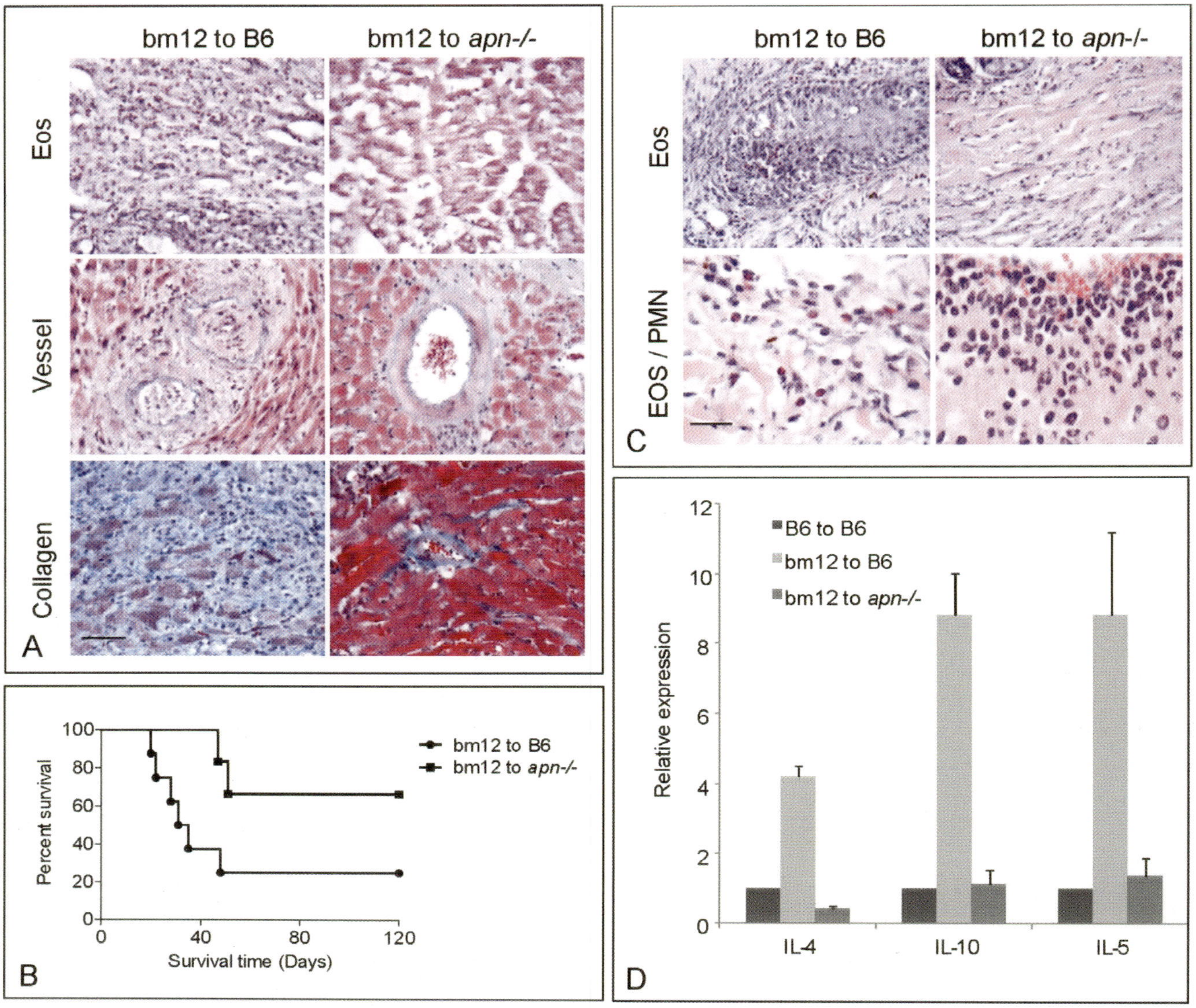

Figure 1. Effect of adiponectin in mouse MHC class II mismatched cardiac and skin transplantation. A. Heterotopic cardiac transplantation with bm12 mice as donors, B6 (left panel, n = 6) and Apn−/− (right panel, n = 5) as the recipients. The grafts were examined after the heart beat had ceased. The tissue sections were stained for eosinophils (Eos), vessel occlusion and tissue fibrosis. B. Cardiac graft survival curves in bm12 mice to B6 or Apn−/− mice. C. Skin transplantation was performed and the tissues were collected at 7 days after operation. The sections were stained and analyzed. For observation of neutrophil infiltration, the high magnification (1,000 x) was used in HE stained section (Eos/PMN left) in compared with eosinophils (Eos/PMN right). D. Cytokines mRNA expression in heart grafts. The expression of cytokines was measured with quantitative-PCR. One comparable sample each was used for the syngeneic group (B6 to B6), wild type group (bm12 to B6) and Apn−/− group (bm12 to Apn−/−) and the data were present as triplicates for each measurement. Scale Bar = 50 μm.

In this study, with the *apn*−/− mice (B6 background) as recipients the immunomodulatory effects of APN have been investigated in detail both *in vitro* and *in vivo*. There was no chronic rejection, cellular infiltration was minimal and IL-4 expression was reduced in *apn*−/− compared to wild type mice. In mixed lymphocyte reactions (MLRs) the presence of APN enhanced T cell proliferation which was reduced by anti-IL-4 antibody treatment. GATA-3 and p-STAT6 were induced by APN but the induction was blocked by siRNAs specific for APN receptor 1 and 2. Our data here show a direct relationship between APN and IL-4 expression and illustrate cross talk between metabolic pathways and immune regulation.

Materials and Methods

Animals

Inbred male C57BL/6 (B6, H-2^{b}), B6.C-H-2^{bm12}KhEg (bm12, H-2^{bm12}), and BALB/c (H2d) mice (6–8 weeks old, weight of 20–25 g) were maintained in the Laboratory Animal Unit, University of Hong Kong. Adiponectin knockout (*apn*−/−) mice were generated in C57BL/6J background as described previously [13]. The serum APN level was examined by ELISA, in *apn*−/− mice it was undetectable compared to 16.5±3.10 μg/ml in B6 mice (*apn*+/+) and in 4.1±0.03 μg/ml heterozygous (*apn*+/−). All experimental protocols were approved by the Committee on the

Table 1. Cellular infiltration, vasculopathy and tissue fibrosis in heart and skin grafts.

Donor: bm12	Heart transplant		Skin transplant	
Recipient:	**B6**	***Apn−/−***	**B6**	***Apn−/−***
CD4	36±2	6±1***	20±2	0***
CD8	11±1	1±0***	30±2	0***
Eos	79±4	0***	26±2	0***
Vessel occlusion (%)	99.5±0.5	7.95±5.8***	ND	ND
Collagen deposit (%)	28.5±2.9	3.5±0.4***	ND	ND

ND: No determined. ***$p<0.001$ compared to B6.

Use of Live Animals in Teaching and Research, University of Hong Kong (Ref: 1591-07).

Reagents and Chemicals

Reagents and chemicals used are described in the Materials S1.

Heterotopic Cardiac Transplantation and Skin Transplantation

Mouse cardiac transplants were performed as previously described[5] using heterotopic cardiac allografts from bm12 mice as donors and C57BL/6 (B6) mice or *Apn−/−* mice as recipients. Standard microsurgical techniques were used for vascularized grafts transplantation. In brief, the donor heart was carefully detached from the thoracic cavity and placed in cold Lactated Ringers solution containing 100 U/ml heparin. The time for the donor operation was less than 20 min. The donor ascending aorta and the pulmonary trunk from the heart graft was anastomosed end-to-side to the recipient abdominal aorta and inferior vena cava, respectively. The time required for revascularization of aortotomy and venotomy was < 50 min. The animals were observed daily and the loss of viability of the grafts was determined by cessation of palpation and confirmed by histological analysis. Skin transplantation was performed as described previously [14]. Briefly, full-thickness donor skin was grafted to the recipients and the graft sites were covered by plaster removed on day 7. Grafts were observed daily and the rejection was determined when no viable skin remained.

Histological and Immunohistochemical Analysis of Grafts Rejection

Both paraffin and frozen sections (4 μm) were analyzed. The morphology was observed with haematoxylin and eosin (HE) staining. $CD4^+$ and $CD8^+$ cells were detected by immunohistochemical staining. Carbol-chromotrope, Victoria blue and Masson's trichrome staining were used to visualize of eosinophil infiltration, blood vessel elastin and tissue collagen deposits respectively and the counting methods used were as published [5].

Table 2. Serum levels of IL-4 at 7 days post-operatively in mice following skin grafting.

	UT	CompC	MET
B6 to B6	8.36±2.83	ND	14.0±0.52*
Apn−/− to *Apn−/−*	0.70±0.27†	ND	4.57±1.25**
bm12 to B6	36.5±7.23†	14.3±0.68‡	ND
bm12 to *Apn−/−*	1.54±0.37	ND	10.6±3.61**

UT: untreated; ND: not determined. n = 6 in each group (†$p<0.01$ compared to B6 to B6; ‡$p<0.001$ compared to UT; *$p<0.05$ and **$p<0.01$ cpmpared to UT).

Serum Level of Cytokines Expression

Serum and supernatants were collected and stored at −80°C. Cytokine levels were measured by standard ELISA methods following the manufacturer's instructions.

Mixed Lymphocyte Reactions

Splenocytes from bm12 and BALB/c mice were used as stimulators and B6 or *Apn−/−* mice as responders. To reduce the effect of adiponectin present in serum the volume of fetal bovine serum added to cell proliferation assays was sequentially diluted and we observed that the addition of 0.5% FBS had minimal effects and therefore was used at that volume in the subsequent experiments (Fig S4 A) Responder splenocytes (1×10^6) were co-cultured with irradiated stimulating cells at a 1:1 ratio in triplicate for 2 days before the ^{3}H-thymidine was added. The cells were cultured for 1 more day and the cell proliferation was measured using a beta counter (PerkinElmer. Inc, MA USA).

In vitro Generation of Dendritic Cells and T Cells Proliferation Assay

DCs were generated from bone marrow using the protocol of Steinman *et al.* with minor modifications.[14] In brief, bone marrow cells were negatively isolated and cultured with granulocyte-macrophage colony-stimulating factor (GM-CSF) for 7 days. Maturation of DCs was induced by adding 100 ng/ml of lipopolysaccharide (LPS) on day 6 to cultures of immature DCs which were then incubated for an additional day. Dynal® CD4 Negative Isolation Kit was used to isolate $CD4^+$T cells from B6 or *Apn−/−* spleens. $CD4^+$T cells (1×10^5cells/well) were stimulated with γ-irradiated (30 Gray) DCs from bm12 mice in 96 well plates. Proliferation was assessed by ^{3}H-thymidine incorporation during the last 24 hrs of 3 day cultures. To determine the amount of IL-4 produced by T cells supernatants were harvested on day 1 of the DC-T MLRs. The AMPK and P38 inhibitors (compound C and SB203580) were dissolved in DMSO and the final volume of DMSO was <0.1%. Their ability to induce apoptosis was tested for by Annexin V staining and sub-apoptotic concentrations were then used the subsequent experiments.

Quantitative-PCR for Analysis Genes Expression Level

The mRNA expression levels were examined using the GoScript™ Reverse Transcription System and quantitative real-time PCR (Q-PCR) with SYBR® Green-Based Detection system. The primers sequences were showed in Table S1. Relative quantification of mRNA expression was normalized with control GAPDH and analyzed by the Delta Delta Ct ($2^{-\Delta\Delta CT}$) method.

Protein Expression Examination with Western Blot

The protein expression levels were determined by Western blotting. 30 μg of protein was denatured and separated by electrophoresis. After electro-transferred onto PVDF-membranes and blocking with 5% low-fat milk TBST, the primary antibodies were added and incubated overnight at 4°C and then incubated with horseradish peroxidase (HRP)-conjugated secondary antibody. The signals were developed using ECL chemi-luminescence (Amersham). The membranes were stripped and reprobed with an anti-actin antibody. Rat anti-mouse GATA-3 (1:1000), rabbit anti-

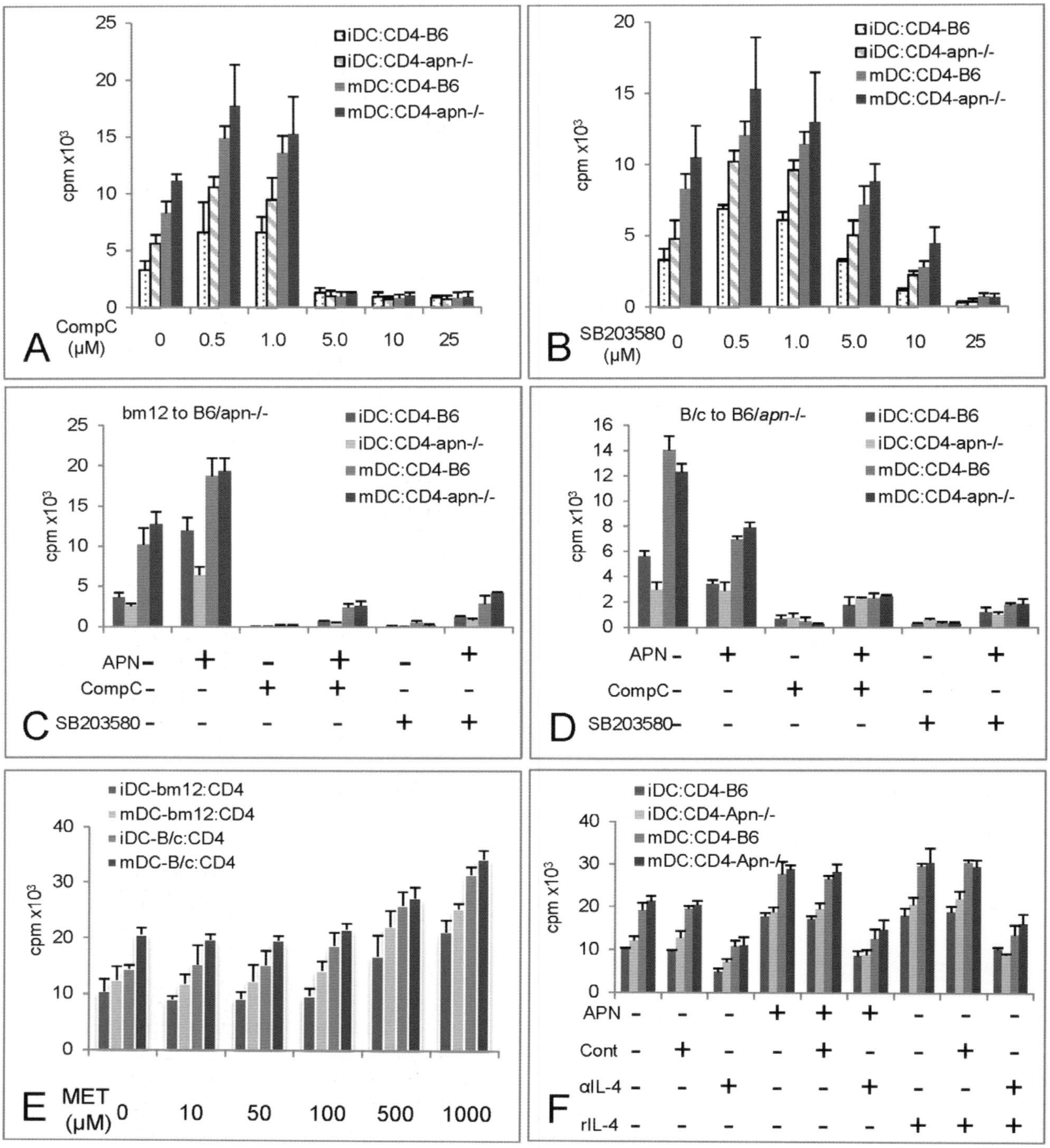

Figure 2. Effects of adiponectin and its signaling pathways on dendritic cell (DC) induced T cell function. Bone marrow derived dendritic cells from bm12 mice were used as stimulator cells and CD4+ T cells from B6 or Apn−/− mice as responder cells. Cell proliferation was measured by ^{3}H-thymidine incorporation. Immature DCs were treated with LPS for an additional 24 h to induce maturation. n = 4 and one representative graph is presented. The APN signaling inhibitors, Compound C (CompC) for AMPK (A) and SB203580 for p38 MAPK (B) were added at different concentrations. The effect of APN and signaling inhibitors on T cell proliferation in MLRs of DCs from bm12 and T cells from apn−/− was measured. APN (5 μg/ml) was added to MLRs for 24 h in the presence or absence of CompC or SB203580 (C). Similarly the compounds were tested in MLRs with DCs from Balb/c (B/c) mice (D). Effect of Metformin (MET) on T cell proliferation was assessed. DCs were obtained from either bm12 or B/c and the T cells were isolated from B6. MET was added to MLRs and the T cell proliferation was measured as above (E). The effect of IL-4 on APN induced proliferation was evaluated. APN (5 μg/ml), anti-IL-4 antibody (αIL-4, 50 μg/ml) and mouse recombinant IL-4 (rIL-4, 50 ng/ml) were added to the MLRs and T cells proliferation were measure as described as above (F).

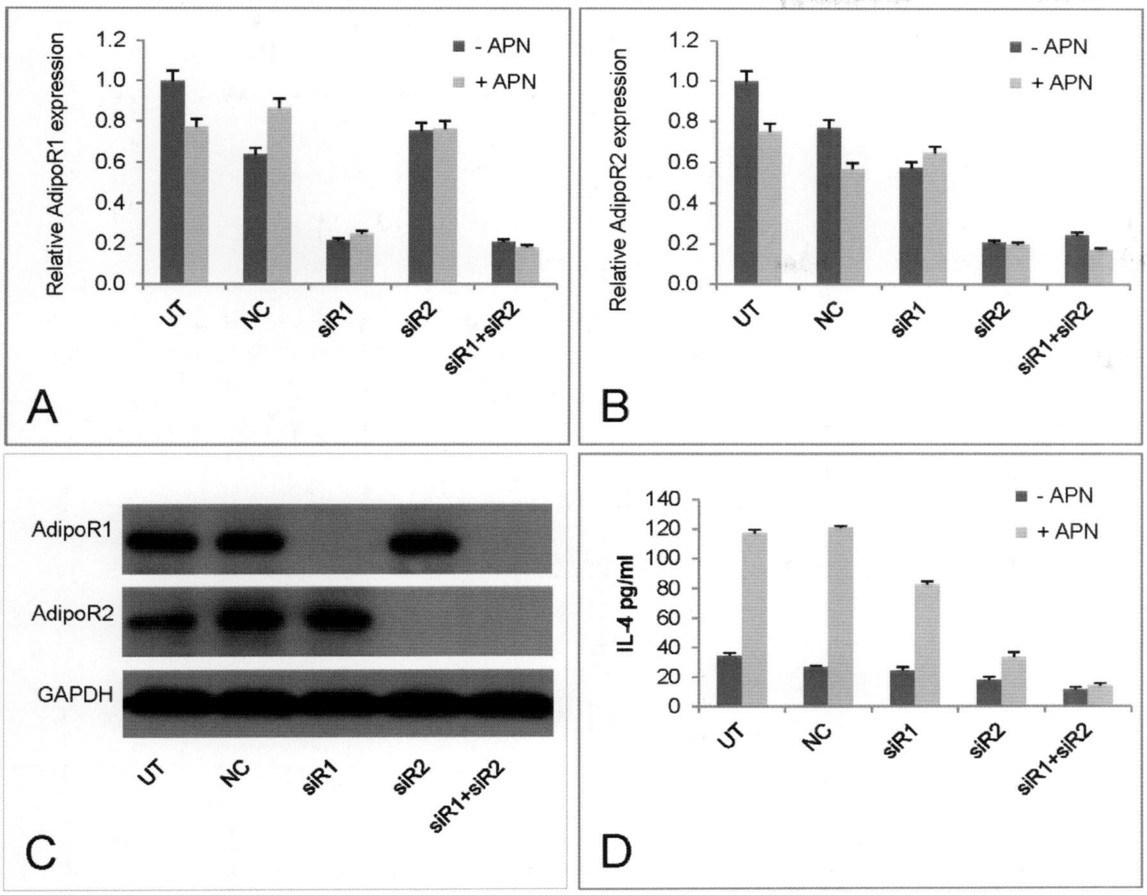

Figure 3. IL-4 production in response to adiponectin receptor AdipoR1 and AdipoR2 knockdown using siRNA. EL-4 cells were transfected with siRNA for AdipoR1 and AdipoR2 for 24 or 48 hours together with control siRNA (n = 2). The effects of siRNA were detected both with Q-PCR and Western blot with specific antibodies. Supernatants were collected for the measurement of IL-4 production.

mouse p38 (1:1000) and p-p38 (1:1000), rabbit anti-mouse STAT6 (1:1000) and p-STAT6 (1:500), goat anti-mouse GAPDH (1:5000), rabbit anti-mouse Histone3 (1:5000), rabbit anti-mouse AdipoR1 and 2 (1:500) were used in experiments.

Inhibition of Gene Expression with siRNAs

Specific synthetic siRNAs were obtained from Invitrogen Hong Kong Ltd. Lipofectamin was used to transfect cells following the manufacturer's instructions. In brief, 2×10^5 EL4 cells were cultured to 50% confluence before the RNAi duplex-Lipofectamine^{TM} RNAiMAX complexes were added. The transfection was repeated after 24 hours. The success of inhibition effect was measured by quantitative (Q)-PCR analysis with AdipoR1 and AdipoR2 primers (Table S1) and further confirmed by Western blotting.

Statistical Analysis

Kaplan-Meier method and the log-rank test were used to analyze graft survival. Mann Whitney test or Dunn's Multiple Comparison Test were used to compare two or three sets data respectively. $p<0.05$ was considered significant. All cell cultures were performed in triplicate and error bars represent the standard error of mean (SEM). Statistical analysis was performed with Prism software (GraphPad Software, La Jolla, CA).

Results

Absence of Chronic Rejection in bm12 to apn–/– Heterotopic Transplants

In bm12 to B6 mice heterotopic cardiac transplants extensive eosinophil infiltration is a hallmark of chronic rejection. Compared to wild type controls (B6) when *apn–/–* mice were the recipient only minimal cellular infiltration was observed (Fig. 1A). $CD4^+$ and $CD8^+$ T cell infiltration was reduced by 90% compared to bm12 to B6 grafts and no eosinophils were observed in graft tissue sections (Fig. 1A, Table1 and Fig. S1). Blood vessel occlusion was also significantly reduced. Similarly, collagen deposition was 8 fold reduced (Fig. 1A and Table1). Concomitantly, graft survival was prolonged with the median survival time of 33 days increasing to >120 days. The mean rejection time was extended from 31 days to 49 days and only 2/8 WT mice survived >120 days compared to 4 of 6 *apn–/–* mice (Fig. 1B). In skin transplants at 7 days, minimal numbers of eosinophils, $CD4^+$, and $CD8^+$ T cells were detected in the grafts in *apn–/–* compared to B6 mice (Fig. 1C, Table1 and Fig. S2), whereas in the *apn–/–* mice a larger number of neutrophils were present in the infiltrate (Fig. 1C).

Expression of Cytokines in Allografts and Serum

Chronic rejection in MHC class II histoincompatible transplantation is driven by Th2 cytokines with IL-4 expression key to

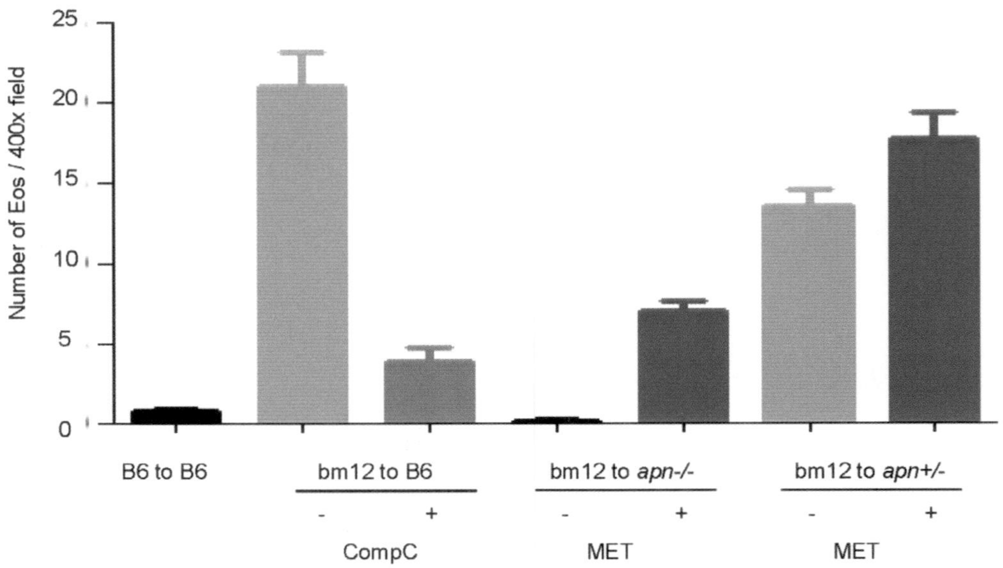

Figure 4. Effect of adiponectin signaling pathway inhibitors and agonist on MHC class II mismatched skin transplantation. For skin transplantation bm12 mice were used as donors and B6, Apn–/– or APN+/- mice as recipients (n = 6 each). The animals were treated with Compound C (CompC, 5 mg/kg/day), Metformin (MET, 250 mg/kg/day) and the grafts were obtained at day 7 after transplantation. The number of eosinophil was counted the average is shown.

the initiation of the immune response. IL-4 expression in both grafts and serum were examined by Q-PCR and ELISA. Compared to B6 transcripts for the Th2 cytokines IL-10, IL-4 and IL-5 were reduced in the *apn–/–* mice (Fig. 1D). In serum of skin transplant recipients at days 7 post-operatively low levels of IL-4 were found in *apn–/–* to *apn–/–* grafted mice. IL-4 production was increased 4 fold in B6 recipients compared to syngeneic group, but only 2 fold in *apn–/–* recipients (Table 2), suggesting that IL-4 up-regulation in *apn–/–* mice in response to skin grafts might be dysregulated. We also observed that mRNA expression of the Th1 cytokines, IL-2 and IFN-γ in grafts was reduced in the *apn–/–* compared to B6 recipients. Furthermore, IL-17 and PD-L1 were reduced in the cardiac transplants whereas expression of the APN receptors AdipoR1 and AdipoR2 was increased in *apn–/–* (Fig S3). Serum levels of Th1 cytokines showed no significant difference although slight increase of IFN-γ was observed (Table S2).

Effect of Inhibition of APN Signaling on Mixed Lymphocytes Reactions (MLRs)

To test the effect of inhibiting APN signaling on T cell proliferation in B6 or *apn–/–* mice, bone marrow derived DCs from bm12 mice were cultured for 7 days and then treated with LPS to induce DC maturation (Fig. S5B and 5C). For comparison, DCs from BALB/c (B/c) mice were used in some experiments. T cells isolated from B6 or *apn–/–* spleens were used as responder cells. Both immature and mature DCs were analyzed in MLRs at DC to T cell ratios of 1:10 (Fig. S5A). Dose dependent inhibition with both CompC and SB203580 was observed with CompC being the more potent inhibitor which at 5 μM completely inhibited T cells proliferation but 25 μM in SB203580. At these concentrations SB203580 induced apoptosis but CompC did not (Fig S4 B & C). Mature DCs significantly increased the proliferation of both B6 and *apn–/–* derived T cells. Although a higher response to bm12 DCs stimulation was induced in *apn–/–* compared to B6 T cells there was no statistical significant between the two ($p>0.05$; Fig. 2A.and 2B).

APN alone amplified the proliferative response of both B6 and *apn–/–* T cells to bm12 DCs which was inhibited by the treatment with CompC or SB203580 (Fig. 2C). The addition of APN to MLRs with BALB/c derived DCs as stimulator cells inhibited T cell proliferation (Fig. 2D). CompC and SB203580 could not fully inhibit proliferation in the present of exogenous APN and their inhibitory were only partially reversed by APN.

As APN signals mainly through AMPK we further investigated if enhancement of AMPK activity modulated T cells proliferation. Metformin (MET) is an AMPK agonist and addition of this compound induced a dose dependent increase in T cell proliferation in B6 and *apn–/–* T cells but with no obvious difference between the two. At doses of 500 μM ($p<0.05$) and 1000 μM ($p<0.001$) the increase in T cell proliferation was significant but was similar both in B6 and in *apn–/–* groups (Fig. 2E).

As the effect on T cell proliferation might relate to IL-4 production an anti-IL-4 neutralizing antibody was added. The anti-IL-4 antibody alone effectively inhibited bm12 induced T cell proliferation when either immature DC or mature DCs were present in the cultures ($p<0.01$). APN enhanced T cell proliferation was also suppressed by the anti-IL-4 antibody when either immature DC or mature DCs were used as stimulator cells ($p<0.01$ and 0.001 respectively), suggesting that proliferation was partially mediated by IL-4 (Fig. 2F).

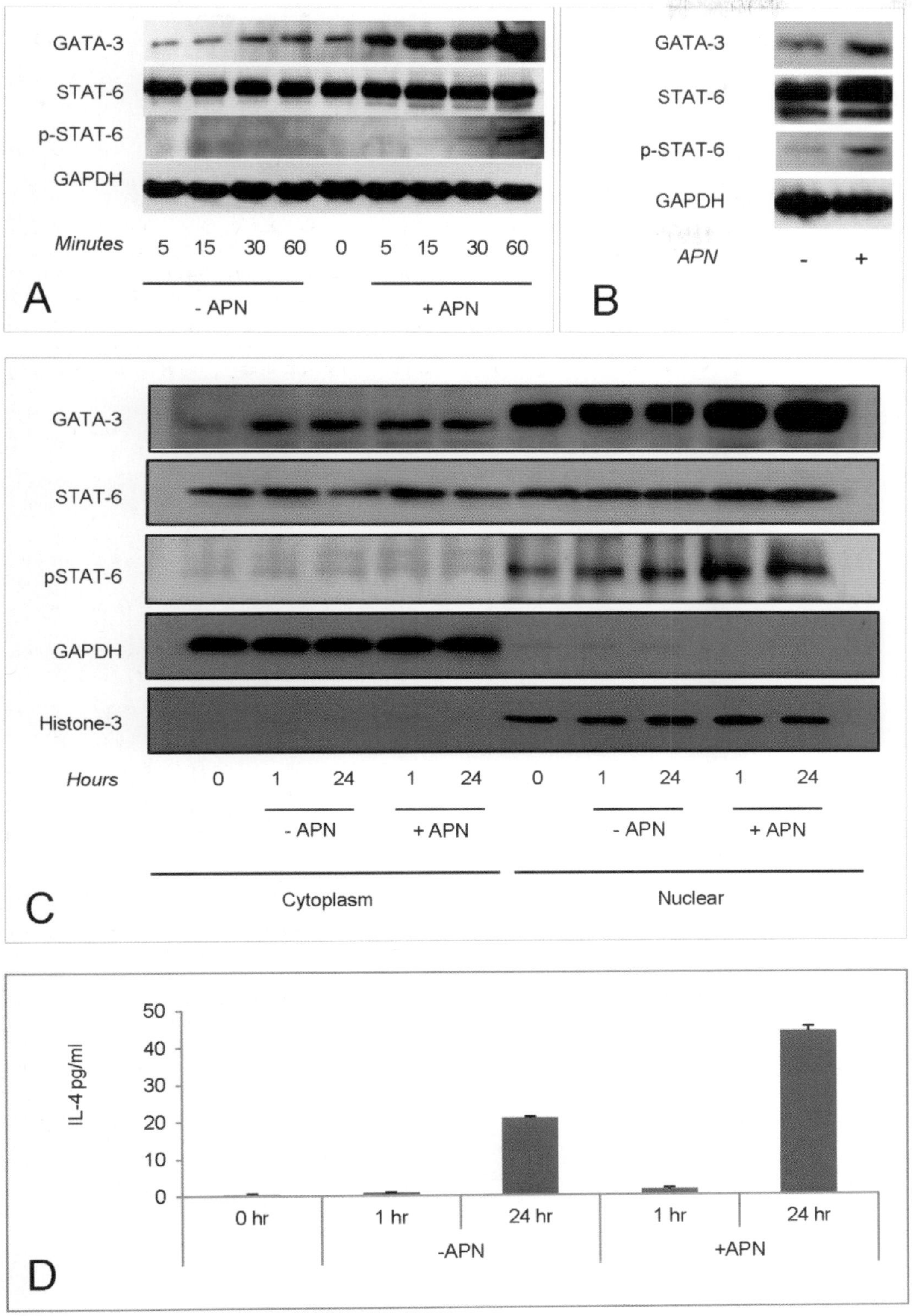

Figure 5. GATA-3 and STAT6 expression in response to Adiponectin (APN). Intracellular signaling pathways for IL-4 production were detected using the IL-4 producing T cell line EL-4. Cells were cultured in RBMI medium with 2.5% fetal bovine serum. The APN (5 μg/ml) was added and the samples were collected with the indicated time points (n = 3). The expression of GATA-3 and STAT6 was detected in whole lysates (A and B) or separated cytoplasmic and nuclear parts (C and D) using Western blot. The expression of IL-4 was detected in supernatants with ELISA.

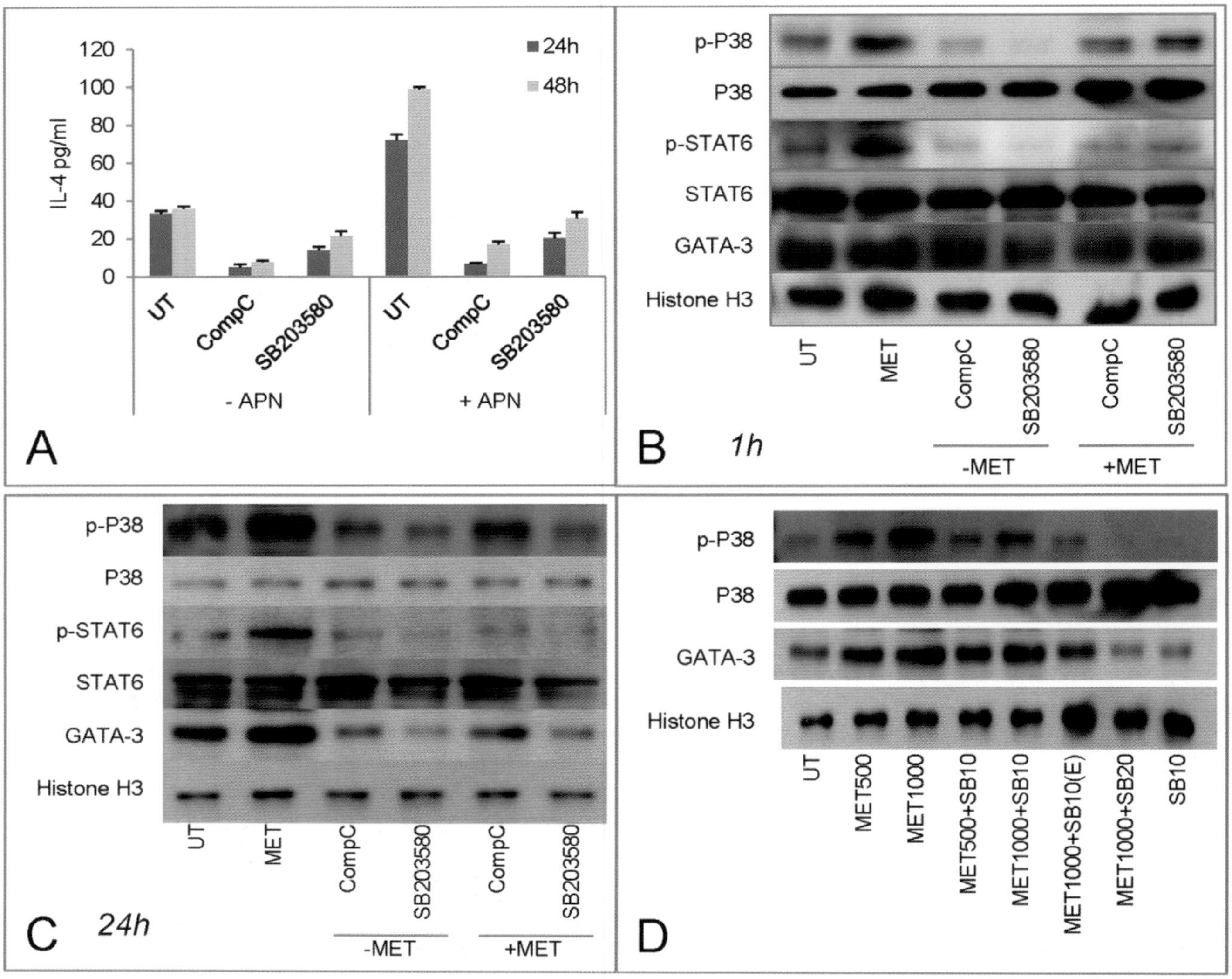

Figure 6. Functions of AMPK and p38 in IL-4 expression in response to Metformin (MET) treatment. A. EL-4 cells were cultured with APN (5 μM), Compound C (CompC, 10 μM) and SB203580 (10, 20 μM) for 1 h and 24/48 h and supernatants were collected for IL-4 detection (n = 3). B and C. Nuclear proteins were obtained for intracellular signaling pathway molecules detection using Western blots. D. MET induced up-regulation of p-p38 was inhibited by increasing the dose of SB203580 or reducing that of MET or by pre-treating with SB203580 for 1 h (E) by Western blots.

The Effect of Target Specific Inhibition of APN Signaling on IL-4 Production

To investigate the contribution of APN signaling on IL-4 production specific siRNAs for APN receptors AdipoR1 and AdipoR2 were used and the outcomes measured by Q-PCR and protein expression. Compared to control or irrelevant siRNAs, which induced a maximum of 24% reduction in receptor expression in the presence of APN, specific siRNAs for AdipoR1 and AdipoR2 resulted in 65 to 73% inhibition. When the two siRNAs were added together expression of AdipoR1 and AdipoR2 mRNA was inhibited >80% (Fig. 3A and 3B). Modified AdipoR1 and AdipoR2 protein expression was confirmed by Western blotting (Fig. 3C). Specific inhibition of AdipoR1 and AdipoR2 reduced APN induced IL-4 production by 31.7 and 72.2% respectively, in case of double inhibition, 88.5% of APN induced IL-4 production was suppressed (Fig. 3D). Thus APN plays an important role in IL-4 production directly through its action on AdipoR1 and R2 with activation of the latter being more efficient.

Effect of Modulating APN Signaling on bm12 to B6 or apn–/– Skin Transplantation

Since targeting APN could inhibit or enhance T cell proliferation and IL-4 production *in vitro* we extended these studies to determine possible *in vivo* effects on the survival of skin grafts. Eosinophil infiltration is characteristic of the immune response in bm12 to B6 skin grafts therefore we evaluated the number of eosinophils in bm12 grafts in B6 or *apn−/−* mice treated *in vivo* with CompC or MET (Fig 4). On day 7 the number of eosinophils was greatly reduced following treatment with CompC compared to untreated control group with B6 mice as the recipients (4 ± 3 vs. 21 ± 9, $p<0.001$), whereas eosinophil infiltration was reversed in bm12 grafts in *apn–/–* recipients receiving MET (7 ± 3 vs. 0, $p<0.01$). These results were confirmed using *apn+/–* heterozygote mice in which the number of eosinophils was lower than in B6 ($p>0.05$) but higher than in *apn–/–* ($p<0.001$) recipients and eosinophil infiltration was further increased following treatment with MET (Fig. 4). IL-4 production was also measured in B6 recipients treated with CompC and a 61% reduction in serum IL-4 was observed. When compared to *apn–/–* as recipients treatment with MET increased IL-4 in serum by 5.8 fold these effects of MET on IL-4 production were also observed in syngeneic group (Table 2).

APN Treatment Increased Nuclear GATA-3 and p-STAT6 Expression Levels

To explore further APN effects on IL-4 production expression levels of GATA-3 and STAT6 were measured in the IL-4 producing T cell line, EL4. In the presence of APN the expression of GATA-3 in whole cell lysates was increased within 60 min and maintained at 24 h. No induction of STAT6, which is constitutively expressed, was observed (Fig. 5A and B) however there was a marginal increase in phosphorylated-STAT6 (p-STAT6) at 1 h which was more obvious at 24 h (Fig. 5B). GATA-3 was mainly located in nucleus and its expression was increased by APN treatment. STAT-6 could be found both in cytoplasm and nucleus and nuclear expression of p-STAT6 was enhanced by APN (Fig. 5C). APN treatment increased the level of IL-4 expression in EL4 cell supernatants (Fig. 5D).

Relationship of AMPK and p38 MAPK in IL-4 Production

APN induced IL-4 expression in EL4 cells was inhibited by CompC and SB203580 suggesting both APN activated AMPK and p38 influence IL-4 production (Fig. 6A). Based on studies in skeletal muscle cells it seems that p38 is a downstream target of AMPK [15], whether or not this is the case for T cells is not clear. Treatment with MET increased phosphorylated p38 (p-p38) levels in the nuclear protein extracts both at 1 h and 24 h time points. Enhanced expression of p-p38 was inhibited by CompC treatment implying that the effect was mediated by AMPK (Fig. 6B and 6C). However, at 1 h SB203580 had no inhibitory effect on p-P38 but at 24 h the effect had a similar magnitude to that of MET. This was confirmed by the increasing the dose of SB203580 or lowering the dose of MET with same dose of SB203580 (Fig. 6D). These results suggest that the effect of APN mediated AMPK induction of IL-4 might be through p38 activation.

Discussion

In this study we have investigated APN signaling in the regulation of IL-4 using mouse models of MHC class II mismatched transplantation in which the alloreactive immune response is initiated by IL-4 and dominated by Th2 cytokines. When *apn–/–* (B6) mice were used as recipients for bm12 cardiac grafts the survival was increased and accompanied by reduced IL-4 in the grafts and serum. The findings reported here advance our understanding of adiponectin in DC and T cell interactions in Th2 cytokine dominant environments. Low APN levels reduced IL-4 expression which is consistent with previous observations that *apn–/–* mice M1 macrophages are expanded at the expense of M2 cells, which are dependent on IL-4 for their differentiation [16]. In DSS induced intestinal inflammation, the absence of APN reduced tissue damage also similar to that in IL-4 deficiency mice [17] again implying a role for APN in IL-4 production. Furthermore, the upregulation of APN signaling by MET increased eosinophils in skin transplants which supports our previous observation that the PPAR-γ agonist rosiglitazone promotes eosinophil recruitment in heart grafts and suggests that reducing APN could be beneficial in graft survival in MHC class II mismatched grafts rejection. We also noted that chronic rejection in our model (bm12 to C57BL/6) was more pronounced than some previous reports in the literature [18] which might in part relate to the genetic background of the mice used in our study. The C57BL/6 both wild type and *apn–/–* are derived from C57BL/6N and the bm12 obtained from Jackson Laboratory was on a C65BL/6J background. In 6J to 6N strain combination of skin transplantation, a 2 fold increase in IFN-γ and IL-2 in the serum was observed in wild type as well as *apn–/–* compared to the syngeneic controls (Table S2) but there was no significant difference between chronic rejection groups. However, in comparison levels of IL-4 were altered (>4 fold increase in the wild type group, Table1). These observations demonstrate that genetic background can modify qualitative aspects of responses in the same disease model [19]. Our results on graft rejection are contrary to those in which *apn–/–* mice were also used as transplant recipients [20] and this may be due to variations between different strains of *apn–/–* mice as suggested, for example, by the differential response of *apn–/–* mice to DSS induced intestinal inflammation [21,22]. The underlying differences between of these *apn–/–* mice remain unclear but may relate to the knockout procedure in gene manipulation and/or background as illustrated by the variations in their insulin resistance and glucose intolerance [23].

T cells from *apn–/–* and wild type B6 mice exhibited similar *in vitro* proliferative responses to bm12 splenocytes or bone marrow derived DCs indicated no defect in T cell development or activation. APN enhanced T cell proliferation in bm12 to B6 or *apn–/–* combinations but reduced proliferation when BALB/c derived cells were used as the donor demonstrating the presence or absence of APN is a key factor in T cell proliferation in the MHC class II disparate or fully mismatched combination. The marginally higher T cell proliferation and IL-4 production in *apn–/–* cells to bm12 stimulation is due to elevated expression of the APN receptors especially AdipoR2 (Fig S6). The loss of grafts in *apn–/–* in the absence of alloreactivity suggests that tissue repair is deficient due to ischemia reperfusion, which causes myocardium damage in *apn–/–* mice [24].

One of APN intracellular signaling pathways is p38 [15]. Here we observed a dose dependent of inhibition of T cell proliferation in B6 and *apn–/–* mice with SB203580. CD28 mediated T cell proliferation was through p38 [25] and B7-CD28 co-stimulation is essential in immune rejection of bm12 and B6 combinations [26]. Our data confirmed previous observations that inhibition of p38 reduces T cell proliferation in MLRs of bm12 to B6 [25]. AMPK is another downstream target of APN. Inhibition of T cell proliferation by an AMPK inhibitor was observed in MLRs of bm12 or BALB/c to B6 or *apn–/–* as donors and recipients respectively. In the presence of APN the inhibitory effect of the AMPK inhibitor was incomplete indicating that APN may have an effect in restricting the inhibition effect of CompC. Unlike the direct effects of p38 on antigen presentation it appears that AMPK activation is not essential for activation and expression of effecter molecules following immune stimulation but for their response to metabolic stress [27]. However, others report that AMPK knockdown modulates DC maturation through TLR related metabolic changes [28] which highlights the complexity of AMPK signaling in immune responses need to further investigate.

Regarding IL-4 expression inhibition of AMPK reduced basal levels of IL-4 whereas treatment with the AMPK agonist Metformin enhanced IL-4 production. Metformin also increased phospho-p38 and the effect was further rescued by AMPK inhibition implying that MET induced p38 activation was AMPK dependent and the effect of MET on IL-4 production was through p38 pathway. At higher doses or by pre-treating cells SB203580 had an inhibitory effect of GATA-3 and p-STAT6 confirmed that p38 was involved in MET induced IL-4 expression through AMPK.

In conclusion, our data provide direct evidence that APN aids in promoting IL-4 production that can enhance eosinophil infiltration and contribute to graft rejection and therefore treatment with an APN inhibitor promotes graft survival. The application of APN inhibitors in other Th2 cytokine dominant immune reactions remains to be investigated.

Supporting Information

Figure S1 Immunohistochemical analysis of cardiac transplantation grafts. Sections were stained with Hematoxylin and Eosin (HE), rat anti-mouse CD4 and CD8 antibodies and bm12 to B6 grafts are compared to bm12 to APM−/− grafts. The samples were obtained from the grafts which the heart beating was stopped.

Figure S2 Immunohistochemical analysis of cellular infiltration. The tissue sections were stained with rat anti-mouse F4/80, rat anti-mouse CD4 and CD8 antibodies to illustrate the containing of macrophages, CD4+ and CD8+ cells in skin transplantation with bm12 as the donor to B6 or Apn−/− as the recipients.

Figure S3 Expression the cytokines mRNA in grafts. Th1, Th17, co-stimulatory molecule PD-L1, APN and its receptors in grafts of bm12 as donor and B6 or Apn−/− as recipient by Q-PCR were analyzed. One sample was used in each B6 and Apn−/− group.

Figure S4 A Determination of serum FBS concentration used in MLRs containing splenocytes. **B** and **C** Effect of Compound C and SB203580 treatment on splenocyte apoptosis using Annexin V staining.

Figure S5 Mixed lymphocytes reaction (MLR). A Bone marrow derived dendritic cells from bm12 as the stimulator cells and T cells isolated from spleen of B6 or Apn−/− mice as the responder cells. The cells were mixed at different ratios and proliferation was measured with 3H-thymidine incorporation. **B** and **C** The maturation of dendritic cells from bm12 or B/c. Bone marrow cells were isolated and cultured for 7 days in present of IL-4 and GM-CSF, the cells was added LPS (100 µg/ml) for 1 more day to induce the maturation. CD80, CD86 and MHC class II were used as maturation markers.

Figure S6 Expression of AdipoR1 and AdipoR2 on T cells isolated from spleen of B6 and Apn−/− mice. The T cells were isolated with Dynal® CD4 Negative Isolation Kit and total RNA was extracted. The mRNA expression levels were determined by quantitative Q-PCR.

Table S1 The primers used in Quantitative real-time PCR (Q-PCR). The primers were synthesized by Invitrogen Hong Kong Ltd.

Table S2 Serum levels of IFN-γ and IL-2 at 7 days post-operatively in mice following skin grafting. n = 6 in each group (†$p<0.01$ compared to B6 to B6; ††$p<0.001$ compared to *Apn−/−* to *Apn−/−*; ‡‡$p<0.01$ compared to B6 to B6 and ‡$p<0.05$ compared to *Apn−/−* to *Apn−/−*).

Materials S1

Author Contributions

Conceived and designed the experiments: DL JL PT YC. Performed the experiments: DL JYST JP DH YKC JZ VL. Analyzed the data: DL JYST JL PT YC. Contributed reagents/materials/analysis tools: AX VL. Wrote the paper: DL JYST JL PT YC.

References

1. Yokota T, Oritani K, Takahashi I, Ishikawa J, Matsuyama A, et al. (2000) Adiponectin, a new member of the family of soluble defense collagens, negatively regulates the growth of myelomonocytic progenitors and the functions of macrophages. Blood 96: 1723–1732.
2. Park PH, Huang H, McMullen MR, Bryan K, Nagy LE (2008) Activation of cyclic-AMP response element binding protein contributes to adiponectin-stimulated interleukin-10 expression in RAW 264.7 macrophages. J Leukoc Biol 83: 1258–1266.
3. Folco EJ, Rocha VZ, Lopez-Ilasaca M, Libby P (2009) Adiponectin inhibits pro-inflammatory signaling in human macrophages independent of interleukin-10. J Biol Chem 284: 25569–25575.
4. Mandal P, Pratt BT, Barnes M, McMullen MR, Nagy LE (2011) Molecular mechanism for adiponectin-dependent M2 macrophage polarization: link between the metabolic and innate immune activity of full-length adiponectin. J Biol Chem 286: 13460–13469.
5. Chen Y, Li D, Tsang JY, Niu N, Peng J, et al. (2011) PPAR-gamma signaling and IL-5 inhibition together prevent chronic rejection of MHC Class II-mismatched cardiac grafts. J Heart Lung Transplant 30: 698–706.
6. Wilk S, Scheibenbogen C, Bauer S, Jenke A, Rother M, et al. (2011) Adiponectin is a negative regulator of antigen-activated T cells. Eur J Immunol 41: 2323–2332.
7. Tsang JY, Li D, Ho D, Peng J, Xu A, et al. (2011) Novel immunomodulatory effects of adiponectin on dendritic cell functions. International immunopharmacology 11: 604–609.
8. Chen Y, Liu Y, Yuan ZW, Tian LN, Dallman MJ, et al. (2007) Rosiglitazone suppresses cyclosporin-induced chronic transplant dysfunction and prolongs survival of rat cardiac allografts. Transplantation 83: 1602–1610.
9. Kosuge H, Haraguchi G, Koga N, Maejima Y, Suzuki J, et al. (2006) Pioglitazone prevents acute and chronic cardiac allograft rejection. Circulation 113: 2613–2622.
10. LaRosa DF, Rahman AH, Turka LA (2007) The innate immune system in allograft rejection and tolerance. J Immunol 178: 7503–7509.
11. Goldman M, Le Moine A, Braun M, Flamand V, Abramowicz D (2001) A role for eosinophils in transplant rejection. Trends Immunol 22: 247–251.
12. Buonocore S, Flamand V, Goldman M, Braun MY (2003) Bone marrow-derived immature dendritic cells prime in vivo alloreactive T cells for interleukin-4-dependent rejection of major histocompatibility complex class II antigen-disparate cardiac allograft. Transplantation 75: 407–413.
13. Ma K, Cabrero A, Saha PK, Kojima H, Li L, et al. (2002) Increased beta -oxidation but no insulin resistance or glucose intolerance in mice lacking adiponectin. The Journal of biological chemistry 277: 34658–34661.
14. Tsang JY, Tanriver Y, Jiang S, Xue SA, Ratnasothy K, et al. (2008) Conferring indirect allospecificity on CD4+CD25+ Tregs by TCR gene transfer favors transplantation tolerance in mice. J Clin Invest 118: 3619–3628.
15. Yoon MJ, Lee GY, Chung JJ, Ahn YH, Hong SH, et al. (2006) Adiponectin increases fatty acid oxidation in skeletal muscle cells by sequential activation of AMP-activated protein kinase, p38 mitogen-activated protein kinase, and peroxisome proliferator-activated receptor alpha. Diabetes 55: 2562–2570.
16. Ohashi K, Parker JL, Ouchi N, Higuchi A, Vita JA, et al. (2010) Adiponectin promotes macrophage polarization toward an anti-inflammatory phenotype. J Biol Chem 285: 6153–6160.
17. Stevceva L, Pavli P, Husband A, Ramsay A, Doe WF (2001) Dextran sulphate sodium-induced colitis is ameliorated in interleukin 4 deficient mice. Genes and immunity 2: 309–316.
18. Schenk S, Kish DD, He C, El-Sawy T, Chiffoleau E, et al. (2005) Alloreactive T cell responses and acute rejection of single class II MHC-disparate heart allografts are under strict regulation by CD4+ CD25+ T cells. Journal of Immunology 174: 3741–3748.
19. Rosenberg DW, Giardina C, Tanaka T (2009) Mouse models for the study of colon carcinogenesis. Carcinogenesis 30: 183–196.
20. Okamoto Y, Christen T, Shimizu K, Asano K, Kihara S, et al. (2009) Adiponectin inhibits allograft rejection in murine cardiac transplantation. Transplantation 88: 879–883.

21. Fayad R, Pini M, Sennello JA, Cabay RJ, Chan L, et al. (2007) Adiponectin deficiency protects mice from chemically induced colonic inflammation. Gastroenterology 132: 601–614.
22. Nishihara T, Matsuda M, Araki H, Oshima K, Kihara S, et al. (2006) Effect of adiponectin on murine colitis induced by dextran sulfate sodium. Gastroenterology 131: 853–861.
23. Gibson F, Froguel P (2004) Genetics of the APM1 locus and its contribution to type 2 diabetes susceptibility in French Caucasians. Diabetes 53: 2977–2983.
24. Shibata R, Sato K, Pimentel DR, Takemura Y, Kihara S, et al. (2005) Adiponectin protects against myocardial ischemia-reperfusion injury through AMPK- and COX-2-dependent mechanisms. Nat Med 11: 1096–1103.
25. Schafer PH, Wadsworth SA, Wang L, Siekierka JJ (1999) p38 alpha mitogen-activated protein kinase is activated by CD28-mediated signaling and is required for IL-4 production by human CD4+CD45RO+ T cells and Th2 effector cells. J Immunol 162: 7110–7119.
26. Yang J, Riella LV, Boenisch O, Popoola J, Robles S, et al. (2009) Paradoxical functions of B7: CD28 costimulation in a MHC class II-mismatched cardiac transplant model. Am J Transplant 9: 2837–2844.
27. Mayer A, Denanglaire S, Viollet B, Leo O, Andris F (2008) AMP-activated protein kinase regulates lymphocyte responses to metabolic stress but is largely dispensable for immune cell development and function. Eur J Immunol 38: 948–956.
28. Krawczyk CM, Holowka T, Sun J, Blagih J, Amiel E, et al. (2010) Toll-like receptor-induced changes in glycolytic metabolism regulate dendritic cell activation. Blood 115: 4742–4749.

Ex Vivo Expanded Human Regulatory T Cells Delay Islet Allograft Rejection via Inhibiting Islet-Derived Monocyte Chemoattractant Protein-1 Production in CD34^{+} Stem Cells-Reconstituted NOD-*scid IL2rγ*^{null} Mice

Fang Xiao[1], Liang Ma[1¤], Min Zhao[2], Guocai Huang[2], Vincenzo Mirenda[1], Anthony Dorling[1], Robert Lechler[1❡], Giovanna Lombardi[1*❡]

1 Medical Research Council (MRC) for Transplantation, King's College London, London, United Kingdom, **2** Department of Diabetes & Endocrinology, King's College London, London, United Kingdom

Abstract

Type 1 diabetes mellitus (T1DM) is an autoimmune disease caused by immune-mediated destruction of insulin-secreting β cells of the pancreas. Near complete dependence on exogenous insulin makes T1DM very difficult to control, with the result that patients are exposed to high blood glucose and risk of diabetic complications and/or intermittent low blood glucose that can cause unconsciousness, fits and even death. Allograft transplantation of pancreatic islets restores normoglycemia with a low risk of surgical complications. However, although successful immediately after transplantation, islets are progressively lost, with most of the patients requiring exogenous insulin within 2 years post-transplant. Therefore, there is an urgent requirement for the development of new strategies to prevent islet rejection. In this study, we explored the importance of human regulatory T cells in the control of islets allograft rejection. We developed a pre-clinical model of human islet transplantation by reconstituting NOD-*scid IL2rγ*^{null} mice with cord blood-derived human CD34^{+} stem cells and demonstrated that although the engrafted human immune system mediated the rejection of human islets, their survival was significantly prolonged following adoptive transfer of *ex vivo* expanded human T_{regs}. Mechanistically, T_{regs} inhibited the infiltration of innate immune cells and CD4^{+} T cells into the graft by down-regulating the islet graft-derived monocyte chemoattractant protein-1. Our findings might contribute to the development of clinical strategies for T_{reg} therapy to control human islet rejection. We also show for the first time that CD34^{+} cells-reconstituted NOD-*scid IL2rγ*^{null} mouse model could be beneficial for investigating human innate immunity *in vivo*.

Editor: Paolo Fiorina, Children's Hospital Boston/Harvard Medical School, United States of America

Funding: The research was funded by the National Institute for Health Research (NIHR) Biomedical Research Centre based at Guy's and St Thomas' NHS Foundation Trust and King's College London. The views expressed are those of the authors and not necessarily those of the NHS, the NIHR or the Department of Health. The authors acknowledge financial support from Guy's and St Thomas' Charity Trust (R070723), Medical Research Council in the UK (MR/J006742/1), and British Heart Foundation in the UK (RG/08/005/25303). The funders had no role in study, data collection and analysis, decision to publish, or preparation of the manuscript.

Competing Interests: The authors have declared that no competing interests exist.

* E-mail: giovanna.lombardi@kcl.ac.uk

¤ Current address: Heart Centre, William Harvey Research Institute, Queen Mary, University of London, London, United Kingdom

❡ These authors contributed equally to this work.

Introduction

Type 1 diabetes mellitus (T1DM) is a chronic autoimmune disease in which insulin-secreting pancreatic β cells are destroyed by autoreactive T cells. It is characterized by dysregulation of blood glucose caused by β -cell insufficiency. Among the available treatments, human islet transplantation has emerged as a promising approach that restores glycemic stability even if full discontinuation of insulin treatment is not practical [1–3]. Transplanted islets, which consist of small clusters of cells containing insulin-producing β-cells, however provoke the same immunological responses as solid organ transplants, and necessitate immunosuppressive therapy to reduce immune-mediated rejection [4]. Immunosuppressive drugs have severe side effects, and they are toxic to β-cells as well as being ineffective at preventing late-stage allograft rejection [5,6]. To achieve durable success in islet transplantation, there is a need to develop applicable strategies for immunomodulation in order to suppress T cell-mediated alloimmune responses [7–10].

CD4^{+}CD25^{hi}FoxP3^{+} regulatory T cells (T_{regs}) have been shown to be important for the control of autoimmunity and maintenance of allograft tolerance [7]. In humans, normally only 5–10% of peripheral blood CD4 T cells are natural-occurring regulatory T cells [11] and thus large-scale *ex vivo* expansion is required for therapeutic application [12]. We and others have recently shown that large-scale *ex vivo* expanded human T_{regs} maintain their immunosuppressive capacity and are stable *in vitro* and *in vivo* under inflammatory conditions and are safe for clinical use [13–16]. This raises the possibility that T_{regs} may be used in islet transplantation to protect human grafted islets from alloimmune rejection without the side effects of systemic immunosuppression.

The recent development of 'humanized' mice has allowed the *in vivo* investigation of human immune responses [17–20]. In transplantation models, we and others have demonstrated that *ex vivo* expanded human T_{regs} can prevent the development of transplant arteriosclerosis [21] and skin allograft rejections [22] in peripheral blood mononuclear cells (PBMC)-reconstituted humanized mouse models [23]. The protective function of adoptively transferred human T_{regs} has also been investigated in PBMC-reconstituted humanized mouse transplanted with porcine islets. More recently, Douglas *et al.* have shown that human T_{regs} can prevent human islet transplant rejection by inhibiting T cell differentiation in PBMC-reconstituted Balb/cRag2$^{-/-}\gamma c^{-/-}$ mouse model [24]. In the present study, we adoptively transferred *ex vivo* expanded human T_{regs} into CD34$^+$ stem cells-reconstituted NOD-*scid IL2rγ*^{null} (NSG) mice to determine whether T_{regs} can protect grafted human islets from immune-mediated rejection, focusing primarily on the effects of T_{regs} on the innate immune responses.

Materials and Methods

Ethics statements

Use of human peripheral blood from healthy volunteers (REC Ref: 09/H0707/86), cord blood from full-term deliveries (REC Ref: 08/H0802/160) and islets from cadaveric donors (REC Ref: 05/MER09/48) has been approved by the National Research Ethics Service Committee London - Westminster, UK. Blood donors and the relatives of islet donors gave written informed consent for scientific use of the human materials. All consent procedures were approved by the National Research Ethics Service Committee London - Westminster, UK.

All animal experiments were conducted in accordance with UK Research Councils' and Medical Research Charities' guidelines on Responsibility in the Use of Animals in Bioscience Research, and the Home Office Animals Scientific Procedures Act (1986) under a UK Home Office license. Anesthetics and analgesics were administered to minimize or eliminate the pain and distress appropriately.

Isolation of CD34$^+$ stem cells from human umbilical cord blood

Cord blood was supplied by the NHS Cord Blood Bank (Colindale, London, UK). Mononuclear cells were isolated using density gradient centrifugation over Ficoll-Paque (GE Healthcare, Hatfield, UK) and enriched for CD34$^+$ cells by positive immunomagnetic isolation according to the manufacturer's instructions (Miltenyi Biotech, Surrey, UK).

Reconstitution of mice with human stem cells

NSG mice (The Jackson Laboratory) were bred and maintained in the Biological Services Unit of King's College London under specific pathogen-free conditions. Mice of 4–6 week old were irradiated with 240 cGy of γ-rays and received intravenous injection of 2×10^5 CD34$^+$ stem cells within 24 hours (**Fig. 1A**). For simplicity, the CD34$^+$ cells-reconstituted NSG mice are hereafter referred to as hu-NSG mice and NSG mice lacking CD34$^+$ cells injection are referred to as NSG mice.

Preparation of human regulatory T cells

Human leukocyte cones were obtained from the National Blood Transfusion Service (Tooting, London, UK). PBMC were isolated by Lymphocyte (PAA, Austria) density gradient centrifugation. CD4$^+$CD25$^+$ T cells (T_{regs}) were isolated from PBMC using a CD4$^+$CD25$^+$ Regulatory T Cell Isolation Kit (Miltenyi Biotec) according to the manufacturer's instructions. The CD4$^+$CD25$^-$ cells (T_{effs}) were used as autologous responder cells for *in vitro* suppression assays. Isolated T_{regs} were expanded as previously published [14]. Briefly, T_{regs} were cultured in X-vivo 15 medium (Lonza, Slough, UK) supplemented with 5% of human AB male pooled serum (HS, Biosera, London, UK), in the presence of recombinant IL-2 (1000 IU/mL, Proleukin-Novartis, Surrey, UK), rapamycin (100 nM) (Sigma, Surrey, UK) and Human T-Expander CD3/CD28 Dynabeads (CD3/CD28 beads, Invitrogen, Paisley, UK) in a 1:1 cell to bead ratio for three rounds of expansion, 8–10 days each. After the third round of expansion, the beads were removed and the T_{regs} were rested for 5–7 days in medium containing low concentration of IL-2 (20 IU/mL) before being intravenously injected into the mice.

T cell proliferation assay

Cell suspensions (1×10^5) prepared from the spleen of hu-NSG mice were cultured in 10% FBS RPMI-1640 medium in the presence of CD3/CD28 beads at a 1:1 bead to cell ratio. T-cell proliferation was measured after a 72 hour culture by adding ^{3}H thymidine (1 μM) for the last 16 hours. In a mixed lymphocyte reaction (MLR), human CD4$^+$ cells isolated from the spleen of hu-NSG mice immunized by HLA-mismatched PBMC were co-cultured with serial dilutions of irradiated [3000 gray (Gy) for 10 min] PBMC from the same donor (specific PBMC) and the PBMC from an unrelated donor (third-party PBMC). The proliferation assays were performed in a five day culture.

The suppressive activity of expanded T_{regs} was tested by co-culturing responder T cells (CD4$^+$CD25$^-$, T_{effs}) labelled with 5 μM carboxyfluorescein succinimidyl ester (CFSE, Invitrogen) with serial dilutions of *ex vivo* expanded autologous T_{regs} in the presence of CD3/CD28 beads in a 1:1 T_{effs} to bead ratio in RPMI-1640 medium containing 10% of human AB serum for 5 days. Proliferation was analyzed by flow cytometry. The percentage of proliferative T_{effs} in the absence of T_{regs} was taken as 100% proliferation.

Islet transplantation and adoptive transfer of T_{regs}

Hu-NSG and NSG mice were rendered diabetic (blood glucose level≥20 mM) by a single intraperitoneal (i.p.) injection of streptozotocin (STZ), 180 mg/kg body weight. Human islets were obtained from King's Cell Isolation Unit (London, UK). All islets were maintained in CMRL 1066 culture medium (Invitrogen) containing 2.5% human albumin at 37°C in an atmosphere of 95% air 5% CO_2 until transplanted. Human islet equivalents (IEQs, 3000–4000) were then transplanted under the left kidney capsule of diabetic mice that were anesthetized with pentobarbital sodium at 50 mg/kg [25]. After surgery, the mice were given subcutaneously 0.03 mg/ml of Vetergesic Multidose (buprenorphine) (Alstoe Ltd. Animal Health, UK) in 100 μl of sterile saline for post-operative analgesia. A total of 6×10^6 *ex vivo* expanded human T_{regs} expressing the same HLA-DR as the engrafted CD34$^+$ stem cells (**Table S1**) were injected intravenously into recipient mice immediately after islet transplantation. Blood glucose levels in recipient mice were evaluated using a blood glucose sensor (Abbott Diabetes Care Ltd., Witney, Oxon, UK). Loss of graft function was determined by blood glucose values≥20 mM.

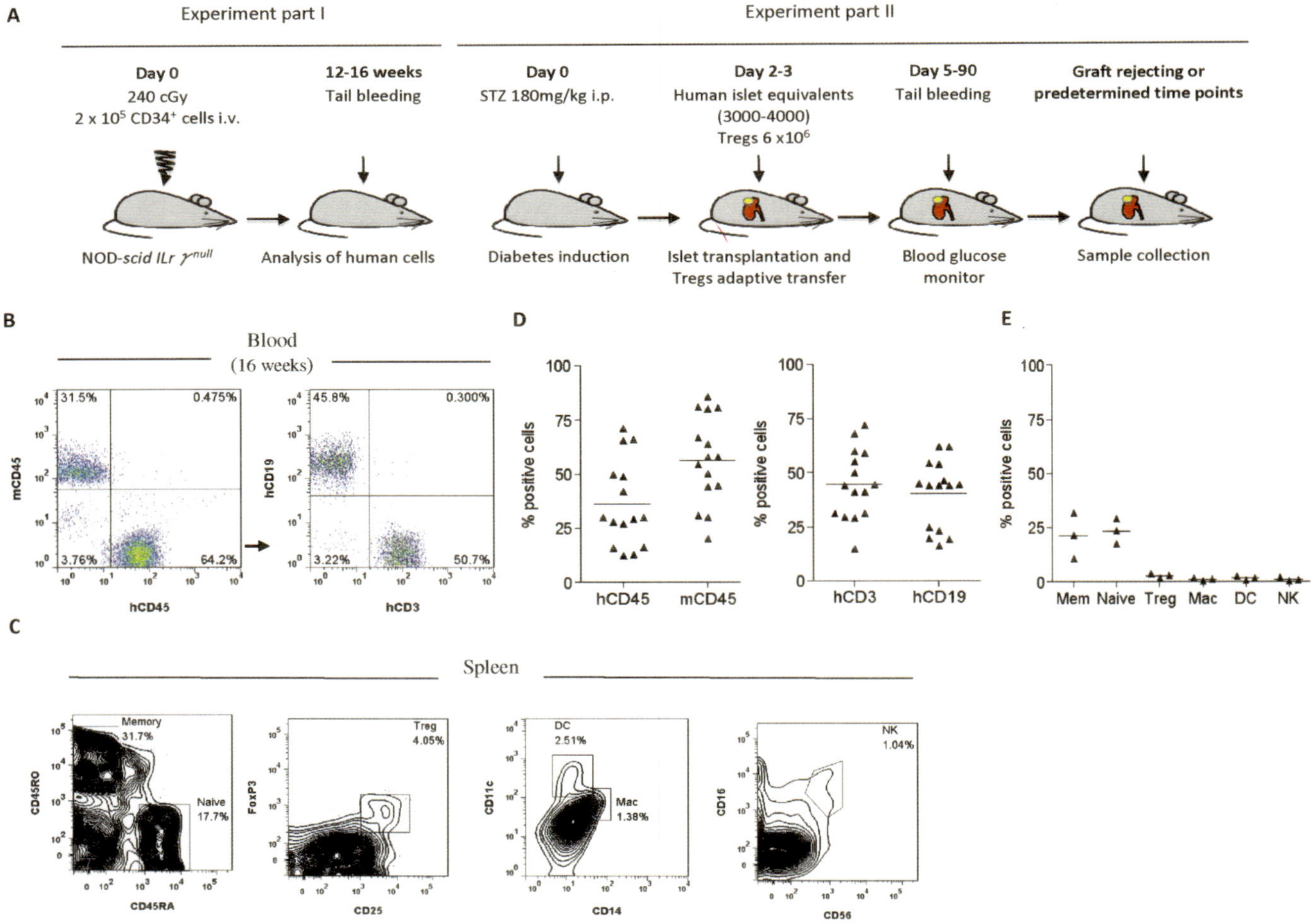

Figure 1. Reconstitution of NSG mice with human CD34$^+$ stem cells. (A) Strategy for generation of humanized mouse model of islet transplantation. (B) A representative FACS profile of human CD45$^+$, human CD19$^+$ and human CD3$^+$ cells in peripheral blood of hu-NSG mice, 12–16 weeks after transfer of CD34$^+$ cells (n = 15). Human CD19$^+$ B cells and CD3$^+$ T cells were identified in the gate for human CD45$^+$ cells. (C) Splenocytes from hu-NSG mice were analyzed by FACS for human CD45RA$^+$ (naïve T cells), human CD45RO$^+$ (memory T cells), human CD4$^+$CD25$^+$FoxP3$^+$ (Tregs), human CD11c$^+$ (dendritic cells), human CD14$^+$ (macrophages) and human CD16$^+$CD56$^+$ (NK cells) expression. (D–E) Data are summarized. Plotted lines represent the mean (n = 15, D; n = 3, E).

Nephrectomy

Selected mice with successful islet transplants were subjected to unilateral left nephrectomy to evaluate a return to hyperglycemic states. Anaesthetized mice were placed in a lateral decubitas position and a 2 cm incision was made over the left flank. The kidneys were extracorporealized. The renal artery was ligated together with the vein and ureter, prior to kidney resection. All animals were monitored closely postoperatively, and blood glucose was measured every 24 hours for 5 days.

Flow cytometric analysis

Flow cytometric analysis of human antigens in human T_{regs} and leukocytes was performed as previously described [26]. Fluorochrome-coupled antibodies specific for human CD45, CD3, CD19, CD45RA, CD45RO, CD4, CD25, FoxP3, CD14, CD11C, CD16 and CD56 were used for analysis of the human cell engraftment in hu-NSG mice. An APC-conjugated antibody against human monocyte chemoattractant protein-1 (MCP-1) was used for the detection of MCP-1 expression in islet cells. Single cell suspensions from the draining lymph nodes (left renal) and spleens were prepared from the islet-transplanted hu-NSG mice at the time of rejection (islets alone group) or at 21 days post-transplantation (islets+T_{regs} group), and stained with antibodies against human CD4, CD25 and FoxP3. Flow cytometric data were acquired using a FACS Calibur (BD Biosciences, San Jose, CA, USA) and analyzed using FlowJo 7.5 software (TreeStar Inc.).

Co-culture of human islets and T_{regs}

The human islets were dissociated into single cells with 0.05% trypsin-EDTA. The single cells (0.5 million cells) were cultured with or without 1 million *ex vivo* expanded T_{regs} in the presence of CD3/CD28 beads in 10% HS RPMI-1640 medium for 48 hours. LPS (1 μg/mL) was then added to the cultures for an additional 24 hours. As a control, the islets were co-cultured with autologous T_{effs} under the same conditions. After the incubation period, T_{regs} or T_{effs} were positively isolated using CD4 Dynabeads (Invitrogen). The eluted fraction was used for flow cytometric analysis and real-time RT-PCR for expression of MCP-1.

Real-time RT-PCR

PCR primers specific for human MCP-1 were designed as previously published [27] and RNA was extracted from islet grafts harvested at the time of rejection (islets alone group) or at 21 days post-transplantation (islets+T_{regs} group) and from cultured single islet cells using RNeasy Mini Kit (Qiagen). Real-time RT-PCR was performed using Brilliant SYBR Green QRT-PCR Master Mix Kit, following the manufacturer's protocol (Agilent Technologies, UK).

Enzyme-linked immunosorbent assay (ELISA) for human IgG, IgM, insulin and complement 3 (C3)

Human IgM and IgG were measured in the serum of hu-NSG mice over 12–16 weeks after the $CD34^+$ stem cells injection, and then anti-keyhole limpet hemocyanin (KLH) IgM and IgG were measured two weeks after hu-NSG mice were immunized with KLH whole protein (Sigma), using standard ELISA protocols (11).

Mouse sera taken from islet-transplanted hu-NSG mice at the time points when blood glucose was 7, 20 and 28 mM were assessed for human insulin and sera taken at the time of islet allograft rejection (blood glucose>20 mM) were determined for human C3 by ELISA kits (Millipore, Watford, UK).

Cytokine detection

Human Th1/Th2 cytokines were determined in the supernatants of $CD4^+$ T cells isolated from the spleen cells of hu-NSG mice after a 3 day stimulation by CD3/CD28 beads, and in the serum samples harvested at the time of rejection (islets alone group) or at 21 days post-transplantation (islets+T_{regs} group). A human Th1/Th2 11plex kit (eBiosciences) was used according to the manufacturer's protocol. Data acquisition was performed on a FACS Calibur (BD Biosciences) and then was analyzed using the BD Cytometric Bead Array software (BD Biosciences). The cytokines detected were IFN-γ, IL-1β, IL-2, IL-4, IL-5, IL-6, IL-8, IL-10, IL-12p70, TNF-α and TNF-β.

Histological and immunohistochemical analysis

Graft-bearing kidneys were harvested, fixed in 10% buffered formalin, and embedded in paraffin at the time of rejection (islets alone group) or at 21 days post-transplantation (islets+T_{regs} group). Sections (5 μm) were conventionally processed and stained with hematoxylin and eosin (H&E). For characterization of cell type-specific expression of antigens, single immunofluorescence staining was used: after antigen retrieval by microwaving for 5 min in 0.01 M citrate buffer (pH 6.0), sections were blocked with 10% goat normal serum for 30 min and then incubated overnight at 4°C with primary antibodies against the following: human CD45 (1:50; Dako, clone 2B11+PD7/26), insulin conjugated with HRP (1:50; Abcam, clone D3E7), complement 3d (C3d) conjugated with HRP (1:60; Dako, polyclonal), human CD4 (1:40; Dako, clone 4B12), human CD8 (1:60; Abcam, clone 14), human CD11b (1:50; eBiosciences, clone ICRF44) and human CD66b (1:50; BioLegend, clone G10F5). Diaminobenzidene and FITC- or TRITC-conjugated secondary antibodies were applied for 2 hours at room temperature. Sections were mounted in ProLong Gold Antifade Reagent with DAPI (Invitrogen). For identification of T_{regs}, slides were double stained with primary antibodies: mouse anti-human CD4 and rabbit anti-human FoxP3 (1:60; both Abcam, polyclonal). FITC-conjugated goat anti-mouse IgG and TRITC-conjugated goat anti-rabbit IgG (both Sigma) were used as secondary antibodies. Negative controls with nonspecific IgG were processed in parallel. Images were acquired using a Cooled Mono14 Bit camera (Q IMAGING, Canada) and Micro-Manager 1.3 software (University of California, USA).

Statistics

All statistical analysis were performed using the two-tailed Student's *t*-test (unpaired) for the group data and log-rank test for the survival data (Prism 4.0; GraphPad Software, USA). Data were presented as means ± SD and *P* values<0.05 were considered significant.

Results

NSG mice reconstituted with human $CD34^+$ stem cells are engrafted with a functional human immune system

A number of humanized mouse models have been generated for the *in vivo* study of human immune responses [28,29]. Here, NSG mice of 4-6 weeks of age were injected with cord blood-derived $CD34^+$ stem cells (**Fig. 1**A). After 3 months, a significant percentage of human cells was identified by flow cytometric analysis in the blood of NSG recipients (36%±5%) with 1:1 ratio of T and B cells (**Fig. 1B and D**). Various subsets of immune cells were present in the spleens of these animals, including naïve T cells ($CD45RA^+$), memory T cells ($CD45RO^+$), T_{regs} ($CD4^+CD25^+$ $FoxP3^+$), macrophages ($CD14^+$), dendritic cells ($CD11c^+$) and NK cells ($CD16^+CD56^+$) (**Fig. 1C and E**).

To validate the function of engrafted T cells, splenocytes from hu-NSG mice were stimulated *in vitro* with anti-CD3/CD28 beads. T cells responded to polyclonal stimulation (**Figure S1** (A)) and the cytokines IL-2, TNF-α, TNF-β, IL-8 and IL-1β were detected in culture supernatants (**Table 1**). Next, human $CD4^+$ T cells from the spleens of hu-NSG mice that had been immunized *in vivo* with allogeneic PBMC (specific PBMC) (**Figure S1** (B)) were re-stimulated *in vitro* with specific PBMC or with third party PBMC. These $CD4^+$ T cells showed significant responses to the specific PBMC, but not to third party PBMC (**Figure S1** (B)).

The function of B cells in hu-NSG mice was also evaluated and both IgM and IgG were detected in sera (IgM: 76.67±1.45 μg/mL; IgG: 44.39±9.4 μg/mL) (**Figure S2** (A)) and in supernatants after culturing B cells *in vitro* in the presence of IL-2 and IL-21 (IgM: 0.37±0.013 μg/mL; IgG: 0.99±0.21 μg/mL) (**Figure S2** (A)). Furthermore, KLH-specific IgM responses, but not IgG, were induced *in vivo* after KLH immunization (**Figure S2** (B)), as previously observed [26,30].

Table 1. Cytokine production by human CD4 T cells from hu-NSG mice *in vitro*.

	Spl:CD4		AdPBMC:CD4	
Pg/mL	**Control**	**CD3/CD28**	**Control**	**CD3/CD28**
IFN-γ	ud*	ud	ud	168.5±97.27
IL-2	ud	298.58±20.26	ud	1750.18±223.93
TNF-α	ud	62.30±6.86	ud	1197.47±192.22
TNF-β	7.75±2.62**	118.62±21.35	5.98±2.45	510.9±89.35
IL-10	ud	ud	ud	201.91±39.45
IL-8	101.83±34.39	150.41±9.21	73.54±22.63	1871.14±318.04
IL-1β	2.52±1.45	0.63±0.36	3.17±1.83	10.98±6.33

Human $CD4^+$ T cells were stimulated with CD3/CD28 beads for three days. Supernatants were analyzed by cytometric bead array for cytokine production (n=3). Cytokines IL-4, IL-5, IL-6 and IL-12p70 were not detectable in the supernatants. Spl:CD4 denotes CD4 cells from the spleen of a hu-NSG mouse. AdPBMC:CD4 indicates CD4 cells from PBMC of a healthy donor.
*: undetectable. **: mean ± SD.

Human islet allografts stimulate immune responses in hu-NSG mice

Having confirmed that hu-NSG mice had a functional adaptive immune response, although partially impaired [26,30,31], mice with successful human cell engraftment (human $CD45^+$ cells>15%) were rendered diabetic. They were then transplanted with human IEQs (3000-4000) under the kidney capsule. This resulted in immediate establishment of normoglycemia (blood glucose<13.8 mM) [24,32]. Islet allograft rejection, as evidenced by a rise in blood glucose above 20 mM, was observed in all hu-NSG mice by day 17 post-transplantation while normoglycemia remained stable over an observation of 90 days in NSG mice (6 animals for each group) (**Fig. 2A**). In order to demonstrate the functionality of transplanted islets *in vivo*, six mice with successful islet transplantations were selected to undergo unilateral left nephrectomy, which restored a hyperglycemic state within 24 hours (**Figure S3**). Human insulin levels in the sera from islet transplanted-hu-NSG mice correlated negatively with the levels of blood glucose (**Fig. 2B**).

Immune responses stimulated by islet allografts were analyzed in the sera and by histology at the time of rejection. Significant amounts of human C3 were detected in the sera of hu-NSG mice with islet transplants, but not in hu-NSG mice lacking islet transplants or in NSG mice with or without islet transplants (**Fig. 3A**). Human cytokines, including IFN-γ, IL-4 and IL-1β, were detected at pg/mL levels in the sera from the islet transplanted-hu-NSG mice but not in the hu-NSG without islet transplants (**Fig. 3B**). Histological analysis revealed damaged islet-structures with fewer insulin positive cells in mice with rejecting allografts (**Fig. 4c and g**). A large number of graft-infiltrating mononuclear cells (**Fig. 4e, f and i**) and human $CD45^+$ cells (**Fig. 4h**) were detected in hu-NSG recipients, but not in NSG mice (**Fig. 4a, b and d**). A significant number of macrophages ($CD11b^+$), neutrophils ($CD66b^+$) and $CD4^+$ T cells were recruited into the graft-bearing kidney tissue in hu-NSG mice (**Fig. 4l, m and j**). Very few, if any, $CD8^+$ T cells were identified in hu-NSG mice (**Fig. 4k**). C3d deposition in the islet grafts was also observed (**Fig. 4n**). Altogether these results indicate that hu-NSG mice mount both innate and adaptive immune responses against transplanted human islet allografts.

Ex vivo polyclonally expanded human Tregs delay human islet allograft rejection

Next, we investigated the impact of T_{regs} on the modulation of human islet allograft rejection. Human T_{regs} ($CD4^+CD25^+$) were isolated and expanded *in vitro* in the presence of rapamycin and IL-2 [14]. The T_{reg} lines were characterized phenotypically and functionally, prior to adoptive transfer into recipient mice. Flow cytometric analysis revealed that greater than 98% of CD4-gated T_{regs} expressed high levels of CD25 and FoxP3 (**Figure S4** (A)). T_{regs} displayed a marked suppressive ability as measured by CFSE dilution (**Figure S4** (B) and (C)).

T_{reg} lines (6×10^6) were then injected intravenously into hu-NSG mice at the time of islet transplant. Islet graft survival was monitored by measuring blood glucose levels in the sera of the mice. The results demonstrated that the transfer of *ex vivo* expanded T_{regs} prolonged the survival of islets (median survival time T_{regs}-treated mice 32 days versus 17 days in mice receiving islets alone) (n = 15 for islets alone group; n = 10 for islets+T_{regs} group; **Fig. 5A**). To confirm that the prolonged graft survival was the result of T_{reg}-mediated suppression, islet grafts were harvested at the time of graft-rejection for T_{reg}-untreated recipients and at day 21 post-transplantation (animals with grafts undergoing rejection were excluded) for T_{reg}-treated recipients. Histological analysis demonstrated that surviving grafts contained densely packed insulin-producing cells and intact islet structures, whereas grafts undergoing rejection exhibited destroyed lobular structure of islets with few remaining insulin positive-staining cells (**Fig. 5B**). The numbers of macrophages ($CD11b^+$), neutrophils ($CD66b^+$) and $CD4^+$ T cells infiltrating the grafts were markedly reduced in T_{reg}-treated animals, compared with T_{reg}-untreated recipients (n = 3 for each group) (**Fig. 5B and C**). These results suggest a potent suppression of innate and $CD4^+$ T cell-mediated immune responses by T_{regs}. The improved histology correlated with the presence of T_{regs} ($CD4^+FoxP3^+$) in the graft of T_{reg}-treated animals (**Fig. 5D**) and higher numbers of T_{regs} in the draining lymph nodes (**Fig. 6A**). Lower numbers of total $CD4^+$ T cells were observed in the spleens and draining lymph nodes of these mice compared to T_{reg}-untreated mice (**Fig. 6B and C**), whereas no significant differences were found in the number of

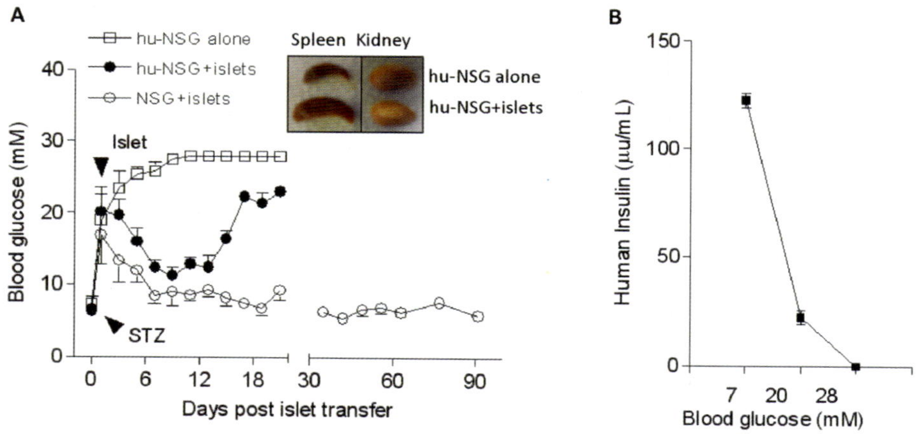

Figure 2. Diabetic hu-NSG mice reject the grafted human islets. (A) The function of grafted human islets was evaluated by measuring blood glucose levels. As a control, NSG mice without $CD34^+$ cell reconstitution remained normoglycemic after islet transplantation. The insert shows a representative image of a kidney and a spleen from hu-NSG mice that received (bottom) or did not receive (top) islet transplants (n = 6). STZ: streptozotocin. (B) Serum samples from hu-NSG mice that were grafted with human islets were measured by ELISA for human insulin when blood glucose was 7, 20 and 28 mM (n = 3).

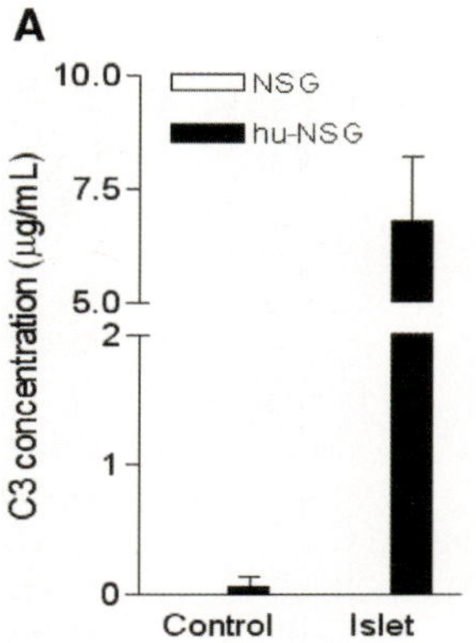

B

Pg/mL	Control	Islet
IFN-γ	ud*	8.85 ± 0.7
IL-2	34.36 ± 11.28**	7.73 ± 6.66
IL-4	ud	49.34 ± 1.45
IL-10	0.42 ± 0.12	3.10 ± 0.37
IL-8	1.7 ± 0.49	11.16 ± 9.2
IL-1β	ud	0.79 ± 0.14

Figure 3. Human innate and adaptive immune responses mediate islet rejection in the hu-NSG mice. (A) Sera were analyzed by ELISA for human C3 levels in hu-NSG mice with/without human islet transplants or NSG mice with/without transplants (n = 3). Control: no islet transplant. (B) Sera were collected at the time of graft rejection. Cytokines were measured by cytokine bead array (n = 3). Control: sera from hu-NSG mice without islet transplant. *: undetectable. **: mean ± SD.

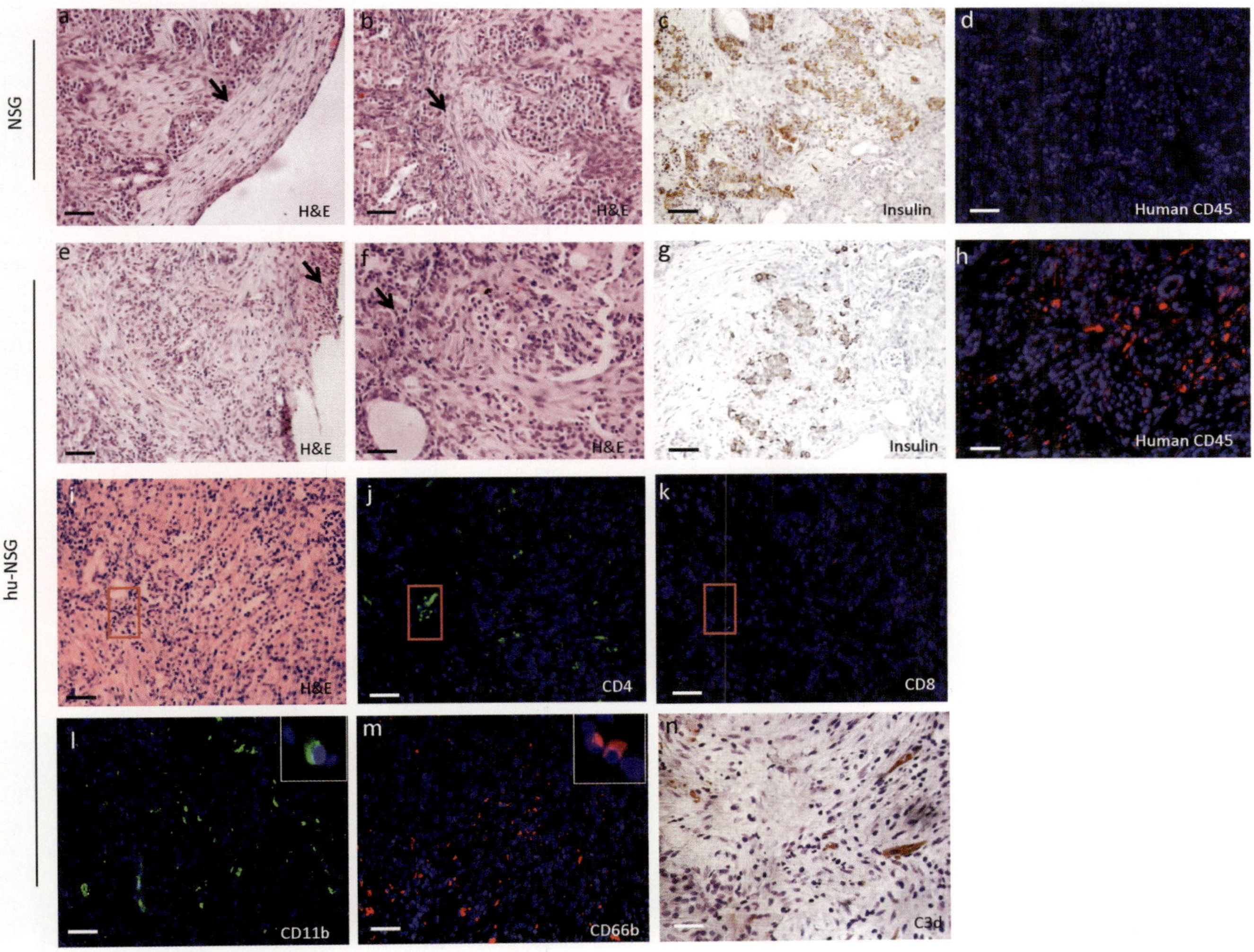

Figure 4. Infiltration of immune cells and C3 deposit in the grafted human islets. Tissue samples of islet allograft bearing kidney in hu-NSG mice were collected at the time of islet allograft rejection. Sections were stained with H & E (**a–b, e–f and i**) and antibodies to human antigens: insulin (**c** and **g**, brown), CD45 (**d and h**, green), CD4 (**j**, green), CD8 (**k**, red), CD11b (**l**, green), CD66b (**m**, red), and C3d (**n**, brown). Arrow indicates the kidney capsule or the area around islet grafts. Red square indicates the site of the infiltration. Scale bar: 100 μm.

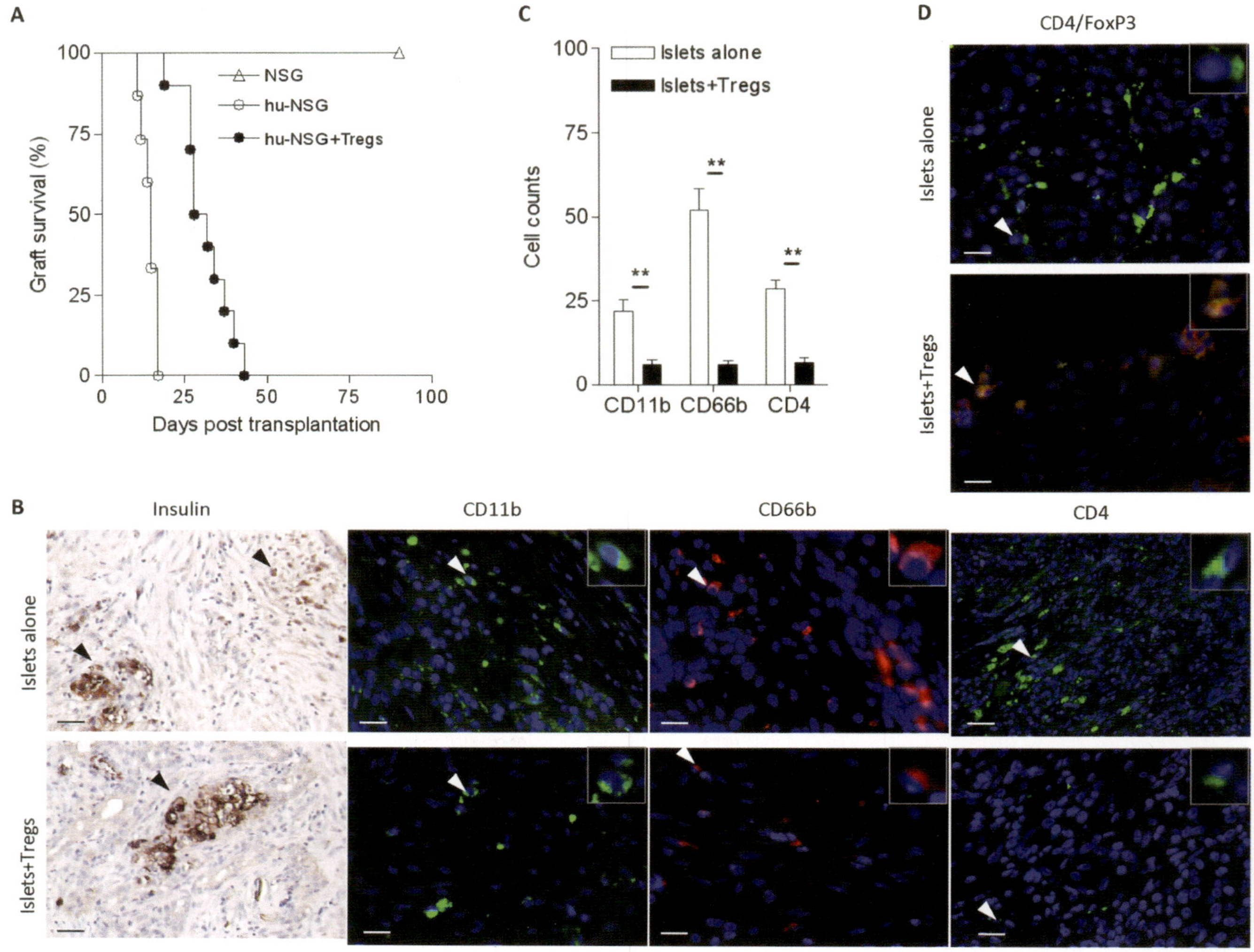

Figure 5. Adoptive transfer of *ex vivo* expanded T_{regs} protects human islet allograft from rejection. (A) Percentage graft survival in hu-NSG mice with or without T_{reg}-treatments (n = 15 for islets alone group; n = 10 for T_{regs}-treated group; Log-rank test, p = 0.0004). (B) Histological examination of islet grafts determined by immunostaining with antibodies for human antigens: insulin (brown), CD11b (green), CD66b (red), and CD4 (green). Nuclei were stained with DAPI (blue). Tissues were harvested at the time of islet allograft rejection in T_{regs}-untreated animals and at day 21 post-islet transfer in T_{reg}-treated animals. (C) Quantitative data analysis of islet graft immunostaining. Data represent results from three individual mice per group. (D) Identification of T_{regs} in the islet grafts. The harvested grafts were double-stained with FITC-conjugated CD4 (green) and TRITC-conjugated FoxP3 (red). CD4/FoxP3 double-positive cells are shown by yellow colour. Inset images show enlarged area indicated by a white arrow. Black arrow indicates islets grafts. **: $p<0.01$. Scale bar: 50 μm.

$CD4^+CD25^+FoxP3^+$ cells in the spleens between the two groups of mice (**Fig. 6A**).

Ex vivo expanded human Tregs down regulate MCP-1 expression by islets

Having observed a decreased infiltration of macrophages ($CD11b^+$) and neutrophils ($CD66b^+$) in the islet grafts of hu-NSG mice and an increase in T_{regs} in the draining lymph nodes following adoptive transfer of T_{regs}, we chose to focus on the mechanisms behind the regulation of innate cell infiltration. Specifically, we investigated the possibility that T_{regs} exhibited suppression of innate cells by regulating the expression of MCP-1, which is secreted by islet cells and is responsible for macrophage/neutrophil recruitment [33,34]. Islet allografts were harvested at the time of rejection in the T_{reg}-untreated group and at day 21 post-transplantation in the T_{reg}-treated group. RT-PCR analysis showed that the level of MCP-1 gene transcription in T_{reg}-treated animals was reduced by 71% compared with T_{reg}-untreated animals (**Fig. 7A**). To test the direct effect of T_{regs} on MCP-1 production by islets, T_{regs} were co-cultured with freshly isolated single islet cells *in vitro*. Consistent with the *in vivo* findings, T_{regs} reduced MCP-1 transcription in the cultured islet cells (**Fig. 7B**). In contrast, autologous T_{effs} co-cultured with islet cells had no effect on MCP-1 expression (**Fig. 7B**). Flow cytometric analysis confirmed that T_{regs} significantly decreased the number of MCP-1 positive cells in islet cells (**Fig. 7C and F**) and the expression of MCP-1 by islet cells during co-culture with T_{regs} (**Fig. 7D and E**). Interestingly, when the cytokine profile was analyzed in the sera of T_{reg}-treated animals, IFN-γ was remarkably increased while IL-4 was significantly decreased (**Fig. 8**). Compared with controls, IL-8 was significantly elevated in serum of islet-transplanted hu-NSG mice (**Fig. 8**).

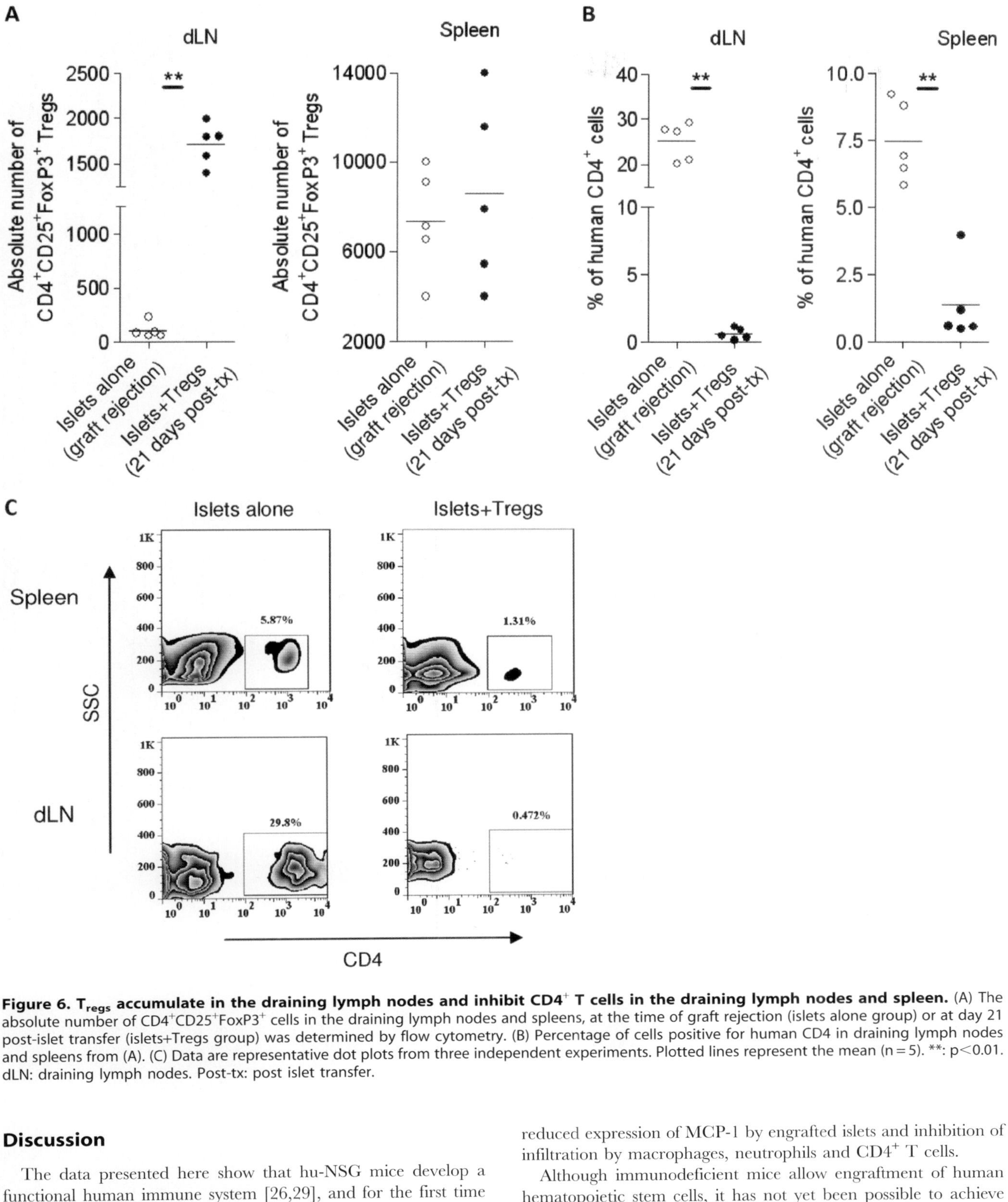

Figure 6. T_{regs} accumulate in the draining lymph nodes and inhibit $CD4^+$ T cells in the draining lymph nodes and spleen. (A) The absolute number of $CD4^+CD25^+FoxP3^+$ cells in the draining lymph nodes and spleens, at the time of graft rejection (islets alone group) or at day 21 post-islet transfer (islets+Tregs group) was determined by flow cytometry. (B) Percentage of cells positive for human CD4 in draining lymph nodes and spleens from (A). (C) Data are representative dot plots from three independent experiments. Plotted lines represent the mean (n = 5). **: $p<0.01$. dLN: draining lymph nodes. Post-tx: post islet transfer.

Discussion

The data presented here show that hu-NSG mice develop a functional human immune system [26,29], and for the first time we demonstrate the utility of hu-NSG mice for studying innate immune responses to human islet allografts. Our study provides evidence that *ex vivo* expanded human T_{regs} delay human islet allograft rejection in hu-NSG mice, via a mechanism involving reduced expression of MCP-1 by engrafted islets and inhibition of infiltration by macrophages, neutrophils and $CD4^+$ T cells.

Although immunodeficient mice allow engraftment of human hematopoietic stem cells, it has not yet been possible to achieve completely normal human hematopoiesis in any of the currently available immunodeficient mouse strains [28,29]. The hu-NSG mice generated in this study were approximately 30% chimeric with human cells ($CD45^+$ cells) including T- and B-cells and subsets of various immune cells that are present in the spleen: these

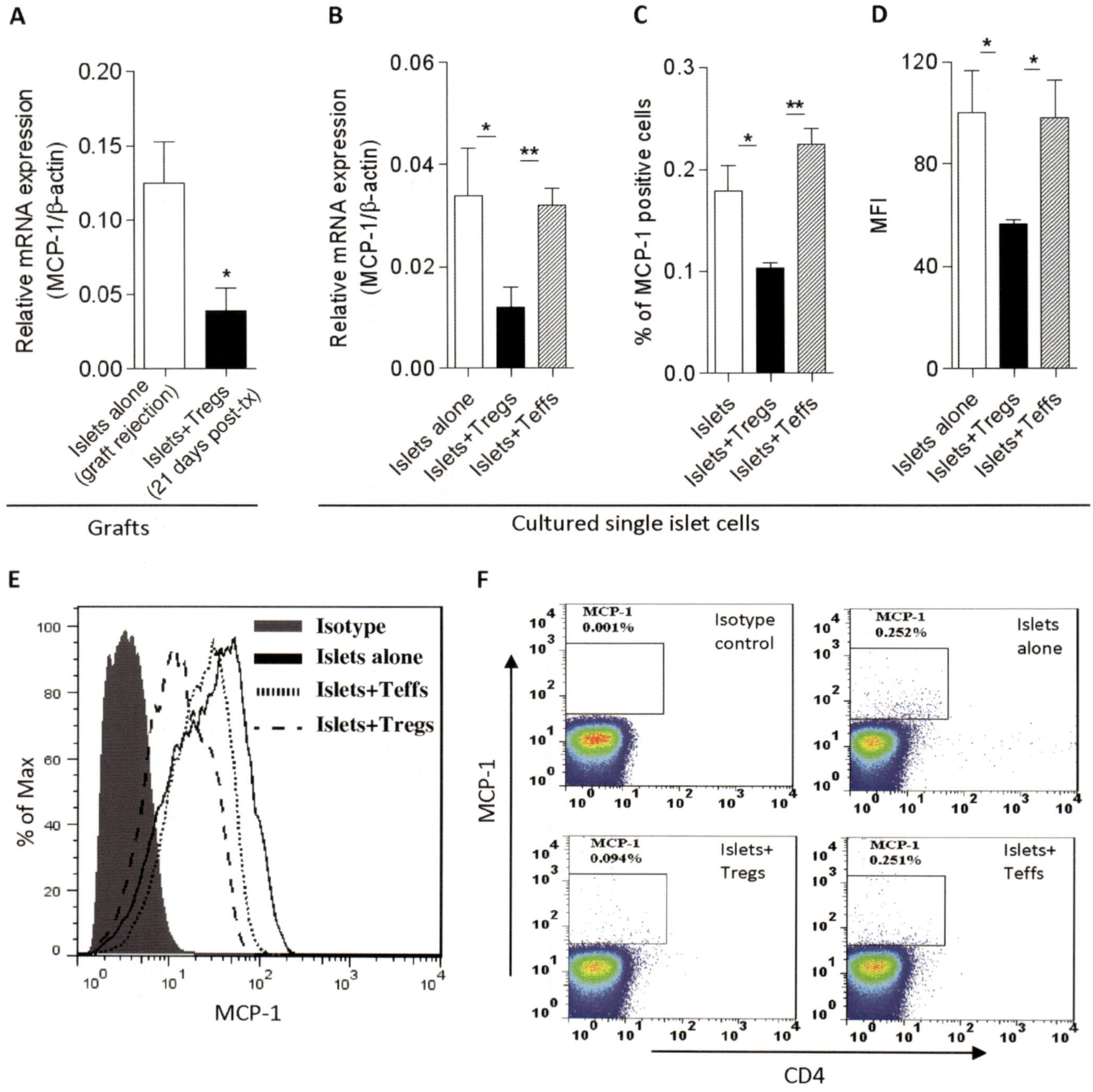

Figure 7. T_{regs} reduced MCP-1 production *in vitro* and *in vivo*. (A) MCP-1 expression in islet grafts at the time of rejection (islets alone group) or at day 21 post-islet transfer (islets+T_{regs} group) was measured by real-time RT-PCR (n = 5). β-actin was used as the endogenous control. (B) The expression of mRNA was analyzed by real-time RT-PCR in islet cells co-cultured with T_{regs} for three days. (C–D) Cumulative data (mean ± SD) for MCP-1 expression in cultured islet cells. MFI: mean fluorescence intensity. (E–F) Representative plots from 4 independent experiments are shown. *: $p<0.05$; **: $p<0.01$. Post-tx: post islet transfer.

include T_{regs} ($CD4^+CD25^+FoxP3^+$), monocytes/macrophages ($CD14^+$), DC ($CD11c^+$) and NK cells ($CD56^+CD16^+$), indicating reconstitution of human lymphohematopoiesis in these mice. We noted human CD3 T cells engraftment in hu-NSG mice 12-16 weeks after $CD34^+$ cell transfer, which was earlier than other reports [35]. This may be due to differences in experimental conditions and protocols used to engraft human stem cells, including the choice of recipient age and source of human $CD34^+$ cells [35].

The engrafted human T cells in our system were able to produce cytokines including IL-2, TNF-α, TNF-β, IL-8 and IL-1β and to respond to polyclonal CD3/CD28 stimulation, although less efficiently than in adult blood, suggesting partial function of engrafted T cells [26,29–31,36,37]. Confirming published work [26,30,31,36–38], an impaired B cell response was also observed

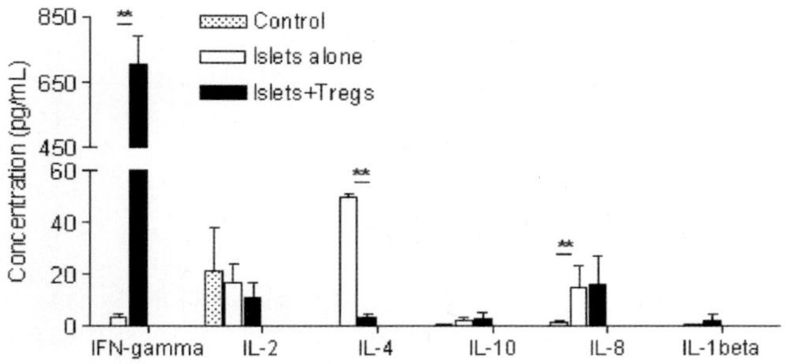

Figure 8. T_{regs} regulate human cytokine production in islet-transplanted hu-NSG mice. Sera were collected at the time of rejection (islets alone group) or at day 21 post-islet transfer (islets+T_{regs} group). Cytokines were measured by cytokine bead array (n = 3). Control: sera from hu-NSG mice without islet transplant. **: $p<0.01$.

in these animals, showing inefficient production of antigen-specific IgG. This is believed to be due to defective interaction between human B and T cells [26,30,31,36–38], resulting from a lack of human leukocyte antigen (HLA) expression in the mouse thymus [26,38]. This possibility has been supported by the improved antigen-specific human T cell and antibody responses achieved when human $CD34^+$ cells were injected in immunodeficient mice that expressed HLA molecules either by transgenesis [38,39] or following transplantation of human thymus [40]. Nevertheless, although NSG mice receiving $CD34^+$ cells failed to develop efficient antigen-specific immune responses [26,30,31,36,37], we found that, following immunization, engrafted human T cells responded to alloantigens, as shown by ^{3}H-thymidine incorporation in an *in vitro* culture of $CD4^+$ cells from the spleen. These findings do not exclude the possibility that other antigen recognition pathways exist [28], thus there remains a need to assess the major histocompatiblity complex (MHC) restriction of human T cells in this animal model.

The importance of the innate immune system is currently poorly understood in this model of human allograft rejection. The presence of C3d deposition and infiltration of macrophages ($CD11b^+$) and neutrophils ($CD66b^+$) into rejecting islet allografts in these animals supports the idea that our system might be useful for the study of innate immune responses to allografts. This view is further strengthened by the detection of human C3 in the sera of the islet-transplanted hu-NSG mice generated in this study, which we speculate was locally produced by infiltrating human inflammatory cells [41,42]. Indeed, local immune cell-derived production of complement emerges as a key mediator of complement's impact on adaptive immune responses [42].

One of the advantages of $CD34^+$ cells-reconstituted humanized mice is that they lack graft-versus-host disease (GvHD) [43]. By rendering mice diabetic before islet transplantation, we have been able to monitor the islet allograft rejection spontaneously mediated by hu-NSG mice, evidenced by raising blood glucose. This contrasts with PBMC-reconstituted NSG (huPBL-NSG) mice, which died from GvHD within the first 30 days and provided only 4-5 week window of opportunity of the human immune responses [32]. As a consequence, in the huPBL-NSG mice, rejection is often determined *post-facto* by histopathology, making the huPBL-NSG mouse model difficult to use for interventional studies [32]. In keeping with blood glucose data, histological examination showed a significant human $CD45^+$ leukocytes infiltrate and islet destruction in islet allograft, suggesting human immune-mediated rejection in our system. These data are inconsistent with the experiments using human $CD34^+$ cells-reconstituted Balb/cRag2$^{-/-}\gamma c^{-/-}$ mice [44]. The explanation for this discrepancy might lie in the difference in the mouse strains [45,46]. Indeed NSG mice, with NOD (nobese diabetic) background, allow better hematopoietic engraftment than do Balb/cRag2$^{-/-}\gamma c^{-/-}$ mice because the NOD variant of signal regulatory protein-α (SIRP-α) binds human CD47, whereas Balb/cRag2$^{-/-}\gamma c^{-/-}$ mouse SIRP-α does not [18]. Binding of SIRP-α expressed on mouse macrophages to human CD47 is critical for the development of human hematopoiesis *in vivo* and *Sirpa* polymorphism has been identified as a new genetic determinant of human hematopoietic stem cell engraftment [18].

We have here tested for the first time the impact of *ex vivo* expanded human T_{regs} on the innate immune responses to human islet allograft in the humanized mice. Several groups have developed an optimal protocol for expanding T_{regs} for therapeutic use [47–49]. T_{regs} used in current study were expanded in the presence of CD3/CD28 beads and rapamycin as we previously published [14]. Rapamycin prevents outgrowth of contaminating non-regulatory cells, enhances T_{reg} survival and expands the most stable subpopulation of T_{regs} [49]. In the current study, we observed that in T_{regs}-treated group, islet rejection was delayed for 15 days. Histological analysis demonstrated that there was significantly less infiltrating macrophages, neutrophils and $CD4^+$ T cells with preservation of islet structure in the grafts from T_{reg}-treated animals, suggesting that suppressive properties of T_{regs} are not limited to effects on T-cell responses but also include inhibition of pathology mediated by cells of the innate immune system system [50,51]. Our demonstration is in agreement with recent findings suggesting that expanded human T_{regs} can prevent rejection of porcine islet xenograft in huPBL-NSG mice [52] and human islet allograft in PBMC-reconstituted Balb/cRag2$^{-/-}\gamma c^{-/-}$ mice [24]. Similar results were also observed in the study of capacity of T_{regs} to interfere with the innate immune responses from other groups, including ours [53], in murine models of infectious diseases [54], skin transplantation [53] and islet engraftment [50]. Whether the inhibition of $CD4^+$ T cell recruitment to the islet allograft was due to a direct effect of T_{regs} on T cells or the consequence of the action of T_{regs} on the innate immune system, as recently suggested [50], needs further investigation.

Our data also showed that T_{regs} detected by double staining of CD4 and FoxP3 were not present in a large numbers in the graft at day 21 post-transfer in T_{regs}-treated group, suggesting that they may have had an initial effect on the islet, and then migrated to draining lymph nodes [50] [24]. This speculation was confirmed by our findings that the absolute numbers of T_{regs} was significantly higher in draining lymph nodes, along with significant decrease of $CD4^+$ T cells in spleen and draining lymph nodes from T_{reg}-treated animals when compared with in T_{regs}-untreated animals. In line with our findings, T_{regs} have been demonstrated to sequentially migrate from the site of tissue inflammation to the draining lymph nodes to suppress alloimmune responses in a mouse islet allograft model [55].

The ability of T_{regs} to inhibit a range of immune responses and target a variety of cells suggests that they use multiple different effector mechanisms [56]. In our study, T_{regs} directly interacted with pancreatic islets, in the absence of effect T-cells, and inhibited the innate responses of islets for chemokine MCP-1 production *in vitro*. Consistent with our *in vitro* data, adaptive transfer of T_{regs} resulted in decreased expression of MCP-1 on islet graft *in vivo*. This finding may partly explain the mechanism underlying inhibiting of infiltration by T_{regs} in the graft. Furthermore, elevated serum levels of IFN-γ in the T_{regs}-treated animals suggest the contribution of IFN-γ to regulation of T_{regs} as previously published [57], although additional work needs to be done to prove that IFN-γ is essential to the delay of islet rejection [57]. IFN-γ is secreted by Th1 cells and conventionally thought to be responsible for driving cell-mediated immune responses. However, in recent years the promoting effects of IFN-γ on the development of Th1-controlling T_{regs} has drawn attention from various groups [58,59]. The early production of IFN-γ by induced T_{regs} following reencounter with antigen has been demonstrated to prevent the initiation of aggressive immune responses, including graft rejection, by controlling T-cell effector mechanisms [60]. In contrast to our findings, one report showed decreased IFN-γ levels in the sera from T_{regs}-treated mice [52]. The difference in IFN-γ levels might be the different type of human hematopoietic cells engrafted through reconstitution with either $CD34^+$ cells or PBMC [52]. In addition, IL-4, which can up-regulate MCP-1 expression in a variety of cells [61], was remarkably decreased in T_{reg}-treated animals. These data suggest that the balance between these two cytokines might contribute to the regulation of cellular MCP-1 expression [62].

In conclusion, the present study provides evidence that *ex vivo* expanded human T_{regs} prolong islet allograft survival via inhibiting infiltration of macrophages, neutrophils and $CD4^+$ T cells possibly through a MCP-1-dependent mechanism. These data may contribute to the development of clinical strategies for the generation of T_{reg} therapy to control human islet rejection. Also, we reveal for the first time that $CD34^+$ stem cells-reconstituted NSG mouse model might offer a tool for pre-clinical evaluation of human innate immune responses to human allografts.

Supporting Information

Figure S1 Assessment of human T cell function in hu-NSG mice. (A) Splenocytes from hu-NSG mice and PBMC from healthy donors (AdPBMC) were stimulated with CD3/CD28 beads for 3 days. T cell function was determined by ^{3}H-thymidine uptake (n = 6). (B) Human $CD4^+$ T cells isolated from hu-NSG mice immunized with 10^7 PBMC (specific) were cultured with the same PBMC and with third party PBMC for 5 days. T cell function was assessed in MLRs (n = 3). The insert shows the spleens from a representative immunized (left) and non-immunized mouse (right).

Figure S2 Production of human immunoglobins by human B cells in hu-NSG mice. (A) Human IgM and IgG were determined by ELISA in sera from hu-NSG mice 12–16 weeks after $CD34^+$ cell reconstitution and in supernatants of B cells cultured in the presence of IL-2 and IL-21. (B) Keyhole limpet haemocyanin (KLH)-specific human IgM or IgG were determined in the sera from hu-NSG mice immunized with KLH. Sera from non-immunized hu-NSG mice were used as control. (n = 3). For the B cell culture, a representative result of three independent cultures is shown. NSG: sera from NSG mice without $CD34^+$ cell reconstitution; Nil: supernatant from the B cell culture in the absence of IL-2 and IL-21.

Figure S3 Assessment of grafted human islet in hu-NSG mice. Human islet equivalents (IEQs, 3000–4000) were transplanted into the kidney capsule of chemically-induced diabetic mice and blood glucose was measured. The islets were removed via unilateral nephrectomy when establishment of normoglycemia (blood glucose<13.8 mM) had been confirmed in hu-NSG mice and at day 30 post-islet transfer in NSG mice. The function of human islet grafts was evaluated by measuring blood glucose levels. All mice returned rapidly to a hyperglycemic state. Data shown are representative examples from 3 animals in each group. STZ: streptozotocin.

Figure S4 The phenotype and functional analysis of *ex vivo* expanded human T_{regs}. (A) Representative flow cytometric analysis of the expression of CD25 and FoxP3 molecules by T_{regs} (cells were gated on human CD4 expression). Data are from one out of three independent experiments with T_{regs} derived from three individual donors. (B) CFSE–labelled $CD4^+CD25^-$ cells (responders) were co-cultured with serial dilutions of expanded autologous T_{regs} in the presence of anti-CD3/CD28 beads for 5 days. Flow cytometric analysis was performed to assess cellular proliferation by CFSE dilution. (C) Quantitative analysis of T_{regs} suppressive function. The data shown are representative of three independent experiments.

Table S1 HLA typing.

Acknowledgments

We thank C. Scotta for advice on T_{reg} expansion; GP Vinson (The School of Biological and Chemical Sciences, Queen Mary, University London, UK) and MP Gordge (Department of Biomedical Science, University of Westminster) for help in the preparation of the manuscript.

Author Contributions

Conceived and designed the experiments: FX LM VM RL GL. Performed the experiments: FX LM. Analyzed the data: FX LM. Contributed reagents/materials/analysis tools: MZ GH. Wrote the paper: FX. GH and AD Helped in designing the experiments: GH AD. Reviewed/edited the manuscript: LM AD RL GL.

References

1. Shapiro AM, Ricordi C, Hering BJ, Auchincloss H, Lindblad R, et al. (2006) International trial of the Edmonton protocol for islet transplantation. N Engl J Med 355: 1318–1330.
2. Ryan EA, Paty BW, Senior PA, Bigam D, Alfadhli E, et al. (2005) Five-year follow-up after clinical islet transplantation. Diabetes 54: 2060–2069.
3. Fiorina P, Secchi A (2007) Pancreatic islet cell transplant for treatment of diabetes. Endocrinol Metab Clin North Am 36: 999–1013; ix.
4. Harlan DM, Kenyon NS, Korsgren O, Roep BO (2009) Current advances and travails in islet transplantation. Diabetes 58: 2175–2184.
5. Lamb KE, Lodhi S, Meier-Kriesche HU (2011) Long-term renal allograft survival in the United States: a critical reappraisal. Am J Transplant 11: 450–462.
6. Maffi P, Bertuzzi F, De Taddeo F, Magistretti P, Nano R, et al. (2007) Kidney function after islet transplant alone in type 1 diabetes: impact of immunosuppressive therapy on progression of diabetic nephropathy. Diabetes Care 30: 1150–1155.
7. Wood KJ, Bushell A, Hester J (2012) Regulatory immune cells in transplantation. Nat Rev Immunol 12: 417–430.
8. Vergani A, D'Addio F, Jurewicz M, Petrelli A, Watanabe T, et al. (2010) A novel clinically relevant strategy to abrogate autoimmunity and regulate alloimmunity in NOD mice. Diabetes 59: 2253–2264.
9. Fiorina P, Voltarelli J, Zavazava N (2011) Immunological applications of stem cells in type 1 diabetes. Endocr Rev 32: 725–754.
10. Vergani A, Fotino C, D'Addio F, Tezza S, Podetta M, et al. (2013) Effect of the purinergic inhibitor oxidized ATP in a model of islet allograft rejection. Diabetes 62: 1665–1675.
11. Baecher-Allan C, Brown JA, Freeman GJ, Hafler DA (2001) CD4+CD25high regulatory cells in human peripheral blood. J Immunol 167: 1245–1253.
12. Tang Q, Lee K (2012) Regulatory T-cell therapy for transplantation: how many cells do we need? Curr Opin Organ Transplant 17: 349–354.

13. Di Ianni M, Del Papa B, Zei T, Iacucci Ostini R, Cecchini D, et al. (2012) T regulatory cell separation for clinical application. Transfus Apher Sci 47: 213–216.
14. Scotta C, Esposito M, Fazekasova H, Fanelli G, Edozie FC, et al. (2013) Differential effects of rapamycin and retinoic acid on expansion, stability and suppressive qualities of human CD4+CD25+FOXP3+ T regulatory cell subpopulations. Haematologica 98: 1291–1299.
15. Afzali B, Edozie FC, Fazekasova H, Scotta C, Mitchell PJ, et al. (2013) Comparison of regulatory T cells in hemodialysis patients and healthy controls: implications for cell therapy in transplantation. Clin J Am Soc Nephrol 8: 1396–1405.
16. Tresoldi E, Dell'Albani I, Stabilini A, Jofra T, Valle A, et al. (2011) Stability of human rapamycin-expanded CD4+CD25+ T regulatory cells. Haematologica 96: 1357–1365.
17. Brehm MA, Racki WJ, Leif J, Burzenski L, Hosur V, et al. (2012) Engraftment of human HSCs in nonirradiated newborn NOD-scid IL2rgamma null mice is enhanced by transgenic expression of membrane-bound human SCF. Blood 119: 2778–2788.
18. Takenaka K, Prasolava TK, Wang JC, Mortin-Toth SM, Khalouei S, et al. (2007) Polymorphism in Sirpa modulates engraftment of human hematopoietic stem cells. Nat Immunol 8: 1313–1323.
19. Watanabe S, Ohta S, Yajima M, Terashima K, Ito M, et al. (2007) Humanized NOD/SCID/IL2Rgamma(null) mice transplanted with hematopoietic stem cells under nonmyeloablative conditions show prolonged life spans and allow detailed analysis of human immunodeficiency virus type 1 pathogenesis. J Virol 81: 13259–13264.
20. Shultz LD, Ishikawa F, Greiner DL (2007) Humanized mice in translational biomedical research. Nat Rev Immunol 7: 118–130.
21. Nadig SN, Wieckiewicz J, Wu DC, Warnecke G, Zhang W, et al. (2010) In vivo prevention of transplant arteriosclerosis by ex vivo-expanded human regulatory T cells. Nat Med 16: 809–813.
22. Issa F, Hester J, Goto R, Nadig SN, Goodacre TE, et al. (2010) Ex vivo-expanded human regulatory T cells prevent the rejection of skin allografts in a humanized mouse model. Transplantation 90: 1321–1327.
23. Sagoo P, Ali N, Garg G, Nestle FO, Lechler RI, et al. (2011) Human regulatory T cells with alloantigen specificity are more potent inhibitors of alloimmune skin graft damage than polyclonal regulatory T cells. Sci Transl Med 3: 83ra42.
24. Wu DC, Hester J, Nadig SN, Zhang W, Trzonkowski P, et al. (2013) Ex Vivo Expanded Human Regulatory T Cells Can Prolong Survival of a Human Islet Allograft in a Humanized Mouse Model. Transplantation.
25. Zhao M, Christie MR, Heaton N, George S, Amiel S, et al. (2002) Amelioration of streptozotocin-induced diabetes in mice using human islet cells derived from long-term culture in vitro. Transplantation 73: 1454–1460.
26. Watanabe Y, Takahashi T, Okajima A, Shiokawa M, Ishii N, et al. (2009) The analysis of the functions of human B and T cells in humanized NOD/shi-scid/gammac(null) (NOG) mice (hu-HSC NOG mice). Int Immunol 21: 843–858.
27. Huang SJ, Schatz F, Masch R, Rahman M, Buchwalder L, et al. (2006) Regulation of chemokine production in response to pro-inflammatory cytokines in first trimester decidual cells. J Reprod Immunol 72: 60–73.
28. Hu Z, Yang YG (2012) Human lymphohematopoietic reconstitution and immune function in immunodeficient mice receiving cotransplantation of human thymic tissue and CD34(+) cells. Cell Mol Immunol 9: 232–236.
29. Garcia S, Freitas AA (2012) Humanized mice: current states and perspectives. Immunol Lett 146: 1–7.
30. Ishikawa F, Yasukawa M, Lyons B, Yoshida S, Miyamoto T, et al. (2005) Development of functional human blood and immune systems in NOD/SCID/IL2 receptor {gamma} chain(null) mice. Blood 106: 1565–1573.
31. Traggiai E, Chicha L, Mazzucchelli L, Bronz L, Piffaretti JC, et al. (2004) Development of a human adaptive immune system in cord blood cell-transplanted mice. Science 304: 104–107.
32. King M, Pearson T, Shultz LD, Leif J, Bottino R, et al. (2008) A new Hu-PBL model for the study of human islet alloreactivity based on NOD-scid mice bearing a targeted mutation in the IL-2 receptor gamma chain gene. Clin Immunol 126: 303–314.
33. Piemonti L, Leone BE, Nano R, Saccani A, Monti P, et al. (2002) Human pancreatic islets produce and secrete MCP-1/CCL2: relevance in human islet transplantation. Diabetes 51: 55–65.
34. Ehrnfelt C, Kumagai-Braesch M, Uzunel M, Holgersson J (2004) Adult porcine islets produce MCP-1 and recruit human monocytes in vitro. Xenotransplantation 11: 184–194.
35. Brehm MA, Cuthbert A, Yang C, Miller DM, DiIorio P, et al. (2010) Parameters for establishing humanized mouse models to study human immunity: analysis of human hematopoietic stem cell engraftment in three immunodeficient strains of mice bearing the IL2rgamma(null) mutation. Clin Immunol 135: 84–98.
36. Matsumura T, Kametani Y, Ando K, Hirano Y, Katano I, et al. (2003) Functional CD5+ B cells develop predominantly in the spleen of NOD/SCID/gammac(null) (NOG) mice transplanted either with human umbilical cord blood, bone marrow, or mobilized peripheral blood CD34+ cells. Exp Hematol 31: 789–797.
37. Baenziger S, Tussiwand R, Schlaepfer E, Mazzucchelli L, Heikenwalder M, et al. (2006) Disseminated and sustained HIV infection in CD34+ cord blood cell-transplanted Rag2-/-gamma c-/- mice. Proc Natl Acad Sci U S A 103: 15951–15956.
38. Shultz LD, Saito Y, Najima Y, Tanaka S, Ochi T, et al. (2010) Generation of functional human T-cell subsets with HLA-restricted immune responses in HLA class I expressing NOD/SCID/IL2r gamma(null) humanized mice. Proc Natl Acad Sci U S A 107: 13022–13027.
39. Danner R, Chaudhari SN, Rosenberger J, Surls J, Richie TL, et al. (2011) Expression of HLA class II molecules in humanized NOD.Rag1KO.IL2RgcKO mice is critical for development and function of human T and B cells. PLoS One 6: e19826.
40. Jaiswal S, Pazoles P, Woda M, Shultz LD, Greiner DL, et al. (2012) Enhanced humoral and HLA-A2-restricted dengue virus-specific T-cell responses in humanized BLT NSG mice. Immunology 136: 334–343.
41. Li K, Sacks SH, Zhou W (2007) The relative importance of local and systemic complement production in ischaemia, transplantation and other pathologies. Mol Immunol 44: 3866–3874.
42. Kolev M, Le Friec G, Kemper C (2013) The role of complement in CD4(+) T cell homeostasis and effector functions. Semin Immunol 25: 12–19.
43. McCune JM, Namikawa R, Kaneshima H, Shultz LD, Lieberman M, et al. (1988) The SCID-hu mouse: murine model for the analysis of human hematolymphoid differentiation and function. Science 241: 1632–1639.
44. Jacobson S, Heuts F, Juarez J, Hultcrantz M, Korsgren O, et al. (2010) Alloreactivity but failure to reject human islet transplants by humanized Balb/c/Rag2gc mice. Scand J Immunol 71: 83–90.
45. Sun Z, Denton PW, Estes JD, Othieno FA, Wei BL, et al. (2007) Intrarectal transmission, systemic infection, and CD4+ T cell depletion in humanized mice infected with HIV-1. J Exp Med 204: 705–714.
46. Hofer U, Baenziger S, Heikenwalder M, Schlaepfer E, Gehre N, et al. (2008) RAG2-/- gamma(c)-/- mice transplanted with CD34+ cells from human cord blood show low levels of intestinal engraftment and are resistant to rectal transmission of human immunodeficiency virus. J Virol 82: 12145–12153.
47. Miyara M, Yoshioka Y, Kitoh A, Shima T, Wing K, et al. (2009) Functional delineation and differentiation dynamics of human CD4+ T cells expressing the FoxP3 transcription factor. Immunity 30: 899–911.
48. Putnam AL, Brusko TM, Lee MR, Liu W, Szot GL, et al. (2009) Expansion of human regulatory T-cells from patients with type 1 diabetes. Diabetes 58: 652–662.
49. Battaglia M, Stabilini A, Migliavacca B, Horejs-Hoeck J, Kaupper T, et al. (2006) Rapamycin promotes expansion of functional CD4+CD25+FOXP3+ regulatory T cells of both healthy subjects and type 1 diabetic patients. J Immunol 177: 8338–8347.
50. Chen D, Zhang N, Fu S, Schroppel B, Guo Q, et al. (2006) CD4+ CD25+ regulatory T-cells inhibit the islet innate immune response and promote islet engraftment. Diabetes 55: 1011–1021.
51. Harrison OJ, Powrie FM (2013) Regulatory T cells and immune tolerance in the intestine. Cold Spring Harb Perspect Biol 5.
52. Yi S, Ji M, Wu J, Ma X, Phillips P, et al. (2012) Adoptive transfer with in vitro expanded human regulatory T cells protects against porcine islet xenograft rejection via interleukin-10 in humanized mice. Diabetes 61: 1180–1191.
53. Tanriver Y, Martin-Fontecha A, Ratnasothy K, Lombardi G, Lechler R (2009) Superantigen-activated regulatory T cells inhibit the migration of innate immune cells and the differentiation of naive T cells. J Immunol 183: 2946–2956.
54. Maloy KJ, Salaun L, Cahill R, Dougan G, Saunders NJ, et al. (2003) CD4+CD25+ T(R) cells suppress innate immune pathology through cytokine-dependent mechanisms. J Exp Med 197: 111–119.
55. Zhang N, Schroppel B, Lal G, Jakubzick C, Mao X, et al. (2009) Regulatory T cells sequentially migrate from inflamed tissues to draining lymph nodes to suppress the alloimmune response. Immunity 30: 458–469.
56. Schmidt A, Oberle N, Krammer PH (2012) Molecular mechanisms of treg-mediated T cell suppression. Front Immunol 3: 51.
57. Sawitzki B, Kingsley CI, Oliveira V, Karim M, Herber M, et al. (2005) IFN-gamma production by alloantigen-reactive regulatory T cells is important for their regulatory function in vivo. J Exp Med 201: 1925–1935.
58. Hall AO, Beiting DP, Tato C, John B, Oldenhove G, et al. (2012) The cytokines interleukin 27 and interferon-gamma promote distinct Treg cell populations required to limit infection-induced pathology. Immunity 37: 511–523.
59. Koch MA, Thomas KR, Perdue NR, Smigiel KS, Srivastava S, et al. (2012) T-bet(+) Treg cells undergo abortive Th1 cell differentiation due to impaired expression of IL-12 receptor beta2. Immunity 37: 501–510.
60. Wood KJ, Sawitzki B (2006) Interferon gamma: a crucial role in the function of induced regulatory T cells in vivo. Trends Immunol 27: 183–187.
61. Lee YW, Hennig B, Toborek M (2003) Redox-regulated mechanisms of IL-4-induced MCP-1 expression in human vascular endothelial cells. Am J Physiol Heart Circ Physiol 284: H185–192.
62. Chen P, Zhang Z, Chen Q, Ren F, Li T, et al. (2012) Expression of Th1 and Th2 cytokine-associated transcription factors, T-bet and GATA-3, in the eutopic endometrium of women with endometriosis. Acta Histochem.

15

Improved Clinical Outcomes of High Risk β Thalassemia Major Patients Undergoing a HLA Matched Related Allogeneic Stem Cell Transplant with a Treosulfan Based Conditioning Regimen and Peripheral Blood Stem Cell Grafts

Vikram Mathews*, Biju George, Auro Viswabandya, Aby Abraham, Rayaz Ahmed, Abhijeet Ganapule, Eunice Sindhuvi, Kavitha M. Lakshmi, Alok Srivastava

Department of Haematology, Christian Medical College, Vellore, India

Abstract

Improving clinical outcomes among high risk Class III β thalassemia major patients (Class IIIHR) receiving an allogeneic SCT remains a challenge. From October, 2009 a treosulfan based regimen (TreoFluT) was used for all consecutive Class III patients (n = 50). The clinical outcomes were compared with the historical conventional busulfan (BuCy) based regimen (n = 139). Use of TreoFluT was associated with a significantly reduced incidence of sinusoidal obstruction syndrome (SOS) among Class IIIHR cases (78% to 30%; P = 0.000) and early TRM (46% to 13%; p = 0.005). There was also a trend towards better engraftment in the Class IIIHR subset (P = 0.055). However, the use of bone marrow (BM) as source of stem cells along with the TreoFluT regimen was associated with 50% early mixed chimerism which reduced to 8.5% with the use of a peripheral blood stem cell graft (PBSC). Use of a PBSC graft was not associated with a significant increase in the incidence of acute or chronic graft versus host disease (GVHD). The overall and event free survival was significantly better among the Class IIIHR subset with the use of TreoFluT Vs. BuCy (86.6±7.3 Vs. 39.4±6.8%; P = 0.002 and 77.8±8.8 Vs. 32.4±6.5%; P = 0.003 respectively). A TreoFluT conditioning regimen with a PBSC graft can significantly improve clinical outcomes of Class IIIHR patients.

Editor: Wilbur Lam, Emory University/Georgia Insititute of Technology, United States of America

Funding: The authors have no support or funding to report.

Competing Interests: The authors have declared that no competing interests exist.

* E-mail: vikram@cmcvellore.ac.in

Introduction

Allogeneic stem cell transplantation (SCT) remains the only curative option for patients with β thalassemia major. The correction of this disorder by an allogeneic stem cell transplant was first described by Thomas et al [1]. Subsequently, a myeloablative conditioning regimen of busulfan and cyclophosphamide was established and has been the standard of care for stem cell transplantation in this condition [2]. The current risk stratification [3,4] of patients with β thalassemia major undergoing a myeloablative allogeneic stem cell transplantation (SCT) has significant limitations and fails to recognize a very high risk group. Prior to stem cell transplant patients who were ≥7 years old and had a liver size ≥5 cms constitute what we previously defined as a very high risk subset of a conventional high risk Class III group (Class III high risk or Class IIIHR) [5]. The adverse impact of age and liver size was further validated by an international collaborative analysis which was recently reported [6]. Class III and more specifically Class III high risk (HR) subset have a high risk of graft rejection and regimen related toxicity especially sinusoidal obstruction syndrome (SOS) leading to multi-organ failure and death. The poor clinical outcome in this subset of older patients with very poor pre-transplant medical therapy, as reported by us, is not reflected in the Western literature due to the use of adequate blood transfusion and chelation support prior to transplant. However, when such a population is transplanted even in a developed country with expertise in such transplants the rejection rate is as high as 34% [7].

This has lead to the evaluation of a number of novel conditioning regimens in this group [3,4,8,9,10,11]. Treosulfan (dihydroxybusulfan), in the recent past, has attracted a lot of attention as an agent to replace busulfan in view of its favorable toxicity profile [12]. It is especially attractive in the context of an allogeneic SCT for high risk β thalassemia major because of its reported low hepatic toxicity profile and consistent pharmacokinetic profile which are both significant problems with conventional busulfan in this population [5,13,14]. Bone marrow has been the preferred choice of stem cells to reduce the risk of graft versus host disease (GVHD) in this non malignant condition, though the incidence of both acute and chronic GVHD in this predominantly pediatric population is low [14,15]. Recently a similar low incidence of acute and chronic GVHD with a PBSC graft in the setting of matched unrelated transplants has been reported from China [16].

We report our experience of allogeneic SCT in Class III and the Class IIIHR subset and the impact of the use of a previously reported reduced toxicity Treosulfan based regimen [11,17] modified by the use of peripheral blood stem cell (PBSC) graft.

Materials and Methods

This is a retrospective analysis of anonymous patient data. All data was taken from patient records at the Christian Medical College and Hospital, and this study was approved by the ethical review board of Christian Medical College.

All consecutive transfusion dependant β thalassemia patients with a HLA identical related donor or a ≥9 of 10 high resolution HLA matched unrelated donor who underwent an allogeneic SCT at our centre from October, 1991 to February, 2012 were included in this analysis.All patents and donors underwent the procedure after getting written and informed consent. The consent forms and consent procedure was approved by the institutions review board. Hard and soft copies of the consent form and all the data generated from the transplant procedure on patients and donors is filed permanently in our department.

Pre-transplant evaluation

All patients were evaluated with a complete blood count (CBC), biochemical profile and serology for HIV, HBV, HCV and CMV. Pre-transplant a liver biopsy was performed at the time of Hickman catheter insertion.

Conditioning

Conditioning regimensin the majority was a myeloablative regimen consisting of a combination of busulfan and cyclophosphamide (BuCy) as previously reported by us [14]. From October, 2009 till to date, in an effort to reduce the treatment related morality (TRM) and graft rejection in our high risk cases, the conditioning regimen was modified. This involved the use of a Treosulfan based conditioning regimen as previously reported [11,17]and consisted of administering thiotepa 8 mg/kg on day -6, fludarabaine 30 mg/m^2/day×4 days from day-5 to -2 and treosulfan 14 gm/m^2×3 days from day-5 to -3 (TreoFluT).

Bone Marrow Harvest

Until the introduction of a TreoFluT conditioning regimen in October 2009 the stem cell source was bone marrow (BM) alone for the majority of patients (98.7%). Bone marrow was harvested under general anesthesia from the iliac crest and the target cell dose was 6×10^8 nucleated cells/Kg body weight of the recipient. The harvest was collected in ACD with preservative free heparin using one-liter harvest bags. For major ABO mismatched transplants, red cell depletion was achieved with 6% hydroxyethyl starch and gravity sedimentation. After the introduction of the treosulfan conditioning regimen in October, 2009 the stem cell source initially continued to be BM until October, 2010. Due to increased concerns of early mixed chimerism and graft rejection the stem cell source was changed PBSC for all Class III patients who were conditioned with a TreoFluT based regimenfrom November, 2010. The stem cell products were administered soon after harvest or processing.

GVHD prophylaxis

Cyclosporine and short course methotrexate was used as GVHD prophylaxis; cyclosporine was administered at a dose of 2.5 mg/Kg intravenously over four hours twice daily starting on day –4 and changed to oral administration at 5 mg/Kg twice daily when mucositis had resolved. Cyclosporine levels were monitored and the dose adjusted to achieve a target level of 100–300 ng/ml. The methotrexate dose was 10 mg/m^2 on day +1 and 7 mg/m^2 on day 3, 6 and 11. Acute GVHD was treated with dexamethasone or methyl prednisone. Steroid refractory GVHD was treated as per the discretion of the treating physician.

Chimerism Analysis

Analysis of chimerism and quantification of recipient and donor in samples was done by polymerase chain reactionamplification of informative STR or VNTR followed by gene scan analysis as has been previously reported by us [18].

Supportive care

All patients were nursed in a positive pressure HEPA filtered transplant unit. None of the patients received prophylactic antibiotics or underwent gut decontamination. Prophylactic acyclovir was administered for the first 100 days; it was continued beyond day 100 if patient had GVHD and required additional immuno-suppression. Trimethoprim-sulphamethoxazole and oral penicillin prophylaxis was initiated after stable engraftment and continued for a year. At the end of one year all patients who did not have evidence of GVHD and were off all immunosuppressive drugs were vaccinated against polio, diphtheria, tetanus, hemophilus influenza and pneumococcus.

Definitions

Incidence and severity of GVHD was defined as per established criteria [19]. Hepatic sinusoidal obstruction syndrome (SOS) was diagnosed according to Baltimore criteria [20]. Mixed chimerism for the purpose of this study was defined as ≤95% donor cell percentage. Event free survival (EFS) was defined from the time of transplant to an event; an event was primary graft rejection, death or recurrence of transfusion dependence. Stable mixed chimerism with transfusion independence was not considered an event for this analysis. Overall survival (OS) was defined as time from transplant to death due to any cause.

Statistical analysis

The $\chi 2$, t test or fisher exact test and Mann Whitney U test were used to compare differences between groups. Probabilities of event free survival (EFS) and overall survival (OS) following transplant were estimated by the Kaplan-Meier method and the significance assessed by log-rank test. The relationships of clinical features to outcome were analyzed by Cox proportional hazard model.Significance levels were set at 0.05. Statistical analysis was done using SPSS version 11.0.

Results

Demographic and Clinical Characteristics

A total of 362 patients with transfusion dependent β thalassemia underwent an allogeneic SCT between January, 1991 and February, 2012 at our centre. 358 (98.8%) of these transplants were from related donors and of the related donors 348 (97.2%) were HLA identical. The median age of this cohort was 7±4.4 years and there were 227 males (62.7%). There were 16(4.4%), 144 (39.8%) and 202 (55.8%) transplants in Lucarelli Class I, II and III respectively.

Of the 202 Class III patients, 82 (40.5%) were classified as Class IIIHR (Age≥7 years and liver size≥5 cms). The conditioning regimen used for the Class III patients was BuCy in 139 (68.8%) and TreoFluT in 50 (24.7%). Similarly, the 82 cases identified as Class IIIHR were conditioned with BuCy in 54 (65.8%) and TreoFluT in 24 (29.2%). The baseline characteristics and clinical outcomes of Class III and Class IIIHR patients conditioned with BuCy and TreoFluTregimens are summarized in Tables 1 and 2 respectively.With the exception of the significantly higher use of PBSC grafts among those conditioned with the TreoFluT regimen there were no other significant differences in baseline characteristics among patients conditioned with these regimens among the entire Class III (Table 1) and the Class IIIHR subset (Table 2).

Engraftment and day28 chimerism analysis

The proportion of patients who engrafted post-transplant was higher with the TreoFluT based conditioning regimen (Table 1) and this tended to statistical significance in the Class IIIHR subset (Table 2: 78% Vs. 96% in favor of the TreoFluT group; P-value0.055). The time to achieve a platelet count $>20\times10^9$/Lt was significantly shorter with the TreoFluT conditioning regimen for the entire Class III and the Class IIIHR subset (Table 1 and 2). This was predominantly contributed by the use of a PBSC graft in patients conditioned with TreoFluT as illustrated in Table 3. This faster engraftment translated into significantly lower number of platelet and packed red cell units (PRC) transfused in the peri-transplant period (Table 1). Among patients conditioned with a TreoFluT regimen the use of PBSC grafts was also associated with significant reduction in peri-transplant platelet and PRC units

Table 1. Baseline characteristics, supportive care and clinical outcomes of Class III patients receiving different conditioning regimens.

Variable	Bu/Cy[a] (n = 139) n(%)/Median (range)/Mean ± SD	TreoFluT[b] (n = 50) n(%)/Median (range)/Mean ± SD	P-value
Age	9 (2–24)	11 (2–21)	0.108
Sex: Male	87 (63)	30 (60)	0.738
Female donor to Male recipient (F>M)	50 (36)	14 (28)	0.384
HBsAg positive	5 (4)	1 (2)	1.000
HCV positive	28 (20)	7 (14)	0.401
CMV IgG positive	130 (96)	47 (94)	0.448
Liver Size (cms)	4.6±1.7	4.6±1.8	0.907
Splenectomy	30 (22)	8 (16)	0.537
ALT[*] (IU/Lt)	80 (10–357)	54 (8–230)	0.031
AST (IU/Lt)	56 (15–199)	45 (14–186)	0.143
Serum Ferritin (ng/ml)	4096 (681–13600)	4380 (1449–10950)	0.397
Number of packed cells transfused pre-transplant	120 (20–450)	119.5 (22–280)	0.653
Stem cell source:			
BM[@]	128 (92)	13 (26)	
G-CSF primed BM	9 (7)	-	0.000
PBSC[#]	2 (1)	37 (74)	
CD34 ($\times10^6$/kg)	6.7 (2.64–15.9)	11.4 (2–30)	0.000
Engraftment	122 (88)	47 (94)	0.289
Engraftment (days):			
Time to ANC$>0.5\times10^9$/Lt	16.9±4.1	16.1±3.2	0.242
Time to platelet$>20\times10^9$/Lt	32.7±17.6	18.8±8.0	0.000
Peri-transplant support:			
(up to day 100)			
Platelet units transfused	23 (5–92)	13 (1–76)	0.000
PRC[θ] units transfused	19 (0–357)	13 (1–91)	0.003
Sinusoidal obstruction syndrome	92 (66)	11 (22)	0.00
Graft Rejection	16 (12)	4 (8)	0.599
Graft versus host disease:			
Acute GVHD[©]	55 (44)	17 (35)	0.305
Chronic GVHD[©]	17 (18)	4 (11)	0.430
Treatment related mortality(<day 100)	39 (28)	6 (12)	0.021
Overall Survival 3 yrs[∞]	63.6±4.2	87.4±4.8	0.011
Event free survival 3 yrs[∞]	57.3±4.3	78.8±6.0	0.041

[a]BuCy: Busulfan + Cyclophosphamide; *ALT: Alanine aminotransferase.
[b]TreoFluT: Treosulfan, fludarabine and thiotepa; ˆAST: Aspartate aminotransferase.
[@]BM: Bone marrow; #PBSC: Peripheral blood stem cells.
[θ]PRC: Packed red cell units; ©GVHD: graft versus host disease.
[∞]3 yrs. 3 years Kaplan-Meier estimate±1SE%.

Table 2. Baseline characteristics, supportive care and clinical outcomes of Class IIIHR (High Risk) group receiving different conditioning regimens.

Variable	Bu/Cy[a](n = 54) n(%)/Median (range)/Mean ± SD	TreoFluT[b] (n = 24) n(%)/Median (range)/Mean ± SD	P-value
Age	12 (7–24)	12 (3–21)	0.565
Sex: Male	31 (57)	16 (67)	0.466
Female donor to Male recipient (F>M)	19 (35)	5 (21)	0.289
HBsAg positive	3 (6)	-	0.549
HCV positive	11 (20)	5 (21)	1.000
CMV IgG positive	52 (96)	22 (92)	0.097
Liver Size (cms)	6.2±1.4	6.1±1.2	0.770
Splenectomy	22 (41)	7 (29)	0.448
ALT*(IU/Lt)	106 (20–309)	49 (8–230)	0.008
AST^ (IU/Lt)	65 (18–199)	43.5 (14–186)	0.048
Serum Ferritin (ng/ml)	4537 (1528–11885)	4591 (1838–10710)	0.799
Number of packed cells transfused pre-transplant	152 (72–450)	150 (26–280)	0.422
Stem cell source:			
BM[@]	52 (96)	7 (29)	
G-CSF primed BM	2 (4)	-	0.000
PBSC[#]	-	17 (71)	
CD34 ($\times 10^6$/kg)	5.8 (2.9–14.8)	9.95 (2–30)	0.001
Engraftment	42 (78)	23 (96)	0.055
Engraftment (days):			
Time to ANC>0.5×10^9/Lt	17.0±5.1	15.8±3.4	0.503
Time to platelet>20×10^9/Lt	35.4±12.9	20±10.2	0.000
Peri-transplant support:			
(upto day 100)			
Platelet units transfused	21 (5–92)	16.5 (1–76)	0.063
PRC[θ] cell units transfused	18 (5–357)	13.5 (1–88)	0.020
Sinusoidal obstruction syndrome	42 (78)	7 (30)	0.000
Graft Rejection	7 (13)	2 (8)	0.713
Graft versus host disease:			
Acute GVHD[©]	23 (55)	8 (35)	0.194
Chronic GVHD[©]	6 (21)	2 (11)	0.445
Treatment related mortality(<day 100)	25 (46)	3 (13)	0.005
Overall Survival 3 yrs[∞]	39.4±6.8	86.6±7.3	0.002
Event free survival 3 yrs[∞]	32.4±6.5	77.8±8.8	0.003

[a]BuCy: Busulfan + Cyclophosphamide; *ALT: Alanine aminotransferase.
[b]TreoFluT: Treosulfan, fludarabine and thiotepa; ^AST: Aspartate aminotransferase.
[@]BM: Bone marrow; #PBSC:Peripheral blood stem cells.
[θ]PRC: Packed red cell units; [©]GVHD: graft versus host disease.
[∞]3 yrs. 3 years Kaplan-Meier estimate±1SE%.

transfusedin comparison to those that received a BM graft (Table 3).

The early experience with the TreoFluT regimen using a BM graft (n = 13) resulted in 6 (50%) of evaluated patients (one died prior to day 28) having mixed chimerism. For recipients with mixed chimerism intervention with rapid withdrawal of cyclosporine and donor lymphocyte infusion was considered when serial chimerism values showed a downward trend with no evidence of graft versus host disease (GVHD) or if the recipient became transfusion dependent in the absence of evidence of post-transplant pure red cell aplasia. Of the 6 cases with mixed chimerism 2 went on to complete rejection (day 74 and day 76) while 4 were salvaged with these interventions (2 received DLI). Following this experience the graft source was changed to PBSC for Class III patients conditioned with TreoFluT. With the use of PBSC (n = 37), mixed chimerism was seen in 3 (8.5%) of the 35 patients evaluated (2 died prior to day 28). Of these three, one patient was a 20 year old man who underwent a 9/10 MUD transplant. This patient had a documented parvovirus B19 infection on day 15 and went on to have a primary graft failure with autologous recovery. The remaining two cases were salvaged with rapid tapering of immunosuppression and infusion of DLI. Figure 1A summarizes the day 28 chimerism data among patients receiving a TreoFluT conditioning regimen. The number of cases

Table 3. Comparison of Class III patients who received TreoFluTconditioning with either a bone marrow or peripheral blood source of stem cells.

Variable	BM@ (n = 13) n(%)/Median range)/Mean ± SD	PBSC# (n = 37) n(%)/Median (range)/Mean ± SD	P-value
Age	9 (6–14)	11 (2–21)	0.001
Sex: Male	10 (77)	20 (54)	0.197
Female donor to Male recipient (F>M)	4 (31)	10 (27)	1.000
CD34 ($\times 10^6$/kg)	8.8 (2.1–24.4)	12.5 (2–30)	0.000
Engraftment	12 (92)	35 (95)	1.000
Engraftment (days):			
Time to ANC>0.5×10^9/Lt	16.4±2.6	16.0±3.4	0.051
Time to platelet>20×10^9/Lt	26.2±8.8	16.5±6.3	0.000
Chimerism:			
Evaluated on Day 28:	12 (92.3)	35 (94.5)	0.720
Percentage donor cells	97.5 (52–100)	100 (0–100)	0.004
Mixed chimerism	6 (50%)	3 (8.5%)	0.005
Graft Rejection	2 (15)	2 (5)	0.275
Peri-transplant support:			
(upto day 100)			
Platelet units transfused	20 (10–31)	13 (1–76)	0.000
PRC$^\theta$ units transfused	17 (8–65)	12 (1–91)	0.001
Sinusoidal obstruction syndrome	5 (39)	6 (17)	0.133
Graft versus host disease			0.498
Acute GVHD©	3 (23)	14 (39)	1.000
Chronic GVHD©	1 (9)	3 (12)	
Treatment related mortality(<day 100)	2 (15)	4 (11)	0.643
Overall Survival 3 yrs$^\infty$	72.2±2.7	87.3±5.4	0.717
Event free survival 3 yrs$^\infty$	65.9±2.8	73.9±11.2	0.309

@BM: Bone marrow; #PBSC: Peripheral blood stem cells.
$^\theta$PRC: Packed red cell units; ©GVHD: graft versus host disease.
$^\infty$3 yrs. 3 years Kaplan-Meier estimate±1SE%3.

with mixed chimerism was higher and the median day 28 chimerism was significantly lower in patients receiving a BM graft (Figure 1A).

Sinusoidal obstruction syndrome

There was significant reduction in incidence of SOS in Class III patients (Table 1: P-value = 0.000) and Class IIIHR patients (Table 2: P-value = 0.000)conditioned with a TreoFluTregimen. Among Class IIIHR cases, those conditioned with BuCy had a 78% incidence of SOS while those conditioned with the TreoFluT regimen it was 30%. Of the 7(30%) Class IIIHR cases conditioned with TreoFluT that had a documented SOS, it was mild self-limiting and managed conservatively in 6 and in only one case did it result in multi-organ failure leading to death. In contrast among Class IIIHR cases conditioned with a BuCy regimen in 10 (24%) of the 42 cases documented to have SOS this was the major contributory cause of death. The low incidence of SOS and other regimen related toxicity translated to a significantly lower day 100 treatment related mortality (TRM) among Class IIIHR patient conditioned with TreoFluT (Table 2: 13% Vs. 46%; P-value-0.005).

Graft versus host disease

There was no significant difference in the incidence of acute or chronic GVHD among Class III or Class IIIHR cases conditioned with either regimens (Table 1 and 2 respectively). Among Class III patient's conditioned with a TreoFluT regimen who received either a BM or a PBSC graft Grade 2–4 acute GVHD was seen in 3 (23%) Vs. 10 (27%)respectively while Grade 3–4 acute GVHD was seen in none Vs. 3 (8.1%) respectively (Table 3). Of the 3 patients who developed Grade 3–4 acute GVHD among those who received a PBSC graft, one patient responded to therapy and has complete resolution of GVHD while the other two succumbed to it.Among the 3 (12%) that developed chronic GVHD after a TreoFluT conditioning regimen and PBSC graft(Table 3) it was extensive in one while it was limited in the other two.

Survival

After excluding patients who had early TRM (<100 days) the actuarial median follow up of this cohort was 42 months (range: 3–254). The 3 year Kaplan-Meier estimate of OS and EFS of the entire Class III cohort was 67.4±3.5% and 58.9±3.7% respectively. Among the Class III patients use of a TreoFluT regimen was associated with a significant improvement in OS and EFS (as illustrated in Figure 1C and 1D) respectively. Similarly, the OS and EFS were significantly superior in the Class IIIHR subset that was conditioned with a TreoFluT regimen (illustrated in Figure 1E and 1F respectively).

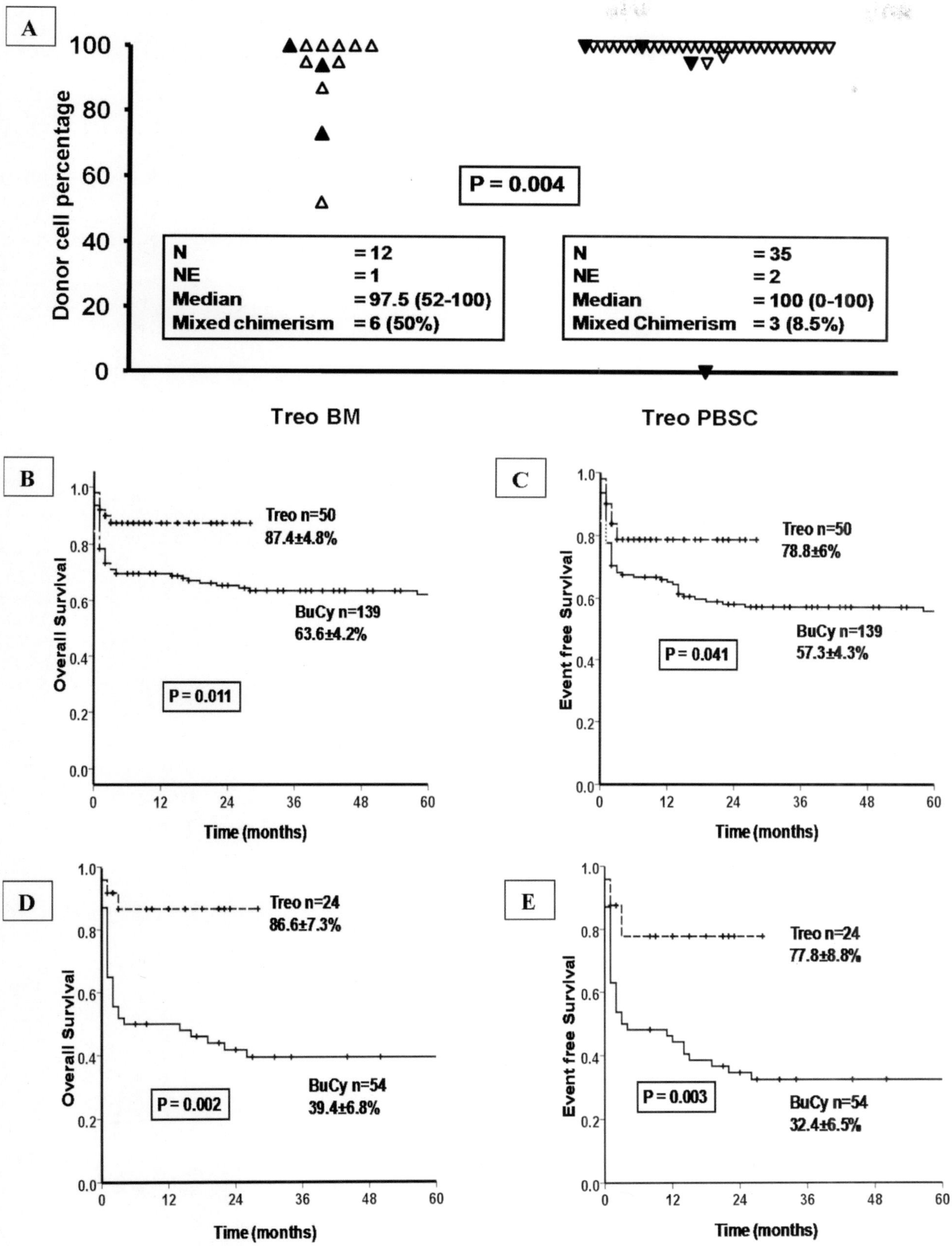

Figure 1. Analysis of day 28 chimerism and survival in different subsets. (A) Day 28 chimerism comparing patients conditioned with aTreoFluT regimen and receivingeither a bone marrow graft (Treo BM) or a peripheral blood stem cell graft (Treo PBSC); NE = not evaluated; indicates cases that had died prior to day 28 and were hence: not evaluated. ▲ Filled triangles indicates cases that had an event defined as either graft rejection or death. △ Empty triangles indicate cases that did not have an event defined as either graft rejection or death (B) Overall survival of all Class

III patients conditioned with either a TreoFluT (Treo) or a busulfan based regimen (Bu/Cy) (C) Event free survival of all Class III patients conditioned with either a TreoFluT (Treo) or a busulfan based regimen (Bu/Cy) (D) Overall survival of all Class IIIHR patients conditioned with either a TreoFluT (Treo) or a busulfan based regimen (Bu/Cy) (E) Event free survival of all Class IIIHR patients conditioned with either a TreoFluT (Treo) or a busulfan based regimen (Bu/Cy).

Cause of deaths

Among the Class III patients 39 (28%) of the cases conditioned with a Bu/Cy regimen died while 6 (12%) of those conditioned with a TreoFluT regimen died. Table 4 summarizes the major contributory cause of death among these two groups. As illustrated in table 4, SOS was a major contributing factor for death when Bu/Cy was the conditioning regimenand was significantly lower when a TreoFluT regimen was used. Deaths beyond day 100 was seen in 12 (8.6%) of cases conditioned with Bu/Cy and the major contributory cause was infections. Among those conditioned with TreoFluT there were 2 (4%) deaths beyond day 100, both were related to graft rejection and both had received a BM graft.

Discussion

Improving clinical outcomes of Class III and the Class IIIHR [5] β thalassemia major following an allogeneic SCT remains a challenge. We had previously reported the poor clinical outcome of our newly recognized Class IIIHR subset following allogeneic SCT using a conventional myeloablative Bu/Cy regimen [5].

The major contributory factors for the poor clinical outcome in these patients were a combination of high risk for graft rejection and regimen related toxicity (RRT) [5]. Early attempts to reduce RRT in a similar cohort of cases were done by reducing the cumulative dose of busulfan and cyclophosphamide. Experience from such an approach, as reported by the Pesaro group, suggested that a reduction in TRM was achieved but there was a significantly higher risk of graft rejection [10]. While other regimens have been reported to improve the clinical outcome of Class III thalassemia patients undergoing an allogeneic SCT [9] we would argue that most published data does not address the very high risk subset as defined by us [5]. The clinical outcome of a similar cohort reported from a developed country center would suggest that one could anticipate a graft rejection close to 34% [7] with intravenous busulfan in spite of pharmacokinetic monitoring and appropriate dose modifications.

Table 4. Comparison of major contributory cause of early death (death <100 days post transplant) among Class III patients.

Variable	Bu/Cy[a] n = 139	Treo[b] n = 50	P-value
Died < day 100	39 (28%)	6 (12%)	0.001
Rejection	5 (3.6%)	-	0.581
Sinusoidal obstruction syndrome	17 (12.1%)	1 (2%)	0.035
Infection	7 (5%)	2 (4%)	0.768
DAH[#]	2 (1.4%)	-	0.394
Cardiac failure	2 (1.4%)	1 (2%)	0.798
Hemorrhagic cystitis	1 (0.7%)	-	0.548
GVHD[©]	2 (1.4%)	2 (4%)	0.281
Intra-cerebral bleed	3 (2.1%)	-	0.295

[a]BuCy Busulfan + Cyclophosphamide.
[b]TreoFluT Treosulfan, fludarabine and thiotepa.
[#]DAH Diffuse alveolar hemorrhage.
[©]GVHD Graft versus host disease.

We were particularly attracted to the treosulfan based regimen due to the low hepatotoxicity profile of this agent [12] and the reported low incidence of SOS in patients with thallasemia major [11,17]. Hepatic SOS was a major problem with a conventional myeloablative regimen in our Class IIIHR patients with 78% of cases developing this complication and in 24% of such cases it lead to multi-organ failure and death.

Our initial experience with this TreoFluT regimen with a BM graft in this cohort at a very high risk for graft rejection was concerning, with 6 (50%) having early mixed chimerism. Our experience and reported data would suggest that early mixed chimerism, unlike late stable mixed chimerism, usually predicts secondary graft rejection in up to 50% of these cases [21]. Four of these initial 6 cases of mixed chimerism were salvaged with rapid taper of immune-suppression (2 of these required additional DLI to restore transfusion independence). The regimen itself was very well tolerated. We then opted to use a PBSC graft source with the same conditioning regimen. This approach resulted in greater consistency of early complete chimerism and was associated with additional benefits such as faster engraftment and significantly reduced peri-transplant transfusion support. Use of a PBSC graft did not result in a significantly higher incidence of acute or chronic GVHD compared to a BM graft with the same regimen. Chronic GVHD remains a concern with the use of a PBSC graft and this is one of the reasons why we have restricted the use of this regimen along with a PBSC graft to Class III patients.

Unfortunately, in resource constrained environments, such as ours and many other developing countries, it is not uncommon for a majority of patients with β thalassemia major to present late for transplantation. The body mass index (BMI) of our Class III patients is reflective of the poor clinical condition of a majority of these patients with the median BMI being 14.9 (range: 10.2–23.8) (figure S1). Only 22 (10.9%) of our Class III patients had a BMI in the normal range.

This retrospective data analysis is limited by the comparison of the use of TreoFluT regimen with a historical control spanning more than two decades. However, as illustrated in figure S2 the clinical outcome analyzed by 5 year intervals since the start of our transplant program reflects that there has been marginal, statistically not significant, improvement in the event free survival of our Class III or Class IIIHR cases over this time period. This illustrates that improvements in techniques and supportive care cannot explain the improved outcome seen with this treosulfan based regimen in our center.

In summary, this data suggests that even in a very high risk group of β thalassemia major patients undergoing an allogeneic SCT the benefits of this TreoFluT regimen along with a PBSC graft outweighs the risks and can significantly improve the overall and event free survival.

Author Contributions

Conceived and designed the experiments: VM. Performed the experiments: VM BG AV RA AG ES AS AA. Analyzed the data: VM KML BG AS. Contributed reagents/materials/analysis tools: ES. Wrote the paper: VM BG AS.

References

1. Thomas ED, Buckner CD, Sanders JE, Papayannopoulou T, Borgna-Pignatti C, et al. (1982) Marrow transplantation for thalassaemia. Lancet 2: 227–229.
2. Lucarelli G, Polchi P, Galimberti M, Izzi T, Delfini C, et al. (1985) Marrow transplantation for thalassaemia following busulphan and cyclophosphamide. Lancet 1: 1355–1357.
3. Lucarelli G, Galimberti M, Polchi P, Angelucci E, Baronciani D, et al. (1990) Bone marrow transplantation in patients with thalassemia. N Engl J Med 322: 417–421.
4. Lucarelli G, Galimberti M, Polchi P, Angelucci E, Baronciani D, et al. (1992) Bone marrow transplantation in adult thalassemia. Blood 80: 1603–1607.
5. Mathews V, George B, Deotare U, Lakshmi KM, Viswabandya A, et al. (2007) A new stratification strategy that identifies a subset of class III patients with an adverse prognosis among children with beta thalassemia major undergoing a matched related allogeneic stem cell transplantation. Biol Blood Marrow Transplant 13: 889–894.
6. Sabloff M, Chandy M, Wang Z, Logan BR, Ghavamzadeh A, et al. (2010) HLA-matched sibling bone marrow transplantation for beta-thalassemia major. Blood 117: 1745–1750.
7. Chiesa R, Cappelli B, Crocchiolo R, Frugnoli I, Biral E, et al. (2010) Unpredictability of intravenous busulfan pharmacokinetics in children undergoing hematopoietic stem cell transplantation for advanced beta thalassemia: limited toxicity with a dose-adjustment policy. Biol Blood Marrow Transplant 16: 622–628.
8. Lawson SE, Roberts IA, Amrolia P, Dokal I, Szydlo R, et al. (2003) Bone marrow transplantation for beta-thalassaemia major: the UK experience in two paediatric centres. Br J Haematol 120: 289–295.
9. Sodani P, Gaziev D, Polchi P, Erer B, Giardini C, et al. (2004) New approach for bone marrow transplantation in patients with class 3 thalassemia aged younger than 17 years. Blood 104: 1201–1203.
10. Lucarelli G, Clift RA, Galimberti M, Polchi P, Angelucci E, et al. (1996) Marrow transplantation for patients with thalassemia: results in class 3 patients. Blood 87: 2082–2088.
11. Bernardo ME, Zecca M, Piras E, Vacca A, Giorgiani G, et al. (2008) Treosulfan-based conditioning regimen for allogeneic haematopoietic stem cell transplantation in patients with thalassaemia major. Br J Haematol 143: 548–551.
12. Danylesko I, Shimoni A, Nagler A (2012) Treosulfan-based conditioning before hematopoietic SCT: more than a BU look-alike. Bone Marrow Transplant 47: 5–14.
13. Srivastava A, Poonkuzhali B, Shaji RV, George B, Mathews V, et al. (2004) Glutathione S-transferase M1 polymorphism: a risk factor for hepatic venoocclusive disease in bone marrow transplantation. Blood 104: 1574–1577.
14. Chandy M, Balasubramanian P, Ramachandran SV, Mathews V, George B, et al. (2005) Randomized trial of two different conditioning regimens for bone marrow transplantation in thalassemia–the role of busulfan pharmacokinetics in determining outcome. Bone Marrow Transplant 36: 839–845.
15. Rajasekar R, Mathews V, Lakshmi KM, George B, Viswabandya A, et al. (2009) Cellular immune reconstitution and its impact on clinical outcome in children with beta thalassemia major undergoing a matched related myeloablative allogeneic bone marrow transplant. Biol Blood Marrow Transplant 15: 597–609.
16. Li C, Wu X, Feng X, He Y, Liu H, et al. (2012) A novel conditioning regimen improves outcomes in beta-thalassemia major patients using unrelated donor peripheral blood stem cell transplantation. Blood 120: 3875–3881.
17. Bernardo ME, Piras E, Vacca A, Giorgiani G, Zecca M, et al. (2012) Allogeneic hematopoietic stem cell transplantation in thalassemia major: results of a reduced-toxicity conditioning regimen based on the use of treosulfan. Blood.
18. Sellathamby S, Balasubramanian P, Sivalingam S, Shaji RV, Mathews V, et al. (2006) Developing an algorithm of informative markers for evaluation of chimerism after allogeneic bone marrow transplantation. Bone Marrow Transplant 37: 751–755.
19. Glucksberg H, Storb R, Fefer A, Buckner CD, Neiman PE, et al. (1974) Clinical manifestations of graft-versus-host disease in human recipients of marrow from HL-A-matched sibling donors. Transplantation 18: 295–304.
20. Jones RJ, Lee KS, Beschorner WE, Vogel VG, Grochow LB, et al. (1987) Venoocclusive disease of the liver following bone marrow transplantation. Transplantation 44: 778–783.
21. Lucarelli G, Andreani M, Angelucci E (2002) The cure of thalassemia by bone marrow transplantation. Blood Rev 16: 81–85.

Macrophage/Epithelium Cross-Talk Regulates Cell Cycle Progression and Migration in Pancreatic Progenitors

Kristin Mussar[❾], **Andrew Tucker**[❾], **Linsey McLennan, Addie Gearhart, Antonio J. Jimenez-Caliani, Vincenzo Cirulli, Laura Crisa***

Department of Medicine, Institute of Stem Cell and Regenerative Medicine, University of Washington, Seattle, Washington, United States of America

Abstract

Macrophages populate the mesenchymal compartment of all organs during embryogenesis and have been shown to support tissue organogenesis and regeneration by regulating remodeling of the extracellular microenvironment. Whether this mesenchymal component can also dictate select developmental decisions in epithelia is unknown. Here, using the embryonic pancreatic epithelium as model system, we show that macrophages drive the epithelium to execute two developmentally important choices, i.e. the exit from cell cycle and the acquisition of a migratory phenotype. We demonstrate that these developmental decisions are effectively imparted by macrophages activated toward an M2 fetal-like functional state, and involve modulation of the adhesion receptor NCAM and an uncommon "paired-less" isoform of the transcription factor PAX6 in the epithelium. Over-expression of this PAX6 variant in pancreatic epithelia controls both cell motility and cell cycle progression in a gene-dosage dependent fashion. Importantly, induction of these phenotypes in embryonic pancreatic transplants by M2 macrophages *in vivo* is associated with an increased frequency of endocrine-committed cells emerging from ductal progenitor pools. These results identify M2 macrophages as key effectors capable of coordinating epithelial cell cycle withdrawal and cell migration, two events critical to pancreatic progenitors' delamination and progression toward their differentiated fates.

Editor: Kathrin Maedler, University of Bremen, Germany

Funding: L. Crisa was supported by NIH RO1 HL075270, LSDF Program Project grant, and JDRF grant #17-2011-620. V. Cirulli was supported by ADA Basic Research Award 1-11-BS-28 and JDRF Research Grants #1-2005-1084 and #17-2011-620, and LSDF Program Project grant. The funders had no role in study design, data collection and analysis, decision to publish, or preparation of the manuscript.

Competing Interests: The authors declared that no competing interests exist.

* E-mail: lcrisa@uw.edu

❾ These authors contributed equally to this work.

Introduction

The cross-talk between the mesenchyme and epithelia is critical to both the growth of epithelial organs during development as well as tissue regenerative processes in post-natal life [1]. The identification of the cellular mediators of these effects is subject of substantial research efforts in the field of regenerative medicine, as it may lead to uncover signals that could be targeted to restore loss of tissue function in degenerative diseases, organ autoimmunity or injury.

Among mesenchymal cell types that dynamically populate both developing and injured tissues are cells of the innate immune system, namely macrophages. Hence, high numbers of macrophages colonize virtually all epithelial tissues early in embryogenesis [2], and key trophic effects of this immune cell subset have been inferred by the severely impaired growth of epithelial organs displayed by animal models deficient in macrophages or macrophage-dependent functions [3–7]. Recruitment of myeloid cell populations from the bone marrow to the periphery continues to be essential in adulthood for the maintenance of tissue integrity, since, in their absence, tissue repair and regenerative events following injury are critically blunted [8–13]. To date, experimental evidence indicate that macrophages may primarily influence the growth and/or regeneration of epithelial organs indirectly, i.e. by supporting functions such as clearance of dying cells [4,14], angiogenesis [15–17] and remodeling of extracellular matrices [18]. Whether macrophages can directly dictate select developmental options in epithelia remains presently unclear.

During pancreatic development, at E14.5–15.5 gestational age, epithelial progenitors emerge from a rudimentary ductal tree through a regulated sequence of events that includes withdrawal from the cell cycle, delamination into the surrounding mesenchyme and differentiation into endocrine or exocrine cell types [19–21]. As such, while providing a pool of progenitors competent to execute specific developmental steps and make divergent lineage choices, the E14.5/E15.5 pancreas represents a valuable model to study how such epithelial programs might be impacted on by other exogenous cellular cues. In this regard, *in vivo* and *in vitro* studies have provided evidence that, over-imposed to a hierarchy of transcription factors expressed by the epithelium [19–21], interactions of the epithelium with the pancreatic mesenchyme govern the balance between the exocrine and the endocrine developmental fate of progenitors [22,23] and are required for the growth of the pancreatic epithelial compartment as a whole [24]. At present, few studies have reported the presence of tissue macrophages within the pancreatic mesenchyme and noted reduced growth of endocrine cells in their absence [25,26]. However, the possible role of macrophages as regulators of select developmental events in the pancreatic epithelium remains unknown.

A corollary to this question is whether diverse states of activation of tissue macrophages differentially affect pancreatic developmental programs. Indeed, macrophages resident within tissues may adopt a spectrum of functional states. At the extreme of this spectrum are classically (M1) and alternatively activated (M2) macrophages [27]. M1 phenotypes are acquired by macrophages upon encounter with pathogens, and lead to the production of high levels of pro-inflammatory mediators and reactive nitrogen intermediates that contribute to pathogen clearance. Conversely, "alternative" or M2 activation states are characterized by the production of lower levels of pro-inflammatory cytokines, synthesis of decoy anti-inflammatory receptors, little or no nitrogen derivatives, as well as production of mediators of tissue remodeling. As such, M2 macrophages have immune-regulatory functions that dampen inflammation and promote repair during wound healing. Stimulation of macrophages with cytokines such as IFNγ/LPS or IL4 polarize them toward M1- and M2-like activation states, respectively [28,29], providing an approach to study *in vitro* effector functions related to these states.

Interestingly, the M2-like phenotype is the predominant activation state of macrophages resident in embryonic tissues [30]. The M2 phenotype is also induced in response to tissue damage during the resolution phase of wound healing, implying that, during tissue repair, a window of opportunity exists for M2 macrophages to recapitulate, post-natally, fetal-like inductive functions on epithelia. Hence, animal models of wound healing, in which such polarized macrophages are present in high numbers, may provide ideal *in vivo* systems to assess the functional impact of M2 macrophages on developing pancreatic epithelia. In this regard, we have previously described a mouse model in which the tissue microenvironment at site of wound healing is enriched for cells of the macrophage lineage [31]. In these mice, inactivation of Id1 and Id3 genes results in functional defects of vascular and hemopoietic cell lineages, leading to impaired engraftment of tissue transplants. However, reconstitution of Id1+/−Id3−/− mice with wild type bone marrow (BM) rescues the engraftment defects and results in the enhanced recruitment of BM-derived vasculogenic and myeloid cells at sites of tissue repair [31–33]. Importantly, using microarray gene expression profiling, we demonstrated that myeloid cells isolated from tissue grafts in BM-reconstituted Id1+/−Id3−/− mice are functionally skewed toward M2 immune responses [31].

In the present study, using both *in vivo* studies in Id1/Id3-deficient mice and *in vitro* organ cultures, we uncover a role of M2 macrophages in instructing the pancreatic epithelium to acquire a motile phenotype and negatively regulate cell cycle progression. Induction of these phenotypes in transplants of embryonic pancreatic epithelium is associated with an increased frequency of cells committed to the endocrine lineage emerging from the ductal pool. We demonstrate that macrophages mediate these effects through modulation of the adhesion receptor NCAM and up-regulation of an uncommon isoform of PAX6 in a subset of ductal cells.

Matherials and Methods

Mouse breeding and bone marrow reconstitution

All mice strains were bred and housed at the University of Washington pathogen-free facility. Id1$^{+/-}$Id3$^{+/-}$ heterozygous breeders, Id1$^{+/-}$Id3$^{-/-}$ experimental and WT mice were genotyped as described previously [31]. WT mice were used as bone marrow donors. Bone marrow (BM) cells were flushed from femurs with RPMI-10% FCS, and injected intravenously (5–10×10^6) in 6- to 8-week-old lethally irradiated WT and Id1$^{+/-}$Id3$^{-/-}$ mice (1,200 rads). Eight to 12 weeks post-BM reconstitution, mice were transplanted with embryonic pancreatic explants. All procedures were approved by the Institutional Animal Care and Use Committee of the University of Washington (Protocol number 4231-01). All surgical procedures were performed under anesthesia and all efforts were undertaken to minimize suffering.

Embryonic pancreas dissection, collagenase digestion and transplantation of epithelium- enriched fractions

Time-dated pregnant WT females were used as donors of E14.5–E15.5 embryos. Embryonic pancreatic tissue was dissected and digested for 1 hour at 37°C in HBSS/0.1% collagenase A/20 µg/ml DNase. To facilitate dissociation of the mesenchyme from the epithelial component of the pancreas, the tissue was pipetted at 15 minutes intervals during digestion. Following this step, the resulting epithelial clusters were separated from the mesenchymal fraction through 3 rounds of gravity sedimentations on sterile medium. This procedure consistently resulted in >80% enrichment of epithelial cells, as measured by immunostaining and flow cytometric analysis of cell suspensions for the epithelial marker E-cadherin. Epithelial cell clusters were then transplanted as a cell pellet under the kidney capsule of naive, BM-reconstituted Id1$^{+/-}$Id3$^{-/-}$, or WT mice. Each transplant recipient routinely received pancreatic epithelial clusters derived from 5–6 embryos.

Histology and morphometric analysis

Two weeks post-transplantation, mice were euthanized and kidneys carrying the grafts harvested, fixed in 4% PFA and embedded in OCT for histology. Seven-micron cryostat sections were cut and processed for immunofluorescence. Briefly, after citrate antigen retrieval, sections were permeabilized in 0.05% Triton-X 100, blocked in 50 mM Glycine for 10′ at RT followed by incubation in 1% BSA/2% donkey serum for 1 hour at RT. Primary antibodies used for immunostaining were: mouse anti-E-cadherin (BD Biosciences, Clone36/E-cadherin), goat anti-PDX-1 (kind gift of Dr. M. Sander, UCSD), sheep anti-insulin (The Binding Site), mouse anti-glucagon (clone 79bB10, Sigma), mouse anti-PCNA (clone PC10, Santa Cruz antibodies), rabbit anti-somatostatin (Dako), rabbit anti-PP (Invitrogen), rabbit anti-alpha-amylase (Sigma), rabbit anti-NCAM (kind gift of Dr. K. Crossin, TSRI), rabbit anti-PAX6 and mouse-anti-P27^{Kip} (Chemicon). Secondary antibodies (Jackson Immuno-Research Lab) were species-specific Fab^2 fragments Rhodamine-Red conjugated donkey anti-mouse IgG, FITC-conjugated donkey anti-goat IgG, Cy5-conjugated donkey anti-sheep IgGs, Cy5 or FITC conjugated-donkey anti-rabbit IgGs. In situ immuno-detection of P27^{Kip} was obtained by tyramide amplification using the TSA kit #2 (Molecular Probes) as per manifacturer's instructions. Apoptotic cells were detected using the ApoTag-Fluorescein in Situ Apoptosis Detection Kit (Millipore) in combination with immunostaining for E-cadherin. After staining, sections were mounted and visualized at a NIKON Eclipse-800 microscope, equipped with a Spot II CCD camera or at a Zeiss Axiovert microscope equipped with a scanning laser confocal attachment (Nikon A1). Morphometric analysis was performed on ~20–30 sections per graft, collected at 100-µm intervals until exhaustion of the grafts, using the Spot Advanced and ImageProPlus software. Collectively morphometric analysis was performed on a total of 150–240 sections per group.

RNA isolation and Real-time PCR

RNA was isolated using the RNAeasy Kit (Qiagen), treated with DNase (Ambion) for 30 minutes at 37°C, and purified by phenol/chloroform extraction and ethanol precipitation. Purified RNA was retro-transcribed into cDNA using oligo dT primers and the Superscript III reverse transcriptase (Invitrogen). Expression of specific genes was assayed by either standard semi-quantitative PCR or in triplicates by real time PCR using either the SensiMix SYBR green PCR master mix (Bioline) or the iTaq SYBR green amplification system (Biorad). The following mouse-specific primer pairs were used: *18S* forward GTAACCCGTTGAACCCCATT and reverse CCATCCAATCGGTAGTAGCG; *E-cadherin* forward ACTGTGAAGGGACGGTCAAC and reverse TGTfCCCGGGTATCATCATCT; *PDX-1* forward GAAATCCACCAAAGCTCACG and reverse TTCAACATCACTGCCAGCTC; *Ngn3* forward GAGGCTCAGCTATCCACTGC and reverse TTGGAACTGAGCACTTCGTG; *Neuro-D1* forward GCTCCAGGGGTTATGAGATCG and reverse CTCTGCATTCATGGCTTCAA; *NKX6.1* forward GACGGAGAGTCAGGTCAAGG and reverse AGAGTTGGGTCCAGAGGTT; *NKX2.2* forward TCTACGACAGCAGCGACAAC and reverse TTGTCATTGTCCGGTGACTC; *INS-1* forward CAGCCCTTAGTGACCAGC and reverse GCTCCCCACACACCAGGTA; *Glucagon* forward GATGAACACCAAGAGGAA and reverse TCCAAGTAAGAACTCACAT ; *PAX6* (isof1+5a) forward CAGCTTGGTGGTGTCTTTGT and reverse ACTTGGACGGGAACTGACAC ; *ΔPD-PAX6* forward CAAAACTCTTGACAGGAAGGAGGG and reverse GCCTCAATCTGCTCTTGGGTAA.

Primers for the amplification of human transcripts were: *E-cadherin* forward GAACGCATTGCCACATACAC and reverse ATTCGGGCTTGTTGTCATTC; *PDX-1* forward CCTTTCCCATGGATGAAGTC and reverse GGAACTCCTTCTCCAGCTCT; *NG3* forward CTATTCTTTTGCGCCGGTAG and reverse ACTTCGTCTTCCGAGGCTCT; *NKX2.2* forward GAACCCCTTCTACGACAGCAG and reverse TTGTCATTGTCCGGTGACTC; *NKX6.1* forward ATTCGTTGGGGATGACAGAG and reverse CCGAGTCCTGCTTCTTCTTG; *MAF-B* forward CCTGGCTTTCTGAACTTTGC and reverse ACGTTCTCTATGCGGTTTGG; *Insulin* forward GGGGAACGAGGCTTCTTCTA and reverse CACAATGCCACGCTTCTG; *Glucagon* forward GAATTCATTGCTTGGCTGGT and reverse CGGCCAAGTTCTTCAACAAT; *Somatostatin* forward CACTCTCCAGCTCGGCTTTC and reverse AGTACTTGGCCAGTTCCTGC; *PP* forward CGCTGTCCATCGTCCTGG and reverse GTACTTGGCCAGTTCCTGCT; *NCAM* forward GCTGGACAAAGATGGGGAACA (specific to exon6-exon7 boundary from RefSeq NG-032036.1) and reverse CGCCAGCCTTGTTCTCAGCAAT.

Conditions for standard PCR were: 95°C for 5 minutes, followed by 95°C for 30 seconds, 57°C for 30 seconds and 72°C for 30 seconds for 36 cycles, with a final extension at 72°C for 5 minutes

Real time amplification conditions for mouse primers were 95°C for 15 seconds and 60°C for 45 seconds, for 40 cycles. Conditions for human NCAM real time PCR were 95°C for 15 seconds, 58°C for 30 seconds and 72°C for 20 seconds, for 40 cycles. For each primer combination, amplification efficiency was consistently >95%. Threshold cycle numbers (*Ct*) were determined using the SDS 2.3 software (Applied Biosystems) and analyzed using the $\Delta\Delta Ct$ method. All real time PCR reactions were performed using either the 7900HT Real Time PCR system (Applied Biosystems) or the CFX96 real Time PCR system (Biorad).

Construction of lenti-viral vectors, virus production and cell transduction

cDNA from E15.5 mouse brain was used as template to amplify an open reading frame of the ΔPD-PAX6 mRNA using the Expand High Fidelity Taq polymerase (Roche) and the following primers: forward AAAACTCTTGACAGGAAGGAG and reverse CCTGAATACCCAACTGCTGT. The resulting blunt-ended product was 3′ A-tailed with *Taq* DNA polymerase, ligated into the pcDNA2.1/TOPO-TA vector (Invitrogen) and sequenced. For expression in mammalian cells, an EcoR1 fragment of the TOPO vector containing the ΔPD-PAX6 insert was cloned into the EcoR1 site of the HIV vector ROVER downstream of a human CMV promoter and upstream of an IRES sequence driving a GFP reporter [34]. This HIV vector was VSV-G pseudotyped by packaging in HEK-293T cells transfected with the transgene plasmid and the packaging plasmids pMD.G (VSV-G), pMDLg/p.RRE (*gag* and *pol*), and pRSV-Rev (*rev*). Viral supernatants were harvested after 48 h, concentrated by ultracentrifugation and viral titers, defined as transducing units/ml or multiplicity of infection (MOI), estimated by transduction of 293T-cells and flow cytometric analysis of GFP^+ cells. Viral preparations were used to transduce cell lines at either 5 or 30 MOI by overnight incubation in the presence of 5 μg/ml polybrene. Transduction was verified 72 hours later by flow cytometric analysis of GFP^+ cells and Western blotting analysis of cell lysates for ΔPD-PAX6.

Macrophage derivation and macrophage/epithelial cell co-cultures

Mouse BM cells, obtained by flushing femurs and tibias, were deprived of endogenous fibroblasts through a 1 hour incubation at 37°C on tissue-culture treated dishes. Non-adherent cells were recovered and cultured for 6 days in RPMI 10% FCS in the presence of M-CSF (20 ng/ml, Peprotech). Purity of macrophage cultures was verified by flow cytometric analysis for F4/80 and Gr1. M1 and M2 macrophage polarization was further induced by culturing the resulting macrophages in the presence of LPS (100 ng/ml) and IFNγ (500 U/ml) (M1) or IL4 (20 ng/ml, Peprotech) (M2) for 48 hours.

For epithelium/macrophages co-cultures, epithelial cell clusters isolated from embryonic pancreata as described above were seeded into V-shaped 96 well plates in 200 microliters of RPMI-5% FCS-5×10^{-5} M β-mercaptoethanol. In experiments using sorted cell subsets, cell clusters were dissociated into single cell suspensions using non-enzymatic dissociation medium (Sigma), labeled with anti-E-cadherin antibody and sorted by flow cytometry according to the expression levels of E-cadherin, using a FACS Aria cell sorter (Beckton Dickinson). Cell equivalents of one embryonic pancreas were seeded per well; 50×10^3 M1 or M2 macrophages were then added to each well and cultures incubated for 72 hours at 37°C in a humidified incubator.

Cell lines, flow cytometry and migration assays

The pancreatic ductal lines SU-86 (ATCC), G3LC (a sub-clone of SU.86 derived in our laboratory), and PANC-1 (ATCC) were maintained in RPMI-10% FCS-22 mM glucose, 100 mM pen/strep. For co-cultures with polarized macrophages, 0.5×10^6 epithelial cells were seeded into a 10 cm dish in growth medium. Macrophages (1×10^6) were added 8 hours later, and cultures continued over a 48-hour period. Cells were then harvested, labeled with PERCP-conjugated anti-mouse CD45 and FITC-conjugated anti-NCAM Ab and sorted by flow cytometry as $CD45^-NCAM^+$ and $CD45^-NCAM^-$ subsets. For quantification of DNA content, epithelial cell cultures that had reached 50—60% confluency were pulsed for 6 hours with BrDU (10 µg/ml), harvested by trypsinization and fixed in 70% cold ethanol over-night at 4°C followed by incubation with 50 µg/ml RNase A at 37°C for 30 min. After digestion with DNase (Ambion) for 1 hour at 37C and immunostaining with PE-conjugated anti-BRDU antibody (clone Bu20a, Biolegend), cells were labeled with the dye 7AAD and DNA content analyzed at a FACScalibur flow cytometer (Becton Dickinson) using the Flow JO software.

Cell migration was assayed using a two-chamber Trans-well system (24 well plate format, Costar). In preliminary experiments we established that Collagen IV-coated (5 µg/ml) 5 µm-pore filters and Matrigel-coated (1:30 dilution) 8 µm-pore filters provided optimal adhesive substrates and migration conditions for G3LC and SU86 cells, respectively. For cell migration, G3LC and SU86 cell lines were serum-starved for 6 hours in RPMI-0.5% BSA, trypsinized and seeded in duplicates on the top chamber of the Trans-wells at 40,000 per well in M199/0.5% BSA/4 mM $MnCl_2$. Six hundred microliters of the same medium containing 20% FCS or HGF/SF (100 ng/ml) was then placed in the bottom chamber as chemoattractant. Trans-wells were incubated at 37°C for either 3 hours (G3LC) or 5 hours (SU86). Cultures were fixed in 4% PFA, and stained with a solution of 1% Crystal Violet/ 10 mM Borate/10%ethanol for 30 minutes. After removing the cells from the top surface of the filters with a cotton swab, cells that had migrated to the bottom side of the membrane were visualized at a light microscope (Olympus). Migrating cells were counted in 5 consecutive fields across the Trans-wells using a 10× objective.

Western Blotting

Cell cytoplasmic and nuclear extracts were prepared using the NE-PER cell extraction Kit (Pierce) in the presence of a proteases inhibitors cocktail (Complete, Roche), and PMSF (1 mM). Protein concentration of lysates was determined by the BCA protein assay (Pierce). Equal amounts of protein (5–10 µg) were then separated under reducing conditions onto 4–12% polyacrilamide gels (Nu-Page, Invitrogen) and transferred by Western blotting onto PVDF membranes (Immobilon, Millipore). After blocking of the membranes in 1% dry milk −0.1% Tween-20 over-night at 4C, the membranes were probed with rabbit anti-PAX6 Ab (Millipore), anti-$p21^{Cip}$ (SC-397, Santa Cruz antibodies), anti-$p27^{kip}$ (clone DCS7, Calbiochem), anti-Retinoblastoma, anti-cyclin E (Cell Signaling) or anti-β-actin mAb (clone AC-15, Sigma) followed by HRP-conjugated donkey-anti rabbit or donkey-anti-mouse secondary antibodies. Membrane-bound antibodies were detected by chemoluminescence using an ECL-detection kit (Amersham).

Statistical Analysis

Statistical significance of differences observed in experiments of tissue morphometric analysis, real time PCR experiments, and migration assays, was validated by Student T-test or by Anova one-group variance test, using the Statview Software with limit for significance set at $p<0.05$.

Results

Developmental effects of tissue microenvironments enriched in M2 macrophages on the embryonic pancreatic epithelium

To investigate possible developmental effects of M2-polarized macrophages on the embryonic pancreatic epithelium, explants of embryonic pancreata at E14.5–E15.5 were depleted of the fetal mesenchymal component by collagenase digestion followed by >80% enrichment of epithelial cell clusters by gravity sedimentation. Epithelial clusters were then transplanted under the kidney capsule of BM-reconstituted Id1+/−Id3−/− mice or wild type (WT) controls. Two weeks after transplantation, the grafts were harvested and processed for histology. Immunostaining for E-cadherin revealed the development of both ducts and islet-like clusters within the grafts of either BM-reconstituted Id1+/−Id3−/− mice (Fig. 1A–C) or WT mice (Fig. 1D–F). Morphometric analysis of tissue sections collected throughout the grafts of either hosts showed no significant differences in frequency of apoptotic cells (Figure S1), total E-cadherin$^+$ area, or in the E-cadherin$^+$ areas of either ductal or islet-like clusters (Fig. 1G), indicating no overt differential effects of either transplant microenvironments on the engraftment of the pancreatic epithelium as a whole. Total E-cadherin+ areas of the grafted tissues were however significantly lower in non-irradiated, non-BM reconstituted naive Id1+/−Id3−/− controls, as compared to BM-reconstituted mice (Fig. 1G) demonstrating the requirement for reconstitution with WT BM for tissue engraftment, as previously described [31].

Interestingly, two-color immunostaining for PDX-1 and E-cadherin revealed a significant increase in the number of PDX-1$^+$E-cadherin$^+$ cells associated with ductal structures in the grafts from BM-reconstituted Id1+/−Id3−/− mice (Fig. 1A–C and 1H) as compared to WT transplant recipients (Fig. 1D–H). Additional immunostaining for insulin demonstrated an increased frequency of insulin$^+$ cells associated with the ducts in the grafts of BM-reconstituted Id1+/−Id3−/− mice (Fig. 2A and 2C), whereas in WT grafts most insulin$^+$ areas appeared to be organized into islet-like clusters away from the ducts (Fig. 2B). Further immunostaining for markers of cell proliferation demonstrated a ~40% decrease in the number of insulin$^+$PCNA$^+$ cells within islet clusters and ducts (Fig. 2D) in the grafts of BM-reconstituted Id1+/−Id3−/− mice, indicating decreased proliferation of ß-cells. Lastly, glucagon$^+$ areas were increased of ~1.5 folds in the islet clusters engrafted in BM-reconstituted Id1+/−Id3−/− mice, (Fig. 2E), whereas glucagon$^+$ cells associated with the ducts where rare and did not differ from that observed in WT grafts. No significant differences in the frequency of other endocrine cell types (e.g. PP, somatostatin, ghrelin cells) were observed (not shown). In addition, consistent with the prevalent endocrine over exocrine development previously observed in embryonic pancreatic explants depleted of fetal mesenchymal cells [22,23], no exocrine amylase$^+$ developed in the grafts of either hosts (not shown). However, one additional phenotype that we noted in the grafts of BM-reconstituted Id1+/−Id3−/− mice was an increased frequency of duct-associated NCAM$^+$ cells (Fig. 3A–B arrowheads, and D), many of which expressed PDX-1 (Fig. 3C).

These results indicate that transplant environments enriched for M2-polarized macrophages support the accumulation of PDX-1$^+$, NCAM$^+$ and insulin-producing endocrine cells lining within and/ or adjacent to the ductal epithelium. In light of the evidence that induction and sustained expression of NCAM are associated with differentiation of endocrine cell lineages [35,36], and that PDX-1 and insulin expression in duct-associated cells occurs in models of islet neogenesis, [37–42], our results suggest that M2 macrophage-enriched microenvironments support the recruitment of islet progenitors from ductal domains. However, as insulin$^+$ cells emerge from the ductal compartment and organize into islet-like clusters away from the ducts, this environment restricts their proliferative capability.

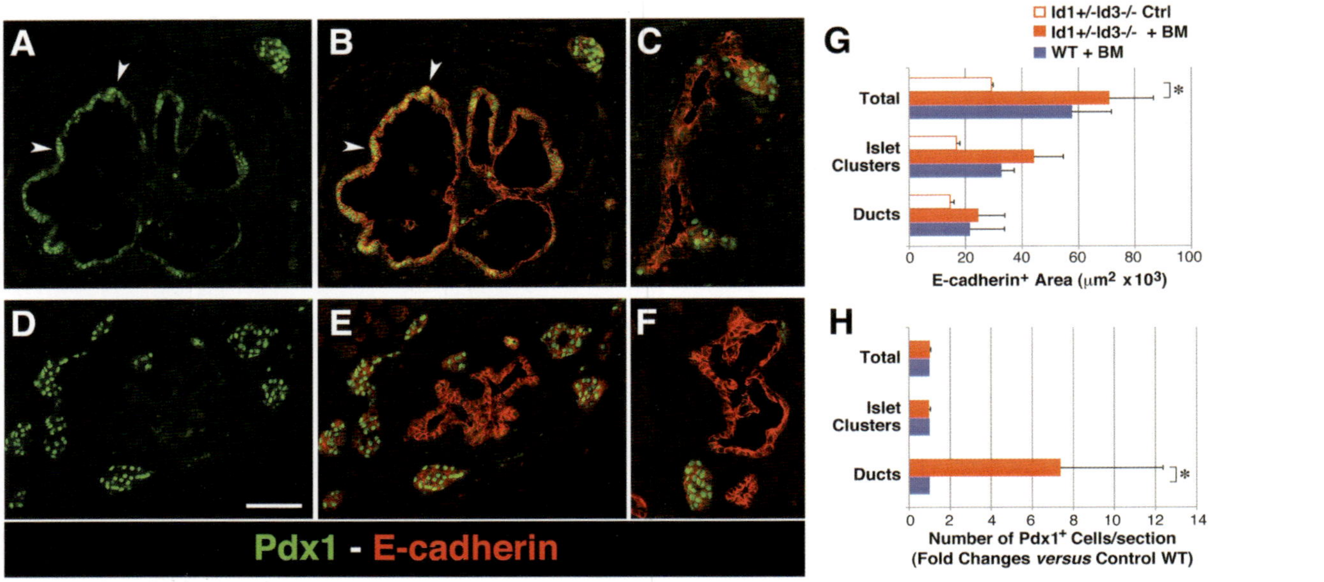

Figure 1. Increased frequency of PDX-1$^+$ pancreatic progenitors emerging from the ducts in transplant microenvironments enriched in M2 macrophages. Tissue sections of E14–15.5 pancreatic epithelial grafts transplanted in BM-reconstituted Id1+/−Id3−/− mice (A–C) or WT controls (D–F), stained by two-color immuno-fluorescence for PDX-1 (green) and E-cadherin (red). Numerous PDX-1$^+$ cells are comprised within or emerge from ductal structures in the grafts of BM-reconstituted Id1+/−Id3−/− mice (arrowheads). (G–H) Morphometric analysis of E-Cadherin$^+$ grafts areas (G) and PDX-1$^+$ cells counted within the grafts (H). Bars represent mean ± SEM of n = 4 experiments including a total of 8 grafts in Id1+/−Id3−/− and 6 grafts in WT mice. Scale bar = 60 μm; * $p \leq 0.001$.

M2 macrophages promote NCAM expression and an uncommon PAX6 transcriptional phenotype in embryonic pancreatic organ cultures

To determine whether M2 macrophages would be sufficient to recapitulate *in vitro* the NCAM$^+$ phenotype observed *in vivo*, embryonic pancreatic explants depleted of their mesenchymal component, were incubated with macrophages in organ cultures. Macrophages used in these co-cultures were differentiated from mouse BM using M-CSF and polarized toward either M1 or M2 immune functions by cytokine treatment [29]. After three days, epithelial cells within these organ cultures were analyzed by flow cytometry. Two color immunostaining for NCAM and the pan-leukocyte marker CD45, followed by gating on the CD45 negative epithelial population, showed that co-culture with M2 polarized macrophages increases the proportion of NCAM$^+$ cells as compared to co-cultures with M1 macrophages or cultures in medium alone (Fig. 4A).

Based on the knowledge that NCAM expression is induced in the islet cell lineage as it develops from ductal progenitors, we sought to determine if the observed NCAM induction was modulated in concert with transcriptional programs regulating islet cell development. Previous reports indicated a role of the transcription factor PAX6 in the regulation of NCAM in neuro-endocrine tissues [43,44], as well as in the development of the islet cell lineage [45–48]. Hence, we set out to analyze expression of PAX6 transcripts in the co-cultures. For this purpose, we used either primers specific for the paired (PD) isoforms of PAX6 (i.e. canonical and 5a variants) [49,50], or the paired-less ΔPD-PAX6, a variant described as selectively expressed in both developing neural and pancreatic tissues [51–53]. We found that while transcription of paired-PAX6 mRNAs is not differentially modulated by M1 *versus* M2 macrophages, the ΔPD-PAX6-specific transcript is significantly up-regulated by about two-folds in M2-macrophages/epithelial cells co-cultures (Fig. 4B). Gene expression of other transcription factors such as NeuroD1, Nkx2.2, Nkx6.1, PDX-1 and Ngn3 was not differentially affected in M2- *versus* M1-marophages/epithelium co-cultures (data not shown).

Further studies were then undertaken to evaluate the expression of ΔPD-PAX6 in the embryonic pancreas. In the developing E14–15.5 pancreas, high levels of E-cadherin and expression of the transcription factor SOX9 characterize pools of ductal progenitors that give rise to both endocrine and exocrine lineages [54,55], whereas relatively low levels of E-cadherin is observed in epithelial cells already committed to either fates [21]. To determine whether PD and ΔPD-PAX6 transcripts were differentially expressed in these epithelial compartments, single cell suspensions of E14–E15.5 fetal pancreata were sorted as E-cadherin high, intermediate and low populations (Fig. 4C) and mRNA transcription assessed by real time PCR. This analysis revealed that levels of ΔPD-PAX6 transcripts are higher in the epithelial E-cadh^{High} as compared to the E-cadh^{Int} or E-cadh^{Low} fractions (Fig. 4D), indicating preferential expression of this transcript in ductal pools. Control PCRs for E-cadherin- and SOX9-specific transcripts in the sorted populations demonstrated progressive increase of these mRNAs from E-cadh^{Low} to E-cadh^{High} subsets (Fig. 4E), validating the cell subset enrichment obtained by sorting.

To investigate whether ΔPD-PAX6 induced in organ cultures by M2 macrophages was also differentially expressed *in vivo* in M2-macrophages-enriched grafts of BM-reconstituted Id1+/−Id3−/− mice *versus* WT controls, the grafts were micro-dissected, lysed and their mRNA was analyzed by real time PCR using primers specific for either PD or ΔPD-PAX6 transcripts. In these experiments, to account for the epithelial component of the grafts, levels of PAX6 transcripts were normalized to E-cadherin mRNA and expressed as fold changes over those detected in freshly isolated epithelial clusters from E14–E15 pancreata. This analysis revealed substantial up-regulation of ΔPD-PAX6 over PD-PAX6 transcripts in the grafts of both hosts (Fig. 5A). Levels of ΔPD-

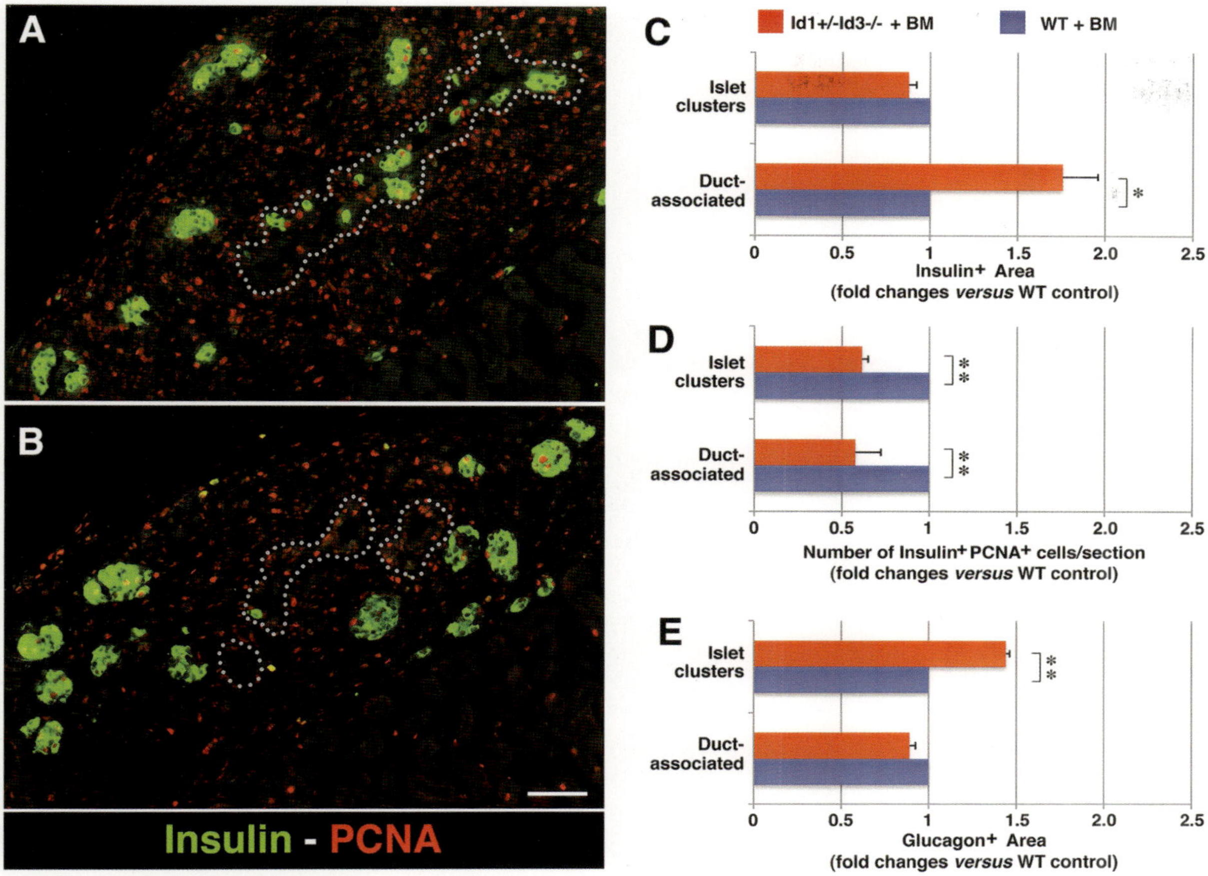

Figure 2. Frequency and proliferative potential of endocrine-committed progenitors in pancreatic transplants. (A–B) Tissue sections of E14–15.5 pancreatic epithelial grafts transplanted in BM-reconstituted Id1+/−Id3−/− mice (A) or WT controls (B), stained by two-color immunofluorescence for Insulin (green) and the proliferation marker PCNA (red). Dotted lines delineate boundaries of ductal structures. (C–E) Morphometric analysis of Insulin$^+$ areas (C), proliferating Insulin$^+$PCNA$^+$ cells (D) and Glucagon$^+$ areas (E), assessed in the grafts. Bars represent mean ± SEM of n = 3 experiments, including a total of 7 grafts in Id1+/−Id3−/− and 5 grafts in WT mice. Scale bar = 120 μm; *$p = 0.01$ and ** $p < 0.002$.

PAX6 up-regulation, however, were most dramatic in the grafts of BM-reconstituted Id1+/−Id3−/− mice (i.e. 80 fold induction) as compared to the grafts of WT mice (i.e. 30 fold induction) (Fig. 5A).

Paired canonical and 5a variants of PAX6 transcripts are translated into 46 and 48 kDa proteins, respectively, whereas ΔPD-PAX6 mRNAs have been described to encode for 30–32 kDa proteins [49–53], herein referred to as p46, p48 and p32. To determine whether ΔPD-PAX6 transcripts induced by M2 macrophages in organ cultures were translated into protein, and investigate the nuclear *versus* cytoplasm subcellular localization of this protein relatively to other PAX6 isoforms, nuclear and cytoplasmic lysates of the organ cultures were analyzed by Western blotting using an anti-PAX6 antibody specific for a COOH terminal peptide common to all PAX6 isoforms. Consistent with the transcript analysis (Fig. 4B), these experiments confirmed that M2 macrophages increase the expression of a p32 form of PAX6 in pancreatic epithelial organ cultures relative to their M1 counterpart (Fig. 5B). Intriguingly, expression of the p32 isoform was not confined to the nucleus; rather, a considerable amount was retained in the cytoplasm. In addition, induction of this isoform was not observed in the presence of M2 macrophage-conditioned media alone (not shown), indicating the requirement of cell-cell interactions. The paired canonical and 5a isoforms of PAX6 were also detected, but their expression levels were not differentially modulated in the presence of M1 and M2 macrophages (Fig. 5B).

The unusually high cytoplasmic localization of p32 PAX6 induced in organ cultures by M2-macrophages prompted us to investigate whether PAX6 cytoplasmic immunoreactivity identifies selected populations of epithelial cells within the grafts. Indeed two-color immunofluorescence for E-cadherin and PAX6 revealed the presence of scattered single cells with a strong PAX6-specific cytoplasmic immunoreactivity in ductal structures (Fig. 5C, left two panels). Ductal cells with this unusual PAX6 expression pattern were frequently comprised within groups of NCAM$^+$ cells (Fig. 5C, right panel) indicating that these two populations were partially overlapping. Unlike the cytoplasmic expression pattern of this unique ductal population, PAX6 immunoreactivity in the islet clusters away from the ducts was predominantly nuclear (Fig. 5D)

Taken together, these results indicate that M2 macrophages recapitulate in organ cultures the induction of NCAM observed in the Id1/Id3 KO transplantation model. They further identify the ΔPD-PAX6 isoform as a hallmark of M2 macrophage inductive functions on the developing pancreatic epithelium.

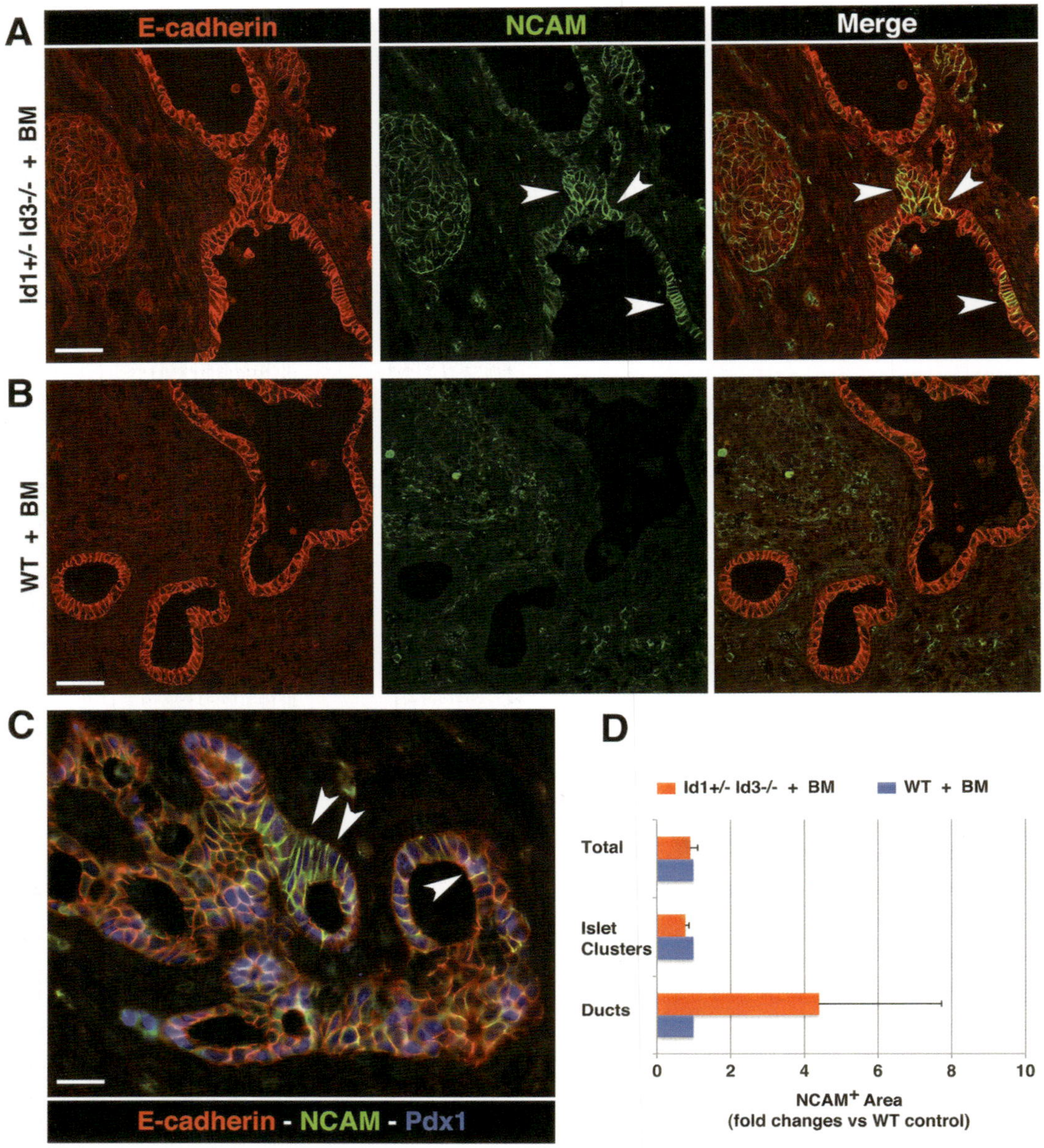

Figure 3. Modulation of NCAM expression in the ductal epithelium of embryonic pancreatic transplants. (A–B) Tissue sections of E14–15.5 pancreatic grafts transplanted in BM-reconstituted Id1+/−Id3−/− mice (A) or WT (B) hosts, immuno-stained for NCAM (green) and E-cadherin (red). Numerous patches of NCAM$^+$ epithelial cells are present in ductal structures of grafts from Id1+/−Id3−/− mice (arrowheads) but not in those from WT hosts. C) NCAM$^+$E-cadherin$^+$ ductal domains comprise PDX-1$^+$ progenitors (blue, arrowheads). D) Morphometric analysis of NCAM$^+$ areas measured in the grafts. Bars represent mean ± SEM of n = 3 experiments, including a total of 7 grafts in Id1+/−Id3−/− and 5 grafts in WT mice. Scale bars = 90 μm in A–B and 45 μm in C.

NCAM induction in ductal epithelia by M2 macrophages marks cells with a highly migratory phenotype

The enhanced expression of NCAM and ΔPD-PAX6 induced in embryonic pancreatic epithelia by M2-macrophages raised the question as to the functional significance of these cellular responses.

Over-expression of NCAM in epithelia has been associated with the acquisition of cell motility [56–58]. To investigate whether NCAM expression induced by cell-cell interactions with M2 macrophages imparts similar functions on pancreatic ductal epithelia, we turned to ductal epithelial cell lines as a model system. Co-culture of M2 but not M1 macrophages with the pancreatic lines SU86 and G3LC induced NCAM expression on a small, but discrete, subset of cells (Fig. 6A). Hence, in this model system, M2 macrophages recapitulate the induction of NCAM expression observed with the pancreatic embryonic epithelium in organ cultures and *in vivo*. Nevertheless, competence to generate this cell subset was line-specific, since the PANC-1 line did not show the emergence of a significant number of NCAM$^+$ cells. As for ΔPD-PAX6, M2 macrophage conditioned media alone did not induce NCAM expression in neither lines (not shown). Although the precise mechanism of NCAM protein up-regulation remains to be fully elucidated, qPCR analysis of epithelial cells co-cultured with M2 macrophages did not reveal increased expression of

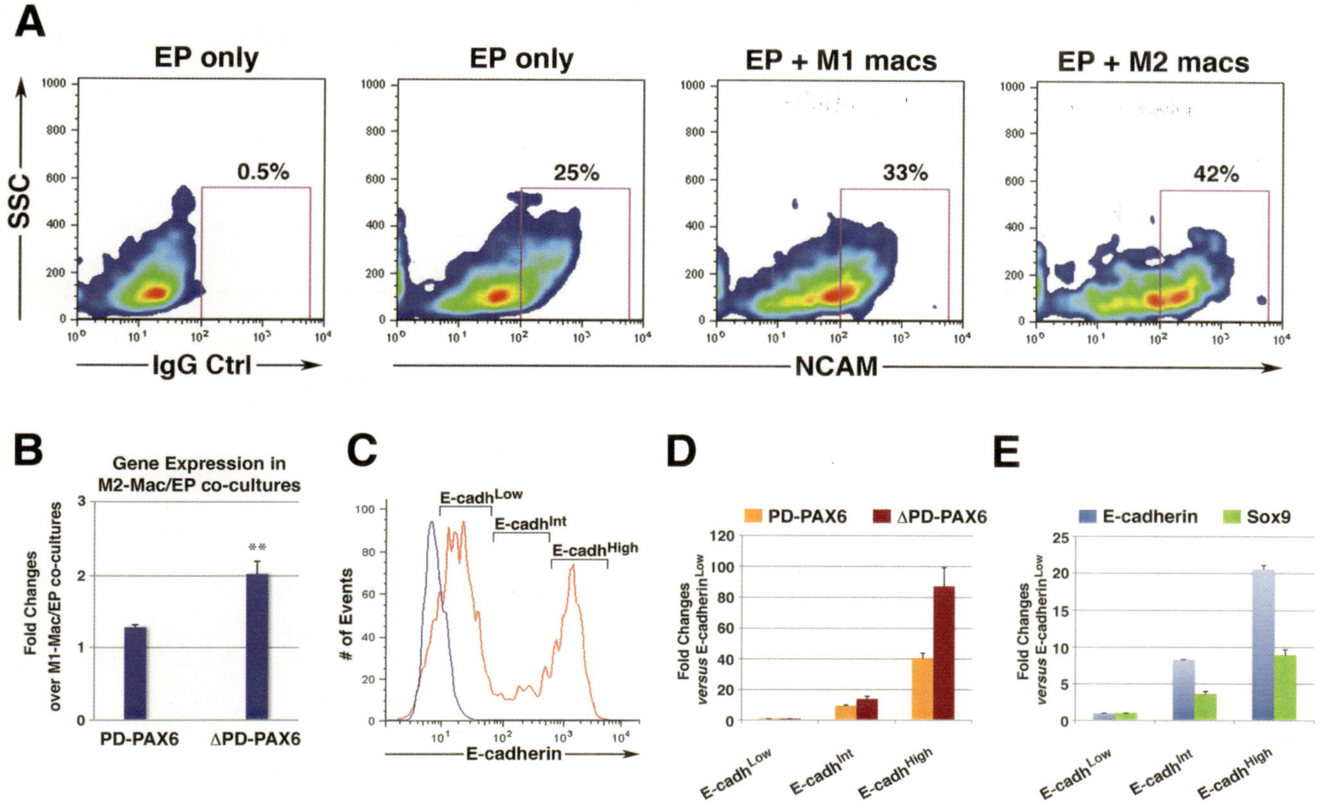

Figure 4. Differential induction of NCAM and PAX6 by M2 versus M1 macrophages in organ cultures, and in select pancreatic epithelial subpopulations. A) E14–15.5 pancreatic epithelial cells, cultured for 3 days in medium alone (Ep) or in the presence of M1- (Ep+M1 macs) or M2- (Ep+M2 macs) macrophages, were immuno-stained for NCAM and the pan-leukocyte marker CD45. Flow cytometric contour plots of cells gated as CD45 negative (i.e. epithelial cells only) are shown, and percentages of NCAM^{+} cells are indicated in the right quadrants. Representative of n = 4 experiments. B) qPCR analysis of the indicated gene transcripts detected in macrophage/embryonic epithelium organ cultures. Values from each experimental condition were normalized to E-cadherin mRNA. Bars are mean ± SEM of n = 4 experiments; ** $p<0.01$. C) Flow cytometric hystogram of epithelial cells from E14–E15.5 pancreata stained for E-cadherin (red) or IgG control (blue). The sorting windows used for the isolation of E-cadherin High, Intermediate and Low populations are shown. (D–E) qPCR analysis of E-cadherin, SOX9 and PAX6-specific transcripts expressed in the indicated sorted populations. Representative of 2 experiments, each from a pool of 28–30 embryos with values presented as mean ± SEM of triplicate samples.

NCAM-specific transcripts as compared to the levels detected in the parental lines (Figure S2), suggesting a post-transcriptional regulation of NCAM expression.

To determine whether NCAM^{+} G3LC ductal cells generated in co-culture with M2 macrophages had acquired an enhanced migratory phenotype, cell cultures were labeled for CD45 and NCAM and sorted as CD45^{Neg}NCAM^{Pos} and CD45^{Neg}NCAM-^{Neg}. The two subsets were then used in chemotactic migration assays. These experiments revealed that NCAM^{Pos} cells exhibited significantly higher migratory responses to chemotactic stimuli provided by FCS than their NCAM^{Neg} counterparts (Fig. 6B,). Further Western blotting analysis of cell lysates from the sorted populations, revealed that the NCAM^{Pos} but not the NCAM^{Neg} cells expressed a 32 kDa protein specifically detected by the anti-PAX6 antibody, consistent with the expression of a ΔPD-PAX6 isoform within the highly migratory NCAM^{Pos} subset (Fig. 6C). PD-PAX6 was also down-regulated in this latter fraction.

These results show that induction of NCAM on the ductal epithelium by functionally polarized M2 macrophages selects for cells with enhanced competency to respond to exogenous migratory cues. The data further show that NCAM and ΔPD-PAX6 are induced within the same cell population.

Low levels of expression of ΔPD-PAX6 are sufficient to impart a migratory phenotype in pancreatic ductal epithelia

The *in vivo* and *in vitro* studies presented above indicate that induction of NCAM and ΔPD-PAX6 by M2-macrophages are overlapping phenotypes, suggesting a possible functional relationship of NCAM and ΔPD-PAX6 expression. To date, no biological functions have been attributed to the ΔPD-PAX6 isoform.

To shed light into the functions mediated by this PAX6 isoform, we amplified this variant mRNA from mouse fetal brain cDNA using PCR primers spanning the exon3/8 boundary and the 3′ UTR of PAX6, as described [52], and cloned the resulting cDNA product into a lenti-viral vector carrying constitutive expression of a GFP reporter. Viral transduction of HEK-293T or G3LC cells and Western blotting analysis of cell protein extracts confirmed that the cloned cDNA is expressed in epithelial cells as a stable protein of ~32 kDa, with both a nuclear and cytoplasmic localization (Figure S3). Following these experiments, G3LC and SU86 cells were infected at 5 and 30 MOI, and transduced GFP^{+} cells were sorted by flow cytometry to generate ΔPD-PAX6^{Low} and ΔPD-PAX6^{High} sub-lines. Phenotypic characterization of these lines demonstrated that expression of ΔPD-PAX6 at the

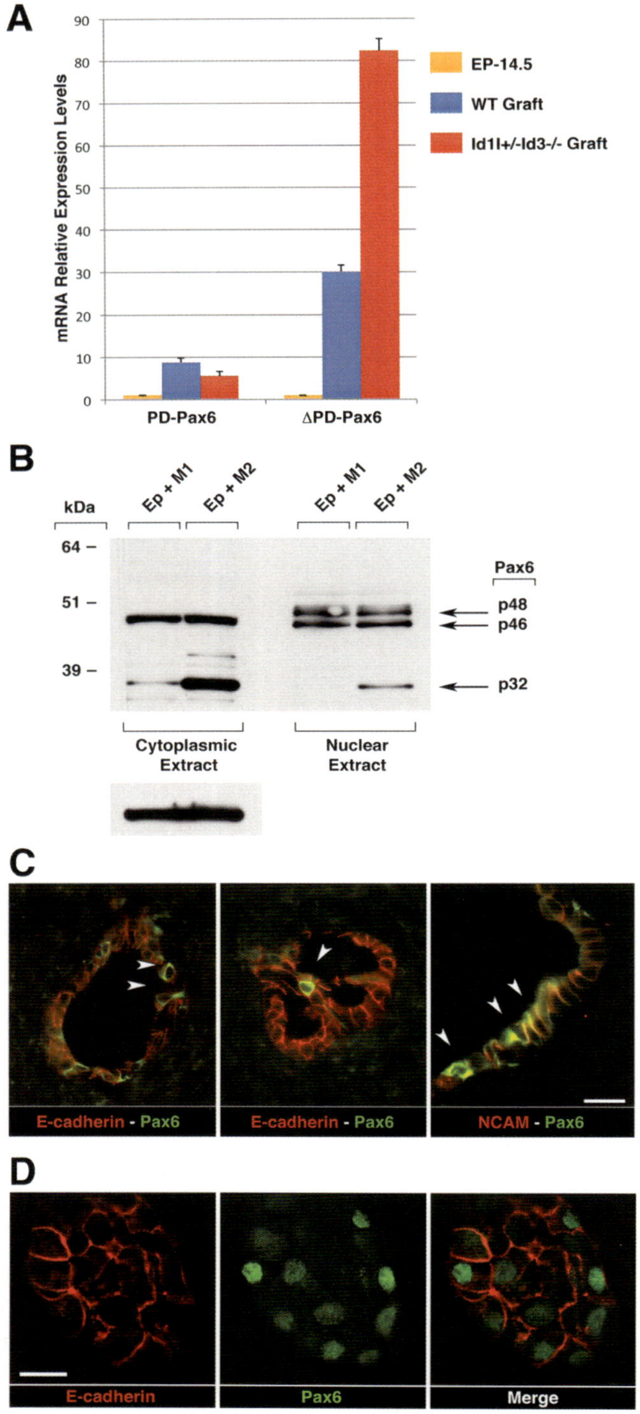

Figure 5. Expression of PAX6 transcripts and protein isoforms in the grafts and cultures of embryonic pancreatic epithelium. (A) qPCR analysis of paired (PD) and paired-less (ΔPD) PAX6 transcripts detected in epithelial grafts from WT or Id1+/−Id3−/− hosts 2 weeks post-transplant, as compared to those detected in epithelial clusters isolated from E14.5 pancreata. Bars represent mean ± SEM of triplicate values normalized to E-cadherin mRNA. Representative of n = 2 experiments. (B) Western blotting analysis of cytoplasmic and nuclear cell lysates from organ cultures of E14.5–15.5 pancreatic epithelium with M1 (EP+M1) or M2 (EP+M2) macrophages. Membranes were probed with an anti-PAX6 antibody or with an anti-β-actin antibody, as loading control. Representative of n = 3 experiments. (C–D) Tissue sections of E14–15.5 pancreatic grafts transplanted in BM-reconstituted Id1+/−Id3−/− mice, immuno-stained for PAX6 (green) and either E-cadherin or NCAM (red). Scale bars = 25 μm in C and 15 μm in D. (C) PAX6 immunoreactivity in ductal structures is observed in individual E-cadherin^{+} cells, within NCAM^{+} ductal domains and with a prevalent cytoplasmic pattern (arrowheads). (D) In contrast, PAX6 immunoreactivity in islet-like cell clusters shows a predominant nuclear localization.

levels achieved in these transduction experiments does not induce NCAM (Fig. 7A). However, ΔPD-PAX6^{Low} but not ΔPD-PAX6^{High} lines exhibited enhanced migratory responses to chemotactic stimuli provided by either FCS or HGF/SF as compared to mock-transduced control lines (Fig. 7B–C).

These results demonstrate that the ΔPD-PAX6 isoform does not influence NCAM protein expression in ductal epithelia; however, at low levels, it is sufficient to increase cell motility. Collectively, the data identify induction of NCAM and regulation of ΔPD-PAX6 expression as two distinct phenotypes elicited by M2 macrophages, which co-operate to enhance cell motility in ductal epithelial cells.

Over-expression of ΔPD-PAX6 modulates epithelial cell cycle progression in a dose dependent fashion and is associated with the acquisition of islet progenitor phenotypes

Another effect we have observed in the M2 macrophage-enriched transplantation model is a negative regulation of epithelial cell proliferation in islet cell clusters, as measured by a decreased frequency of Insulin^{+}PCNA^{+} cells (Fig. 2D). To investigate whether induction of ΔPD-PAX6 alone in pancreatic epithelial cells could influence cell cycle progression, we performed cell cycle analysis of ΔPD-PAX6^{Low} and ΔPD-PAX6^{High} lines. This analysis revealed that transduction of ΔPD-PAX6 results in a decreased proportion of cells in S phase and accumulation of cells in G2/M phase (Fig. 8A, Regions 2 and 3, respectively) indicating a blockage at this latter checkpoint of the cell cycle. Notably, this effect on cell cycle progression was most dramatic in the ΔPD-PAX6^{High} lines, indicating a dosage dependent effect of ΔPD-PAX6. Accordingly, growth curves of either ΔPD-PAX6^{High} SU86 and G3LC lines demonstrated a ~50% and 30% decrease in cell numbers, respectively, at 5 days of culture (Fig. 8B). Further Western blotting analysis of modulators of the cell cycle demonstrate that expression of ΔPD-PAX6 is associated with up-regulation of the cell cycle brake p27^{kip} in the nuclear fraction, in a fashion proportional to the levels of ΔPD-PAX6 expression. In contrast no significant changes in the expression levels and/or sub-cellular distribution of p21^{cip} and cyclin E were detected (Fig. 8C). Based on these results, we investigated the pattern of expression of p27^{kip} in the embryonic pancreatic transplants. These studies revealed that in WT hosts p27^{kip}-specific immunoreactivity is predominantly localized in the cytoplasm, with few scattered cells exhibiting nuclear staining, whereas grafts in Id1/Id3-deficient hosts displayed both cytoplasmic and nuclear immunoreactivity (Figure S4).

We further analyzed ΔPD-PAX6-transduced G3LC and SU.86 lines for the expression of markers of islet lineages (e.g. NKX6.1, NKX2.2, PDX-1, Ngn3, MAF-B) and pancreatic hormones (e.g. insulin, glucagon, somatostatin and PP). PCR analysis of these transcripts in the linear range of amplification revealed that ΔPD-PAX6 transduction in these lines does not result in detectable expression of islet hormones (Figure S5). However, these studies showed that both G3LC ΔPD-PAX6^{Low} and ΔPD-PAX6^{High} cells up-regulate the expression of transcription factors activated during

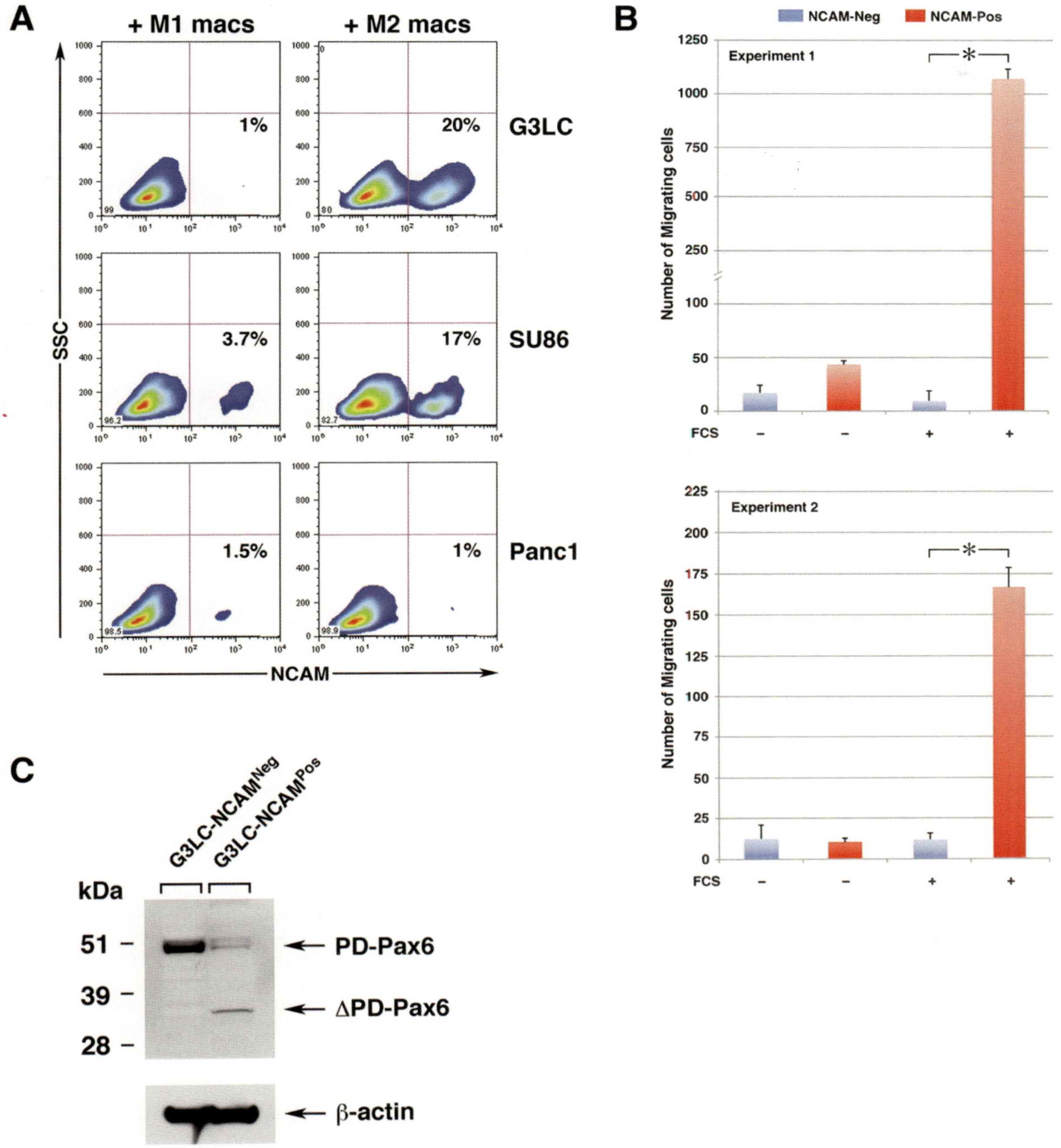

Figure 6. Induction of NCAM and ΔPD-PAX6 by M2 macrophages are overlapping phenotypes associated with enhanced migration. (A) Flow cytometric analysis of G3LC, SU86 and PANC-1 cell lines co-cultured with either M1 (M1 macs) or M2 (M2 macs) macrophages, immunostained for NCAM and the pan-leukocyte marker CD45. The contour plots shows cells gated as $CD45^{neg}$ (i.e. epithelial cells only), and the percentage of $NCAM^{+}$ cells are indicated in the right lower quadrant. (B) Migration of G3LC cells sorted from co-cultures with M2 macrophages as $CD45^{neg}NCAM^{Neg}$ and $CD45^{neg}NCAM^{Pos}$ subsets, in response to 20% FCS. Bars represent the mean ± SD of duplicate samples in each experiment. **p*<0.001. (C) Western blotting analysis of PAX6 isoforms expressed in cytoplasmic cell lysates from sorted $NCAM^{Neg}$ and $NCAM^{Pos}$ G3LC cells derived from the M2 macrophages co-cultures shown in panel A.

islet cell lineage development, i.e. NKX6.1, NKX2.2, PDX-1 and MAF-B. NKX6.1 and MAF-B, but not NKX2.2, were also up-regulated in SU86 ΔPD-$PAX6^{High}$ cells as compared to the parental line (Figure S5).

Taken together, these results provide novel evidence for a functional link between modulation of ΔPD-PAX6 and activation of cellular pathways involved in epithelial cell growth arrest. They further indicate the potential of ΔPD-PAX6 to positively regulate the progression of pancreatic ductal epithelia toward endocrine progenitor cell fates.

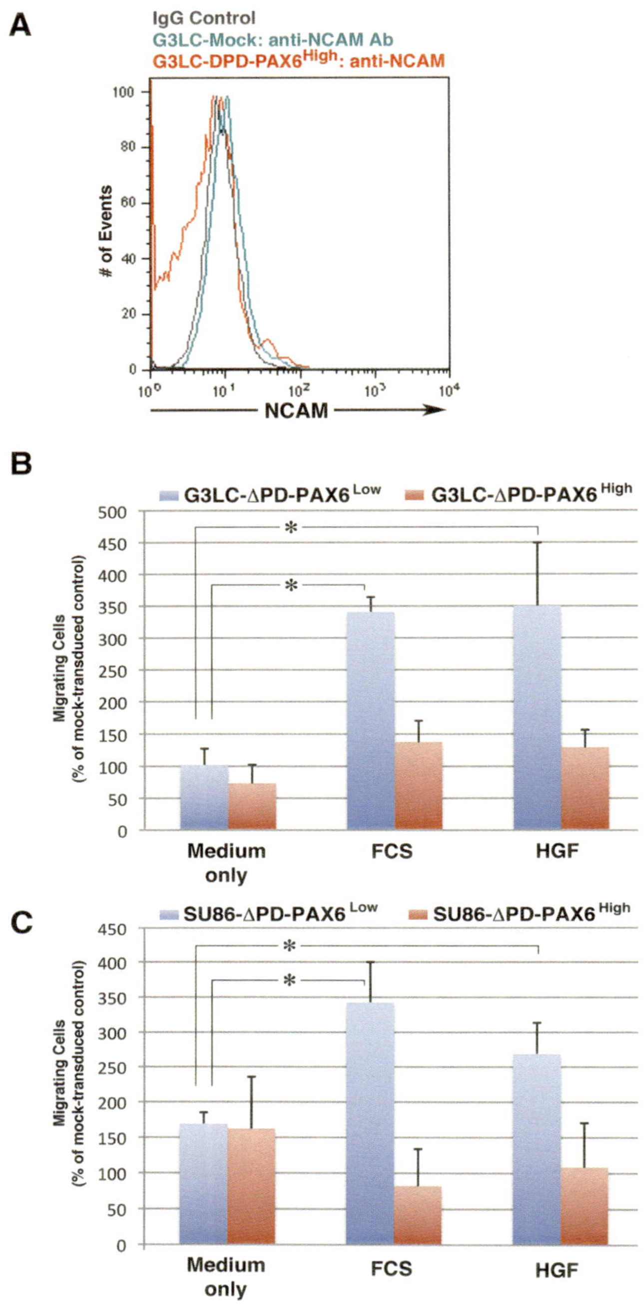

Figure 7. Over-expression of ΔPD-PAX6 enhances migration of pancreatic epithelial cells but does not induce NCAM. (A) Flow cytometric analysis of G3LC cells transduced with either empty (G3LC-Mock) or ΔPD-PAX6 expressing lenti-viruses at 30 MOI (G3LC-ΔPD-PAX6^{High}) immunostained for NCAM. Over-expression of ΔPD-PAX6 is not sufficient to induce NCAM expression. (B–C) Migratory responses of Low (ΔPD-PAX6^{Low}) and High (ΔPD-PAX6^{High}) ΔPD-PAX6 expressors, generated by lentivirus transduction at 5 and 30 MOI, respectively, in response to chemotactic stimuli provided by FCS and HGF/SF as compared to medium alone. Bars represent mean ± SEM of n = 3 experiments. * $p \leq 0.001$.

Discussion

In the developing pancreas, the migration of epithelial progenitors from ductal compartments into the surrounding mesenchyme and its coordination with differentiative events are thought to be critical to the development of both the exocrine and the endocrine compartments of this organ. Enhanced progenitor delamination and islet neogenesis from putative duct associated precursors have also been invoked in models of pancreatic tissue regeneration associated with inflammation [37–42]. To date, the possible role of macrophages and their functional polarization in these phenomena has remained virtually unexplored.

We found that M2 macrophages/epithelial interactions *in vivo* and *in vitro* result in the expression of NCAM in a subpopulation of ductal cells and that NCAM induction marks cells with migratory capabilities far greater than the NCAM-negative ductal pool. Previous reports have demonstrated a role of NCAM in cell types segregation and tissue patterning during embryogenesis, and shown that its induction in epithelial cells may act as a switch of cell migration by disrupting cadherin-mediated cell adhesion and/ or regulating FGF receptor signaling [56–58]. Collectively, these observations suggest that macrophages may be involved in modulating epithelial cell migration not only by remodeling the extracellular environment, as previously described [18], but also by directly regulating the expression of select motogenic adhesion receptors such as NCAM in the epithelium itself. This migratory phenotype may be relevant to the segregation of islet progenitors from ductal domains. Consistent with this possibility, we observed that the NCAM$^+$ ductal epithelium comprises PDX-1$^+$ and insulin$^+$ cells, a pattern previously described in models of islet neogenesis [37–42].

In searching for putative inductive functions of macrophages on pancreatic transcriptional programs [19–21,59–65], we found that the interaction of embryonic pancreatic epithelium with M2 macrophages *in vitro* and *in vivo* results in the up-regulation of a truncated isoform of PAX6. Previous studies have shown that activation of the PAX6 locus in vertebrates results in three main PAX6 transcripts encoding distinct proteins with variations in their functional domains. These include the "canonical" and the "5a variant" of PAX6, both containing a "paired" (PD) and a "paired-type" homeodomain for DNA binding, as well as a "paired-less" or ΔPD-PAX6 variant lacking the paired domain but maintaining the homeodomain [49–53]. Studies in animal models bearing mutations that disrupt the expression of PD-PAX6 isoforms have shown their critical role in modulating the balance of developing glucagon- *versus* insulin-producing islet cells, as well the expression of genes required for endocrine secretory functions [45–48]. Much less is known on how expression of ΔPD-PAX6 is regulated and what its function(s) might be. Previous studies have reported a spatially and temporally restricted expression of this PAX6 variant in the embryonic retinas, olfactory epithelium and pancreas [51,66,67], suggesting functions linked to the development of these tissues [68].. Our data provide novel evidence that induction of ΔPD-PAX6 in the embryonic pancreatic epithelium occurs upon interaction with M2 macrophages, uncovering one potential cellular mechanism regulating its expression. We further show significant up-regulation of ΔPD-PAX6 during tissue healing, suggesting that this isoform may be implicated not only in developmental events, but also in repair responses of this tissue.

We found that expression of ΔPD-PAX6 transcripts is enriched in ductal epithelia of the fetal pancreas. It was reported that the PAX6 gene locus can be activated in the primitive pancreatic duct at E9.5 [45,47,69], and in scattered duct-associated epithelial cells in models of islet neogenesis [39]. Nevertheless, our finding of a ΔPD-PAX6 variant in embryonic ductal cells uncovers a previously unrecognized complexity in patterns of PAX6 isoforms expressed in distinct pancreatic populations. Importantly, the proposed role of embryonic ductal compartments as source of

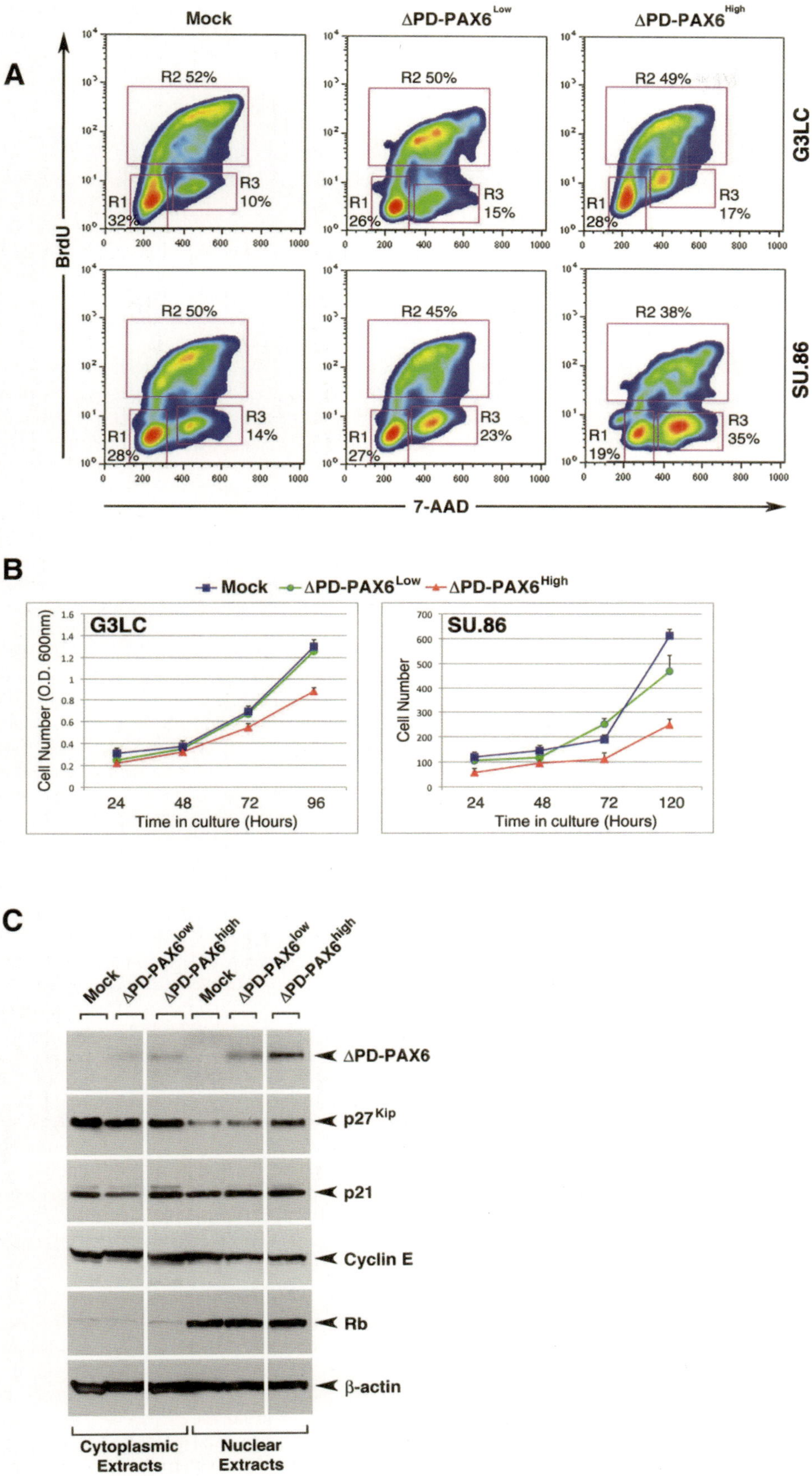
A
Mock
ΔPD-PAX6 Low
ΔPD-PAX6 High
G3LC
SU.86
BrdU
7-AAD
R2 52%
R1 32%
R3 10%
R2 50%
R1 26%
R3 15%
R2 49%
R1 28%
R3 17%
R2 50%
R1 28%
R3 14%
R2 45%
R1 27%
R3 23%
R2 38%
R1 19%
R3 35%
B
Mock
ΔPD-PAX6 Low
ΔPD-PAX6 High
G3LC
SU.86
Cell Number (O.D. 600nm)
Cell Number
Time in culture (Hours)
C
Mock
ΔPD-PAX6 low
ΔPD-PAX6 high
ΔPD-PAX6
p27 Kip
p21
Cyclin E
Rb
β-actin
Cytoplasmic Extracts
Nuclear Extracts

Figure 8. Modulation of epithelial cell cycle progression by ΔPD-PAX6. (A) Cell cycle analysis of mock-transduced, Low (ΔPD-PAX6^{Low}) and High (ΔPD-PAX6^{High}) ΔPD-PAX6 G3LC, and SU.86 cells, as measured by flow cytometric analysis of DNA content and BrdU incorporation. In each plot, percentages of cells in G0/G1, S and G2/M are indicated in regions R1, R2 and R3 respectively. Representative of n = 2 experiments. (B) Growth curves of G3LC and SU86 lines as a function of ΔPD-PAX6 expression levels. Representative of n = 3 experiments. (C) Western blotting analysis of PAX6, p27^{kip}, p21^{cip}, cyclin E, Retinoblastoma (Rb) protein and β-actin expressed in cell lysates obtained from Mock, Low (ΔPD-PAX6^{Low}) and High ΔPD-PAX6 (ΔPD-PAX6^{High}) G3LC. Representative of n = 2 experiments.

multipotent progenitors [70] implies that ΔPD-PAX6 may function, at least in part, by regulating early developmental events rather than terminal endocrine maturation, as ascribed to canonical full-length PAX6 [47]. Indeed, we found that over-expression of ΔPD-PAX6 in ductal epithelial cells is associated with up-regulation of early markers of islet cell lineages, including PDX-1, NKX2.2, NKX6.1 and MAF-B. Concomitantly, ΔPD-PAX6 over-expression enhances cell migration and induces cell cycle withdrawal, two functions required for progenitor delamination and differentiation, prior to terminal maturation. Intriguingly, there is a clear gene dosage effect of ΔPD-PAX6 on these cellular responses in such a way that while low levels of expression are permissive for enhancing cell migration, high levels are most effective at inducing cell cycle exit. These results suggest a stepwise model (Fig. 9) by which cell-cell interactions of proliferating ductal epithelial cells with M2 macrophages results initially in induction of NCAM and high levels of ΔPD-PAX6 expression, thereby providing signals for both facilitating sorting out from the ductal compartment and exiting the cell cycle. Thereafter, as levels of ΔPD-PAX6 decline, delamination and migration of such progenitors into the surrounding mesenchyme is promoted. Ultimately, release from M2 macrophages interactions triggering ΔPD-PAX6 up-regulation may be required for endocrine-committed progenitors to resume cell proliferation away from the ducts in response to other mesenchymal cues and expand into islet cell clusters [22,24]. This expectation is consistent with our results in the Id1/Id3 deficient mouse, showing that embryonic epithelial transplants exposed to a strong M2 macrophage inflammatory milieu exhibit enhanced frequency of endocrine committed cells emerging from the ducts, but decreased proliferation of their progeny in the islet clusters.

The mechanisms underlying enhanced cell migration and slow down of the cell cycle induced by ΔPD-PAX6 warrant further studies. This is a complex undertaking because there is evidence that, depending on the cellular context, ΔPD-PAX6 may either enhance or repress several pathways by establishing intermolecular interactions with other transcriptional regulators [52,71–74]. These include binding to regulators of the cell cycle (e.g. retinoblastoma) as well as to other PAX6 isoforms [72,73]. In this regard, it is noteworthy that some target genes of canonical PAX6 itself include mediators of cell migration [75,76], and that developmental effects of canonical PAX6 in neuronal lineages are also gene-dosage dependent [77]. Hence it is possible that ΔPD-PAX6 acts as cell-context dependent modulator of distinct effectors to coordinate epithelial cell cycle withdrawal, migration, and differentiation. Beyond its relevance to embryonic development, the observed effects of ΔPD-PAX6 induction on cell cycle progression in pancreatic cell lines identify a mechanism potentially critical to the control of pathological tissue growth, such as pancreatic tumor progression. Given the fact that the PAX6 locus can be abnormally activated in tumors of many branched epithelial organs [75,78], this finding may have implications for the regulation of cell growth in other tumor cell types as well.

Previous reports have provided evidence pro-proliferative effects of pancreatic fibroblasts on the developing epithelium [22,24]. Our finding that M2 macrophages, through up-regulation of ΔPD-PAX6, may actually slow down the progression of pancreatic epithelia through the cell cycle, suggests that similarly polarized macrophages populating the developing pancreas could function to counter-regulate mesenchymal pro-proliferative cues. This is further supported by the observation that the blockade in cell cycle progression is accompanied by increased nuclear localization of p27^{kip}, a cyclin-dependent kinase inhibitor shown to be expressed in pancreatic epithelia that have exited the cell cycle and committed to differentiation [79,80]. Our results are also consistent with the observation that pancreatic tissue developing in the absence of macrophages exhibits an increased proliferation of ductal compartments and a decreased endocrine cell mass [25,26]. Taken together, these observations are consistent with functionally opposing effects of M2 macrophages and mesenchymal fibroblasts on cell cycle progression of pancreatic epithelia, and argue that in the developing pancreas, a spatially restricted positioning and/or activation of M2 macrophages must be present to allow for their anti-proliferative effects to take place on progenitors delaminating from the ductal compartment, but not on their islet cell progeny.

Collectively, our studies uncover a novel role of macrophages in their M2 state of activation as positive regulators of pancreatic progenitors recruitment and differentiation toward the islet cell lineage, as well as modulators of islet cell cycle progression. Although the molecular effectors of these macrophage-driven functions remain to be identified, our findings point to a cellular mechanism that could be exploited in pancreatic tissue regeneration. Hence, in light of these results it may be important to test whether brakes on islet regenerative responses *in vivo* following injury and/or degeneration may be modulated by targeting the anti-proliferative effects of M2 macrophages. In addition, the functional properties of macrophages identified here may be harnessed for the development of improved protocols of *in vitro* directed differentiation of islet cells from either ESC or iPSC preparations [81–83]. Hence, macrophages with distinct states of functional activation may be exploited to promote either expansion or differentiation of stem cell/progenitor cell populations.

Supporting Information

Figure S1 Frequency of apoptotic cells in grafts of embryonic pancreatic epithelium. Morphometric analysis of apoptotic cells detected by TUNEL assay within E-cadherin^{+} areas of grafts retrieved from BM-reconstituted WT (blue bar) and Id1/Id3-deficient (red bar) hosts. Bars represent means ± SEM of determinations performed in grafts from WT (n = 3) and Id1/Id3-deficient mice grafts (n = 5). *NS* = not significant.

Figure S2 NCAM mRNA expression in the NCAM^{Pos} and NCAM^{Neg} fractions of ductal epithelium/macrophages co-cultures. Real time qPCR analysis of NCAM-specific transcripts detected in G3LC and SU.86 cells sorted as CD45^{Neg}NCAM^{Neg} (blue bars) and CD45^{Neg}NCAM^{Pos} (red bars) fractions from co-cultures with M2-polarized macrophages. Levels of NCAM transcripts detected in NCAM^{Pos} fractions of either cell lines are not significantly different than those detected in the NCAM^{Neg} fraction, or corresponding parental line (yellow bars).

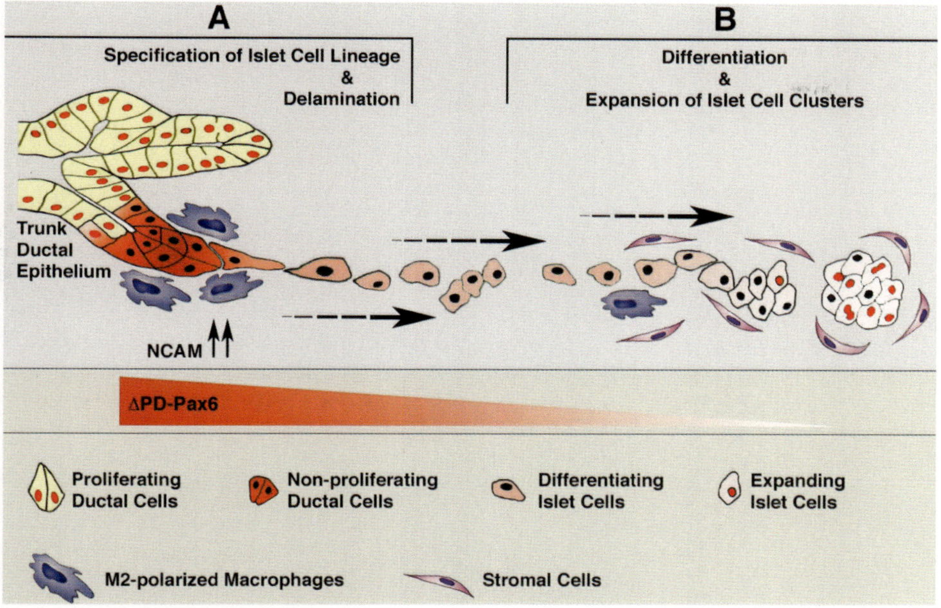

Figure 9. Hypothetical model of macrophages-induced developmental effects on embryonic pancreatic epithelium. (A) Interactions of M2 macrophages with proliferating ductal epithelial cells induce expression of NCAM in delaminating progenitors. Concomitantly, high levels of ΔPD-PAX6 are induced. This latter change results in slowing-down the cell cycle, allowing for the initiation of differentiative events in progenitors committed to endocrine lineages. At the same time, NCAM induction, through disruption of E-cadherin and/or potentiation of FGF signaling, facilitates sorting of committed progenitors out of the ductal lining. (B) Motility of the committed progenitors increases as high levels of ΔPD-PAX6 progressively wear off, allowing their delamination and migration away from the ducts. Eventually, expression of ΔPD-PAX6 returns to very low levels in endocrine-committed cells, permitting migration arrest and resumption of proliferation in response to pro-proliferative cues provided by stromal cells, leading to the formation of islet cell clusters. We suggest that regulation of such ΔPD-PAX6-driven functions, reliant on cell-cell interactions with M2 macrophages and exquisitely sensitive to gene dosage, provides a novel mechanism explaining how cell cycle withdrawal and initiation of cell migration may be functional linked and coordinated in epithelial cells committed to leave ductal progenitor pools.

Bars represent means ± SEM of n = 3 sorting experiments using G3LC cells and n = 1 experiment using SU.86 cells, with each experiment run in triplicate samples.

Figure S3 Transduction of ΔPD-PAX6 in epithelial lines. Western blotting analysis of detergent lysates from HEK-293T and G3LC cells, transduced with empty (mock) or ΔPD-PAX6 expressing lenti-vectors. Blots were probed with either anti-PAX6 antibody or anti-beta actin antibody, as loading control. In both lines, expression of a 32 kDa PAX6 isoform is detectable in nuclear and cytoplasmic lysates. The G3LC line also expresses endogenous paired PAX6 variants (PD-PAX6).

Figure S4 Expression pattern of $p27^{Kip}$ in grafts of embryonic pancreatic epithelium. Tissue sections of E14–15.5 pancreatic epithelial grafts transplanted in BM-reconstituted WT mice (upper panels) or Id1+/−Id3−/− mice (lower panels), stained by two-color immuno-fluorescence for $p27^{Kip}$ (green) and DAPI (blue). Dotted lines delineate boundaries of islet-like cell clusters. Grafts from WT hosts exhibit a predominant cytoplasmic localization of $p27^{Kip}$, whereas grafts from Id1+/−Id3−/− mice reveal both cytoplasmic and nuclear localizations (arrowheads). Scale bar in middle panels = 30 µm; Scale bar in right panels = 5 µm.

Figure S5 Transduction of ΔPD-PAX6 in pancreatic ductal lines results in the expression of islet lineage phenotypes. PCR analysis of the indicated transcripts expressed in Mock (Ctrl), ΔPD-PAX6^{High}, and ΔPD-PAX6^{Low} G3LC and SU.86 lines. A cDNA prepared from human fetal pancreas (Hu-PANC) was used as a positive control. Representative of n = 2 experiments.

Acknowledgments

We are grateful to Drs. René Le Boeuf, John Scott, Michael Schwartz (University of Washington), Lori Sussel (Columbia University), and Chris Rhodes (University of Chicago) for insightful discussions and comments on the manuscript.

Author Contributions

Conceived and designed the experiments: LC. Performed the experiments: KM AT AG A.J.J-C VC LC. Analyzed the data: LC. Contributed reagents/materials/analysis tools: LC VC. Wrote the paper: LC. Responsible for animal breeding, and performed experiments of molecular and cellular biology: LM.

References

1. Stappenbeck TS, Miyoshi H (2009) The role of stromal stem cells in tissue regeneration and wound repair. Science 324: 1666–1669.
2. Morris L, Graham CF, Gordon S (1991) Macrophages in haemopoietic and other tissues of the developing mouse detected by the monoclonal antibody F4/80. Development 112: 517–526.

3. Pollard JW (2009) Trophic macrophages in development and disease. Nat Rev Immunol 9: 259–270.
4. Dai XM, Ryan GR, Hapel AJ, Dominguez MG, Russell RG, et al. (2002) Targeted disruption of the mouse colony-stimulating factor 1 receptor gene results in osteopetrosis, mononuclear phagocyte deficiency, increased primitive progenitor cell frequencies, and reproductive defects. Blood 99: 111–120.
5. Michaelson MD, Bieri PL, Mehler MF, Xu H, Arezzo JC, et al. (1996) CSF-1 deficiency in mice results in abnormal brain development. Development 122: 2661–2672.
6. Van Nguyen A, Pollard JW (2002) Colony stimulating factor-1 is required to recruit macrophages into the mammary gland to facilitate mammary ductal outgrowth. Dev Biol 247: 11–25.
7. Wiktor-Jedrzejczak W, Bartocci A, Ferrante AW Jr, Ahmed-Ansari A, Sell KW, et al. (1990) Total absence of colony-stimulating factor 1 in the macrophage-deficient osteopetrotic (op/op) mouse. Proc Natl Acad Sci U S A 87: 4828–4832.
8. Abe S, Boyer C, Liu X, Wen FQ, Kobayashi T, et al. (2004) Cells derived from the circulation contribute to the repair of lung injury. Am J Respir Crit Care Med 170: 1158–1163.
9. Boulter L, Govaere O, Bird TG, Radulescu S, Ramachandran P, et al. (2012) Macrophage-derived Wnt opposes Notch signaling to specify hepatic progenitor cell fate in chronic liver disease. Nat Med 18: 572–579.
10. Lee S, Huen S, Nishio H, Nishio S, Lee HK, et al. (2011) Distinct macrophage phenotypes contribute to kidney injury and repair. J Am Soc Nephrol 22: 317–326.
11. Pull SL, Doherty JM, Mills JC, Gordon JI, Stappenbeck TS (2005) Activated macrophages are an adaptive element of the colonic epithelial progenitor niche necessary for regenerative responses to injury. Proc Natl Acad Sci U S A 102: 99–104.
12. Saclier M, Yacoub-Youssef H, Mackey AL, Arnold L, Ardjoune H, et al. (2013) Differentially activated macrophages orchestrate myogenic precursor cell fate during human skeletal muscle regeneration. Stem Cells 31: 384–396.
13. Zhang MZ, Yao B, Yang S, Jiang L, Wang S, et al. (2012) CSF-1 signaling mediates recovery from acute kidney injury. J Clin Invest 122: 4519–4532.
14. Henson PM, Hume DA (2006) Apoptotic cell removal in development and tissue homeostasis. Trends Immunol 27: 244–250.
15. Fantin A, Vieira JM, Gestri G, Denti L, Schwarz Q, et al. (2010) Tissue macrophages act as cellular chaperones for vascular anastomosis downstream of VEGF-mediated endothelial tip cell induction. Blood 116: 829–840.
16. Rao S, Lobov IB, Vallance JE, Tsujikawa K, Shiojima I, et al. (2007) Obligatory participation of macrophages in an angiopoietin 2-mediated cell death switch. Development 134: 4449–4458.
17. Stefater JA 3rd, Lewkowich I, Rao S, Mariggi G, Carpenter AC, et al. (2011) Regulation of angiogenesis by a non-canonical Wnt-Flt1 pathway in myeloid cells. Nature 474: 511–515.
18. Condeelis J, Pollard JW (2006) Macrophages: obligate partners for tumor cell migration, invasion, and metastasis. Cell 124: 263–266.
19. Arda HE, Benitez CM, Kim SK (2013) Gene regulatory networks governing pancreas development. Dev Cell 25: 5–13.
20. Oliver-Krasinski JM, Stoffers DA (2008) On the origin of the beta cell. Genes Dev 22: 1998–2021.
21. Pan FC, Wright C (2011) Pancreas organogenesis: from bud to plexus to gland. Dev Dyn 240: 530–565.
22. Gittes GK, Galante PE, Hanahan D, Rutter WJ, Debase HT (1996) Lineage-specific morphogenesis in the developing pancreas: role of mesenchymal factors. Development 122: 439–447.
23. Miralles F, Czernichow P, Scharfmann R (1998) Follistatin regulates the relative proportions of endocrine versus exocrine tissue during pancreatic development. Development 125: 1017–1024.
24. Landsman L, Nijagal A, Whitchurch TJ, Vanderlaan RL, Zimmer WE, et al. (2011) Pancreatic mesenchyme regulates epithelial organogenesis throughout development. PLoS Biol 9: e1001143.
25. Banaei-Bouchareb L, Gouon-Evans V, Samara-Boustani D, Castellotti MC, Czernichow P, et al. (2004) Insulin cell mass is altered in Csf1op/Csf1op macrophage-deficient mice. J Leukoc Biol 76: 359–367.
26. Geutskens SB, Otonkoski T, Pulkkinen MA, Drexhage HA, Leenen PJ (2005) Macrophages in the murine pancreas and their involvement in fetal endocrine development in vitro. J Leukoc Biol 78: 845–852.
27. Sica A, Mantovani A (2012) Macrophage plasticity and polarization: in vivo veritas. J Clin Invest 122: 787–795.
28. Gordon S (2003) Alternative activation of macrophages. Nat Rev Immunol 3: 23–35.
29. Martinez FO, Gordon S, Locati M, Mantovani A (2006) Transcriptional profiling of the human monocyte-to-macrophage differentiation and polarization: new molecules and patterns of gene expression. J Immunol 177: 7303–7311.
30. Rae F, Woods K, Sasmono T, Campanale N, Taylor D, et al. (2007) Characterisation and trophic functions of murine embryonic macrophages based upon the use of a Csf1r-EGFP transgene reporter. Dev Biol 308: 232–246.
31. Miller R, Cirulli V, Diaferia GR, Ninniri S, Hardiman G, et al. (2008) Switching-on survival and repair response programs in islet transplants by bone marrow-derived vasculogenic cells. Diabetes 57: 2402–2412.
32. Lyden D, Hattori K, Dias S, Costa C, Blaikie P, et al. (2001) Impaired recruitment of bone-marrow-derived endothelial and hematopoietic precursor cells blocks tumor angiogenesis and growth. Nat Med 7: 1194–1201.
33. Lyden D, Young AZ, Zagzag D, Yan W, Gerald W, et al. (1999) Id1 and Id3 are required for neurogenesis, angiogenesis and vascularization of tumour xenografts. Nature 401: 670–677.
34. Cirulli V, Zalatan J, McMaster M, Prinsen R, Salomon DR, et al. (2006) The class I HLA repertoire of pancreatic islets comprises the nonclassical class Ib antigen HLA-G. Diabetes 55: 1214–1222.
35. Langley OK, Aletsee MC, Gratzl M (1987) Endocrine cells share expression of N-CAM with neurones. FEBS Lett 220: 108–112.
36. Mayerhofer A, Lahr G, Gratzl M (1991) Expression of the neural cell adhesion molecule in endocrine cells of the ovary. Endocrinology 129: 792–800.
37. Gu D, Sarvetnick N (1993) Epithelial cell proliferation and islet neogenesis in IFN-γ transgenic mice. Development 118: 33–46.
38. Kritzik MR, Jones E, Chen Z, Krakowski M, Krahl T, et al. (1999) PDX-1 and Msx-2 expression in the regenerating and developing pancreas. J Endocrinol 163: 523–530.
39. Kritzik MR, Krahl T, Good A, Krakowski M, St-Onge L, et al. (2000) Transcription factor expression during pancreatic islet regeneration. Mol Cell Endocrinol 164: 99–107.
40. Song SY, Gannon M, Washington MK, Scoggins CR, Meszoely IM, et al. (1999) Expansion of Pdx1-expressing pancreatic epithelium and islet neogenesis in transgenic mice overexpressing transforming growth factor alpha. Gastroenterology 117: 1416–1426.
41. Wang TC, Bonner-Weir S, Oates PS, Chulak M, Simon B, et al. (1993) Pancreatic gastrin stimulates islet differentiation of transforming growth factor alpha-induced ductular precursor cells. J Clin Invest 92: 1349–1356.
42. Xu X, D'Hoker J, Stange G, Bonne S, De Leu N, et al. (2008) Beta cells can be generated from endogenous progenitors in injured adult mouse pancreas. Cell 132: 197–207.
43. Hirsch MR, Valarche I, Deagostini-Bazin H, Pernelle C, Joliot A, et al. (1991) An upstream regulatory element of the NCAM promoter contains a binding site for homeodomains. FEBS Lett 287: 197–202.
44. Holst BD, Wang Y, Jones FS, Edelman GM (1997) A binding site for Pax proteins regulates expression of the gene for the neural cell adhesion molecule in the embryonic spinal cord. Proc Natl Acad Sci U S A 94: 1465–1470.
45. Ashery-Padan R, Zhou X, Marquardt T, Herrera P, Toube L, et al. (2004) Conditional inactivation of Pax6 in the pancreas causes early onset of diabetes. Dev Biol 269: 479–488.
46. Dohrmann C, Gruss P, Lemaire L (2000) Pax genes and the differentiation of hormone-producing endocrine cells in the pancreas. Mech Dev 92: 47–54.
47. St-Onge L, Sosa-Pineda B, Chowdhury K, Mansouri A, Gruss P (1997) Pax6 is required for differentiation of glucagon-producing alpha-cells in mouse pancreas. Nature 387: 406–409.
48. Verbruggen V, Ek O, Georlette D, Delporte F, Von Berg V, et al. (2010) The Pax6b homeodomain is dispensable for pancreatic endocrine cell differentiation in zebrafish. J Biol Chem 285: 13863–13873.
49. Czerny T, Schaffner G, Busslinger M (1993) DNA sequence recognition by Pax proteins: bipartite structure of the paired domain and its binding site. Genes Dev 7: 2048–2061.
50. Epstein JA, Glaser T, Cai J, Jepeal L, Walton DS, et al. (1994) Two independent and interactive DNA-binding subdomains of the Pax6 paired domain are regulated by alternative splicing. Genes Dev 8: 2022–2034.
51. Kim J, Lauderdale JD (2006) Analysis of Pax6 expression using a BAC transgene reveals the presence of a paired-less isoform of Pax6 in the eye and olfactory bulb. Dev Biol 292: 486–505.
52. Mishra R, Gorlov IP, Chao LY, Singh S, Saunders GF (2002) PAX6, paired domain influences sequence recognition by the homeodomain. J Biol Chem 277: 49488–49494.
53. Turque N, Plaza S, Radvanyi F, Carriere C, Saule S (1994) Pax-QNR/Pax-6, a paired box- and homeobox-containing gene expressed in neurons, is also expressed in pancreatic endocrine cells. Mol Endocrinol 8: 929–938.
54. Lynn FC, Smith SB, Wilson ME, Yang KY, Nekrep N, et al. (2007) Sox9 coordinates a transcriptional network in pancreatic progenitor cells. Proc Natl Acad Sci U S A 104: 10500–10505.
55. Seymour PA, Freude KK, Tran MN, Mayes EE, Jensen J, et al. (2007) SOX9 is required for maintenance of the pancreatic progenitor cell pool. Proc Natl Acad Sci U S A 104: 1865–1870.
56. Edelman GM, Jones FS (1998) Gene regulation of cell adhesion: a key step in neural morphogenesis. Brain Res Brain Res Rev 26: 337–352.
57. Francavilla C, Cattaneo P, Berezin V, Bock E, Ami D, et al. (2009) The binding of NCAM to FGFR1 induces a specific cellular response mediated by receptor trafficking. J Cell Biol 187: 1101–1116.
58. Lehembre F, Yilmaz M, Wicki A, Schomber T, Strittmatter K, et al. (2008) NCAM-induced focal adhesion assembly: a functional switch upon loss of E-cadherin. EMBO J 27: 2603–2615.
59. Doyle MJ, Sussel L (2007) Nkx2.2 regulates beta-cell function in the mature islet. Diabetes 56: 1999–2007.
60. Guo S, Dai C, Guo M, Taylor B, Harmon JS, et al. (2013) Inactivation of specific beta cell transcription factors in type 2 diabetes. J Clin Invest.
61. Hart AW, Mella S, Mendrychowski J, van Heyningen V, Kleinjan DA (2013) The developmental regulator Pax6 is essential for maintenance of islet cell function in the adult mouse pancreas. PLoS One 8: e54173.
62. Papizan JB, Singer RA, Tschen SI, Dhawan S, Friel JM, et al. (2011) Nkx2.2 repressor complex regulates islet beta-cell specification and prevents beta-to-alpha-cell reprogramming. Genes Dev 25: 2291–2305.

63. Schaffer AE, Taylor BL, Benthuysen JR, Liu J, Thorel F, et al. (2013) Nkx6.1 controls a gene regulatory network required for establishing and maintaining pancreatic Beta cell identity. PLoS Genet 9: e1003274.
64. Sosa-Pineda B, Chowdhury K, Torres M, Oliver G, Gruss P (1997) The Pax4 gene is essential for differentiation of insulin-producing beta cells in the mammalian pancreas. Nature 386: 399–402.
65. Taylor BL, Liu FF, Sander M (2013) Nkx6.1 is essential for maintaining the functional state of pancreatic beta cells. Cell Rep 4: 1262–1275.
66. Carriere C, Plaza S, Martin P, Quatannens B, Bailly M, et al. (1993) Characterization of quail Pax-6 (Pax-QNR) proteins expressed in the neuroretina. Mol Cell Biol 13: 7257–7266.
67. Kleinjan DA, Seawright A, Childs AJ, van Heyningen V (2004) Conserved elements in Pax6 intron 7 involved in (auto)regulation and alternative transcription. Dev Biol 265: 462–477.
68. Kim J, Lauderdale JD (2008) Overexpression of pairedless Pax6 in the retina disrupts corneal development and affects lens cell survival. Dev Biol 313: 434–454.
69. Sander M, Neubuser A, Kalamaras J, Ee HC, Martin GR, et al. (1997) Genetic analysis reveals that PAX6 is required for normal transcription of pancreatic hormone genes and islet development. Genes Dev 11: 1662–1673.
70. Bonner-Weir S, Toschi E, Inada A, Reitz P, Fonseca SY, et al. (2004) The pancreatic ductal epithelium serves as a potential pool of progenitor cells. Pediatr Diabetes 5 Suppl 2: 16–22.
71. Bruun JA, Thomassen EI, Kristiansen K, Tylden G, Holm T, et al. (2005) The third helix of the homeodomain of paired class homeodomain proteins acts as a recognition helix both for DNA and protein interactions. Nucleic Acids Res 33: 2661–2675.
72. Cvekl A, Kashanchi F, Brady JN, Piatigorsky J (1999) Pax-6 interactions with TATA-box-binding protein and retinoblastoma protein. Invest Ophthalmol Vis Sci 40: 1343–1350.
73. Mikkola I, Bruun JA, Holm T, Johansen T (2001) Superactivation of Pax6-mediated transactivation from paired domain-binding sites by dna-independent recruitment of different homeodomain proteins. J Biol Chem 276: 4109–4118.
74. Yan Q, Gong L, Deng M, Zhang L, Sun S, et al. (2010) Sumoylation activates the transcriptional activity of Pax-6, an important transcription factor for eye and brain development. Proc Natl Acad Sci U S A 107: 21034–21039.
75. Mascarenhas JB, Young KP, Littlejohn EL, Yoo BK, Salgia R, et al. (2009) PAX6 is expressed in pancreatic cancer and actively participates in cancer progression through activation of the MET tyrosine kinase receptor gene. J Biol Chem 284: 27524–27532.
76. Tyas DA, Pearson H, Rashbass P, Price DJ (2003) Pax6 regulates cell adhesion during cortical development. Cereb Cortex 13: 612–619.
77. Hsieh YW, Yang XJ (2009) Dynamic Pax6 expression during the neurogenic cell cycle influences proliferation and cell fate choices of retinal progenitors. Neural Dev 4: 32.
78. Robson EJ, He SJ, Eccles MR (2006) A PANorama of PAX genes in cancer and development. Nat Rev Cancer 6: 52–62.
79. Georgia S, Bhushan A (2006) p27 Regulates the transition of beta-cells from quiescence to proliferation. Diabetes 55: 2950–2956.
80. Rachdi L, Balcazar N, Elghazi L, Barker DJ, Krits I, et al. (2006) Differential effects of p27 in regulation of beta-cell mass during development, neonatal period, and adult life. Diabetes 55: 3520–3528.
81. Hebrok M (2012) Generating beta cells from stem cells-the story so far. Cold Spring Harb Perspect Med 2: a007674.
82. Otonkoski T, Gao R, Lundin K (2005) Stem cells in the treatment of diabetes. Ann Med 37: 513–520.
83. Pagliuca FW, Melton DA (2013) How to make a functional beta-cell. Development 140: 2472–2483.

17

Tacrolimus Inhibits the Revascularization of Isolated Pancreatic Islets

Ryuichi Nishimura[1], Sho Nishioka[2], Ikuma Fujisawa[2], Hitoshi Shiku[2], Miki Shimada[3], Satoshi Sekiguchi[1], Keisei Fujimori[1], Akira Ushiyama[4], Tomokazu Matsue[5], Noriaki Ohuchi[1], Susumu Satomi[1], Masafumi Goto[1,6*]

1 Division of Advanced Surgical Science and Technology, Tohoku University, Sendai, Japan, **2** Graduate School of Environmental Studies, Tohoku University, Sendai, Japan, **3** Department of Pharmaceutical Sciences, Tohoku University Hospital, Sendai, Japan, **4** Department of Environmental Health, National Institute of Public Health, Wako, Japan, **5** WorldPremier InternationalResearch Center Initiative Advanced Institute for Materials Research, Tohoku University, Sendai, Japan, **6** New Industry Creation Hatchery Center, Tohoku University, Sendai, Japan

Abstract

Aims: Immunosuppressive drugs could be crucial factors for a poor outcome after islet allotransplantation. Unlike rapamycin, the effects of tacrolimus, the current standard immunosuppressant used in islet transplantation, on graft revascularization remain unclear. We examined the effects of tacrolimus on islet revascularization using a highly sensitive imaging system, and analyzed the gene expression in transplanted islets by introducing laser microdissection techniques.

Methods: Islets isolated from C57BL/6-Tg (CAG-EGFP) mice were transplanted into the nonmetallic dorsal skinfold chamber on the recipients. Balb/c athymic mice were used as recipients and were divided into two groups: including a control group (n = 9) and tacrolimus-treated group (n = 7). The changes in the newly-formed vessels surrounding the islet grafts were imaged and semi-quantified using multi-photon laser-scanning microscopy and a Volocity system. Gene expression in transplanted islets was analyzed by the BioMark dynamic system.

Results: The revascularization process was completed within 14 days after pancreatic islet transplantation at subcutaneous sites. The newly-formed vascular volume surrounding the transplanted islets in the tacrolimus-treated group was significantly less than that in the control group ($p<0.05$). Although the expression of *Vegfa* ($p<0.05$) and *Ccnd1* ($p<0.05$) was significantly upregulated in the tacrolimus-treated group compared with that of the control group, no differences were observed between the groups in terms of other types of gene expression.

Conclusions: The present study demonstrates that tacrolimus inhibits the revascularization of isolated pancreatic islets without affecting the characteristics of the transplanted grafts. Further refinements of this immunosuppressive regimen, especially regarding the revascularization of islet grafts, could improve the outcome of islet allotransplantation.

Editor: Kathrin Maedler, University of Bremen, Germany

Funding: This study has been supported by grants from the Japanese Grant-in-Aid for Scientific Research (B), the Takeda Science Foundation, the Mochida Memorial Foundation for Medical and Pharmaceutical Research, and the Japanese Ministry of Health, Welfare and Labor (20120101). The funders had no role in study design, data collection and analysis, decision to publish, or preparation of the manuscript.

Competing Interests: The authors have declared that no competing interests exist.

* E-mail: gotokichi@aol.com

Introduction

Pancreatic islet transplantation is an emerging and promising therapy for type 1 diabetes. However, at least two donor pancreata are needed to reverse hyperglycemia, and substantial number of islet grafts fail within 5 years [1]. Although several factors may contribute to a progressive decline in the function of islet transplants, the main reason for this problem is still uncertain. Pancreatic islet autotransplantation, despite the use of a lower beta-cell mass, shows good results and improves insulin-independence rates in comparison to the islet allotransplantation [2]. Pancreatic islet allografts are affected by various factors, including relatively long cold ischemia times before pancreatic islet isolation [3,4], the need for a purification procedure, and the use of immunosuppressive drugs to regulate the alloimmune responses to the islet grafts.

The inhibitory effects of rapamycin, a key component of the immunosuppressive regimen in the Edmonton protocol, on tumor angiogenesis or pancreatic islet revascularization have recently been clarified [5,6,7,8,9]. However, the inhibitory effects of tacrolimus, which is one of the standard immunosuppressants in both pancreatic islet transplantation and whole pancreas transplantation, on revascularization has been poorly studied, although Turgut et al. reported the prevention of corneal neovascularization by the systemic and topical administration of tacrolimus [10].

Therefore, this study sought to evaluate the effect of tacrolimus on the islet revascularization process using a highly sensitive imaging system combined with the dorsal skinfold chamber (DSC) technique and multi-photon laser-scanning microscopy (MPLSM). This new system enabled repeated observation of the time-dependent changes of islet grafts and surrounding vessels in identical animals without histological sectioning [11]. Spier et al. introduced the anterior chamber of the eye for monitoring revascularization of the islet grafts by using MPLSM [12,13]. Although the anterior chamber of the eye is a breakthrough model, it is not realistic for clinical application. In contrast, the subcutaneous space is an ideal site for islet transplantation due to the minimal invasion and easy access. The liver, which is the current standard transplant site, is often associated with procedure-related complications including hemorrhage, thrombosis, and the strong innate immune response such as the instant blood-mediated inflammatory reaction (IBMIR) [14,15], thus the current model could be a useful and practical tool to analyze the revascularization process of islet grafts.

Hence, the present study examined the effect of tacrolimus on islet revascularization using a highly sensitive imaging system. Furthermore, this study attempted to analyze the state of gene expression in transplanted islet grafts *per se* by introducing laser microdissection techniques.

Materials and Methods

Mouse models

All animals used in this study were handled in accordance with the Guide for the Care and Use of Laboratory Animals published by the National Institutes of Health [16]. The animal studies were approved by the Animal Care and Use Committee of the Tohoku University (approved protocol ID: 2011 NICHe-Animal-13). All surgeries were performed under anesthesia, and all efforts were made to minimize suffering. Male C57BL/6-Tg (CAG-EGFP) mice (9–12 weeks of age; Japan SLC Inc., Shizuoka, Japan) were used as islet donors.

The dorsal skinfold chamber (DSC), which is composed of polyacetal resin (generally known as Duracon; grade M90-44, Polyplastics Co.,Ltd., Tokyo, Japan) [17], was introduced into the recipient mice [11] (Fig. 1A). This nonmetallic chamber is approximately 40% lighter in weight than metallic chamber used traditionally, subjecting mice to less stress. DSC was implanted into male Balb/c nu/nu mice (8–12 weeks of age; Japan SLC Inc.). This model, unlike wild type Balb/c mice, allowed observation for a relatively long preservation period and also to focus on the influence of immunosuppressive chemicals on engraftment without any interference from the specific immune responses.

All animals were bred and maintained in a pathogen-free environment with free access to laboratory chow and water and exhibited no signs of discomfort.

Pancreatic islet isolation and culture

C57BL/6-Tg (CAG-EGFP) mice were anesthetized with the inhalation of isoflurane (Abbott Japan Co., Ltd., Tokyo, Japan). The bile duct was identified and clamped at the papilla Vateri. Four milliliters of cold Hank's balanced salt solution (HBSS) containing 1 g/L collagenase (Sigma type V; Sigma Chemicals, St. Louis, MO, USA) was injected into the common bile duct leading to the pancreas under a stereomicroscope. The pancreas was removed and incubated in a water bath at 37°C for 16 min. The pancreas was digested, the cell suspension was washed two times in HBSS and centrifuged for 1 min. Density-gradient centrifugation was performed for 10 min using Histopaque-1119 (Sigma Diagnostics, St. Louis, MO, USA) and Lymphoprep^{TM} (Nycomed Pharma AS, Oslo, Norway) to isolate pancreatic islets. The islets were cultured in RPMI-1640 containing 5.5 mmol/L glucose and 10% fetal bovine serum at 37°C in 5% CO_2 and humidified air for approximately 3 hours before examination.

Islet transplantation into the dorsal skinfold chamber

Balb/c nu/nu mice underwent islet transplantation into the DSC under isoflurane (Abbott Japan Co., Ltd.) anesthesia. Two to ten of isolated islets were transplanted into each DSC by means of the hand-picking method. The space between skin flap and the cover glass was filled with saline to remove air bubbles. The recovery rate of the grafts at the end of the observation period was almost same between the tacrolimus and control groups.

Experimental groups

The recipient mice with transplanted pancreatic islets were divided into two groups: the control group (n = 9) and the tacrolimus (Astellas, Deerfield, IL)-treated group (0.5 mg/kg/day; n = 7, two of seven islets were observed up to 11 days after transplantation due to technical trouble of DSC.) [18]. Tacrolimus was administered to mice via subcutaneous implanted MICRO-OSMOTIC PUMP (Model 1002, Alzet, Cupertino, CA) for 14 days. The control mice were also implanted with a MICRO-OSMOTIC PUMP and treated with vehicle.

Measurement of tacrolimus concentrations in the whole blood

Blood samples were obtained via the inferior vena cava at 7 days after the initial administration of tacrolimus. Blood samples were stored at −80°C until use. Tacrolimus concentrations in the whole blood were measured by using Dimension TACRO (Siemens Healthcare Diagnostics, Inc., Newark, DE, USA).

In vivo imaging of islets transplanted into the dorsal skinfold chamber

A 0.1 mL sample of Texas Red (10 mg/mL; Invitrogen, Leek, The Netherlands) was injected intravenously via the tail vein. The mice were anesthetized using the inhalation of isoflurane and then were positioned in an acrylic resin tube with an inner diameter of 26 mm. The tube was fixed on an acrylic resin plate and then placed on the microscope stage (Fig. 1B). A multiphoton laser-scanning microscope (MPLSM; FluoView FV1000MPE; OLYMPUS, Tokyo, Japan) equipped with water-dipping lenses (OLYMPUS XLPLN25XWMP NA1.05; OLYMPUS) was used to image the transplanted islet grafts. Distilled water was used as immersion liquid. MPLSM imaging was performed under the minimum required laser-power and scan-time necessary. No signs of photo-damage in islet cells or blood vessels were observed throughout the whole study. I processed images and measured newly-formed vascular volume surrounding the islets using a Volocity 3D system (PerkinElmer, Waltham, MA, USA) to evaluate islet revascularization. The newly-formed vascular volume surrounding the islets at each time point was calculated by the increasing rate against day 1 after transplantation. GFP and Texas Red were excited at 890 nm and separated and collected emission light onto two non-descanned detectors using a dichroic mirror (FV10-MRG/R:DM570) and emission filters (FV10-MRG/R:BA495-540HQ and BA575-630) [12,13].

Laser microdissection

The samples were divided into three groups: 1) islets before transplantation(n = 6), 2) islets in the control group(n = 6), 3) islets in the tacrolimus-treated group(n = 6). Tissues containing pancreatic islets, except for pancreatic islets before transplantation,

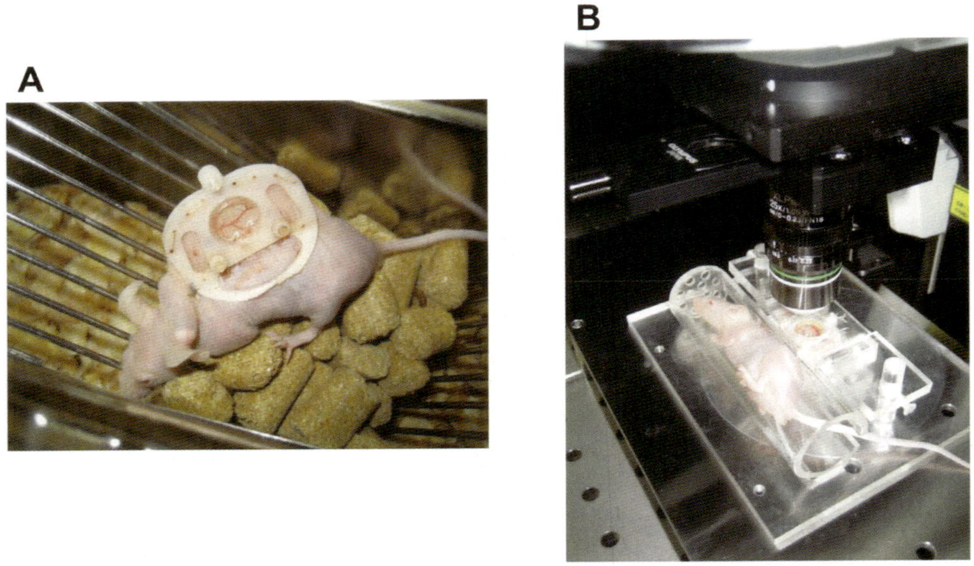

Figure 1. Mice bearing the dorsal skinfold chamber (A). Mice during microscopic observation (B). The mice were positioned in an acrylic resin tube during microscopic observation. The tube was fixed on an acrylic resin plate and then placed on the microscope stage.

were harvested at 7 days after transplantation, frozen with liquid nitrogen and stored at −80°C until use. Ten µm frozen sections were prepared from each of these samples. Frozen prepared sections were fixed with acetone for 30 seconds, and then dehydrated and air dried immediately before performing laser microdissection (LMD). LMD was performed using LMD 7000 (Leica, Bensheim, Germany). The cell lysate was added, and the tube containing the micro-dissected islets was frozen with liquid nitrogen and stored at −80°C.

Quantitative real-time PCR analysis

The total RNA was extracted using the RNeasy Micro Kit (Qiagen, Tokyo, Japan) according to the manufacturer's protocol. The reverse transcription reaction was carried out to synthesize first strand cDNA according to the protocols for the QuantiTect Reverse Transcription kit (Qiagen) at 42°C for 30 min (RT reaction) followed by 95°C for 3 min (deactivation of RTase). The synthesized cDNA samples were stored at −30°C.

Gene expression was analyzed using the BioMark 48.48 dynamic gene expression system (Fluidigm, South San Francisco, CA, USA). Preamplified cDNA was diluted with RNase-free water (1:5) and used for quantitative PCR array analysis. A total of 33 genes were analyzed by the use of BioMark Real-Time PCR Analysis Software Version 2.0 (Fluidigm; Table S1). Actin, cytoplasmic 1 (Beta-actin) (*Actb*) was used as housekeeping gene.

Statistical analyses

All data are expressed as the means ± SEM. Statistical significance was determined using Student's *t*-test, or a one- and two-factor analysis of variance (ANOVA). The Bonferroni correction was used as a post-hoc test when the data were determined to be significant by ANOVA. *P* values less than 0.05 was considered to be significant.

Results

The time-dependent changes of newly-formed vascular volume surrounding the islets

Capillary sprout formation made an appearance at 4 days after transplantation, and these sprouts were interconnected at day 7. The newly-formed microvascular network gradually got bigger. The newly-formed vascular volume surrounding the islet grafts increased until Day 14, and subsequently reached a growth plateau (Figs. 2 and 3).

Tacrolimus concentrations in the whole blood

The blood concentrations of tacrolimus in the tacrolimus-treated group were 7.9±0.4 ng/mL (n = 6).

Inhibition of islet revascularization by administration of tacrolimus

The newly-formed vascular volume surrounding the transplanted islets in the tacrolimus-treated group was less than that in the control group (Fig. 3, $p<0.05$; Fig. 4). The increasing rate of newly-formed vascular volume surrounding the islets on day 14 was also significantly higher in the control group than in the tacrolimus-treated group ($p<0.05$; Fig. 5). The blood glucose levels in tacrolimus-treated group were maintained normoglycemic during the whole study period.

The time-dependent changes of islet graft volume

The islet graft volume was almost identical throughout the whole study period in both groups (Fig. 6).

Gene expression in the transplanted islets

The expression of 33 genes related to inflammation, metabolism, cell cycle, and angiogenesis in the transplanted islets was analyzed. In comparison to the islets before transplantation, the expression of vascular endothelial growth factor A (*Vegfa*) ($p<0.01$), mitogen-activated protein kinase 14 (*Mapk14*) ($p<0.05$), tissue factor (*F3*) ($p<0.01$), G1/S-specific cyclin-D1 (*Ccnd1*), and cell

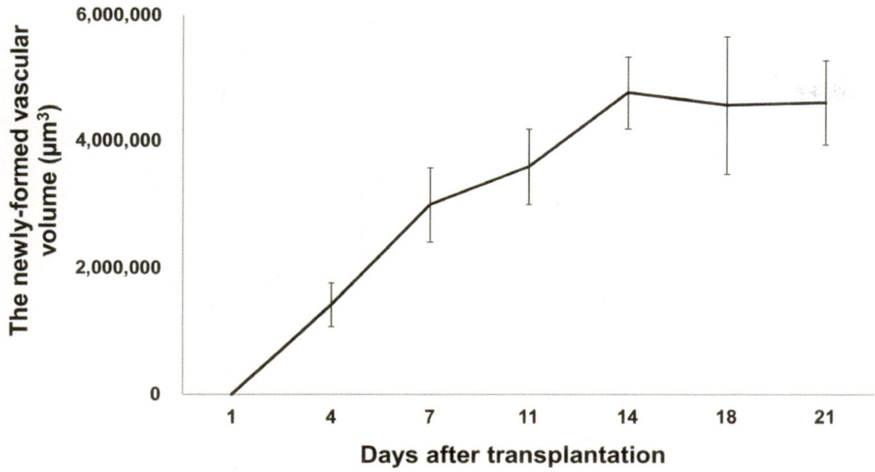

Figure 2. The time-dependent changes of newly-formed vascular volume for the transplanted pancreatic islets. Newly-formed vascular volume surrounding the islets at 4, 7, 11, 14, 18, and 21 days after transplantation was measured by using a Volocity system. All values are expressed as the means ± SEM.

division protein kinase 4 (*Cdk4*) ($p<0.01$) was suppressed in the transplanted islet grafts (control group) (Fig. 6). In contrast, the expression of matrix metalloproteinase-14 (*Mmp14*) ($p<0.01$) was upregulated in the transplanted islet grafts. Although the expression of *Vegfa* ($p<0.05$) and Ccnd1 ($p<0.05$) was significantly upregulated in the tacrolimus-treated group compared with that of the control group, no differences were observed between the tacrolimus-treated and control groups in terms of other types of gene expression (Fig. 7).

Discussion

The outcome of islet allotransplantation is still far inferior to that of islet autotransplantation [2], despite the recent dramatic technical progress in the isolation of islets [3,19,20,21]. Although several factors might contribute to this issue, the use of immunosuppressive drugs in islet allotransplantation could be one of the crucial factors. Tacrolimus is thought to have only marginal adverse effects on islet grafts, and consequently is used as the standard drug in both pancreatic islet and whole pancreas transplantation [22,23]. Unlike whole pancreas transplantation, islet grafts are rendered avascular after enzymatic isolation and must become revascularized after pancreatic islet transplantation. However, the effects of tacrolimus on revascularization have been poorly studied. Therefore, the current study investigated the effect of tacrolimus on islet revascularization using a highly sensitive imaging system and found, for the first time, that tacrolimus substantially abrogates revascularization of transplanted islet grafts.

The present study introduced a highly sensitive imaging system by combining the DSC technique and MPLSM in order to observe the time-dependent changes of newly-formed vessels surrounding the islet grafts [11]. This system allowed the

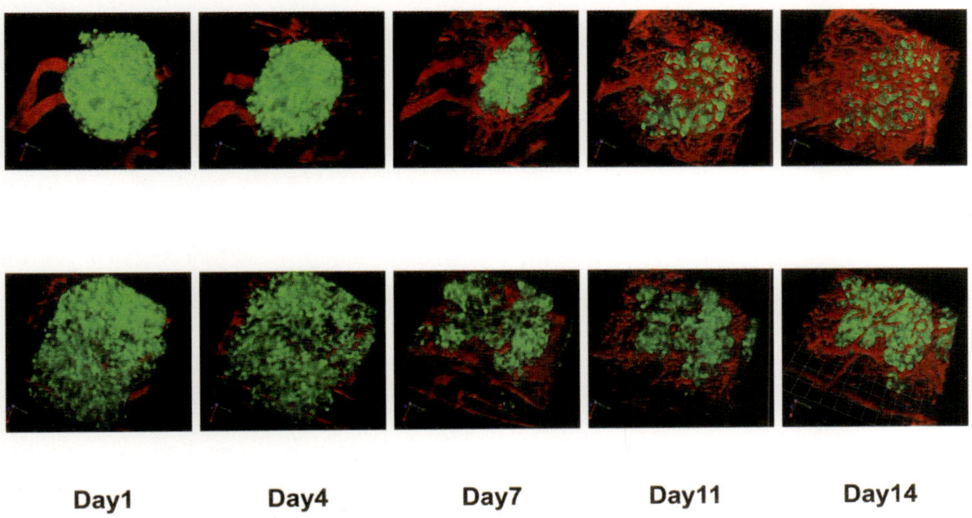

Figure 3. Imaging of the transplanted islets and surrounding blood vessels. Overlay of GFP fluorescence (pancreatic islets) and Texas Red fluorescence (blood vessels). Upper row: islets in the control group, Lower row: islets in the tacrolimus-treated group. GFP and Texas Red were excited at 890 nm. The scale bar indicated 51.0 μm/unit.

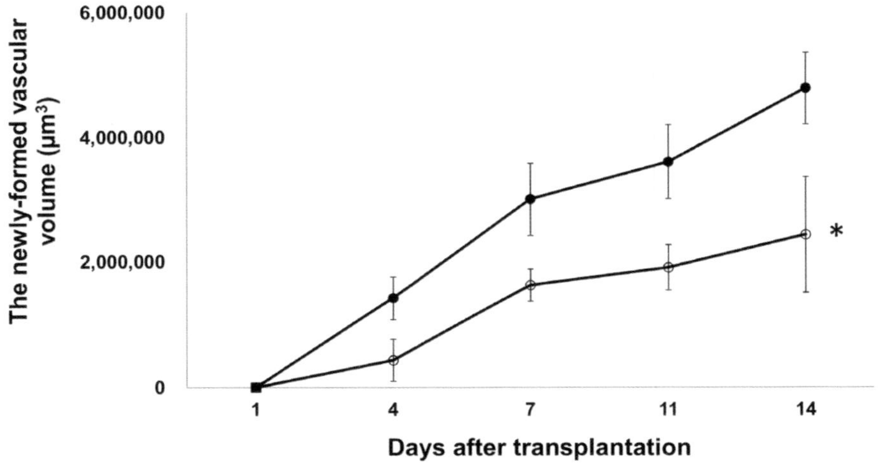

Figure 4. The time-dependent changes of newly-formed vascular volume surrounding the transplanted islets with and without tacrolimus. The newly-formed vascular volume in the control group (closed circles) and the tacrolimus-treated group (open circles). All values are expressed as the means ± SEM. *P<0.05 in comparison to the control group.

observation of the same islet grafts repetitively in identical recipient animals without histological sectioning. Moreover, the use of athymic mice as recipients allowed the revascularization process to be monitored for a longer observation period. This system demonstrated that the revascularization process is completed within 14 days after pancreatic islet transplantation. This finding is consistent with several previous reports [24,25,26,27,28,29] performed by histological sectioning, thus indicating that this observation is accurate and also the established system was confirmed to be a useful tool to analyze the revascularization process of pancreatic islets.

This study further introduced the laser microdissection technique followed by real-time polymerase chain reaction (PCR) assay to analyze the state of gene expression in transplanted islet grafts *per se*. These combined methods using the highly sensitive imaging system and the laser microdissection technique together with real-time PCR assay allowed the simultaneous evaluation of the effect of immunosuppressive drugs not only on the revascularization process but also on the islet grafts *per se*. Notably, this elegant system could also be applicable for studying the angiogenesis and the engraftment in cancer cells and various stem cells.

The expression of *Vegfa*, *Mapk14*, *F3*, *Ccnd1* and *Cdk4* was suppressed in the islets transplanted without tacrolimus, in comparison to the islets prior to transplantation. However, unexpectedly, no difference was seen in hypoxia-inducible

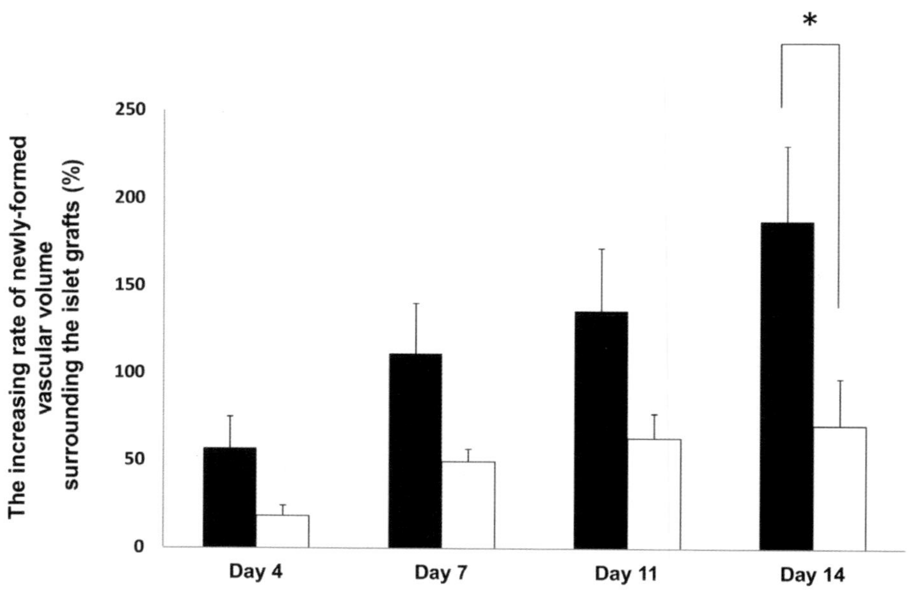

Figure 5. The increasing rate of newly-formed vascular volume surrounding the transplanted islets with and without tacrolimus. The increasing rate (against day 1) of newly-formed vascular volume surrounding the islets at 4, 7, 11, and 14 days after transplantation in the control group (black bar) and the tacrolimus-treated group (white bar) was calculated. All values are expressed as the means ± SEM. *P<0.05 in comparison to the control group.

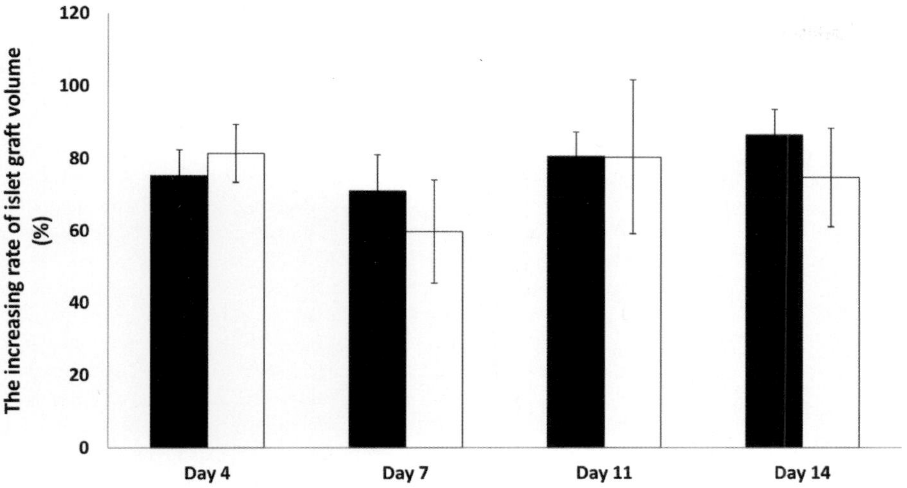

Figure 6. The increasing rate of islet graft volume with and without tacrolimus. The increasing rate (against day 1) of islet graft volume at 4, 7, 11, and 14 days after transplantation in the control group (black bar: n = 9) and the tacrolimus-treated group (white bar: n = 4) was calculated. All values are expressed as the means ± SEM.

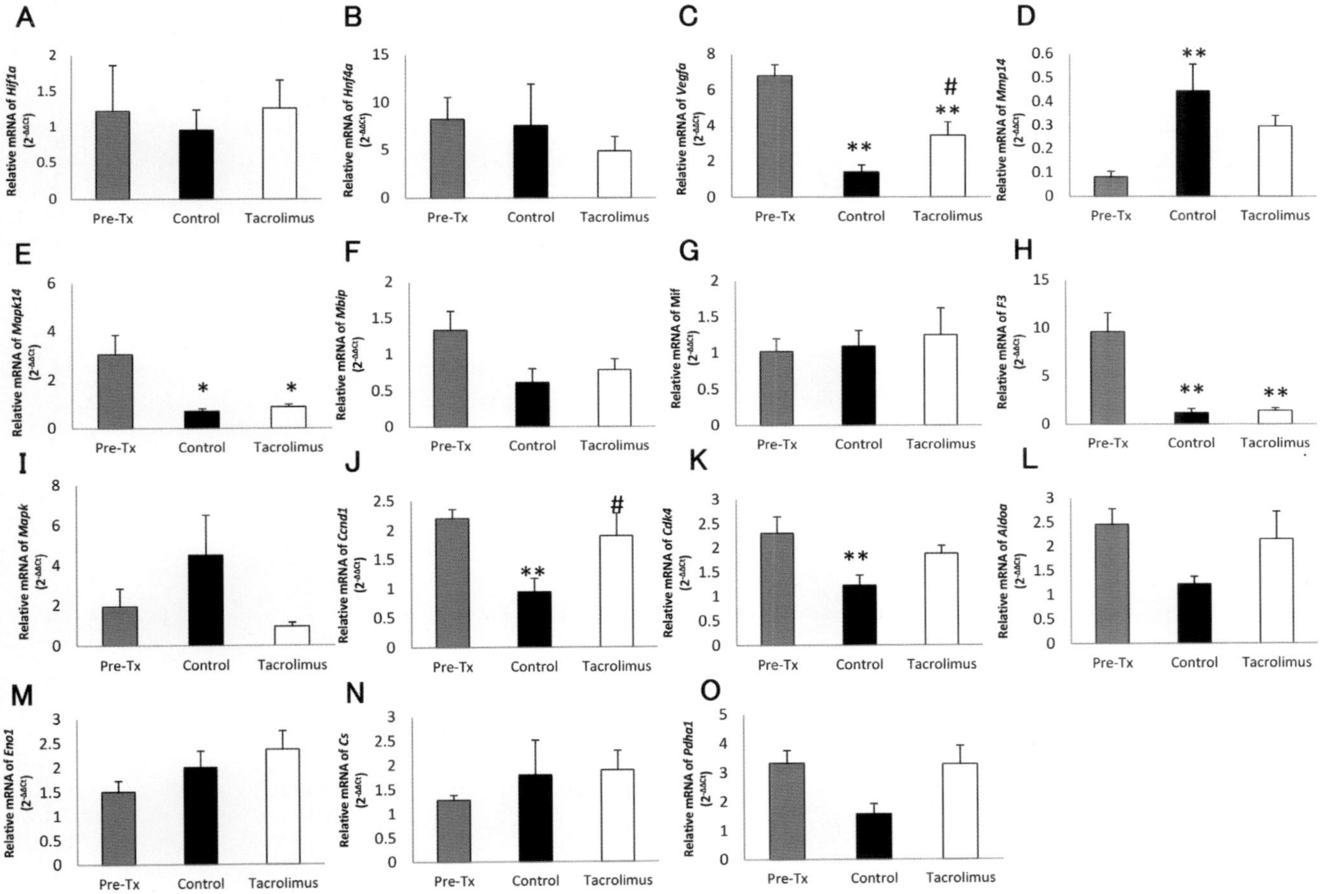

Figure 7. Relative gene expression in the transplanted pancreatic islets with and without tacrolimus. Relative gene expression of *Hif1a* (A), *Hnf4a* (B), *Vegfa* (C), *Mmp14* (D), *Mapk* (E), *Mbip* (F), *Mif* (G), *F3* (H),*Il1b* (I), *Ccnd1* (J), *Cdk4* (K), *AldoA* (L), *Eno1* (M), *Cs* (N), and *Pdha1* (O) in islets before transplantation (gray bar), the control group (black bar), and the tacrolimus-treated group (white bar). The values in the control and tacrolimus treated-group were represented as the ratio to the values in islets before transplantation. *P<0.05 in comparison to the islets before transplantation, **P<0.01 in comparison to the islets before transplantation, and #P<0.05 in comparison to the control group.

factor-1α (*Hif1a*) which is induced by hypoxia. These data suggest that the subcutaneous space might not be as hypoxic as expected. One possible explanation is that only revascularized islets survived and were observed in the present study. Another possible explanation is that only a few islets were transplanted into the DSC, and thus there were enough spaces for angiogenesis surrounding the islet grafts.

The islets transplanted with tacrolimus showed a significantly different expression of *Vegfa* and ccnd1 in comparison to the islets transplanted without tacrolimus, but no differences were observed between the tacrolimus-treated and control groups in terms of other gene expression. Since the expression of *Vegfa*, which is a major stimulator of revascularization by inducing proliferation and migration of endothelial cells and tube formation [30,31,32], was upregulated, it could be speculated that a stimulator of revascularization such as transforming growth factor-β1 and macrophage-colony stimulating factor was released from transplanted islets in response to inhibition of revascularization induced by tacrolimus. However, *Mmp14*, which promotes angiogenesis through extracellular matrix degradation and improves revascularization of transplanted islets [33], was not upregulated in the present study, although Deryugina et al. have reported that *Mmp14* expression can be associated with an upregulation of *Vegf* production [34]. A possible explanation for this discrepancy might be a transplant model, but the detailed mechanism remains uncertain. Therefore, further investigations on the relevance of other growth factors derived from donor islets such as hepatocyte growth factor (HGF) and basic fibroblast growth factor (bFGF) [35,36] are also required in future studies. Considering that no suppression of analyzed gene expression and no reduction of islet graft volume were observed in the tacrolimus-treated group compared with the control group, the inhibitory effect of tacrolimus on islet revascularization may not be mediated by direct damage to the islet grafts. This also suggests a relatively lesser role for donor islet endothelial cells in revascularization process of islet grafts as shown by previous reports [27,37]. Although rapamycin was reported to have deleterious effects on islet viability and growth factor-induced cell cycle regulation [38,39], the present study suggests that tacrolimus appears to have no inhibitory effects on cell cycle regulation.

The dose of tacrolimus in the present study was determined according to previous studies. Lopez-Talavera et al. showed that the administration of tacrolimus at a dose of 0.5 mg/kg/day corresponds to a trough level of 6.0±1.5 ng/mL in rodents, which is similar to the dose used in the Edmonton protocol for humans [18]. Therefore, this dose was used for the tacrolimus-treated group. Islet revascularization was significantly inhibited after the administration of a clinical relevant dose of tacrolimus. Furthermore, Shapiro et al. reported that the portal C_{max} of immunosuppressive drugs was more than two times higher than the systemic C_{max} [40]. Therefore, the detrimental effect of tacrolimus on islet revascularization could be further enhanced when the islet grafts are transplanted into the liver, which is the current standard transplant site. As a result, the optimization of immunosuppressive drugs is of great importance for successful islet allotransplantation. FTY720, a sphingosine 1-phosphate analog, may be potentially useful and effective since previous studies have thus far shown it to effectively suppress immune responses in islet transplantation [41,42]. The established new evaluation system in the present study could be a useful screening tool for optimizing the protocols of revascularization including the immunosuppressive regimen.

In summary, the present study demonstrated that tacrolimus inhibits the revascularization of isolated pancreatic islets without affecting the characteristics of the transplanted grafts. Further refinements in this immunosuppressive regimen, especially with regard to the revascularization of islet grafts, could therefore improve the outcome of islet allotransplantation.

Acknowledgments

The authors thank Megumi Goto, Toshiki Yanagi, and Masako Osawa for their excellent technical assistance. The authors also thank the Biomedical Research Core of Tohoku University Graduate School of Medicine for giving the opportunity to use MPLSM.

Author Contributions

Conceived and designed the experiments: RN MG. Performed the experiments: RN SN IF S. Sekiguchi KF AU MG. Analyzed the data: RN HS MS MG. Wrote the paper: RN TM NO S. Satomi MG.

References

1. Ryan EA, Paty BW, Senior PA, Bigam D, Alfadhli E, et al. (2005) Five-year follow-up after clinical islet transplantation. Diabetes 54: 2060–2069.
2. Sutherland DE, Gruessner AC, Carlson AM, Blondet JJ, Balamurugan AN, et al. (2008) Islet autotransplant outcomes after total pancreatectomy: a contrast to islet allograft outcomes. Transplantation 86: 1799–1802.
3. Goto M, Eich TM, Felldin M, Foss A, Kallen R, et al. (2004) Refinement of the automated method for human islet isolation and presentation of a closed system for in vitro islet culture. Transplantation 78: 1367–1375.
4. Goto M, Imura T, Inagaki A, Ogawa N, Yamaya H, et al. (2010) The impact of ischemic stress on the quality of isolated pancreatic islets. Transplant Proc 42: 2040–2042.
5. Shapiro AM, Lakey JR, Ryan EA, Korbutt GS, Toth E, et al. (2000) Islet transplantation in seven patients with type 1 diabetes mellitus using a glucocorticoid-free immunosuppressive regimen. N Engl J Med 343: 230–238.
6. Zhang N, Su D, Qu S, Tse T, Bottino R, et al. (2006) Sirolimus is associated with reduced islet engraftment and impaired beta-cell function. Diabetes 55: 2429–2436.
7. Guba M, von Breitenbuch P, Steinbauer M, Koehl G, Flegel S, et al. (2002) Rapamycin inhibits primary and metastatic tumor growth by antiangiogenesis: involvement of vascular endothelial growth factor. Nat Med 8: 128–135.
8. Stallone G, Schena A, Infante B, Di Paolo S, Loverre A, et al. (2005) Sirolimus for Kaposi's sarcoma in renal-transplant recipients. N Engl J Med 352: 1317–1323.
9. Cantaluppi V, Biancone L, Romanazzi GM, Figliolini F, Beltramo S, et al. (2006) Antiangiogenic and immunomodulatory effects of rapamycin on islet endothelium: relevance for islet transplantation. Am J Transplant 6: 2601–2611.
10. Turgut B, Guler M, Akpolat N, Demir T, Celiker U (2011) The impact of tacrolimus on vascular endothelial growth factor in experimental corneal neovascularization. Curr Eye Res 36: 34–40.
11. Nishimura R, Goto M, Sekiguchi S, Fujimori K, Ushiyama A, et al. (2011) Assessment for revascularization of transplanted pancreatic islets at subcutaneous site in mice with a highly sensitive imaging system. Transplant Proc 43: 3239–3240.
12. Speier S, Nyqvist D, Cabrera O, Yu J, Molano RD, et al. (2008) Noninvasive in vivo imaging of pancreatic islet cell biology. Nat Med 14: 574–578.
13. Speier S, Nyqvist D, Kohler M, Caicedo A, Leibiger IB, et al. (2008) Noninvasive high-resolution in vivo imaging of cell biology in the anterior chamber of the mouse eye. Nat Protoc 3: 1278–1286.
14. Goto M, Johansson H, Maeda A, Elgue G, Korsgren O, et al. (2004) Low molecular weight dextran sulfate prevents the instant blood-mediated inflammatory reaction induced by adult porcine islets. Transplantation 77: 741–747.
15. Goto M, Tjernberg J, Dufrane D, Elgue G, Brandhorst D, et al. (2008) Dissecting the instant blood-mediated inflammatory reaction in islet xenotransplantation. Xenotransplantation 15: 225–234.
16. Bayne K (1996) Revised Guide for the Care and Use of Laboratory Animals available. American Physiological Society. Physiologist 39: 199, 208–111.

17. Ushiyama A, Yamada S, Ohkubo C (2004) Microcirculatory parameters measured in subcutaneous tissue of the mouse using a novel dorsal skinfold chamber. Microvasc Res 68: 147–152.
18. Lopez-Talavera JC, Garcia-Ocana A, Sipula I, Takane KK, Cozar-Castellano I, et al. (2004) Hepatocyte growth factor gene therapy for pancreatic islets in diabetes: reducing the minimal islet transplant mass required in a glucocorticoid-free rat model of allogeneic portal vein islet transplantation. Endocrinology 145: 467–474.
19. Mita A, Ricordi C, Messinger S, Miki A, Misawa R, et al. (2010) Antiproinflammatory effects of iodixanol (OptiPrep)-based density gradient purification on human islet preparations. Cell Transplant 19: 1537–1546.
20. Goto M, Eich TM, Stahle M, Malmborg A, Engkvist M, et al. (2005) Technical improvement of human pancreatic islet isolation. Transplant Proc 37: 1313–1314.
21. Ichii H, Pileggi A, Molano RD, Baidal DA, Khan A, et al. (2005) Rescue purification maximizes the use of human islet preparations for transplantation. Am J Transplant 5: 21–30.
22. Reffet S, Thivolet C (2006) Immunology of pancreatic islet transplantation. Diabetes Metab 32: 523–526.
23. Singh RP, Stratta RJ (2008) Advances in immunosuppression for pancreas transplantation. Curr Opin Organ Transplant 13: 79–84.
24. Menger MD, Yamauchi J, Vollmar B (2001) Revascularization and microcirculation of freely grafted islets of Langerhans. World J Surg 25: 509–515.
25. Vajkoczy P, Olofsson AM, Lehr HA, Leiderer R, Hammersen F, et al. (1995) Histogenesis and ultrastructure of pancreatic islet graft microvasculature. Evidence for graft revascularization by endothelial cells of host origin. Am J Pathol 146: 1397–1405.
26. Sandberg JO, Margulis B, Jansson L, Karlsten R, Korsgren O (1995) Transplantation of fetal porcine pancreas to diabetic or normoglycemic nude mice. Evidence of a rapid engraftment process demonstrated by blood flow and heat shock protein 70 measurements. Transplantation 59: 1665–1669.
27. Andersson A, Korsgren O, Jansson L (1989) Intraportally transplanted pancreatic islets revascularized from hepatic arterial system. Diabetes 38 Suppl 1: 192–195.
28. Merchant FA, Diller KR, Aggarwal SJ, Bovik AC (1997) Angiogenesis in cultured and cryopreserved pancreatic islet grafts. Transplantation 63: 1652–1660.
29. Mendola JF, Goity C, Fernandez-Alvarez J, Saenz A, Benarroch G, et al. (1994) Immunocytochemical study of pancreatic islet revascularization in islet isograft. Effect of hyperglycemia of the recipient and of in vitro culture of islets. Transplantation 57: 725–730.
30. Lai Y, Schneider D, Kidszun A, Hauck-Schmalenberger I, Breier G, et al. (2005) Vascular endothelial growth factor increases functional beta-cell mass by improvement of angiogenesis of isolated human and murine pancreatic islets. Transplantation 79: 1530–1536.
31. Zhang N, Richter A, Suriawinata J, Harbaran S, Altomonte J, et al. (2004) Elevated vascular endothelial growth factor production in islets improves islet graft vascularization. Diabetes 53: 963–970.
32. Johansson A, Olerud J, Johansson M, Carlsson PO (2009) Angiostatic factors normally restrict islet endothelial cell proliferation and migration: implications for islet transplantation. Transpl Int 22: 1182–1188.
33. Olsson R, Maxhuni A, Carlsson PO (2006) Revascularization of transplanted pancreatic islets following culture with stimulators of angiogenesis. Transplantation 82: 340–347.
34. Deryugina EI, Soroceanu L, Strongin AY (2002) Up-regulation of vascular endothelial growth factor by membrane-type 1 matrix metalloproteinase stimulates human glioma xenograft growth and angiogenesis. Cancer Res 62: 580–588.
35. Vasir B, Reitz P, Xu G, Sharma A, Bonner-Weir S, et al. (2000) Effects of diabetes and hypoxia on gene markers of angiogenesis (HGF, cMET, uPA and uPAR, TGF-alpha, TGF-beta, bFGF and Vimentin) in cultured and transplanted rat islets. Diabetologia 43: 763–772.
36. Watanabe H, Sumi S, Kitamura Y, Nio Y, Higami T (2003) Immunohistochemical analysis of vascular endothelial growth factor and hepatocyte growth factor, and their receptors, in transplanted islets in rats. Surg Today 33: 854–860.
37. Henriksnas J, Lau J, Zang G, Berggren PO, Kohler M, et al. (2012) Markedly decreased blood perfusion of pancreatic islets transplanted intraportally into the liver: disruption of islet integrity necessary for islet revascularization. Diabetes 61: 665–673.
38. Aronovitz A, Josefson J, Fisher A, Newman M, Hughes E, et al. (2008) Rapamycin inhibits growth factor-induced cell cycle regulation in pancreatic beta cells. J Investig Med 56: 985–996.
39. Cross SE, Richards SK, Clark A, Benest AV, Bates DO, et al. (2007) Vascular endothelial growth factor as a survival factor for human islets: effect of immunosuppressive drugs. Diabetologia 50: 1423–1432.
40. Shapiro AM, Gallant HL, Hao EG, Lakey JR, McCready T, et al. (2005) The portal immunosuppressive storm: relevance to islet transplantation? Ther Drug Monit 27: 35–37.
41. Maeda A, Goto M, Zhang J, Bennet W, Groth CG, et al. (2003) Immunosuppression with FTY720 and cyclosporine A inhibits rejection of adult porcine islet xenografts in rats. Transplantation 75: 1409–1414.
42. Shapiro AM, Lakey JR, Paty BW, Senior PA, Bigam DL, et al. (2005) Strategic opportunities in clinical islet transplantation. Transplantation 79: 1304–1307.

18

Immunophenotyping and Efficacy of Low Dose ATG in Non-Sensitized Kidney Recipients Undergoing Early Steroid Withdrawal

Monica Grafals[1,2], Brian Smith[3], Naoka Murakami[4], Agnes Trabucco[1], Katherine Hamill[1], Erick Marangos[1], Hannah Gilligan[1], Elizabeth A. Pomfret[1], James J. Pomposelli[1], Mary A. Simpson[1], Jamil Azzi[3], Nader Najafian[3,5], Leonardo V. Riella[3]*

1 Department of Transplant Surgery, Lahey Clinic Medical Center, Burlington, Massachusetts, United States of America, **2** Department of Medicine, Georgetown University, Washington, D.C., United States of America, **3** Transplantation Research Center, Renal Division, Brigham & Women's Hospital, Harvard Medical School, Boston, Massachusetts, United States of America, **4** Department of Medicine, Beth Israel Medical Center, New York, New York, United States of America, **5** Department of Nephrology, Cleveland Clinic Florida, Weston, Florida, United States of America

Abstract

Rabbit antithymocyte globulin (ATG) is commonly used as an induction therapy in renal transplant recipients, but the ideal dosage in tacrolimus-based early steroid withdrawal protocols has not been established. The purpose of this pilot study was to determine the immunophenotyping and efficacy of lower dose ATG in low immunological-risk kidney transplant recipients. In this prospective study, 45 patients were randomized (1:1) to our standard dose ATG (total dose 3.75 mg/kg)(sATG) vs. lower dose 2.25 mg/kg (lowATG). All patients underwent early steroid withdrawal within 7 days. The primary end point was biopsy-proven acute rejection at 12 months. Prospective immunophenotyping of freshly isolated PBMCs was performed at baseline, 3, 6, 12 months post-transplant. The rate of acute rejection was 17% and 10% in the sATG and lowATG, respectively. Effector memory T cells, Tregs and recent thymic emigrants T cells had similar kinetics post-transplant in both groups. No statistically significant differences were found in graft survival, patient survival or infections between the two groups, though there was a non-significant increase in leukopenia (43%v s. 30%), CMV (8% vs. 0) and BK (4% vs. 0) infections in sATG group vs. lowATG. In sum, in low immunological risk kidney recipients undergoing steroid withdrawal, low dose ATG seems to be efficacious in preventing acute rejection and depleting T cells with potentially lower infectious complications. A larger study is warranted to confirm these findings.

Editor: Aric Gregson, University of California Los Angeles, United States of America

Funding: Funding for this study was provided by the Robert Weiss Grant (MG) and American Heart Association (LVR). The funders had no role in study design, data collection and analysis, decision to publish, or preparation of the manuscript.

Competing Interests: The authors have declared that no competing interests exist.

* Email: leonardoriella@gmail.com

Introduction

Most kidney transplant centers in the United States utilize induction agents as part of their immunosupression protocols as it is believed that these agents prevent early acute rejection episodes and possibly improve graft survival [1–3]. Rabbit antithymocyte globulin (ATG or Thymoglobulin) is the most common induction agent used in renal transplantation and is used in more than 55% of kidney transplants in the USA, despite not being FDA-approved for this use [2]. ATG causes T-cell depletion by inducing complement-dependent cell lysis. It also modulates cell surface and adhesion molecules that regulate T-cell function and leukocyte endothelial interactions, respectively [1,4,5]. Induction therapy with ATG results in a lower acute rejection rate, but is also associated with a higher risk of infections and malignancies [6–8]. An ATG dosage of 6–10 mg/kg has traditionally been the standard of care in most transplant centers in the USA [5,9–12]. ATG has been widely studied in the cyclosporine and low-dose steroid maintenance era, however the optimal dosage of ATG in the setting of tacrolimus use and steroid withdrawal has not been determined.

Our transplant center utilizes 3.75 mg/kg of ATG as induction in both deceased and living donor renal transplantation. Because of drug acquisition costs, risks of malignancies and infections, it is imperative to find the minimum effective dose of ATG that still allows for minimization of maintenance immunosupression. Moreover, the expansion of steroid withdrawal regimens urges a reassessment of optimal ATG dosage. Our hypothesis is that lower ATG dose is effective and safe in non-sensitized renal transplant recipients undergoing steroid withdrawal. Herein, we report an open-label, single-center prospective randomized pilot study comparing two lower dosage ATG regimens (3.75 mg/kg vs. 2.25 mg/kg) in low immunological risk recipients who underwent steroid withdrawal and maintenance immunosuppression with tacrolimus and mycophenolate mofetil.

Methods

Study design and patient selection

This is a prospective, open-label, single center randomized pilot study in adult renal transplant recipients at Lahey Clinic Medical Center, Burlington, MA. Patients above 18 years of age who were scheduled for a living or deceased donor renal transplant were eligible for enrollment. Exclusion criteria included a multi-organ transplant; a current or historic panel reactive antibody >20%; presence of donor specific anti-HLA antibodies; and contraindication to ATG use. The recruitment time was pre-established for 2 years with one additional year of follow-up. The protocol for this trial and supporting CONSORT checklist are available as supporting information (see Checklist S1 and Protocol S1).

Ethics statement

The study protocol was reviewed and approved by an Institutional Review Board at Lahey Clinic Medical Center and was conducted in full conformance with the principles of the Declaration of Helsinki. All study participants provided signed informed consent previous to randomization. The study is listed on http://clinicaltrials.gov (NCT01280617).

Randomization and treatment

After the screening process, eligible patients were randomized in a 1:1 ratio either to receive standard dose ATG of 1.25 mg/kg×3 doses (3.75 mg/kg total dose) [sATG] or low dose ATG of 0.75 mg/kg×3 doses (2.25 mg/kg total dose) [lowATG] (Figure 1). For obese patients, the maximum weight used in the dose calculation was 100 kg. After patient enrollment by a transplant nephrologist, computer-generated protocols were utilized for randomization (performed by research coordinator and implemented by transplant nephrologist).

Patients on both arm received ATG intraoperatively on day 1, followed by daily administration of ATG on days 2 and 3, at the dosage according to the assignment.

All patients received maintenance immunosuppression with tacrolimus, mycophenolate mofetil (MMF) and a 7-day corticosteroid taper. Tacrolimus was initiated on day 1 at 2 mg twice a day and target blood concentrations were 8–10 ng/ml for the first 6 months post-transplant. MMF was dosed as 1000 mg twice a day in both groups. Methylprednisolone was given intravenously at 500 mg on day 0, 200 mg on day 1 and 100 mg on day 2. Prednisone 20 mg was given by mouth on day 3 and 10 mg was given on day 4, followed by fast taper. No further corticosteroid use was planned after the first post-operative week unless patients were on long-term prednisone prior to transplantation for other reasons.

All patients received trimethoprim 80 mg-sulfamethoxazole 400 mg administered orally daily for six months for bacterial and *Pneumocystis jiroveci* prophylaxis. Inhaled pentamidine monthly for 6 months was given in patients allergic to sulfa products. Valganciclovir 450 mg daily or adjusted dose for renal function was given for cytomegalovirus (CMV) prophylaxis for three months in low-to-intermediate risk patients (seropositive donor and recipient [D+/R+], seronegative donor and recipient [D−/R−] and seronegative donor and seropositive recipient [D−/R+] and for 6 months in high-risk seropositive donor and seronegative recipient [D+/R−] patients.

Endpoints

The primary endpoint was the incidence of biopsy-proven acute rejection (BPAR) at 12 months post-transplant. This was determined by pathological evidence of rejection defined by the Banff '97 criteria. Delayed graft function was defined as the need for dialysis within seven days after transplantation. Leukopenia was defined as a WBC count of 3,500 cells/mm^3 or less. Secondary endpoints included: patient survival, graft survival and function (serum creatinine at 3, 6, 12 month), incidence of infection, leukopenia (defined as WBC<3,500) and cancers.

Peripheral blood mononuclear cells (PBMC) isolation

Peripheral blood samples were obtained from patients pre-transplantation, at 3, 6 and 12 months post-transplant. Samples were all collected between 7–9am and were processed within 4 hours at the Immunological Core Facility at the Transplant Research Center, Brigham and Women's Hospital. PBMCs were isolated by density gradient centrifugation using Ficoll-Paque solution (GE Healthcare Biosciences) spun at 800 *g* for 30 minutes at 20°C.

Flow cytometric analysis

Freshly prepared PBMCs were used for flow cytometric analysis using four-color flow cytometry on a FACS Calibur analyzer (Becton Dickinson, NJ) with cell surface staining using anti-CD45RO-FITC, anti-CD31-FITC, anti-CD25-PE, anti CD4-PerCP, anti-CD4-APC, anti-CD8-PerCP, anti-CD62L-APC, anti-CD45RA-APC (BD Biosciences, San Jose, CA, USA). For intracellular staining of FoxP3, permeabilization solution (eBioscience, San Diego, CA, USA) and anti-Foxp3-FITC (eBioscience, San Diego, CA, USA) were used based on manufacturer's protocol.

Statistical analysis

For this pilot study, we estimated that 40 participants in total were needed [13]. Statistical analysis was performed in GraphPad Prism version 5.0d and Microsoft Excel 2011. Continuous variables were analyzed using two-tailed *t* tests if normally distributed, while nonparametric Mann-Whitney test was used if variable was not normally distributed. Categorical variables were analyzed using chi-square testing, unless expected frequencies were less than five in any group, in which case Fisher's exact test was used. We report means ± SDs. P-values less than 0.05 were considered significant. With the exception of patient survival, all clinical outcomes were censored (patients not followed) beyond the date of graft failure. Thus, analysis of renal function (serum creatinine and eGFR) at various times post-transplant were based on comparing patients who were still alive with functioning grafts at those times.

Results

Study Patients

From the initiation of trial recruitment in November 2010 until the completion of recruitment in April 2013, seventy patients were assessed for eligibility for the study and forty-five patients underwent randomization (Figure 1). Data collection continued until August 2013 with a mean follow-up of 15 months. The two arms were well balanced with no major differences in terms of living versus deceased donor transplant, recipient's gender, age, ethnicity, re-transplant, diabetes, CKD etiology, dialysis time prior to transplant, panel reactive antibody (PRA), donor age and kidney weight (Table 1), with the exception of a slightly higher prevalence of coronary artery disease in the lowATG group compared with sATG (n = 9 vs 4, p = 0.06).

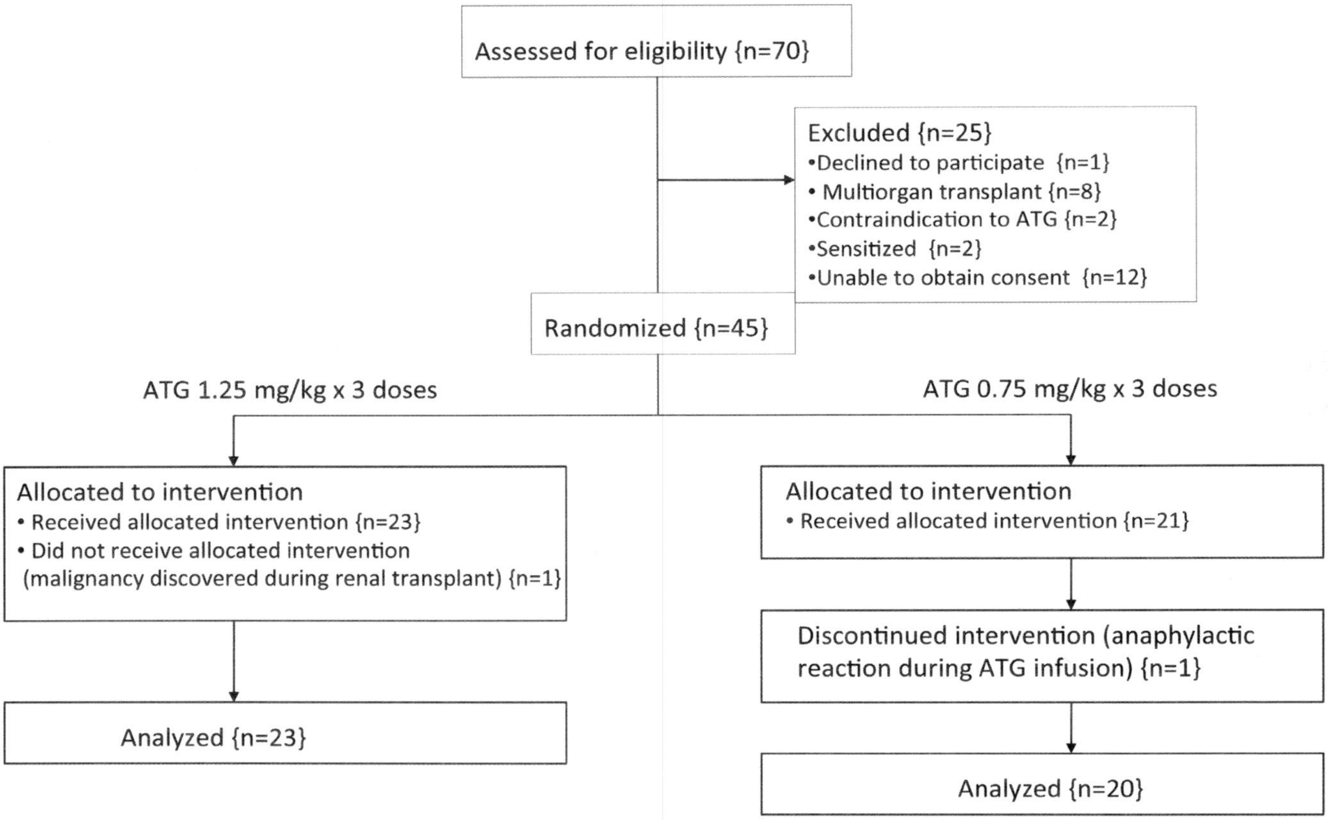

Figure 1. Flow diagram of patients screened and enrolled in the study.

Outcomes

The two arms showed no significant difference at the primary endpoint of biopsy-proven acute rejection (BPAR). The rate of acute rejection in the lowATG group was 10% compared to 17% in the sATG group (p = 0.66) (Table 2). Patient survival at 1 year in the lowATG group was 85% compared with 100% in the sATG (p = 0.11) (Table 2). There were two patient deaths in the lowATG group related to cardiovascular events with a functioning graft. Both patients had been on hemodialysis for more than five years prior to transplantation, had history of coronary artery disease and diabetes, and were long-term smokers. The etiology of the third death was undetermined. Delayed graft function occurred in 40% of patients in the lowATG group compared with 14.3% in the sATG group (p = 0.05). Serum creatinine (sCr) and eGFR were similar between both groups at 1, 6 and 12 months post-transplant (Figure 2). At 12 months post-transplant, the serum creatinine in the lowATG was 1.4±0.44 mg/dl compared with 1.33±0.0.36 in the sATG group (p = 0.56). There were no primary graft failures on either group. There was no significant difference in the tacrolimus trough levels and mycophenolate dosing between the two groups (Table 2).

Adverse events

We observed more leukopenia in the sATG group compared with the lowATG group (43% vs. 30%, p = 0.34) (Table 2). There were two cases of CMV infection in the sATG group and one of these patients also developed BK infection. There were no cases of either BK or CMV in the lowATG group. The incidence of severe infection requiring hospital admission was 13% in the sATG group compared to 10% in the lowATG group (p = 0.55). There was one case of squamous cell cancer on each group and one of prostate cancer in the lowATG group. There was no case of post-transplant lymphoproliferative disorder, Kaposi sarcoma or renal cell carcinoma.

Effects of ATG on peripheral T cells

We compared the kinetics of peripheral blood T cell subsets at baseline and at 3, 6 and 12 months post-transplant between groups (Figure 3, 4). While CD8 T cells were recovered close to baseline after 3 months on both groups, CD4 T cells were persistently lower in both groups up to 12 months post-transplant (20±7.1% lowATG vs. 17±3.6% high ATG compared to baseline 35±3.6% and 37±5.5%, respectively) (Figure 3B). Overall, the percentage of effector memory T cells (CD45RO+CD62Llow) was reduced at 3 months after transplantation but increased after that, reaching its highest percentage at 12 months (Figure 3C). Tregs' percentage slightly increased post-transplant in both groups, though the standard deviations were wide and differences non-significant (Figure 4B).

The ratio of Treg/CD4effmem percentage has been suggested to indicate immune regulation and potentially less risk of rejection [14–16]. We observed a trend towards higher Treg/CD4effmem at 3 months after transplant in the lowATG group, however ratio was similar to baseline at subsequent time points (Figure 4C). We could not identify an association between lower ratio of Treg/CD4effmem and later rejection (data not shown). Recent thymic emigrants (RTE) are a subset of T cells that proliferate in response to IL-7 and in the absence of other costimulation, a property that

Table 1. Baseline characteristics of renal transplant recipients and donors.

	sATG 3.75 mg/kg (n = 23)	lowATG 2.25 mg/kg (n = 20)	P Value
Recipients' characteristics			
Age at transplant (yr)	52.9±12.1	56.6±11.6	0.311
Body weight (kg)	78.5±22.3	88.5 ±21.8	0.148
Body mass index (kg/m^2)	27.6±4.8	29.1±5.9	0.364
PRA (%)	0	0	
Pre-transplant diabetes (%)	11 (47.8)	9 (45)	0.874
Re-transplant (%)	2 (8.6)	1 (5.0)	0.499
Race/ethnicity (%)			0.246
White	13 (56.5)	16 (80)	
Hispanic	6 (26.0)	2 (10)	
African American	2 (8.7)	2 (10)	
Other	2 (8.7)	0 (0)	
Gender (%)			0.456
Males	16 (69.5)	16 (80)	
Females	7 (30.4)	4 (20)	
CKD etiology (%)			0.859
DM	11 (47.8)	9 (45)	
HTN	1 (4.3)	3 (15)	
GN	5 (21.7)	6 (30)	
PKD	4 (17.3)	1 (5)	
Other	2 (8.7)	1 (5)	
Length of dialysis prior to transplant (months)	24.7±23.9	31.2±24.7	0.389
History of CAD	4 (17.4)	9 (45)	0.0591
Average follow up (months)	15.9±6.5	17.8±5.15	0.796
Donors' characteristics (%)			0.392
Females	10 (43.5)	6 (30)	
Males	13 (56.5)	14 (70)	
Type of donors (%)			0.849
Deceased donor	14 (60.8)	12 (60)	
Living donor	9 (39.2)	8 (40)	
Extended-criteria donor	4 (17.4)	6 (30)	0.349
Donor age (yr)	44.4±13.4	47.5±13.5	0.468
CIT (min)	378±332	433±421	0.688
Kidney weight (grams)	213.4±53.5	209.1±51.0	0.809

CKD, chronic kidney disease; CAD, coronary artery disease; CIT, cold ischemia time; GN, glomerular nephritis, ECD, extended-criteria donor; PKD, polycystic kidney disease; PRA, panel reactive antibody.

may help in the reconstitution of T cells after T-cell depletion with ATG [17]. These cells are characterized by the expression of CD4, CD31 and CD45RA. We assessed the kinetics of RTEs after T cell depletion; the percentage of RTEs significantly decreased after ATG on both groups and did not recover back to baseline after that (Figure 4D, E). We did not observe any correlation between the percentage of RTE and the development of leukopenia after ATG.

Cost minimization

Though beyond the scope of this paper, the cost-effectiveness of the different strategies was assessed. ATG costs $600 per 25 mg vial. On an average 80 kg representative patient, the standard dose ATG recipient (3.75 mg/kg total) received 100 mg×3 doses (12 vials), which equals $7,200, while the lowATG recipient (2.25 mg/kg total) received 50 mg×3 doses (6 vials) with a total cost of $3,600. Taking into account the individual weight of patients on this study, the average cost saving was approximately U$2,307 dollars per patient in the lowATG arm compared to sATG.

Discussion

ATG is a potent immune-depleting induction therapy that has significantly reduced the rate of acute rejection in solid organ transplantation. At the same time, however, high dose ATG is associated with increased incidence of leukopenia, malignancy and

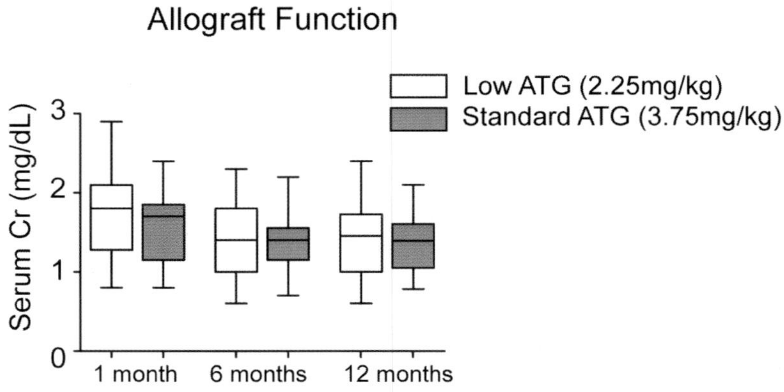

Figure 2. Graft function after transplantation. Serum creatinine was measured at 1, 6, 12 months post-transplantation, as a surrogate of graft function. Means±SD. At each time point, there was no statistically significant difference in serum creatinine between low-dose and high-dose arms by unpaired *t*-test analysis.

infectious complications [6–8]. Despite more than 20 years of clinical use, its optimal dose is still controversial, in particular in the setting of steroid withdrawal.

For the evaluation of efficacy and safety, multiple trials have been conducted to optimize ATG dosage [18]. The initial trials used relatively high cumulative doses of ATG of 10.5 mg/kg with cyclosporine and low-dose steroids maintenance regimen [19,20], followed by efforts to reduce the dosage of ATG. Recently published observational study using ATG induction registry of 2,322 living donor kidney transplants from 49 different centers reported that the mean cumulative dose was 5.29 mg/kg, with 93.6% rejection free survival at 5 years. The registry consisted of a heterogeneous group of patients and the majority of them were receiving low dose steroids long-term [21], leading to difficulties in extrapolating the results to this specific subgroup of patients. Another recent 10-year follow-up study using an early steroid withdrawal reported the use of a total dose 6.25–7.5 mg/kg of thymoglobulin [22]. Wong *et al.* compared different cumulative dosages of thymoglobulin (3.0 mg/kg vs 4.5 mg/kg), and showed no statistically significant difference in acute rejection rate and graft function up to 24 months post transplantation [23]. Though it was relatively small study (7 vs. 9 patients in each arm) and all patients were continued on steroids, this encouraged us to further reduce thymoglobulin dosage in our transplant program.

Our study showed that a lower dose of 2.25 mg/kg of ATG was safe and effective in preventing acute rejection in combination

Table 2. Outcomes and complications after kidney transplantation.

	sATG 3.75 mg/kg (n = 23)	lowATG 2.25 mg/kg(n = 20)	P Value
Rejection	4 (17%)	2 (10%)	0.662
Leukopenia	10 (43%)	6 (30%)	0.342
Severe infection	3 (13%)	2 (10%)	0.556
BK nephropathy	1 (4%)	0 (0)	0.331
CMV infection	2 (8%)	0 (0)	0.487
Patient survival	23 (100%)	17 (85%)	0.106
Delayed graft function (DGF)	3 (14.3%)	8 (40%)	0.0508
sCre post-transplant (mg/dL)			
1 month	1.58±0.10	1.77±0.13	0.267
6 months	1.38±0.08	1.41±0.10	0.853
12 months	1.33±0.07	1.40±0.10	0.563
Trough tacrolimus level (mean±SD; ng/mL)			
3 months	7.24±1.50	7.78±2.56	0.421
6 months	7.60±1.80	6.81±1.99	0.237
12 months	7.20±2.62	5.67±4.05	0.204
Mycophenolate Mofetil dose (mean±SD; mg/day)			
3 months	1730±438	1433±457	0.092
6 months	1535±458	1384±463	0.402
12 months	1354±482	1181±462	0.392

CMV, cytomegalovirus; sCre, serum creatinine.

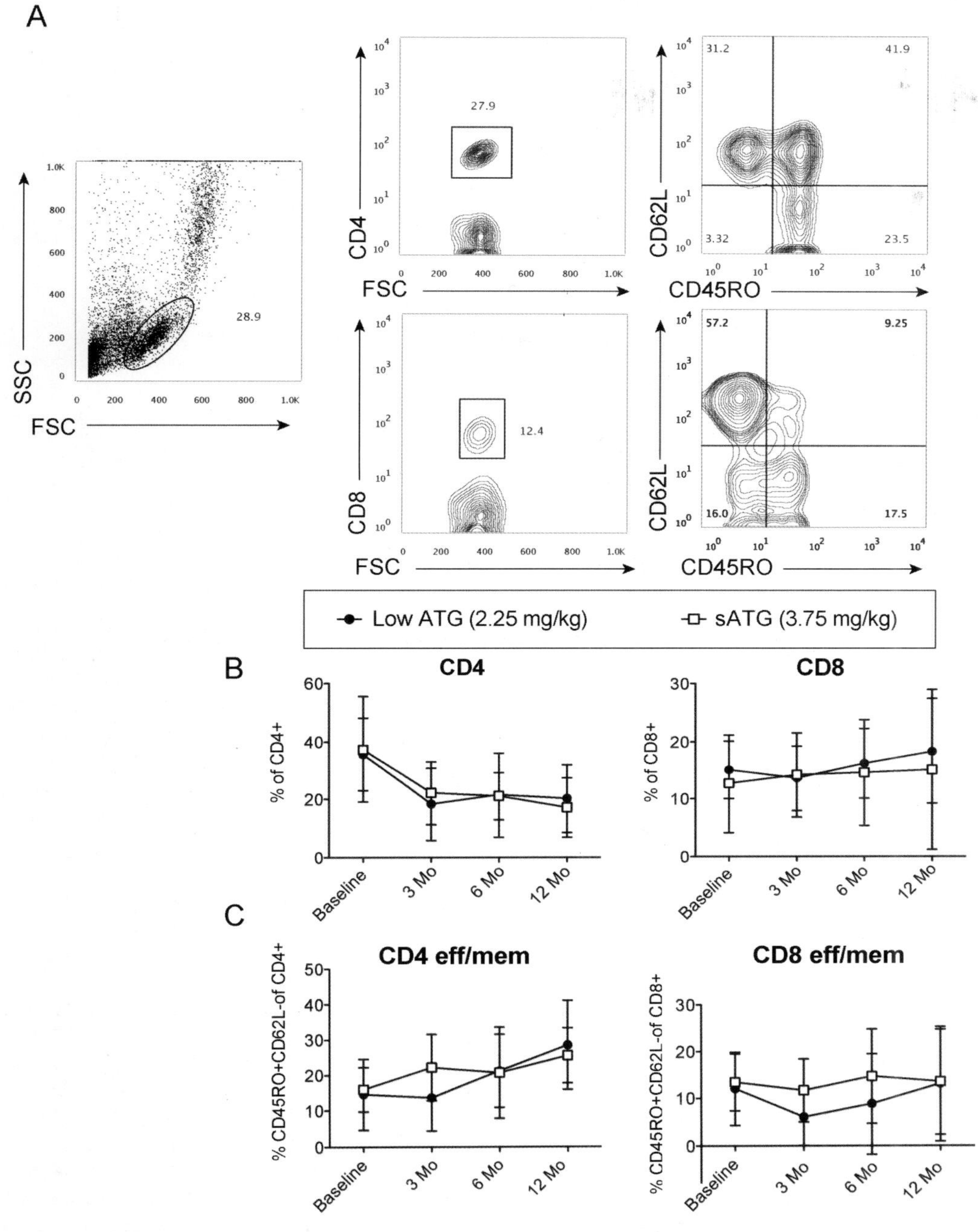

Figure 3. Flow cytometric analyses of peripheral T cells at different time points after transplantation. A, Representative gating strategy of peripheral blood mononuclear cells with live gate, CD4 and CD8 subsets and effector memory T cells ($CD45RO^{+}CD62Llow$). B, Percentage of total CD4 cells and total CD8 cells at 0, 3, 6 and 12 months after transplantation. C, Percentage of $CD4^{+}$ and $CD8^{+}$ effector memory cells after transplantation. Data are expressed as mean and standard deviation (n = 18-20 per group).

with early steroid withdrawal in our non-sensitized kidney transplant cohort. This dose was about 1/3 of the commonly used dose of ATG in most centers. Two cardiovascular deaths with functioning grafts in the lowATG group were likely to have occurred by chance despite randomization, and were unlikely related to difference in ATG dose given. The barely significant increase in CAD history in the low ATG group also supports this hypothesis. In addition, we observed a non-significant reduction in the incidence of leukopenia, CMV and BK infections in lowATG arm, suggesting possible benefit from lower dose ATG. In contrary, DGF was more common in the lowATG group ($p = 0.05$). Reviewing Table 1, we observe a non-significant trend towards higher proportion of ECD kidneys and greater mean cold ischemia time in the lowATG group (30% vs 17% and 433 vs 378 min, $p > 0.05$). Since prior data from larger randomized trials did not show lower DGF in ATG compared to other induction therapies (18), it is hard to conclude the significance of these findings in this smaller cohort. Despite that, the absence of primary graft losses on both groups and the good renal function at 12 months are reassuring. Although this report is an exploratory

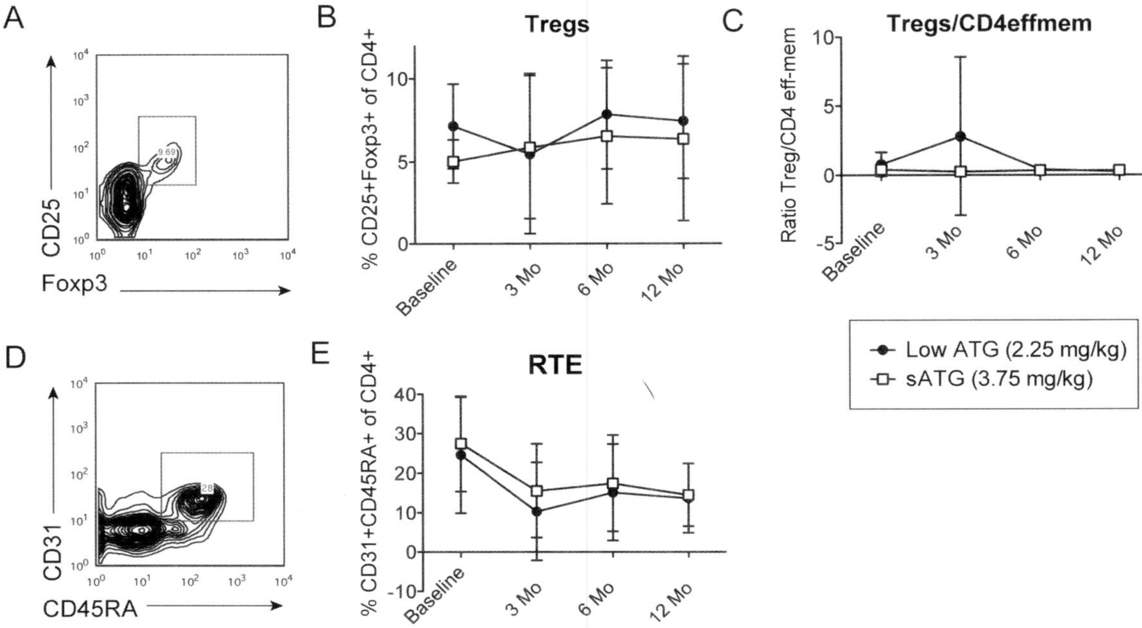

Figure 4. Flow cytometric analyses of Tregs and recent thymic emigrants (RTE) CD4 cells at different time points after transplantation. Representative contour plots of Tregs (A) ($CD25^+Foxp3^+$ of $CD4^+$ cells) and RTEs (D) ($CD45RA^+CD31^+$ of $CD4^+$ cells) cells after gating on $CD4^+$ T cells at different time points after transplantation. Percentage of Tregs (B) and ratio of Tregs related to baseline (C) at different points after transplantation. E, Percentage of RTEs at different points after transplantation. Data are expressed as mean and standard deviation (n = 18-20 per group).

data with small number of cases, these are encouraging results that must be further validated in a larger trial. Since study conclusion, Lahey Clinic has now adopted the lower dose ATG as standard of care in non-sensitized transplant recipients.

Aside from ATG, other induction agents such as basiliximab (anti-IL2 receptor mAb, Novartis) or alemtuzumab (anti-CD52 mAb, Berlex Laboratories) have been used in combination with tacrolimus maintenance and steroid withdrawal. One of the largest prospective trials on steroid withdrawal reported that the rejection rate was higher with basiliximab compared to ATG (24.2% vs 14.4%), though long-term graft outcomes were similar [24]. Alemtuzumab has been tested on a recent randomized controlled trial in patients undergoing steroid withdrawal and was found to be associated with lower rates of acute rejection when compared to basiliximab in low-risk recipients, though late rejections were more common in the alemtuzumab group (1–3 years after transplant) [25]. This is a concern since the follow-up of transplant recipients tends to be less frequent after the first year of transplantation and a rejection episode may go unnoticed for few months.

In face of the increased budget constraints that transplant centers and hospitals are undergoing and the huge expense that ATG accounts for, reduction of ATG dose could have an important financial benefit and a possible cost-reduction of ~U$3,000/patient could be obtained by reducing the ATG dose from our standard protocol (3.75 mg/kg total) to the study dose of 2.25 mg/kg total. Although basiliximab is less expensive (~$4,000 per patient) than ATG, it is a relatively less potent immunosuppressant and is associated with a higher rate of rejection in patients that undergo steroid withdrawal [24]. Alemtuzumab costs less as well ($1,689 for the recommended single dose of 30 mg) and requires shorter hospital stay, given its use as a one-time dose at the time of transplant. However, alemtuzumab is associated with significantly more prolonged T cell depletion, which may require years to recover [18,26]. In addition, Alemtuzumab may promote the development of donor-specific antibodies through its significant effect on B cells subsets [27]. Nevertheless, thymoglobulin and alemtuzumab had similar patient and graft outcomes in recent randomized trials [28,29]. In sum, ATG seems to be the preferred induction agent for patients undergoing steroid withdrawal.

Immune reconstitution after administration of T-cell depletion by thymoglobulin is also of great interest, in particular with experimental evidence suggesting that it may promote tolerance through the induction and expansion of Tregs [14,30]. In children, thymopoiesis plays an important role in the reconstitution of T cells after ATG depletion, while in adults, homeostatic proliferation is dominant due to the progressive atrophy of thymus with age [30,31]. This homeostatic proliferation is predominantly an IL-7 mediated process, enabling T-cell clone which survived depletion to expand. Recent thymic emigrants (RTE) are a subset of T cells that proliferates in response to IL-7 in the apparent absence of other stimulation and may play an important role in the lymphocyte reconstitution after T-cell depletion [17]. Our findings suggest that both higher and lower dose ATG significantly reduce the RTE subset and this subset remains lower than at baseline even 12 months following transplantation, though there was a trend towards greater reduction in the sATG group. This may allude to some long-term consequences of ATG in the homeostasis of T cell subsets and using a lower dose may have potential to limit that. It is clear that immunosuppression has this cumulative effect and once given, it is not possible to take it back and long-term consequences in the immune system are seeing decades to come. In face of our overall prolongation of survival, it is critical to minimize the life-immunosuppression dose.

The limitations of our study include the small number of patients, the predominance of Caucasians, the lack of blinding, the absence of protocol biopsies and the exclusion of sensitized recipients. A longer follow up would also be necessary to fully elucidate the impact of ATG dose on the malignancy rate.

In conclusion, low-dose ATG (2.25 mg/kg) is a promising option as an induction therapy in low-risk patients with no significant differences in acute rejection or graft function when compared to sATG (3.75 mg/kg), and with possibly less leukopenia and infectious complications. In addition, our peripheral blood cell analyses showed similar T cell depletion efficiency with the lower dose ATG. Larger studies are warranted to confirm these findings.

Author Contributions

Conceived and designed the experiments: NN MG AT KH EM HG EAP JJP MAS LVR. Performed the experiments: BS LVR JA. Analyzed the data: NN MG NM LVR. Wrote the paper: LVR MG NM. Patient care: MG AT KH EM HG EAP JJP MAS.

References

1. Halloran PF (2004) Immunosuppressive drugs for kidney transplantation. N Engl J Med 351: 2715–2729.
2. Matas AJ, Smith JM, Skeans MA, Lamb KE, Gustafson SK, et al. (2013) OPTN/SRTR 2011 Annual Data Report: kidney. Am J Transplant 13 Suppl 1: 11–46.
3. Meier-Kriesche HU, Li S, Gruessner RW, Fung JJ, Bustami RT, et al. (2006) Immunosuppression: evolution in practice and trends, 1994–2004. Am J Transplant 6: 1111–1131.
4. Kirk AD (2006) Induction immunosuppression. Transplantation 82: 593–602.
5. Thiyagarajan U, Ponnuswamy A, Bagul A (2013) Thymoglobulin and its use in renal transplantation: a review. American journal of nephrology 37: 586–601.
6. Meier-Kriesche HU, Arndorfer JA, Kaplan B (2002) Association of antibody induction with short- and long-term cause-specific mortality in renal transplant recipients. J Am Soc Nephrol 13: 769–772.
7. Opelz G, Naujokat C, Daniel V, Terness P, Dohler B (2006) Disassociation between risk of graft loss and risk of non-Hodgkin lymphoma with induction agents in renal transplant recipients. Transplantation 81: 1227–1233.
8. Thibaudin D, Alamartine E, Mariat C, Absi L, Berthoux F (2005) Long-term kinetic of T-lymphocyte subsets in kidney-transplant recipients: influence of anti-T-cell antibodies and association with posttransplant malignancies. Transplantation 80: 1514–1517.
9. Brennan D, Daller J, Lake K, Cibrik D, Del Castillo D, et al. (2006) Rabbit antithymocyte globulin versus basiliximab in renal transplantation. The New England journal of medicine 355: 1967–1977.
10. Goggins W, Pascual M, Powelson J, Magee C, Tolkoff-Rubin N, et al. (2003) A prospective, randomized, clinical trial of intraoperative versus postoperative Thymoglobulin in adult cadaveric renal transplant recipients. Transplantation 76: 798–802.
11. Hardinger K, Rasu R, Skelton R, Miller B, Brennan D (2010) Thymoglobulin induction dosing strategies in a low-risk kidney transplant population: three or four days? Journal of transplantation 2010: 957549.
12. Karen LH, Mark AS, Brent M, Jeffrey AL, Surendra S, et al. (2004) Five-Year Follow Up of Thymoglobulin Versus ATGAM Induction in Adult Renal Transplantation. Transplantation 78.
13. Lancaster GA, Dodd S, Williamson PR (2004) Design and analysis of pilot studies: recommendations for good practice. J Eval Clin Pract 10: 307–312.
14. D'Addio F, Boenisch O, Magee C, Yeung M, Yuan X, et al. (2013) Prolonged, low-dose anti-thymocyte globulin, combined with CTLA4-Ig, promotes engraftment in a stringent transplant model. PloS one 8.
15. Krystufkova E, Sekerkova A, Striz I, Brabcova I, Girmanova E, et al. (2012) Regulatory T cells in kidney transplant recipients: the effect of induction immunosuppression therapy. Nephrol Dial Transplant 27: 2576–2582.
16. Zheng XX, Sanchez-Fueyo A, Domenig C, Strom TB (2003) The balance of deletion and regulation in allograft tolerance. Immunol Rev 196: 75–84.
17. Fink PJ (2013) The biology of recent thymic emigrants. Annu Rev Immunol 31: 31–50.
18. Hardinger K, Brennan D, Klein C (2013) Selection of induction therapy in kidney transplantation. Transplant international: official journal of the European Society for Organ Transplantation 26: 662–672.
19. Brennan DC, Flavin K, Lowell JA, Howard TK, Shenoy S, et al. (1999) A randomized, double-blinded comparison of Thymoglobulin versus Atgam for induction immunosuppressive therapy in adult renal transplant recipients. Transplantation 67: 1011–1018.
20. Vincenti F, Schena FP, Paraskevas S, Hauser IA, Walker RG, et al. (2008) A randomized, multicenter study of steroid avoidance, early steroid withdrawal or standard steroid therapy in kidney transplant recipients. Am J Transplant 8: 307–316.
21. Gaber AO, Matas AJ, Henry ML, Brennan DC, Stevens RB, et al. (2012) Antithymocyte globulin induction in living donor renal transplant recipients: final report of the TAILOR registry. Transplantation 94: 331–337.
22. Rizzari MD, Suszynski TM, Gillingham KJ, Dunn TB, Ibrahim HN, et al. (2012) Ten-year outcome after rapid discontinuation of prednisone in adult primary kidney transplantation. Clin J Am Soc Nephrol 7: 494–503.
23. Wong W, Agrawal N, Pascual M, Anderson DC, Hirsch HH, et al. (2006) Comparison of two dosages of thymoglobulin used as a short-course for induction in kidney transplantation. Transpl Int 19: 629–635.
24. Woodle ES, First MR, Pirsch J, Shihab F, Gaber AO, et al. (2008) A prospective, randomized, double-blind, placebo-controlled multicenter trial comparing early (7 day) corticosteroid cessation versus long-term, low-dose corticosteroid therapy. Ann Surg 248: 564–577.
25. Hardinger K, Rhee S, Buchanan P, Koch M, Miller B, et al. (2008) A prospective, randomized, double-blinded comparison of thymoglobulin versus Atgam for induction immunosuppressive therapy: 10-year results. Transplantation 86: 947–952.
26. Kirk AD, Hale DA, Mannon RB, Kleiner DE, Hoffmann SC, et al. (2003) Results from a human renal allograft tolerance trial evaluating the humanized CD52-specific monoclonal antibody alemtuzumab (CAMPATH-1H). Transplantation 76: 120–129.
27. Todeschini M, Cortinovis M, Perico N, Poli F, Innocente A, et al. (2013) In kidney transplant patients, alemtuzumab but not basiliximab/low-dose rabbit anti-thymocyte globulin induces B cell depletion and regeneration, which associates with a high incidence of de novo donor-specific anti-HLA antibody development. J Immunol 191: 2818–2828.
28. Farney AC, Doares W, Rogers J, Singh R, Hartmann E, et al. (2009) A randomized trial of alemtuzumab versus antithymocyte globulin induction in renal and pancreas transplantation. Transplantation 88: 810–819.
29. Hanaway M, Woodle E, Mulgaonkar S, Peddi V, Kaufman D, et al. (2011) Alemtuzumab induction in renal transplantation. The New England journal of medicine 364: 1909–1919.
30. Gurkan S, Luan Y, Dhillon N, Allam S, Montague T, et al. (2010) Immune reconstitution following rabbit antithymocyte globulin. American journal of transplantation: official journal of the American Society of Transplantation and the American Society of Transplant Surgeons 10: 2132–2141.
31. Tchao N, Turka L (2012) Lymphodepletion and homeostatic proliferation: implications for transplantation. American journal of transplantation: official journal of the American Society of Transplantation and the American Society of Transplant Surgeons 12: 1079–1090.

19

Function and Expression of Cystic Fibrosis Transmembrane Conductance Regulator after Small Intestinal Transplantation in Mice

Penghong Song[1], Wenfeng Song[1], Xiaosun Liu[2], Changhai Jin[1], Haiyang Xie[1], Lin Zhou[1], Biguang Tuo[3], Shusen Zheng[1]*

1 Key Laboratory of Combined Multi-organ Transplantation of Ministry of Public Health, First Affiliated Hospital, School of Medicine, Zhejiang University, Hangzhou, China, **2** Department of Surgery, First Affiliated Hospital, School of Medicine, Zhejiang University, Hangzhou, China, **3** Department of Gastroenterology, Affiliated Hospital of Zunyi Medical College, Zunyi, China

Abstract

The secretion function of intestinal graft is one of the most important factors for successful intestinal transplantation. Cystic fibrosis transmembrane conductance regulator (CFTR) mediates HCO_3^- and Cl^- secretions in intestinal epithelial cells. In this study, we made investigation on the expression and function of CFTR in an experimental model of murine small intestinal transplantation. Heterotopic intestinal transplantations were performed in syngeneic mice. The mRNA and protein expressions of CFTR were analyzed by real time PCR and western blot. Murine intestinal mucosal HCO_3^- and Cl^- secretions were examined *in vitro* in Ussing chambers by the pH stat and short circuit current (I_{sc}) techniques. The results showed that forskolin, an activator of CFTR, stimulated jejunal mucosal epithelial HCO_3^- and Cl^- secretions in mice, but forskolin-stimulated HCO_3^- and Cl^- secretions in donor and recipient jejunal mucosae of mice after heterotopic jejunal transplantation were markedly decreased, compared with controls ($P<0.001$). The mRNA and protein expression levels of CFTR in donor and recipient jejunal mucosae of mice were also markedly lower than those in controls ($P<0.001$), and the mRNA and protein expression levels of tumor necrosis factor α (TNFα) were markedly increased in donor jejunal mucosae of mice ($P<0.001$), compared with controls. Further experiments showed that TNFα down-regulated the expression of CFTR mRNA in murine jejunal mucosa. In conclusion, after intestinal transplantation, the function of CFTR was impaired, and its mRNA and protein expressions were down-regulated, which may be induced by TNFα.

Editor: Alejandro Lucia, Universidad Europea de Madrid, Spain

Funding: This work was supported by the National Natural Science Foundation of China (31071015), Qianjiang Talents Project of Science Technology Department of Zhejiang Province (2011R10033), and Education Department of Zhejiang Province (Y200804851). The Project was sponsored by the Scientific Research Foundation for the Returned Overseas Chinese Scholars, State Education Ministry (J20110176) to PS, Science and Technology Innovation Team of Zhejiang Province (2009R50038) to SZ, and the National Natural Science Foundation of China (81160054) to BT. The funders had no role in study design, data collection and analysis, decision to publish, or preparation of the manuscript.

Competing Interests: The authors have declared that no competing interests exist.

* E-mail: shusenzheng@zju.edu.cn

Introduction

Intestinal transplantation is currently accepted as a potential therapeutic option for patients with irreversible intestinal failure, including those with short bowel syndrome, who have life-threatening total parental nutrition complications, e.g. total parental nutrition-related liver dysfunction and difficulty of central venous access. In the past 10 years, the outcomes of intestinal transplantation have been improved dramatically, largely resulting from innovative changes in immunosuppression protocols, surgical advances, improved postoperative care, and accumulated experience. However, the intestinal transplantation continues to be one of the more challenging transplants, with a lower survival compared with that of other solid organ transplants, e.g. liver and renal transplantation [1–4].

The secretion and absorption of intestine is the most important physiological function of intestine. Therefore, the secretion and absorption function of intestinal graft is one of the most important factors for successful intestinal transplantation. The studies have demonstrated that intestinal absorptive function has been impaired following small intestinal transplantation [5,6], and the defects in intestinal absorptive function occur even in nonrejecting small intestinal grafts [7,8]. However, intestinal secretion function after intestinal transplantation is poorly understood. Intestinal secretion not only aids digestion and absorption, but also occurs as a result of some pathophysiologic processes. Intestinal secretion results from the active transports of two principal ions, Cl^- and HCO_3^- [9]. Cystic fibrosis transmembrane conductance regulator (CFTR) is a cAMP-dependent Cl^- channel with Cl^- and HCO_3^- conductance and abundantly expressed in several functionally diverse tissues, such as the pancreas, intestine, kidney, heart, vas deferens, sweat duct and lung [10,11]. In intestinal epithelial cells, CFTR, which mediates Cl^- and HCO_3^- transports, plays an important role in the regulation of intestinal secretion function [9,12].

In the present study, we made an investigation on the function and expression of CFTR in intestinal graft, which is very important for understanding intestinal physiologic function after intestinal transplantation. The process of intestinal transplantation disturbs intestinal physiological function in various ways, including anatomic changes, ischemia–reperfusion injury, acute and chronic graft rejection, and immunosuppressive therapy. In this study, therefore, we used the mode of syngeneic murine heterotopic jejunal transplantation to seek to identify changes in the function and expression of CFTR in the graft, which is exclusive of the confounding effects of pharmacologic immunosuppression, graft rejection, and graft-versus-host reaction.

Materials and Methods

Establishment of Model of Heterotopic Jejunal Transplantation in Mice

Six to ten week male mice with syngeneic C57BL/6 background were used in this study. The mice were purchased from Shanghai Animal Center (Chinese Academy of Science, Shanghai, China) and housed in the experimental animal facility of Zhejiang University under standard care conditions. All animal operative procedure was approved by the Animal Care Committee of Zhejiang University in accordance with the Principles of Laboratory Animal Care (NIH publication 85-23, revised 1985). Murine heterotopic jejunal transplantation was performed according to Zhong et al. [13], with some modifications. Syngeneic C57BL/6 mice were used as donors and recipients. Briefly, after anesthetization by intraperitoneal injection of 50 mg/kg ketamine and 10 mg/kg xylazine, 7 cm donor's upper portion of jejunum was harvested with the Carrel's patches of superior mesenteric artery and portal vein which was stored in ice-cold saline until implantation. Using a 10-0 nylon suture, the donor's Carrel's patches of superior mesenteric artery and portal vein were anastomosed to the recipient abdominal aorta and inferior vena cava, respectively, yielding end-to-side anastomoses in both cases. The proximal end of the graft was closed with 7-0 silk suture, and the distal end of the graft was exteriorized as a stoma. Recipient mice were sacrificed 2 week after transplantation, and graft and host jejunum were used for experiments.

Ussing Chamber Experiments

After brief narcosis with 100% CO_2, the mice were killed by cervical dislocation. The abdomen was opened by midline incision. The jejunal grafts and host jejunums in the experimental mice and jejunums of normal controls were removed and immediately placed in ice-cold iso-osmolar mannitol and indomethacin (1 μmol/L) solution (to suppress trauma-induced prostaglandin release). The jejunums were opened and stripped of external serosal and muscle layers by sharp dissection in the above-mentioned ice-cold iso-osmolar mannitol and indomethacin solution. Ussing chamber experiments were performed as previously described [14]. Briefly, the jejunal mucosae were mounted between two chambers with an exposed area of 0.196 cm^2 and placed in an Ussing chamber. Parafilm "O" ring was used to minimize edge damage to the tissue where it was secured between the chamber halves. The mucosal side was bathed with unbuffered HCO_3^-free modified Ringer's solution circulated by a gas lift with 100% O_2 to facilitate the measurement of HCO_3^- secretion by pH stat method. The serosal side was bathed with modified buffered Ringer's solution (pH 7.4) containing 25 mmol/L HCO_3^- and gassed with 95% O_2/5% CO_2. Each bath contained 10.0 ml of the respective solution maintained at 37°C by a heated water jacket. Experiments were performed under continuous short-circuit conditions to maintain the electrical potential difference at zero, except for a brief period (<2 seconds) at each time point when the open-circuit potential difference was measured. Luminal pH was maintained at 7.40 by the continuous infusion of 0.5 $mmol.L^{-1}$ HCl under the automatic control of a pH-stat system (842 Titrando, pH-Stat Controller, Metrohm). The volume of the titrant infused per unit time was used to quantitate HCO_3^- secretion. These measurements were recorded at 5-minute intervals. The rate of luminal HCO_3^- secretion is expressed as $\mu mol.cm^{-2}.h^{-1}$. The rate of Cl^- secretion was examined by transepithelial short-circuit current (I_{sc}; reported as $\mu Eq.cm^{-2}.h^{-1}$), which was measured via an automatic voltage clamp (Voltage-Current Clamp, EVC-4000; World Precision Instruments, USA). After a 30-minute measurement of basal parameters, forskolin was added to the serosal side of tissue in Ussing chambers. Changes in jejunal HCO_3^- secretion and I_{sc} during the 40-minute period ensuing after the addition of forskolin were determined. The mucosal solution used in Ussing chamber experiments contained the following (in mmol/L): Na^+140, K^+5.4, Ca^{2+}1.2, Mg^{2+}1.2, Cl^- 120, gluconate 25, and mannitol 10. The serosal solution contained (in mmol/L): Na^+140, K^+5.4, Ca^{2+}1.2, Mg^{2+}1.2, Cl^- 120, HCO_3^- 25, HPO_4^{2-} 2.4, $H_2PO_4^-$ 2.4, glucose 10, TTX 0.0001 and indomethacin 0.0001. The osmolalities for both solutions were ~305 mOsm/L.

RNA Extraction and Real-time RT-PCR

Total RNA from the mucosae of jejunal graft, host jejunum, and control jejunum was extracted using Trizol Reagent (Invitrogen) according to the manufacture's instruction. The concentrations of all RNA samples were determined spectrophotometrically. The cDNA was produced from 2 μg of total RNA using M-MLV reverse transcriptase (Promega) according to the manufacturer's instructions. Quantitative real-time RT-PCR was performed on a 7500 Fast Real-Time PCR system (Applied Biosystems, USA) using SYBR® Premix Dimer Eraser (Takara Bio, Dalian, China) following the manufacture's instruction. All samples were run in triplicate and β-actin was used as an internal control. The expression levels of CFTR, solute carrier family 26 member a3 (Slc26a3), solute carrier family 26 member a6 (Slc26a6), tumor necrosis factor α (TNFα), and interferon γ (IFNγ) mRNA were normalized to that of β-actin and were expressed as a ratio relative to β-actin. The primers were as follows: CFTR forward: AAGGCGGCCTATATGAGGTT, reverse: AGGACGATTCCGTTGATGAC; Slc26a3 forward: GAATGCTGATGCAGTTTGCTGAA, reverse: GAGTCCCA GGACAATGGTGAAGA; Slc26a6 forward: TGGTGGTGAA GCTGTTGAATGAC, reverse: ATGTTGCCCACGACATCTA CCTC; TNFα forward: AGCCGATGGGTTGTACCTTG, reverse: GACGGCAGAGAGGAGGTTGA; IFNγ forward: CCT GCGGCCTAGCTCTGAG, reverse: GCCATGAGGAAGAG CTGCA; β-actin forward: TACAGCTTCACCACCACAGC, reverse: TCTCCAGGGAGGAAGAGGAT.

Western Blot Analysis

The mucosae from jejunal graft, host jejunum, and control jejunum were homogenized in lysis buffer (1% Triton X-100, 10 mmol/L Tris, 100 mmol/L NaCl, 1 mmol/L EDTA, 1 mmol/L EGTA, 1% SDS, 0.5% Deoxycholate, 1 mmol/L NaF, 1 mmol/L phenylmethylsulfonyl fluoride, 40 μg of leupeptin/ml, 5 μg of aprotinin/ml, 1 μg of pepstatin/ml) at 4°C. After centrifugation at 14000 rpm for 30 minutes at 4°C, the protein concentrations of supernatants in samples were measured by the BCA protein assay (Pierce, USA). Aliquots of supernatants were used for detecting CFTR, Slc26a3, Slc26a6, TNFα, and INFγ protein using affinity-purified polyclonal antibodies respectively. β-actin was served as internal control. Protein bands were analyzed with image analysis software. Results were expressed as the ratio relative to β-actin.

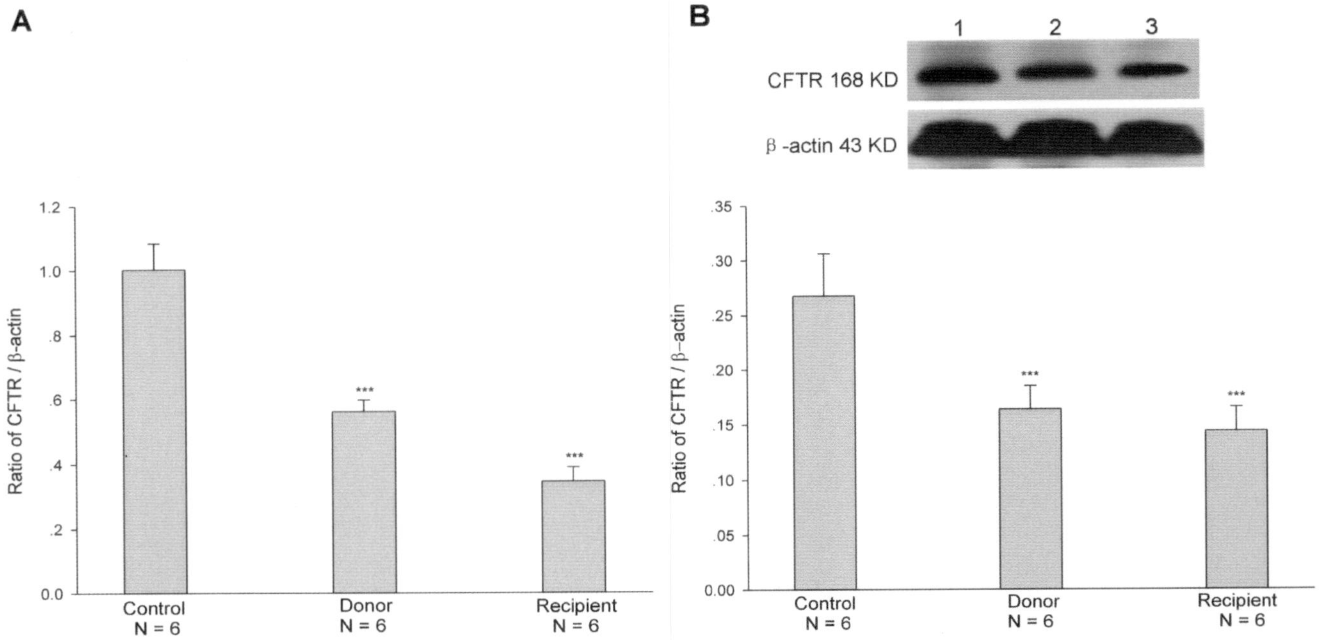

Figure 1. Expressions of mRNA (A) and protein (B) of CFTR in both donor and recipient jejunal mucosae. Upper panel in B is a representative blot graph of CFTR protein. Lane 1: Control; Lane 2: Donor; Lane 3: Recipient. The results are expressed as a ratio to β-actin. Values are mean ± SEM and n = 6 in each series. The mRNA and protein expression levels of CFTR in both donor and recipient jejunal mucosae were markedly lower than those in controls. ***$P<0.001$.

Immunohistochemistry Analysis

Immunohistochemical staining was done on the formalin-fixed and paraffin-embedded tissue blocks as previously described [15]. The tissue blocks were cut into 5 μm sections, deparaffinized, and rehydrated. Antigen retrieval was performed in 10 mmol/L citric acid buffer (pH 6.0) in a 750 W microwave for 15 minutes. Endogenous peroxidase activity was blocked with 0.3% hydrogen peroxide in methanol for 15 minutes. After incubation with anti-TNFα antibody (1:800 dilution, Abcam) overnight at 4°C, the sections were washed in PBS and then incubated with labeled polymer horseradish peroxidase rabbit antibody (Invitrogen) for 1 hour. The sections were rinsed in PBS, incubated with Dako Liquid DAB Large-Volume Substrate-Chromogen System, rinsed gently in distilled water, and counterstained with hematoxylin. Negative controls were also prepared in all assays by replacing anti-TNFα antibody with nonimmune rabbit antiserum. Computer-assisted quantification of the immunostaining was performed as described by Pilette *et al* [16] with an optical microscope (Olympus) equipped with a charge-coupled device (CCD) camera and image analysis software, using a final magnification of 400 ×. Data were collected from an average of 10 randomly selected areas in a random section (average 10 sections) from each examined tissue. Results were expressed as the mean optical density (measured in arbitrary units), representing the mean intensity of staining in the considered area.

Statistics

All results are expressed as mean ± SEM. ΔHCO_3^- and ΔI_{sc} both refer to stimulated peak responses minus basal levels. Data were analyzed by one-way analysis of variance (ANOVA) followed by Newman-Keul's *post-hoc* test or, when appropriate, by the two-tailed student t tests. $P<0.05$ was considered statistically significant.

Results

Expressions of mRNA and Protein of CFTR after Jejunal Transplantation

Intestinal secretion results from the active transports of two principal ions, Cl^- and HCO_3^-. It is well known that CFTR, which mediates intestinal epithelial Cl^- and HCO_3^- transports, plays an important role in the regulation of intestinal secretion function. Therefore, we firstly examined the mRNA and protein expressions of CFTR in both donor and recipient jejunal mucosae after heterotopic jejunal transplantation. As shown in Figure 1, the mRNA and protein expression levels of CFTR in both donor and recipient jejunal mucosae were decreased after heterotopic jejunal transplantation, compared with controls ($P<0.001$). In addition to CFTR, Slc26a3 and Slc26a6 are two major Cl^-/HCO_3^- exchangers and also regulate Cl^- and HCO_3^- transports of intestinal epithelial cells [17]. We further examined the mRNA and protein expressions of Slc26a3 and Slc26a6 in donor and recipient jejunal mucosae after heterotopic jejunal transplantation. As shown in Figure 2 and Figure 3, the mRNA and protein expression levels of both Slc26a3 and Slc26a6 in donor and recipient jejunal mucosae were not significantly altered after heterotopic jejunal transplantation, compared with controls ($P>0.05$). These results indicated that the mRNA and protein expressions of CFTR in intestinal epithelial cells, but not Slc26a3 and Slc26a6, are down-regulated after intestinal transplantation.

CFTR Function after Jejunal Transplantation

The previous studies have demonstrated that forskolin is a CFTR activator in intestinal mucosal epithelial cells [18,19]. We examined the alteration of CFTR function after jejunal transplantation through the application of forskolin. As shown in Figure 4, forskolin-stimulated jejunal mucosal epithelial HCO_3^-

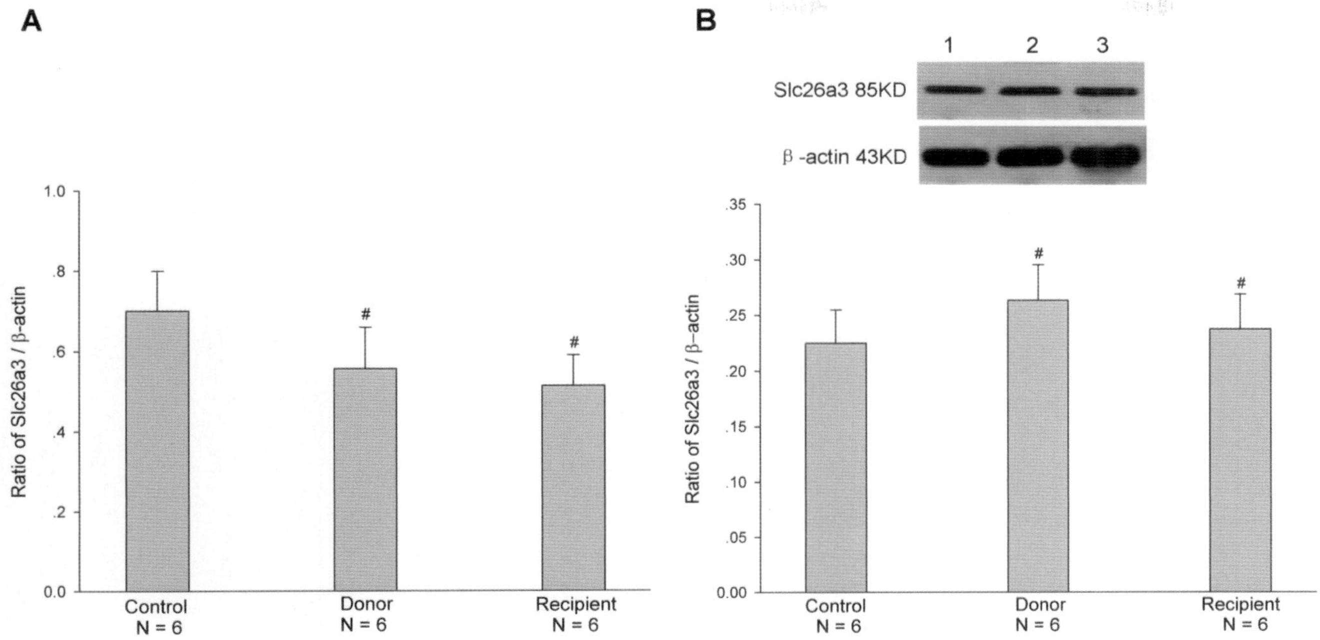

Figure 2. Expressions of mRNA (A) and protein (B) of Slc26a3 in both donor and recipient jejunal mucosae. Upper panel in B is a representative blot graph of Slc26a3 protein. Lane 1: Control; Lane 2: Donor; Lane 3: Recipient. The results are expressed as a ratio to β-actin. Values are mean ± SEM and n=6 in each series. The mRNA and protein expression levels of Slc26a3 in both donor and recipient jejunal mucosae were not altered significantly, compared with controls. $^{\#}P>0.05$.

secretion and I_{sc} were markedly decreased in both donor and recipient jejunums after heterotopic jejunal transplantation, compared with controls. Forskolin-stimulated jejunal mucosal epithelial net peak HCO_3^- secretion and I_{sc} were decreased by 50.35% and 56.83% in donor jejunum (P<0.001) and by 47.97% and 51.66% in recipient jejunum (P<0.001), respectively. The results indicated that CFTR function is impaired in both donor and recipient jejunums after heterotopic jejunal transplantation.

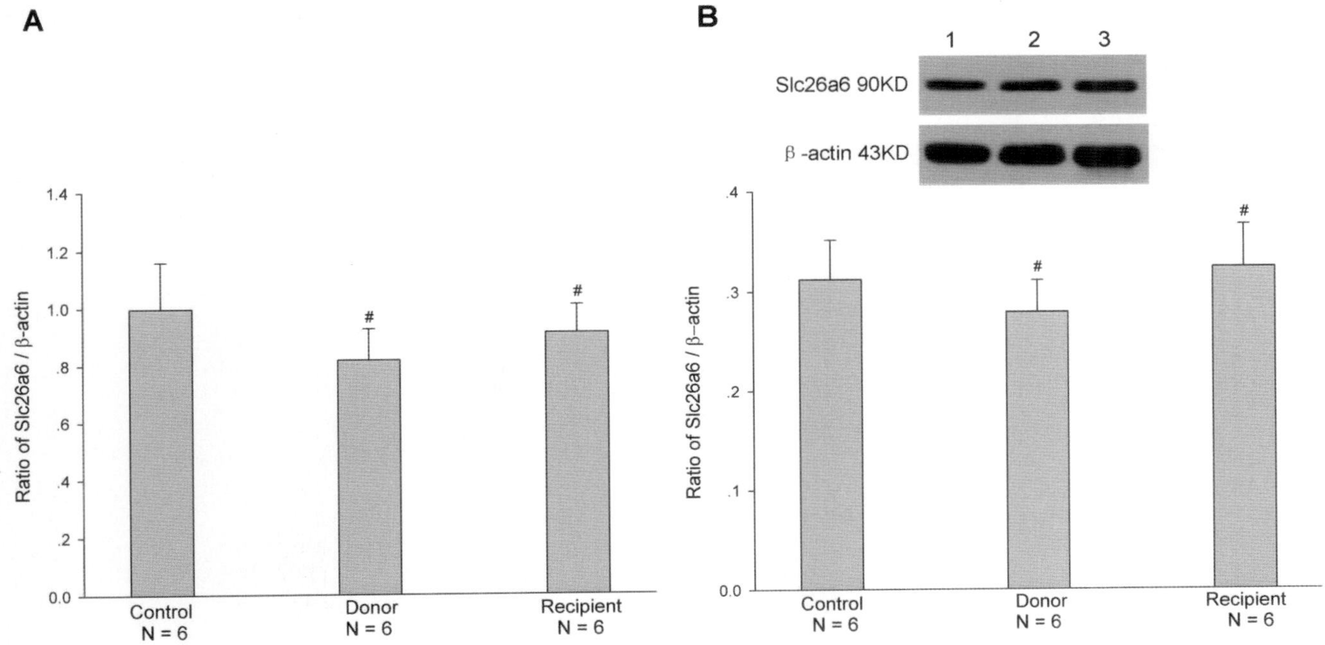

Figure 3. Expressions of mRNA (A) and protein (B) of Slc26a6 in both donor and recipient jejunal mucosae. Upper panel in B is a representative blot graph of Slc26a6 protein. Lane 1: Control; Lane 2: Donor; Lane 3: Recipient. The results are expressed as a ratio to β-actin. Values are mean ± SEM and n=6 in each series. The mRNA and protein expression levels of Slc26a6 in both donor and recipient jejunal mucosae were not altered significantly, compared with controls. $^{\#}P>0.05$.

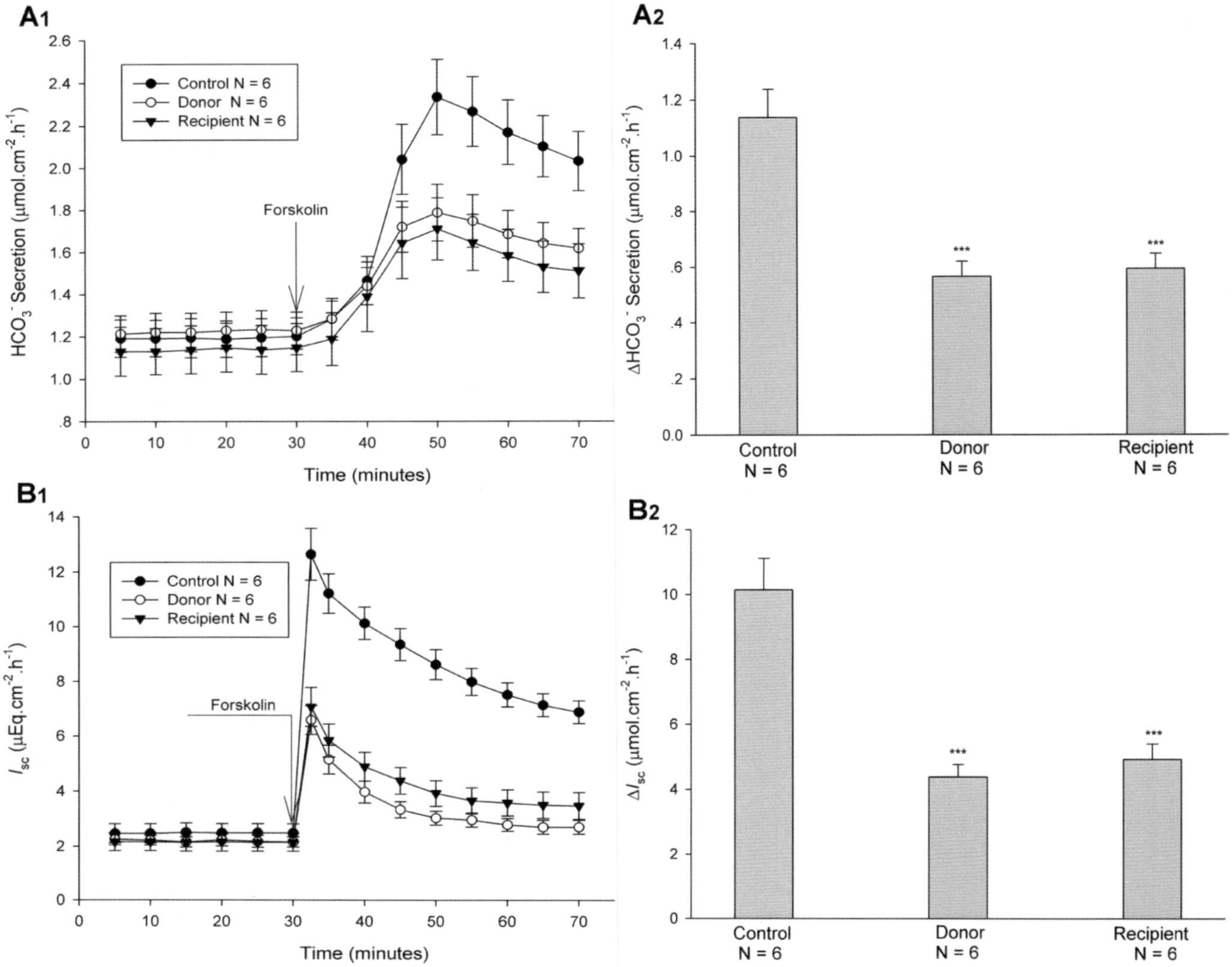

Figure 4. Change of CFTR function after jejunal transplantation in mice. A_1 represents time course of HCO_3^- secretion and A_2 represents ΔHCO_3^-. B_1 represents time course of Cl^- secretion and B_2 represents $\Delta\ Cl^-$. Forskolin (10 µM) was added at the time indicated by the arrow. Values are mean± SEM and n = 6 in each series. Forskolin-stimulated HCO_3^- and Cl^- secretions in both donor and recipient jejunal mucosae were markedly decreased, compared with controls. *** $P<0.001$.

Expressions of mRNA and Protein of Cytokines IFNγ and TNFα after Jejunal Transplantation

The previous studies have shown that cytokines, IFNγ and TNFα, regulated the expression of CFTR in epithelial cells [20-22]. Therefore, we examined the mRNA and protein expressions of cytokines IFNγ and TNFα in both donor and recipient jejunal mucosae after heterotopic jejunal transplantation. The results showed that the mRNA and protein expression levels of IFNγ in both donor and recipient jejunal mucosae were not significantly altered after heterotopic jejunal transplantation, compared with controls (P>0.05, Figure 5). The mRNA and protein expression levels of TNFα in recipient jejunal mucosa were not significantly altered either, compared with controls (P>0.05), but the mRNA and protein expression levels of TNFα in donor jejunal mucosa was markedly increased, compared with controls (P<0.001) (Figure 6). We further examined the expression and location of TNFα in jejunal mucosa by immunohistochemistry. The results showed that TNFα was expressed in the monocytes of intestinal mucosa and there were not the expressions of TNFα in both villous and cryptal epithelial cells of intestinal mucosa, and further confirmed the increased expression of TNFα in jejunal mucosa of donor after transplantation compared with control (Figure 7) (P<0.001).

Effect of TNFα on the mRNA Expression of CFTR in Jejunal Mucosa

We further examined the effect of TNFα on the mRNA expression of CFTR in jejunal mucosa through the experiments *in vitro*. As shown in Figure 8, the mRNA expression level of CFTR in jejunal mucosa was markedly decreased at 1 hour after the incubation of murine jejunal mucosa with TNFα, compared with control (P<0.05), but not time-dependent. The results indicated that TNFα may down-regulate the mRNA expression of CFTR in jejunal mucosa.

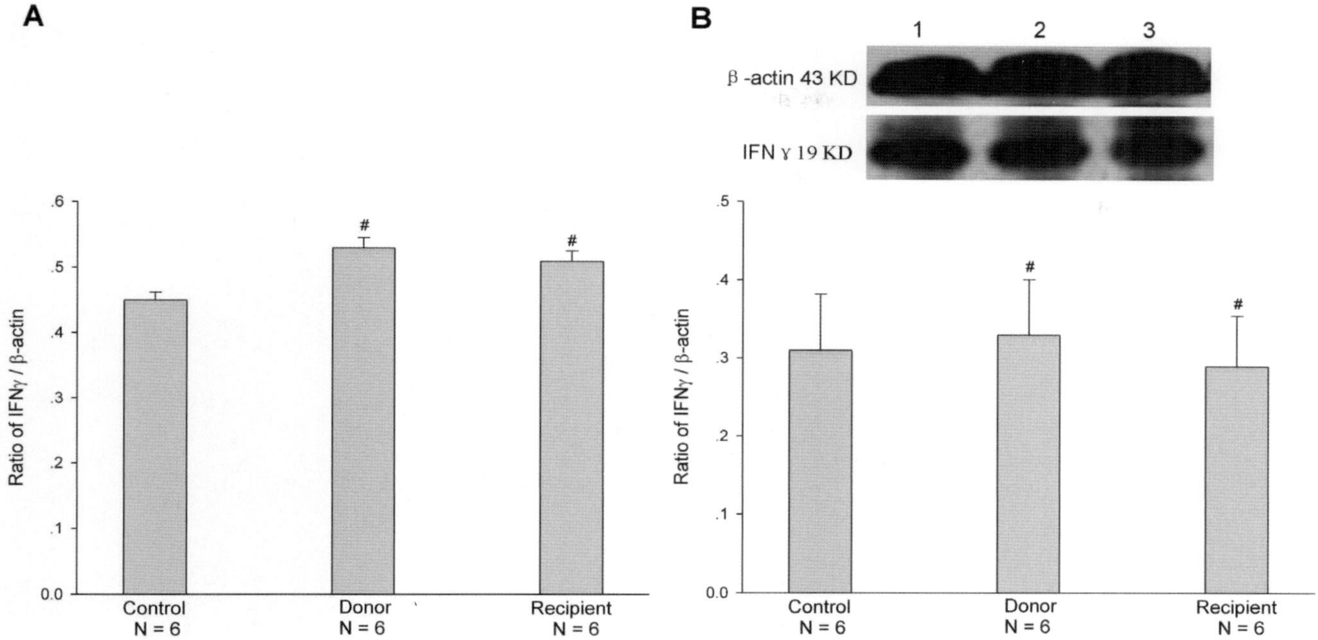

Figure 5. Expressions of mRNA (A) and protein (B) of IFNγ in both donor and recipient jejunal mucosae. Upper panel in B is a representative blot graph of IFNγ protein. Lane 1: Control; Lane 2: Donor; Lane 3: Recipient. The results are expressed as a ratio to β-actin. Values are mean ± SEM and n=6 in each series. The mRNA and protein expression levels of IFNγ in both donor and recipient jejunal mucosae were not significantly altered, compared with controls. #$P>0.05$.

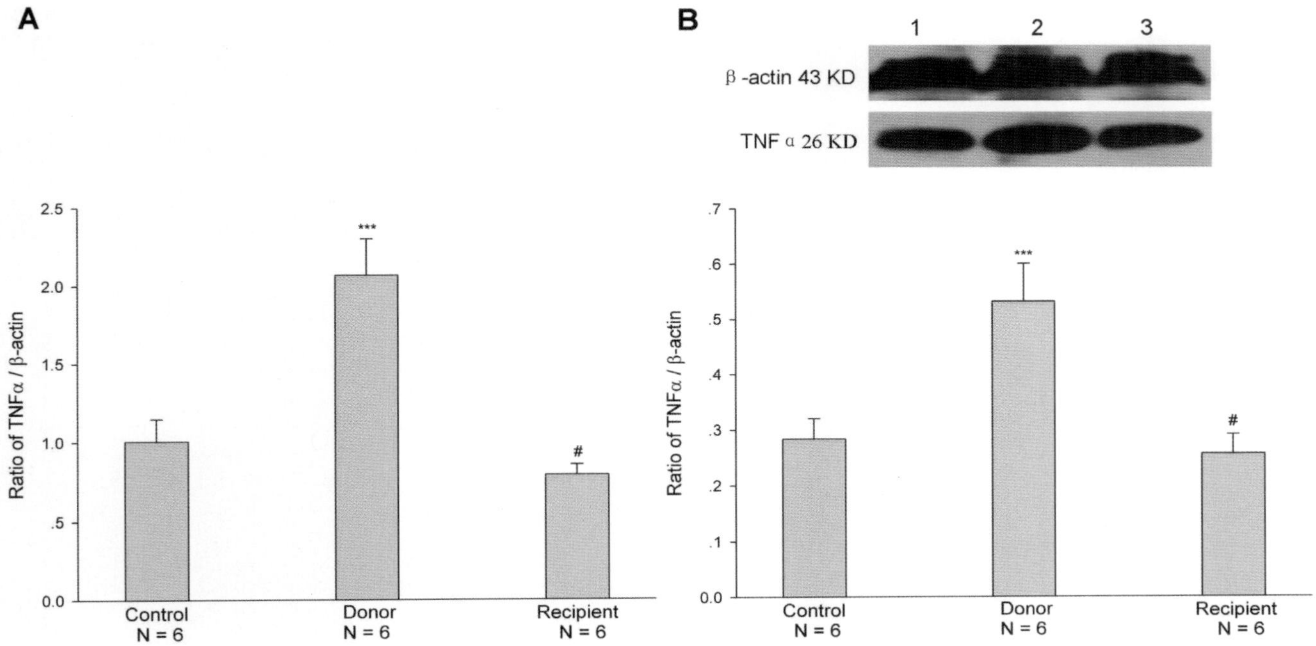

Figure 6. Expressions of mRNA (A) and protein (B) of TNFα in both donor and recipient jejunal mucosae. Upper panel in B is a representative blot graph of TNFα protein. Lane 1: Control; Lane 2: Donor; Lane 3: Recipient. The results are expressed as a ratio to β-actin. Values are mean ± SEM and n=6 in each series. The mRNA and protein expression levels of TNFα in recipient jejunal mucosa were not significantly altered, compared with controls. However, the mRNA and protein expression levels of TNFα in donor jejunal mucosa were markedly higher than those in controls. #$P>0.05$; ***$P<0.001$.

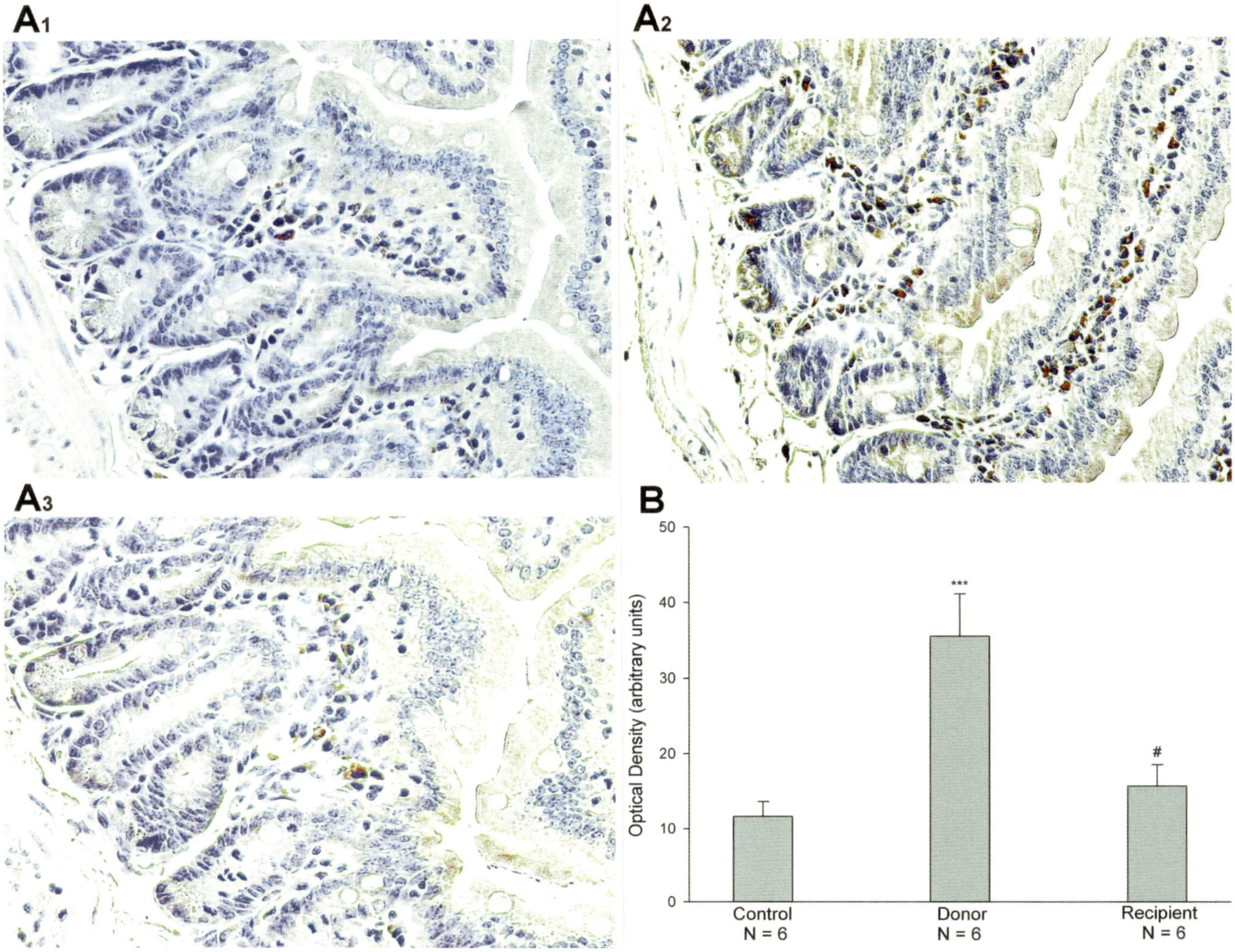

Figure 7. Immunohistochemical analysis of TNFα expression. (A) Representative images for TNFα expressions in the jejunal mucosae of control (A1), donor (A2), and recipient (A3). The brown immunostainings in the cells are TNFα. TNFα is located in the monocytes of intestinal mucosa, and there are not the expressions of TNFα in both villous and cryptal epithelial cells of intestinal mucosa. (B) Expression levels of TNFα in the jejunal mucosae of control, donor, and recipient. The results are expressed as optical density (arbitrary units). Values are mean ± SEM and n = 6 in each series. The expression level of TNFα in the jejunal mucosa of donor was higher markedly than that in control, but there was no significant difference between the expression levels of TNFα in the jejunal mucosae of recipient and control. $^{***}P<0.001$, $^{\#}P>0.05$.

Discussion

In the present study, our results demonstrated that after intestinal transplantation, the function of CFTR was impaired, and its mRNA and protein expressions were down-regulated, which may be induced by TNFα.

Although the outcomes of intestinal transplantation have been improved dramatically in the past 10 years, largely through advances in immunosuppression protocols, improved surgical technique and postoperative care, and accumulated experience, the clinical results are not so satisfactory yet, compared with those of other solid organ transplants, e.g. liver and renal transplantation. The intestine functions as both a secretory and an absorptive organ and is in a dynamic state of secretion and absorption, capable of transporting very large volumes of fluid and electrolytes, which is necessary for digestion and physiologic homeostasis. Therefore, the secretion and absorption function of intestinal graft is a factor that possibly contributes to the clinical success of intestinal transplantation. CFTR is a cAMP-activated epithelial Cl^- channel with Cl^- and HCO_3^- conductance and abundantly expressed in several functionally diverse tissues. In addition to its involvement in epithelial Cl^- and HCO_3^- secretions, CFTR also regulates other plasma membrane proteins, including the outwardly rectifying Cl^- channels, epithelial Na^+ channels, K^+ channels, ATP-release mechanisms, anion exchangers, Na^+-HCO_3^- cotransporters, and aquaporin water channels [23-25]. Thus CFTR might be central in determining transepithelial salt transport, fluid flow, and intracellular ion concentrations. In intestinal epithelial cells, CFTR plays an important role in the regulation of fluid, Cl^-, and HCO_3^- transports [9,12]. Intestinal disease in cystic fibrosis is primarily targeted to the small intestine and is characterized by defective alkalinization of secretions in the proximal small intestine, luminal obstruction by thick mucoid secretions, and malabsorption [26]. However, little is known of the function and expression of CFTR after intestinal transplantation. The previous studies have shown that forskolin stimulates

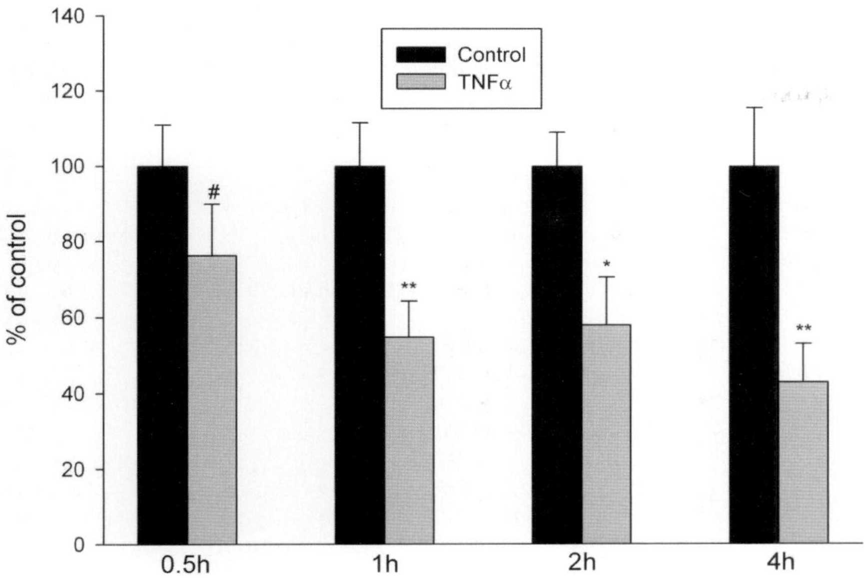

Figure 8. Effect of TNFα on CFTR mRNA expression in jejunal mucosa. The jejunal mucosae in normal mice were treated for different time with TNFα (50 ng/ml) *in vitro*. The RNA extraction and real-time RT-PCR analysis of jejunal mucosae were performed as described in Materials and Methods. The results were expressed as % of control values. Values are mean ± SEM of 6 independent experiments in each series. TNFα markedly increased the mRNA expression level of CFTR in jejunal mocosa after the incubation of 1 hour, but not time-dependent. *$P<0.05$, **$P<0.01$.

intestinal mucosal epithelial HCO_3^- and Cl^- secretions and the deletion of CFTR gene completely abolished forskolin-stimulated intestinal mucosal epithelial HCO_3^- and Cl^- secretions [18,19], strongly demonstrating forkolin induces intestinal mucosal epithelial HCO_3^- and Cl^- secretions through CFTR. In this study, we found that the mRNA and protein expression levels of CFTR, but not Cl^-/HCO_3^- exchanges Slc26a3 and Slc26a6, were markedly decreased in both donor and recipient jejunal mucosae after heterotopic jejunal transplantation compared with controls. The further examination found that forskolin-stimulated jejunal mucosal epithelial HCO_3^- and Cl^- secretions were markedly decreased in both donor and recipient jejunums compared with controls. The results indicated that the CFTR function of intestinal graft is impaired and its mRNA and protein expressions are down-regulated after intestinal transplantation.

What is responsible for the alterations of function and expression of CFTR after intestinal transplantation? The previous studies have shown that TNFα down-regulated CFTR mRNA expression in HT-29 cells, a colon epithelium-derived tumor cell line, in a dose- and time-dependent fashion [22]. IFNγ, but not IFNα or IFNβ, down-regulated CFTR mRNA levels in two colon-derived epithelial cell lines, HT-29 and T84 cells, in a time- and concentration-dependent manner [20]. And TNFα and IFNγ synergistically decreased CFTR mRNA expressions in HT-29 and T84 cells [27]. In addition, TNFα and IFNγ decreased agonist-stimulated CFTR-mediated Cl^- secretion in T84 cells [27,28]. In this study, therefore, we first examined the mRNA and protein expressions of TNFα and IFNγ in donor and recipient jejunums after heterotopic jejunal transplantation. The results showed that the mRNA and protein expression levels of IFNγ in donor and recipient jejunums were not altered significantly compared with controls, and the mRNA and protein expression levels of TNFα in recipient jejunum was not altered significantly either. However, the mRNA and protein expression levels of TNFα in donor jejunum were markedly higher than those in controls. Immunohistochemical results also showed an enhanced expression of TNFα in donor jejunum. The results indicated that it is possible that TNFα induces the alterations of function and expression of CFTR. Our results showed that the alterations of CFTR expression and function occurred in both donor and recipient jejunums, but the alteration of TNFα expression only occurred in the donor jejunum, indicating that TNFα might exert its effect on the recipient jejunum through blood circulation in addition to its local action on the donor jejunum. The further experiments showed that the incubation of jejunal mucosa with TNFα in vitro decreased the mRNA expression level of CFTR in jejunal mucosa. Taken together, these results indicate that TNFα induces the alterations of function and expression of intestinal CFTR after intestinal transplantation.

TNFα is a potent pro-inflammatory cytokine that regulates essential biological functions (e.g., cell differentiation, proliferation, survival, apoptosis) and a broad spectrum of responses to stress and injury, and plays a critical role in the pathogenesis of chronic inflammatory diseases [29,30]. It is primarily produced by immune cells such as monocytes and macrophages, but it can also be released by many other cell types, including acinar cells. The studies in the experiments *in vitro* showed that human colonic epithelial cells might produce a wide range of proinflammatory cytokines, including TNF-α, in response to invasive microbial pathogens [31.32]. In this study, our immunohistochemical results showed that TNFα was located in the monocytes of intestinal mucosa, and there were not the expressions of TNFα in both villous and cryptal epithelial cells of intestinal mucosa. The results indicate that TNFα is primarily produced by the monocytes of intestinal mucosa after the intestinal transplantation.

What induced the increase of TNFα in the mucosa of the intestinal graft? In this study, we used the mode of syngeneic murine heterotopic jejunal transplantation, which is exclusive of the effects of graft rejection and graft-versus-host reaction. In addition, the expression of TNFα was only enhanced in the donor jejunal mucosa, not in the recipient jejunal mucosa, after the heterotopic jejunal transplantation, indicating that it is possible that anatomic changes, including transection of the intestinal wall along with intrinsic neurons, complete extrinsic autonomic denervation, and the disruption of lymphatic drainage, or ischemia–reperfusion injury induced the increase of TNFα in the mucosa of the intestinal graft. Although infection and endotoxemia are potent stimulants of TNFα production, the studies also found that intestinal ischemia–reperfusion increased TNFα levels in the serum and intestinal tissue of rat [33-35]. In addition, enteric nervous system also plays an important role in the regulation of intestinal immune function. The interactions between the enteric nervous system and local immunocytes are responsible for many functional changes, including motility and secretion. Several neuropeptides, such as tachykinins, vasoactive intestinal peptide, somatostatin, and opioids, are involved in both intrinsic and extrinsic innervation but can also affect the release of cytokines and proinflammatory mediators. On the other hand, proinflammatory mediators, such as eicosanoids and cytokines, may activate intrinsic neurons directly or stimulate extrinsic neurons indirectly, releasing neuropeptides which act on intrinsic neurons, smooth muscle cells, or enterocytes [36,37]. In several models of experimental inflammation, intrinsic denervation as well as destruction of sensory C fibres affected the local immune reactions. The functional ablation of sensory neurons by capsaicin pretreatment worsened colitis in rabbit [38]. The vagotomy significantly increased the TNF-α levels in serum and colonic tissue in mice [39,40]. These studies indicate that extrinsic and intrinsic denervations might affect the release of TNF-α in the monocytes of intestinal mucosa.

In conclusion, our study demonstrates that intestinal transplantation impairs the CFTR function and down-regulates the expression of CFTR in intestinal mucosal epithelial cells, even in non-rejecting small intestinal graft. It also implicates that the examination of CFTR mRNA in biopsy specimens following intestinal transplantation may provide useful information for evaluating intestinal graft function.

Author Contributions

Conceived and designed the experiments: PS SZ. Performed the experiments: PS WS XL CJ HX LZ. Analyzed the data: PS WS XL CJ HX LZ BT SZ. Contributed reagents/materials/analysis tools: PS. Wrote the paper: PS BT SZ.

References

1. Fryer JP (2007) Intestinal transplantation: Current status. Gastroenterol Clin N Am 36: 145–159.
2. Fryer JP (2008) The current status of intestinal transplantation. Curr Opin Organ Tran 13: 266–272.
3. Garg M, Jones RM, Vaughan RB, Testro AG (2011) Intestinal transplantation: Current status and future directions. J Gastroenterol Hepatol 26: 1221–1228.
4. Ueno T, Fukuzawa M (2010) Current Status of Intestinal Transplantation. Surg Today 40: 1112–1122.
5. Kim J, Fryer J, Craig RM (1998) Absorptive Function Following Small Intestinal Transplantation. Dig Dis Sci 43: 1925–1930.
6. Watson AJ, Lear PA, Montgomery A, Elliott E, Dacre J, et al. (1988) Water, electrolyte, glucose, and glycine absorption in rat small intestinal transplants. Gastroenterology 94: 863–869.
7. Pakarinen MP, Halttunen J (2000) The physiology of the transplanted small bowel: An overview with Insight into graft function. Scand J Gastroenterol 35: 561–577.
8. Sarr MG (1996) Enteric physiology of the transplanted gut: absorption and motility. Dig Surg 13: 181–193.
9. Banks MR, Farthing MJG (2002) Fluid and electrolyte transport in the small intestine. Curr Opin Gastroenterol 18: 176–181.
10. Bradbury NA (1999) Intracellular CFTR: Localization and function. Physiol Rev 79: S175-S191.
11. Sheppard DN, Welsh MJ (1999) Structure and function of the CFTR chloride channel. Physiol Rev 79: S23-S45.
12. Ameen N, Alexis J, Salas P (2000) Cellular localization of the cystic fibrosis transmembrane conductance regulator in mouse intestinal tract. Histochem Cell Biol 114: 69–75.
13. Zhong R, Zhang Z, Quan D, Duff J, Stiller C, et al. (1993) Development of a mouse intestinal transplantation model. Microsurgery 14: 141–145.
14. Tuo BG, Riederer B, Wang Z, Colledge WH, Soleimani M, et al. (2006) Involvement of the anion exchanger SLC26A6 in prostaglandin E_2- but not forskolin-stimulated duodenal HCO_3^- secretion. Gastroenterology 130: 349–358.
15. Xu J, Xie R, Liu X, Wen G, Jin H, et al. (2012) Expression and functional role of vacuolar H^+-ATPase in human hepatocellular carcinoma. Carcinogenesis 33; 2432–2440.
16. Pilette C, Colinet B, Kiss R, André S, Kaltner H, et al. (2007) Increased galectin-3 expression and intra-epithelial neutrophils in small airways in severe COPD. Eur Respir J 29, 914–922.
17. Dorwart MR, Shcheynikov N, Yang D, Muallem S (2008) The solute carrier 26 family of proteins in epithelial ion transport. Physiology 23: 104–114.
18. Seidler U, Blumenstein I, Kretz A,Viellard-Baron D, Rossmann H, et al. (1997) A functional CFTR protein is required for mouse intestinal cAMP-, cGMP-, and Ca^{2+}-dependent HCO_3^- secretion. J Physiol (Lond) 505: 411–423.
19. Tuo B, Wen G, Seidler U (2009) Differential activation of the CFTR HCO_3^- conductance by genistein and forskolin in murine duodenum. Brit J Pharmacol 158: 1313–1321.
20. Besancon F, Przewlocki G, Baro I, Hongre AS, Escande D, et al. (1994) Interferon-gamma downregulates CFTR gene expression in epithelial cells. Am J Physiol Cell Physiol 267: C1398–C1404.
21. Kulka M, Dery R, Nahirney D, Duszyk M, Befus AD (2005) Differential regulation of cystic fibrosis transmembrane conductance regulator by interferon γ in mast cells and epithelial cells. J Pharmacol Exp Ther 315: 563–570.
22. Nakamura H, Yoshimura K, Bajocchi G, Trapnell BC, Pavirani A, et al. (1992) Tumor necrosis factor modulation of expression of the cystic fibrosis transmembrane conductance regulator gene. FEBS Lett 314: 366–70.
23. Guggino WB, Stanton BA (2006) New insights into cystic fibrosis: molecular switches that regulate CFTR. Nature Rev Mol Cell Biol 7: 426–436.
24. Guggino WB (2004) The cystic fibrosis transmembrane regulator forms macromolecular complexes with PDZ domain scaffolding proteins. Proc Am Thorac Soc 1: 28–32.
25. Riordan JR (2005) Assembly of functional CFTR chloride channels. Annu Rev Physiol 67: 701–718.
26. Eggermont E, De Boeck K (1991) Small-intestinal abnormalities in cystic fibrosis patients. Eur J Pediatr 150: 824–828.
27. Fish SM, Proujansky R, Reenstra WW (1999) Synergistic effects of interferon γ and tumour necrosis factor α on T84 cell function. Gut 45: 191–198.
28. Resta-Lenert S, Barrett KE (2006) Probiotics and commensals reverse TNF-alpha- and IFN-gamma-induced dysfunction in human intestinal epithelial cells. Gastroenterology 130: 731–746.
29. Apostolaki M, Armaka M, Victoratos P, Kollias G (2010) Cellular mechanisms of TNF function in models of inflammation and autoimmunity. Curr Dir Autoimmun 11: 1–26.
30. Croft M (2009) The role of TNF superfamily members in T-cell function and diseases. Nat Rev Immunol 9: 271–285.
31. Eckmann L, Reed SL, Smith JR, Kagnoff MF (1995) Entamoeba histolytica trophozoites induce an inflammatory cytokine response by cultured human cells through the paracrine action of cytolytically released interleukin-1α. J Clin Invest 96: 1269–1279.
32. Jung HC, Eckmann L, Yang SK, Panja A, Fierer J, et al. (1995) A distinct array of proinflammatory cytokines is expressed in human colon epithelial cells in response to bacterial invasion. J Clin Invest 95: 55–65.
33. Arumugam TV, Shiels IA, Margolin SB, Taylor SM, Brown L (2002) Pirfenidone attenuates ischaemia-reperfusion injury in the rat small intestine. Clin Exp Pharmacol Physiol 29: 996–1000.
34. de Arruda MJ, Poggetti RS, Fontes B, Younes RN, Souza Jr AL, et al.(2006) Intestinal ischemia/reperfusion induces bronchial hyperreactivity and increases serum TNF-alpha in rats. Clinics (Sao Paulo) 61: 21–28.
35. Yamamoto S, Tanabe M, Wakabayashi G, Shimazu M, Matsumoto K, et al. (2001) The role of tumor necrosis factor-alpha and interleukin-1beta in ischemia-reperfusion injury of the rat small intestine. J Surg Res 99: 134–141.
36. Bueno L (2000) Neuroimmune alterations of ENS functioning. Gut 47: suppl 4 iv63 - iv65.
37. Straub RH, Wiest R, Strauch UG, Härle P, Schölmerich J (2006) The role of the sympathetic nervous system in intestinal inflammation. Gut 55: 1640–1649.
38. Reinshagen M, Patel A, Sottili M, Nast C, Davis W, et al. (1994) Protective function of extrinsic sensory neurons in acute rabbit experimental colitis. Gastroenterology 106: 1208–1214.
39. Ghia JE, Blennerhassett P, Collins SM (2007) Vagus nerve integrity and experimental colitis. Am J Physiol Gastrointest Liver Physiol 293: G560 - G567.
40. van Westerloo DJ, Giebelen IA, Florquin S, Bruno MJ, Larosa GJ, et al. (2006) The vagus nerve and nicotinic receptors modulate experimental pancreatitis severity in mice. Gastroenterology 130: 1822–1830.

Peroxisome Proliferator-Activated Receptor γ Deficiency in T Cells Accelerates Chronic Rejection by Influencing the Differentiation of CD4+ T Cells and Alternatively Activated Macrophages

Xiaofan Huang[1]⁹, Lingyun Ren[1]⁹, Ping Ye[2], Chao Cheng[1], Jie Wu[1], Sihua Wang[3], Yuan Sun[1], Zheng Liu[1], Aini Xie[4], Jiahong Xia[1,5]*

1 Department of Cardiovascular Surgery, Union Hospital, Tongji Medical College, Huazhong University of Science and Technology, Wuhan, People's Republic of China, **2** Department of Cardiology, Central Hospital of Wuhan, Wuhan, People's Republic of China, **3** Department of Thoracic Surgery, Union Hospital, Tongji Medical College, Huazhong University of Science and Technology, Wuhan, People's Republic of China, **4** Division of Diabetes, Endocrinology and Metabolism, Department of Medicine, Baylor College of Medicine, Houston, Texas, United States of America, **5** Department of Cardiovascular Surgery, Central Hospital of Wuhan, Wuhan, People's Republic of China

Abstract

Background: In a previous study, activation of the peroxisome proliferator–activated receptor γ (PPARγ) inhibited chronic cardiac rejection. However, because of the complexity of chronic rejection and the fact that PPARγ is widely expressed in immune cells, the mechanism of the PPARγ - induced protective effect was unclear.

Materials and Methods: A chronic rejection model was established using B6.C-H-2^{bm12}KhEg (H-2^{bm12}) mice as donors, and MHC II-mismatched T-cell-specific PPARγ knockout mice or wild type (WT) littermates as recipients. The allograft lesion was assessed by histology and immunohistochemistry. T cells infiltrates in the allograft were isolated, and cytokines and subpopulations were detected using cytokine arrays and flow cytometry. Transcription levels in the allograft were measured by RT-PCR. In vitro, the T cell subset differentiation was investigated after culture in various polarizing conditions. PPARγ-deficient regularory T cells (Treg) were cocultured with monocytes to test their ability to induce alternatively activated macrophages (AAM).

Results: T cell-specific PPARγ knockout recipients displayed reduced cardiac allograft survival and an increased degree of pathology compared with WT littermates. T cell-specific PPARγ knockout resulted in more CD4+ T cells infiltrating into the allograft and altered the Th1/Th2 and Th17/Treg ratios. The polarization of AAM was also reduced by PPARγ deficiency in T cells through the action of Th2 and Treg. PPARγ-deficient T cells eliminated the pioglitazone-induced polarization of AAM and reduced allograft survival.

Conclusions: PPARγ-deficient T cells influenced the T cell subset and AAM polarization in chronic allograft rejection. The mechanism of PPARγ activation in transplantation tolerance could yield a novel treatment without side effects.

Editor: Josep Bassaganya-Riera, Virginia Tech, United States of America

Funding: This study was funded by the National Nature Science Foundation of China (Program No: 81070205, 81130056, 81100176 and 81373170). The funders had no role in study design, data collection and analysis, decision to publish, or preparation of the manuscript.

Competing Interests: The authors have declared that no competing interests exist.

* Email: jiahong.xia@mail.hust.edu.cn

⁹ These authors contributed equally to this work.

Introduction

In end-stage heart disease, heart transplantation is becoming the most important clinical treatment [1]. However, even with efficient immunosuppressive therapy to prevent acute rejection in the early stage after transplantation, chronic allograft rejection is the major obstacle to the long-term survival of heart transplant recipients [2]. The principal phenomena causing chronic allograft rejection are coronary allograft vasculopathy (CAV) [3] and leukocytes from recipients infiltrating into allografts [4]. Previous studies have demonstrated that an immune mechanism participates in chronic allograft rejection. Many studies have focused on CD4+ T helper cells and their subsets, such as Th1, Th2, Th17 and regulatory T cells (Treg), in the process of chronic allograft rejection. Th1 and Th17 secrete the pro-inflammatory cytokines interferon (IFN)-γ and IL-17A, which are known to promote chronic allograft rejection [5,6]. Th2 cells secrete IL-4, IL-5, IL-10, and IL-13, whereas Treg have an immunoregulatory function that has protective effects in numerous situations [7,8]. CD4+ T helper cells and their associated cytokines can influence the function and polarization of macrophages [9]. The classically activated macrophage (CAM)/alternatively activated macrophage (AAM) ratio in allografts has been considered to play a key role in the immune response to transplantation [10]. Within the complex mechanism of chronic allograft rejection, both T cells and macrophages participate in the lesion of allografts [3]. These cells are immunotherapy targets in chronic allograft rejection.

Peroxisome proliferator-activated receptor-γ (PPARγ) is a member of a nuclear receptor family that regulates glucose metabolism and lipogenesis. Recently, PPARγ and its agonists were found to have immunoregulatory functions in T cells and macrophages [11–13]. Given the anti-inflammatory effects of PPARγ agonists, we and other researchers have used them to treat both acute and chronic allograft rejection and have observed clear protective effects [14–16]. However, due to the complex pathological process of chronic rejection and the broad effects of PPARγ on multiple immune cells, details regarding the effects of PPARγ on immune cells in chronic allograft rejection are unclear.

To understand the mechanism of PPARγ and its agonists in chronic allograft rejection, we used B6.C-H-2^{bm12}KhEg (H-2^{bm12}) mice as donors and T cell specific PPARγ knockout (PPARγ fl/fl; Lck-Cre$^+$, T-cell-PPARγ^{ko}) mice or wild type (WT) littermates as recipients to establish a single major histocompatibility complex (MHC) class II-mismatched cardiac chronic allograft rejection model. We found that T cell-specific PPARγ deficiency impacted the differentiation of CD4+ T cell subsets and AAM bias in cardiac allografts. The protective effect of PPARγ agonists was eliminated in PPARγ deficiency in T cells.

Materials and Methods

Animals

B6.129-Ppargtm2Rev/J (H-2^b, in short PPARγ fl/fl) mice, B6.Cg-Tg (Lck-cre)548Jxm/J (H-2^b, in short Lck-Cre$^+$) mice and B6.C-H-2^{bm12}KhEg (H-2^{bm12}, in short bm12) mice were purchased from Jackson Laboratories Inc (Bar Harbor, ME, USA). C57BL/6 (H-2^b) mice were purchased from Tongji Medical College of Huazhong University of Science and Technology (HUST) (Wuhan, China). T cell-PPARγ^{ko} mice were generated by crossbreeding and verified by the standard PCR procedure recommended by Jackson Labs. PPARγ fl/fl; Lck-Cre$^+$ T cell-PPARγ^{ko} mice and PPARγ fl/fl; Lck-Cre$^-$ WT littermates were regarded as controls for each other. All of the experimental mice were male and 6 to 8 weeks old (18–25 g body weight). The animals were bred and maintained in a specific pathogen-free (SPF) barrier facility at Tongji Medical College (Wuhan, China). All animal experiments were approved by the Institutional Animal Care and Use Committee of Tongji Medical College. The protocol was approved by the Ethics Committee of Tongji Medical College, Huazhong University of Science and Technology (IORG No: IORG0003571). All surgery was performed under sodium pentobarbital anesthesia, and all efforts were made to minimize suffering.

Cardiac transplantation model and treatment

Heterotopic vascularized cardiac transplantation models were established as described previously [17]. Donor and recipient mice were anesthetized by intraperitoneal injection with ketamine at 1 mg/kg body weight. The donor hearts were transplanted into the abdomens of the recipients; the ascending aorta was connected to the recipient abdominal aorta and the pulmonary artery was sutured with the recipient inferior vena cava. The recipient mice were maintained on a thermal place until recovery from operation. Allograft function was monitored by daily palpation. At the endpoint of experiments, mice were sacrificed by an over dose injection of ketamine and heart grafts were harvested for further detection. Pioglitazone (Ji'nan Zhongke Yitong Chemical Co., Ltd, Ji'nan, China) was provided in the chow (3 mg/kg*d) [15] starting at 1 day prior to the operation.

Histological analyses of allografts

Allografts from recipients were harvested 40 days after the operation. The allograft was embedded in paraffin for hematoxylin and eosin (H&E) and Masson trichrome staining. The severity of each allograft rejection was scored according to graft coronary artery disease (GAD) and parenchymal rejection (PR) grade [18,19]. A portion of the allograft was embedded in OCT (Sakura, Torrance, CA, USA) and subjected to immunohistochemical staining using anti-mouse CD4, CD8, and $\gamma\delta$TCR antibodies (eBioscience, San Diego, CA).

Isolation of infiltrated lymphocytes from allografts and flow cytometry

The infiltrated lymphocytes were isolated as described previously [20]. The allografts were cut into pieces and digested with 2 mg/ml collagenase D (Worthington Bio, Lakewood, NJ) combined with 10% fecal calf serum in RPMI 1640 media for 2 h at 37°C. The suspensions were filtered with cell strainers (40 μm, BD Biosciences, San Diego, CA). The isolated cells were stained with FITC-anti-CD4, APC-Cy7-anti-CD11b, PerCP-Cy5.5-anti-IFN-γ, eFlour660-anti-IL-13, PE-anti-IL-17A, APC-anti-Foxp3, and 7-AAD (eBioscience, San Diego, CA) according to eBioscience's Best Protocols. The cells were assessed with a fluorescence activated cell sorter (FACS) Aria II (BD Biosciences, San Diego, CA) and analyzed using FCS Express 4 Plus (De Novo Software, Los Angeles, CA).

Immunoblots and enzyme-linked immunosorbent assay (ELISA)

To measure the cytokine secretion of the infiltrated CD4+ T cells, lymphocytes were sterilely isolated from allografts using a CD4+ T cell isolation kit (Miltenyi Biotec, Bergisch Gladbach, Germany) and cultured in neutral stimulate with plate-bound anti-CD3 (5 μm/ml, eBioscience) and anti-CD28 (10 μm/ml, eBioscience) antibodies. The supernatants were removed after 48 h, and cytokine levels were analyzed using a mouse cytokine antibody array (RayBiotech Inc., Norcross, GA).

Quantitative real-time PCR

Total RNA was extracted from allografts or cultured cells using TRIzol Reagent (Invitrogen, Carlsbad, CA) following the manufacturer's instructions. cDNA was prepared using the PrimeScript RT Master Mix reverse transcription kit (TaKaRa, Shiga, Japan). The PCR mixture was prepared using SYBR Premix EX Taq (TaKaRa, Shiga, Japan), and transcription levels were detected using a BioRad CFX96 (Bio-Rad Laboratories Inc., Hercules, CA). The relative expression levels were normalized to the expression of GAPDH using the $\Delta\Delta$Ct method. The primers used were as follows: T-bet, forward: 5′-CAACAACCCCTTTGC-GAAAG-3′, reverse: 5′-TCCCCCAAGCAGTTGACAGT-3′; GATA-3, forward: 5′-AGCCACATCTCTCCCTTCAG-3′, reverse: 5′-AGGGCTCTGCCTCTCTAACC-3′; RORγt, forward: 5′-TGCAAGACTCATCGACAAGG-3′, reverse: 5′-AGGGGA-TTCAACATCAGTGC-3′; Foxp3, forward: 5′-ACTGGG-GTCTTCTCCCTCAA-3′, reverse: 5′-GTGGGAAGGTGCAG-AGTAG-3′; iNOS, forward: 5′-GTTCTCAGCCCAACAATAC-AAGA-3′, reverse: 5′-GTGGACGGGTCGATGTCA -3′; Arg1, forward: 5′-CTCCAAGCCAAAGTCCTTAGAG-3′, reverse: 5′-GGAGCTGTCATTAGGGACATC-3′; Mrc1, forward: 5′-AATGAAGATCACAAGCGCTGC-3′, reverse: 5′-TGACACCCAGCGGAATTTCT-3′, GAPDH, forward: 5′-TTCACCACCATGGAGAAGGC-3′, reverse: 5′-GGCATGGACTGTGGTCATGA-3′.

Cell culture and monocyte/Treg coculture

Mouse splenic CD4+ T cells were purified with a CD4+ T cell isolation kit (Miltenyi Biotec, Bergisch Gladbach, Germany) and stimulated with plate-bound anti-CD3 (5 μm/ml, eBioscience) and anti-CD28 (10 μm/ml, eBioscience) antibodies together with IL-12 (10 ng/ml) for Th1 differentiation, IL-4 (10 ng/ml) for Th2 differentiation, TGF-β (5 ng/ml) and IL-6 (20 ng/ml) for Th17 differentiation, and TGF-β (5 ng/ml) alone for Treg differentiation. All cytokines were obtained from eBioscience. Monocytes and Treg were cocultured at a ratio of 2:1 according to a previously reported method [21]. Treg and monocytes were isolated from spleen using a CD4+CD25+ isolation kit or CD11b+ isolation kit (Miltenyi Biotec, Bergisch Gladbach, Germany). The purity of CD11b+ isolated monocytes is greater than 88% by flow cytometry. Cells were cocultured with RPMI 1640 and stimulated by anti-CD3 (5 μm/ml, eBioscience) and LPS (50 ng/ml, Sigma, St Louis, USA) for 36 h.

Statistical analysis

The data are expressed as the mean±SD, and comparisons between groups were conducted using unpaired Student's *t* tests. The allograft survival curve was plotted using the Kaplan-Meier method, and differences were determined using a log-rank test. All data were analyzed using Prism 5.0 (GraphPad Software, La Jolla, CA). P values less than 0.05 were considered statistically significant.

Results

PPARγ-deficient T cells exhibit significant decreases in cardiac allografts survival and aggravate chronic allograft rejection

We established a model of heterotrophic cardiac transplantation using an MHC class II - mismatched model. To investigate the contribution of PPARγ expression in T cells to chronic allograft rejection, we used T cell-PPARγ^{ko} mice as recipients. We evaluated allografts daily by palpation to detect their function. In WT littermates, a median allograft survival (MST) of 67 days was observed after transplantation; however, the MST in T cell-PPARγ^{ko} mice was only 48 days (Figure 1A). To detect lesions of chronic allograft rejection, HE and Masson staining were performed on the allografts 40 days after transplantation. In WT littermates, perivascular leukocytic infiltration, CAV and destruction of the cardiac muscle structure were observed, however, in T cell-PPARγ^{ko} mice, more intensive chronic allograft rejection signs were noted compared with the WT littermates. (Figure 1B). Consistent with these observations, the GAD and PR scores of T cell-PPARγ^{ko} mice were increased compared with WT littermates 40 days after transplantation (Figure 1C). These results suggested that recipients with PPARγ-deficient T cells exhibited decreased allograft survival and aggravated lesions of chronic allograft rejection.

T cell PPARγ deficiency increases CD4+ T cell infiltration in cardiac allografts

Leukocyte infiltration into allografts is a hallmark and pathogenic factor of chronic allograft rejection. Given that we identified more severe lesions in T cell-PPARγ^{ko} mice, we next detected the infiltration of T cell subsets into the allograft 40 days after transplantation. The CD4+, CD8+, and γδTCR+ T cell subsets in allografts were counted per high-power field (HPF) using immunohistochemical staining. Compared with the T cell subsets in the cardiac allografts of WT littermate recipients, a remarkable increase in infiltrated CD4+ T cells was observed in T cell-PPARγ^{ko} mice. In contrast, the numbers of CD8+ and γδTCR+ T cells did not differ between the groups (Figure 2A, B). As T cell-PPARγ^{ko} mice found to have CD4+, CD8+, γδTCR+ T cells and CD11b+ monocytes ratio comparable to those of C57BL/6 and WT littermate initiate before operation (Figure S1).

PPARγ-deficient T cells alter cytokine secretion and the polarization of CD4+ T cells in cardiac allografts

Most studies have focused on Th1 (secreting IFN-γ), Th2 (secreting IL-4/13) and Th17 (secreting IL-17) cells, which were considered the predominant contributors to chronic allograft rejection. Because we found increased CD4+ T cell infiltration in PPARγ-deficient T cell recipients in a previous study, we used a cytokine antibody array to detect cytokine secretion by infiltrated CD4+ T cells *in vitro* under the neutral stimulation conditions with anti-CD3/28 40 days after transplantation. We confirmed that in PPARγ-deficient T cell recipients, CD4+ T cells secreted higher levels of Th1-related IFN-γ and Th17-related IL-17. In contrast, Th2-related IL-5, IL-10 and IL-13 cytokine secretion decreased compared with WT littermates (Figure 3A). We also used RT-PCR to measure the mRNA levels of transcription factors specific for CD4+ T cells in the cardiac allografts. The cardiac allografts from PPARγ-deficient T cell recipients expressed higher levels of Th1- and Th17- related T-bet and RORγt and reduced levels of Th2- and Treg- related GATA-3 and Foxp3 (Figure 3B). The flow cytometry data on the infiltrated CD4+ T cells in the allograft revealed a variation trend consistent with the RT-PCR data (Figure 3C, D).

PPARγ-deficient CD4+ T cells enhance Th1 and Th17 polarization *in vitro*

Previous experiments indicated that CD4+ T cell subsets varied in PPARγ-deficient T cell allografts. We tested whether the PPARγ-deficient T cells exhibited altered polarization into Th1, Th2, Th17, and Treg cells. We isolated CD4+ T cells from the spleens of T cell-PPARγ^{ko} mice or WT littermates and cultured them under Th1/Th2/Th17/Treg-polarizing conditions for 4 days. Cells were then harvested, and intracellular cytokine levels were detected using flow cytometry with intracellular staining for IFN-γ, IL-13, IL-17A, and Foxp3. A remarkable increase in IFN-γ and IL-17A production was observed in the PPARγ-deficient CD4+ T cells. However, the percentage of CD4+IL-13+ and CD4+Foxp3+ T cells did not change (Figure 4A, B). These findings suggested increased differentiation into the Th1 and Th17 subsets in PPARγ-deficient CD4+ T cells. The decreased Th2 and Treg subsets in the allografts were likely attributed to the increase in Th1 and Th17 cells and not to a failure to differentiate.

The effect of T cell PPARγ deficiency on macrophage polarization *in vivo* and *in vitro*

Previous studies have suggested that macrophages participate in chronic allograft rejection and that T cell subsets may influence macrophage polarization [9,10,21]. Therefore, we next examined whether PPARγ-deficient T cells affect macrophage infiltration and polarization in cardiac allografts. Flow cytometry was performed to detect the amount of CD11b+ F4/80+ macrophage

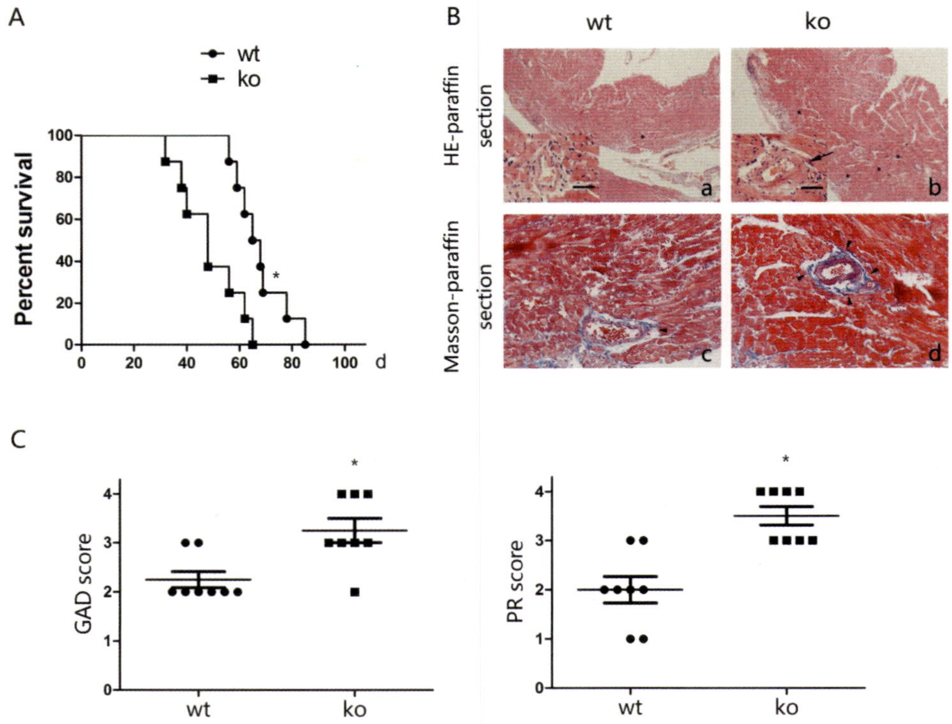

Figure 1. PPARγ-deficient T cells reduce survival and augment lesions associated with chronic rejection. A. The survival time of cardiac allografts in T cell-PPARγ^{ko} mice was significantly shorter than that of reduced compared with WT littermates. B. Cardiac allograft (bm12) sections of lesions 40 days after transplantation from T cell-PPARγ^{ko} mice (ko) or WT littermates. (a, b) HE staining, major view magnification 40×, left bottom view magnification 400×. Scale bars = 100 μm. (c, d) Masson trichrome staining, magnification 400×. T cell-PPARγ^{ko} mice exhibited severe lesions. Arrows indicate obvious intimal hyperplasia, asterisks indicate leukocytic infiltration, and filled arrowheads indicate collagen deposition. C. Graft coronary artery disease (GAD) and parenchymal rejection (PR) scores in T cell-PPARγ^{ko} mice were considerably increased compared with WT littermates. The data are presented as the mean±SD for each group (n = 8), *$p<0.05$.

infiltration at 7, 14, and 40 days after transplantation. In the cardiac allografts from T cell-PPARγ^{ko} mice, the number of macrophages was significantly increased compared with the WT littermates allografts (Figure 5A, B). To identify macrophage polarization into CAM and AAM, we measured the expression of CAM-related-iNOS, AAM-related-Arg1, and Mrc1 using RT-PCR at 7, 14, and 40 days after transplantation. Arg1 and Mrc1 mRNA levels did not increase in T cell-PPARγ^{ko} mice, whereas the levels were significantly elevated in WT littermates on days 14 and 40 post-grafting. In addition, no significant differences in the mRNA levels of CAM-related-iNOS were noted in the two groups. Therefore, in T cell-PPARγ^{ko} recipients mice, macrophages failed to differentiate into AAM in local allografts. Because some studies have demonstrated that Treg can induce AAM polarization, we hypothesized that the PPARγ-deficient Treg failed to induce AAM polarization. We isolated autologous CD4+ CD25+ Treg from the spleens of T cell-PPARγ^{ko} mice or their WT littermates and cocultured these cells with CD11b monocytes from C57BL/6 mice. After 2 days, cells were collected for RT-PCR detection. Arg1 and Mrc1 transcription levels were reduced

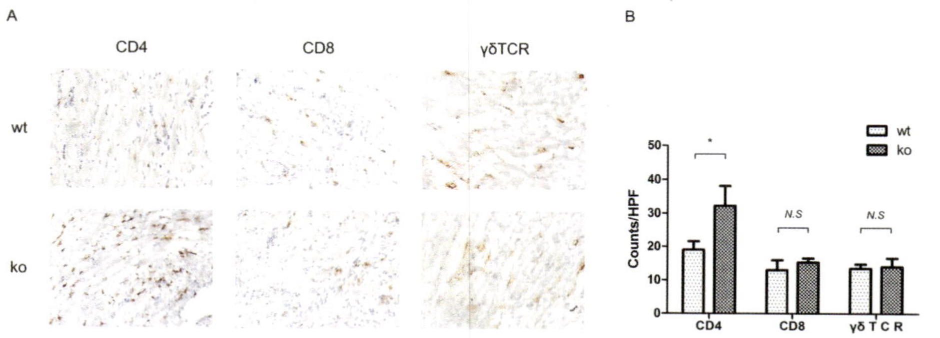

Figure 2. Infiltration CD4+, CD8+, and γδTCR+ cells in donor hearts from T cell-PPARγ^{ko} mice or WT littermates. A. Immunohistochemical staining of CD4+, CD8+, and γδTCR+ cells in allografts 40 days after transplantation. Top, allograft from T cell-PPARγ^{ko} mice (ko); bottom, allograft from WT littermates (wt). B. Quantitative analysis of CD4+, CD8+, and γδTCR+ cells in allografts counted per high power field (HPF). The data are presented as the mean±SD of 8 fields per group, *$p<0.05$.

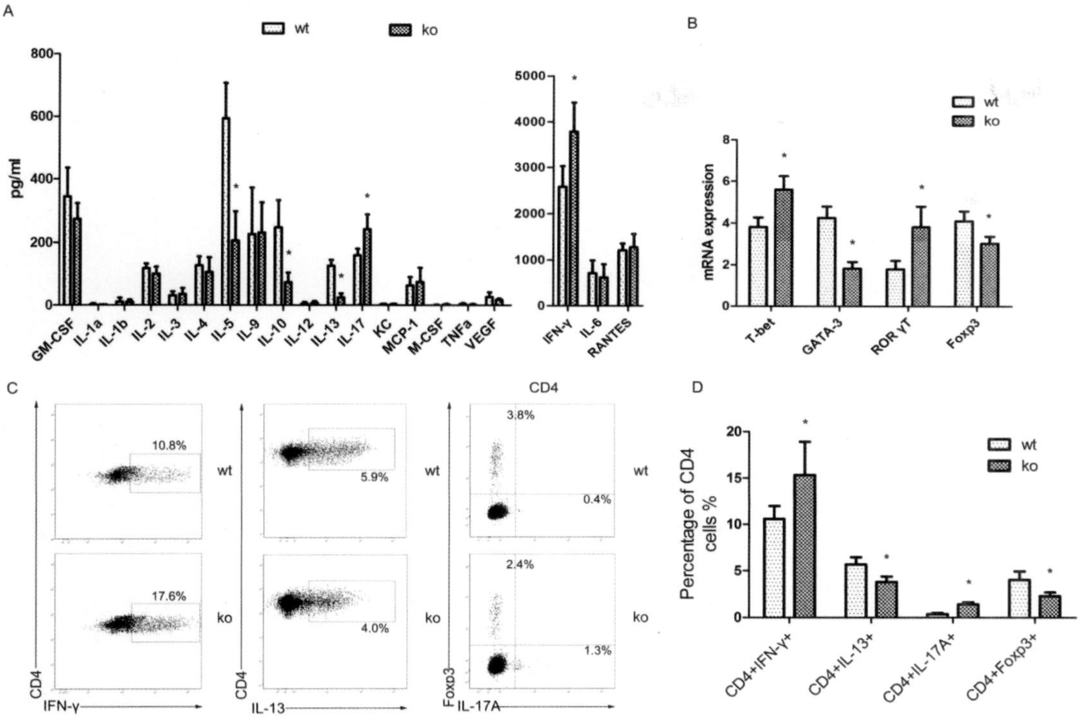

Figure 3. Cytokines and transcription factor expression in infiltrating CD4+ T cells in cardiac allografts. A. Analysis of cytokine secretion by infiltrating CD4+ T cells from T cell-PPARγ^{ko} mice (ko) and WT littermates (wt) using a cytokine antibody array 40 days after transplantation. B. The transcription levels of the transcription factors T-bet, GATA-3, RORγt, and Foxp3 in allografts were measured by RT-PCR 40 days after transplantation. C. Graft-infiltrating CD4+ T cells were isolated 40 days after transplantation. These cells were stained with CD45, CD4, and 7-AAD then intracellularly stained with IFN-γ, IL-13, IL-17A, and Foxp3 for assessment by flow cytometry. D. The percentage of CD4+IFN-γ+/CD4+IL-13+/CD4+IL-17A/CD4+ Foxp3+ cells in infiltrating CD4+ T cells was determined by flow cytometry. The data are presented as the mean±SD for each group (In panels A and B n = 10; in panels C and D n = 5), *$p<0.05$.

in PPARγ-deficient Treg cocultured with monocytes (Figure 6). All of the above results demonstrated that PPARγ-deficient T cells impact AAM polarization *in vivo* and *in vitro*.

PPARγ-deficient T cells abrogate the protective effect of a PPARγ agonist

In our prior study, we demonstrated that PPARγ-deficient T cells reduce the polarization of AAM. Other researchers have observed that PPARγ agonists enhance AAM differentiation [42]. We examined whether PPARγ-deficient T cells neutralize the protective effect of PPARγ agonists in chronic allograft rejection. After treatment with the PPARγ agonist pioglitazone, the median allograft survival significantly decreased in T cell-PPARγ^{ko} mice (Figure 7A). Moreover, Arg1 and Mrc1 transcription levels in allografts significantly decreased in T cell-PPARγ^{ko} groups compared with WT littermates administered pioglitazone 40 days after transplantation (Figure 7B).

Discussion

Several studies have demonstrated the protective role of PPARγ agonists in chronic allograft rejection [15,22,23]. In these studies, the allogeneic reactions of cell infiltration and proinflammatory cytokine secretion are suppressed by PPARγ agonists. However, the details regarding how PPARγ influences the immune response in chronic allograft rejection are unknown. Recent studies have reported that PPARγ plays an important immunoregulatory function in autoimmune diseases, such as experimental autoimmune encephalomyelitis (EAE) [24], allergic airway inflammation [25], trinitrobenzene sulfonic acid-induced colitis [26], and insulin resistance [27]. In these disease models, PPARγ is the key factor promoting the differentiation of CD4+ T cells and macrophages. Our previous study found that PPARγ activation with eicosapentaenoic acid can impact the balance between Th17/Treg cells and protect cardiac allografts [14], consistent with its effect on autoimmune diseases. Therefore, we hypothesize that PPARγ controls T cell subset polarization in chronic allograft rejection and influences tolerance to allografts after transplantation.

In this study, we established a MHC class II-mismatched chronic allograft rejection model. To eliminate confusion due to non-selective PPARγ agonists in the entire immune system, we used B6 background PPARγ fl/fl; Lck-Cre^{+} T cell-specific PPARγ knockout mice and WT littermates as recipients. In the T cell-PPARγ^{ko} group, leukocyte infiltration and CAV were aggravated, and allograft survival decreased compared with WT littermates. These results confirmed that although PPARγ influences both T cells and macrophages [28], in chronic allograft rejection, T cells expressing PPARγ may participate in the primary function of transplant tolerance. Previous studies have suggested that CD4+, CD8+, and γδTCR+ T cells infiltrated into the allografts and contributed to allograft rejection [19,29]. We used immunohistochemical staining to detect infiltrated T cells in cardiac allografts 40 days after transplantation. The number of infiltrated CD4+ T cells was significantly increased in allografts in T cell-PPARγ^{ko} recipients. This result suggested that the infiltration of CD4+ T

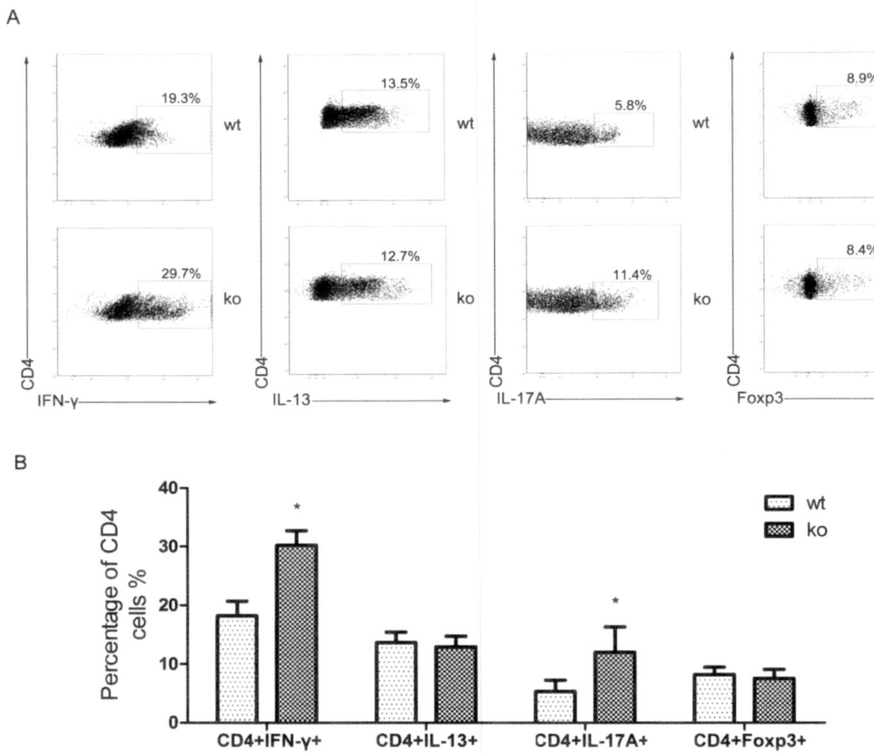

Figure 4. T cell-specific-PPARγ knockout changes CD4+ T cell subsets differentiation. A. CD4+ T cells were isolated from T cell-PPARγ^{ko} mice (ko) and WT littermates (wt) spleens and then cultured in protocols that induce T cell polarization into Th1, Th2, Th17, and Treg. After 4 days of culture, these cells were assessed by flow cytometry. B. The percentage of CD4+IFN-γ+/CD4+IL-13+/CD4+IL-17A/CD4+Foxp3+ cells in each cultured group of total CD4+ cells. The data are presented as the mean±SD for each group (n=5), *$p<0.05$.

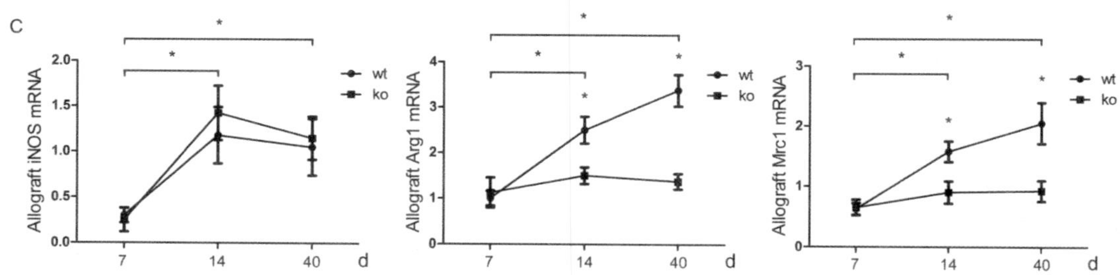

Figure 5. Analysis of macrophage infiltration and polarization in cardiac allografts. A. Flow cytometry analyses of the proportion of CD11b+ F4/80+ macrophages infiltrating cardiac allografts 40 days after transplantation. B. Dynamic analyses of the proportion of infiltrated macrophages in the total mononuclear cells in allografts at 7, 14, and 40 days after transplantation. C. iNOS, Arg1 and Mrc1 transcription levels in allografts were measured by RT-PCR at 7, 14 and 40 days after transplantation. The data are presented as the mean±SD for each group (n=5), *$p<0.05$.

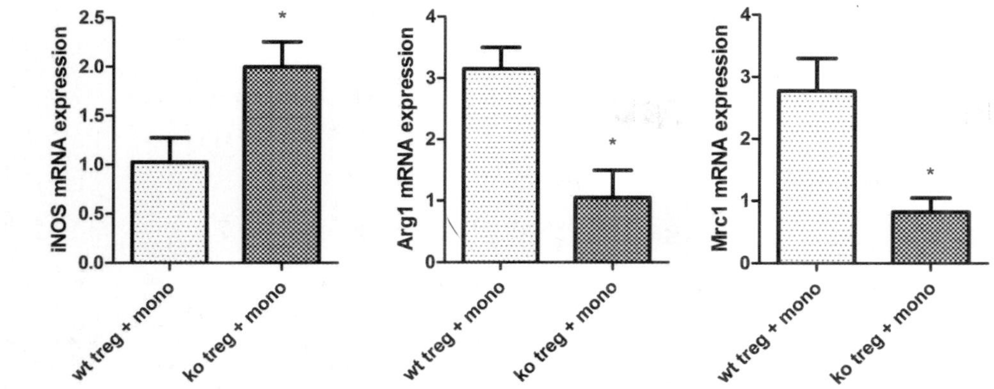

Figure 6. PPARγ^{ko} Treg fail to induce AAM in a monocyte and T cell coculture. CD4+CD25+ T cells were isolated from the spleens of T cell-PPARγ^{ko} mice (ko) and WT littermates (wt) and cocultured with CD11b+ monocytes from PBMC C57BL/6 mice. The transcription level of iNOS, Arg1, and Mrc1 was assessed in monocytes after 48 h of coculture by RT-PCR. The data are presented as the mean±SD for each group (n = 5), *p<0.05.

cells in allografts increased with PPARγ knockout and caused the intensive lesion.

CD4+ T cells and their secretion of various cytokines participate in allogeneic rejection [30]. We isolated infiltrated CD4+ T cells in allografts and examined their secreted cytokines. Based on RT-PCR and flow cytometry, the percentage of Th1 and Th17 increased, whereas Th2 and Treg decreased in the T cell-PPARγ^{ko} group. These results implied that PPARγ knockout altered the subsets of CD4+ T cells. We next examined T cell differentiation *in vitro*. In contrast to the allografts, Th1 and Th17 differentiated more efficiently when PPARγ was knocked out, whereas Th2 and Treg differentiation remained unchanged. These results are consistent with those of previous studies that also used conditional PPARγ knockout mice cells [24,26]. Other laboratories using PPARγ agonists reached similar conclusions. Augstein et al. used the PPARγ agonist troglitazone to reduce T cell production of IFN-γ in an autoimmune diabetes model [31]. In an allergic airway inflammation model, a PPARγ agonist decreased NF-κB activity and reduced IL-17 release [25]. We concluded that the number of Th1 and Th17 cells infiltrated into allografts increased remarkably and led to a relative decrease in Th2 and Treg cells. Th1 is a classic proinflammatory cell and has been shown to be principally responsible for chronic allograft rejection [32]. Yuan et al. demonstrated that Th17 secretion of the proinflammatory cytokine IL-17A resulted in CAV when T-bet was knocked out [6]. Th2 and Treg cells have always been recognized as elements that prolong allograft survival [33,34] and were present at a lower ratio in allografts than in WT littermates. Their protective effect was limited with PPARγ deficiency.

Recent studies have reported that macrophages are a major component in the immune response involved in allograft rejection [35,36]. CAM accelerate the immune response, whereas AAM have repair and anti-inflammatory abilities [37]. Moreover, PPARγ agonists skewed monocytes toward AAM polarization [13]. We have observed that without PPARγ in T cells, PPARγ agonists cannot exert protective function on macrophages. In additional studies, we investigated macrophage polarization in T cell-PPARγ^{ko} mice. Previous studies have indicated that IL-4 and IL-13 binding to IL-4Rα and IL-13Rα1 resulted in downstream phosphorylation of STAT6, thereby causing macrophage polarization [38–40]. More recently, Szanto et al. proposed that PPARγ plays a critical role in these path ways because IL-4 signaling activates PPARγ through STAT6 interactions with PPARγ and promotes their binding to PPRE [41]. Indeed, the IL-4/13-STAT6-KLF4-PPARγ axis is regarded as an essential regulator of CAM/AAM polarization and function [42]. In our experiments, the ratio of Th2 decreased, and Th2-related cytokine production was reduced. The AAM markers Arg1 and Mrc1 were down-regulated after T cell specific knockout of PPARγ. Additionally, Tiemessen et al indicated that Treg have the ability

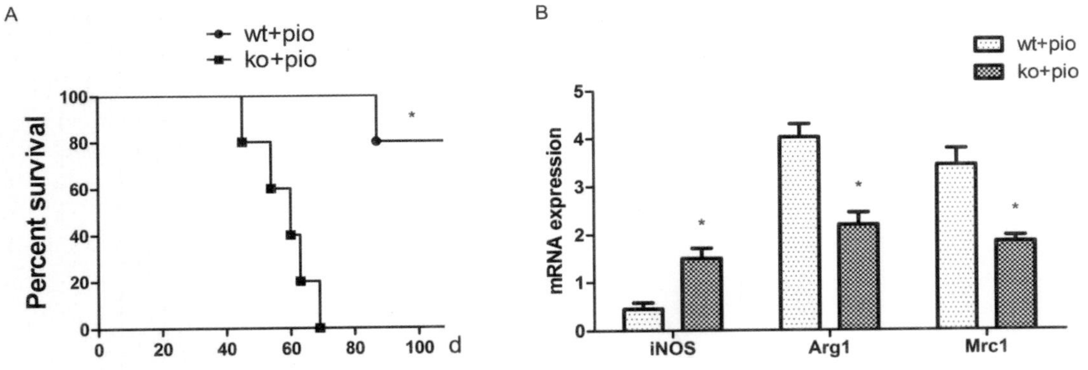

Figure 7. The beneficial effects of pioglitazone on the survival of cardiac allografts were counteracted in T cell-PPARγ^{ko}. A. T cell-PPARγ^{ko} mice (ko) abrogate the protective effect of pioglitazone on the survival curve. B. iNOS, Arg1, and Mrc1 transcription levels in allografts were measured by RT-PCR 40 days after transplantation. The data are presented as the mean±SD for each group (n = 5), *p<0.05.

to induce AAM *in vitro* [21]. Thus, we employed the same method to demonstrate that PPARγ-deficient Treg failed to induce AAM polarization. The reduced Th2-related cytokine release together with the elimination of the ability of Treg to induce AAMs indicated that the decline in number of AAMs in PPARγ-deficient allografts might be the cause of the severity of chronic rejection. To confirm that T cells influenced by PPARγ were the primary cause of AAM polarization in transplantation tolerance, we administered a PPARγ agonist to T-cell-PPARγ^{ko} mice and WT littermate recipients. Indeed, PPARγ-deficient T cells significantly reduced the survival of allografts and suppressed AAM polarization in the pioglitazone-treated groups.

In conclusion, the present study demonstrated that PPARγ expression is important for maintaining subsets of CD4+ T cells and macrophages in transplantation tolerance. The protective effect of a PPARγ agonist in allograft rejection potentially functions through these immune processes. However, one of the remarkable features in chronic rejection is CAV, whose pathologic lesions occasionally appear similar to atherosclerosis but occur through a unique mechanism [43]. Vladimir et al. reported that macrophage-specific PPARγ knockout increased atherosclerosis [44]. PPARγ expression in macrophages requires further investigation. Although PPARγ agonists have effective immunoregulatory capacity in many autoimmune diseases and transplant rejection animal models, the side effects of conventional thiazolidinedione drugs (TZD) have been reported in recent clinical studies [12]. Because the mechanism of the protective effect of PPARγ in chronic rejection has been demonstrated, we expect that PPARγ-targeted therapeutics might serve as a novel method to promote transplant tolerance.

Acknowledgments

The authors of this manuscript have certified that they comply with the Principles of Ethical Publishing.

Author Contributions

Conceived and designed the experiments: XH JW SW AX JX. Performed the experiments: XH LR PY CC. Analyzed the data: XH. Wrote the paper: XH. Revised the manuscript: YS ZL.

References

1. Stehlik J, Edwards LB, Kucheryavaya AY, Benden C, Christie JD, et al. (2012) The registry of the international society for heart and lung transplantation: 29th official adult heart transplant report-2012. J Heart Lung Transplant 31: 1052–1064.
2. Schmauss D, Weis M (2008) Cardiac allograft vasculopathy: recent developments. Circulation 117: 2131–2141.
3. Suzuki J-i, Isobe M, Morishita R, Nagai R (2010) Characteristics of Chronic Rejection in Heart Transplantation. Circ J 74: 233–239.
4. El-Sawy T, Fahmy NM, Fairchild RL (2002) Chemokines: directing leukocyte infiltration into allografts. Curr Opin Immunol 14: 562–568.
5. Piccotti JR, Li K, Chan SY, Eichwald EJ, Bishop DK (1999) Cytokine Regulation of Chronic Cardiac Allograft Rejection: Evidence Against A Role for Th1 in the Disease Process1. Transplantation 67: 1548–1555.
6. Yuan X, Paez-Cortez J, Schmitt-Knosalla I, D'Addio F, Mfarrej B, et al. (2008) A novel role of CD4 Th17 cells in mediating cardiac allograft rejection and vasculopathy. J Exp Med 205: 3133–3144.
7. Tay SS, Plain KM, Bishop GA (2009) Role of IL-4 and Th2 responses in allograft rejection and tolerance. Curr Opin Organ Transplant 14: 16–22.
8. Moraes-Vieira PM, Bassi EJ, Larocca RA, Castoldi A, Burghos M, et al. (2013) Leptin deficiency modulates allograft survival by favoring a Th2 and a regulatory immune profile. [corrected]. Am J Transplant 13: 36–44.
9. Martinez FO, Helming L, Gordon S (2009) Alternative activation of macrophages: an immunologic functional perspective. Annu Rev Immunol 27: 451–483.
10. Mannon RB (2012) Macrophages: contributors to allograft dysfunction, repair, or innocent bystanders? Curr Opin Organ Transplant 17: 20–25.
11. da Rocha Junior LF, Dantas AT, Duarte AL, de Melo Rego MJ, Pitta Ida R, et al. (2013) PPARgamma Agonists in Adaptive Immunity: What Do Immune Disorders and Their Models Have to Tell Us? PPAR Res 2013: 519724.
12. Ahmadian M, Suh JM, Hah N, Liddle C, Atkins AR, et al. (2013) PPARgamma signaling and metabolism: the good, the bad and the future. Nat Med 19: 557–566.
13. Bouhlel MA, Derudas B, Rigamonti E, Dievart R, Brozek J, et al. (2007) PPARgamma activation primes human monocytes into alternative M2 macrophages with anti-inflammatory properties. Cell Metab 6: 137–143.
14. Ye P, Li J, Wang S, Xie A, Sun W, et al. (2012) Eicosapentaenoic acid disrupts the balance between Tregs and IL-17+ T cells through PPARgamma nuclear receptor activation and protects cardiac allografts. J Surg Res 173: 161–170.
15. Kosuge H, Haraguchi G, Koga N, Maejima Y, Suzuki J, et al. (2006) Pioglitazone prevents acute and chronic cardiac allograft rejection. Circulation 113: 2613–2622.
16. Tobiasova Z, Zhang L, Yi T, Qin L, Manes TD, et al. (2011) Peroxisome proliferator-activated receptor-gamma agonists prevent in vivo remodeling of human artery induced by alloreactive T cells. Circulation 124: 196–205.
17. Corry RJ, Winn HJ, Russell PS (1973) Primarily vascularized allografts of hearts in mice. The role of H-2D, H-2 K, and non-H-2 antigens in rejection. Transplantation 16: 343–350.
18. Furukawa Y, Libby P, Stinn JL, Becker G, Mitchell RN (2002) Cold ischemia induces isograft arteriopathy, but does not augment allograft arteriopathy in non-immunosuppressed hosts. The American journal of pathology 160: 1077–1087.
19. Wang S, Xu X, Xie A, Li J, Ye P, et al. (2012) Anti-interleukin-12/23p40 antibody attenuates chronic rejection of cardiac allografts partly via inhibition gammadeltaT cells. Clin Exp Immunol 169: 320–329.
20. Itoh S, Kimura N, Axtell RC, Velotta JB, Gong Y, et al. (2011) Interleukin-17 accelerates allograft rejection by suppressing regulatory T cell expansion. Circulation 124: S187–196.
21. Tiemessen MM, Jagger AL, Evans HG, van Herwijnen MJ, John S, et al. (2007) CD4+CD25+Foxp3+ regulatory T cells induce alternative activation of human monocytes/macrophages. Proc Natl Acad Sci U S A 104: 19446–19451.
22. Chen Y, Liu Y, Yuan Z, Tian L, Dallman MJ, et al. (2007) Rosiglitazone suppresses cyclosporin-induced chronic transplant dysfunction and prolongs survival of rat cardiac allografts. Transplantation 83: 1602–1610.
23. Chen Y, Li D, Tsang JY, Niu N, Peng J, et al. (2011) PPAR-gamma signaling and IL-5 inhibition together prevent chronic rejection of MHC Class II-mismatched cardiac grafts. J Heart Lung Transplant 30: 698–706.
24. Klotz L, Burgdorf S, Dani I, Saijo K, Flossdorf J, et al. (2009) The nuclear receptor PPAR gamma selectively inhibits Th17 differentiation in a T cell-intrinsic fashion and suppresses CNS autoimmunity. J Exp Med 206: 2079–2089.
25. Park SJ, Lee KS, Kim SR, Min KH, Choe YH, et al. (2009) Peroxisome proliferator-activated receptor gamma agonist down-regulates IL-17 expression in a murine model of allergic airway inflammation. J Immunol 183: 3259–3267.
26. Hontecillas R, Bassaganya-Riera J (2007) Peroxisome proliferator-activated receptor γ is required for regulatory CD4+ T cell-mediated protection against colitis. The Journal of Immunology 178: 2940–2949.
27. Odegaard JI, Ricardo-Gonzalez RR, Goforth MH, Morel CR, Subramanian V, et al. (2007) Macrophage-specific PPARgamma controls alternative activation and improves insulin resistance. Nature 447: 1116–1120.
28. Glass CK, Saijo K (2010) Nuclear receptor transrepression pathways that regulate inflammation in macrophages and T cells. Nat Rev Immunol 10: 365–376.
29. Fischbein MP, Yun J, Laks H, Irie Y, Fishbein MC, et al. (2001) CD8+ lymphocytes augment chronic rejection in a MHC class II mismatched model. Transplantation 71: 1146–1153.
30. Liu Z, Fan H, Jiang S (2013) CD4(+) T-cell subsets in transplantation. Immunol Rev 252: 183–191.
31. Augstein P, Dunger A, Heinke P, Wachlin G, Berg S, et al. (2003) Prevention of autoimmune diabetes in NOD mice by troglitazone is associated with modulation of ICAM-1 expression on pancreatic islet cells and IFN-γ expression in splenic T cells. Biochem Biophys Res Commun 304: 378–384.
32. Koglin J, Glysing-Jensen T, Gadiraju S, Russell ME (2000) Attenuated cardiac allograft vasculopathy in mice with targeted deletion of the transcription factor STAT4. Circulation 101: 1034–1039.

33. He XY, Chen J, Verma N, Plain K, Tran G, et al. (1998) Treatment with interleukin-4 prolongs allogeneic neonatal heart graft survival by inducing T helper 2 responses. Transplantation 65: 1145–1152.
34. Ge W, Jiang J, Liu W, Lian D, Saito A, et al. (2010) Regulatory T Cells Are Critical to Tolerance Induction in Presensitized Mouse Transplant Recipients Through Targeting Memory T Cells. Am J Transplant 10: 1760–1773.
35. Wyburn KR, Jose MD, Wu H, Atkins RC, Chadban SJ (2005) The role of macrophages in allograft rejection. Transplantation 80: 1641–1647.
36. Magil AB (2009) Monocytes/macrophages in renal allograft rejection. Transplant Rev (Orlando) 23: 199–208.
37. Gordon S, Martinez FO (2010) Alternative Activation of Macrophages: Mechanism and Functions. Immunity 32: 593–604.
38. Heller NM, Qi X, Junttila IS, Shirey KA, Vogel SN, et al. (2008) Type I IL-4Rs selectively activate IRS-2 to induce target gene expression in macrophages. Sci Signal 1: ra17.
39. Martinez-Nunez RT, Louafi F, Sanchez-Elsner T (2011) The interleukin 13 (IL-13) pathway in human macrophages is modulated by microRNA-155 via direct targeting of interleukin 13 receptor α1 (IL13Rα1). J Biol Chem 286: 1786–1794.
40. Dhakal M, Hardaway JC, Guloglu FB, Miller MM, Hoeman CM, et al. (2013) IL-13Ralpha1 is a surface marker for M2 macrophages influencing their differentiation and function. Eur J Immunol.
41. Szanto A, Balint BL, Nagy ZS, Barta E, Dezso B, et al. (2010) STAT6 transcription factor is a facilitator of the nuclear receptor PPARgamma-regulated gene expression in macrophages and dendritic cells. Immunity 33: 699–712.
42. Liu G, Yang H (2013) Modulation of macrophage activation and programming in immunity. J Cell Physiol 228: 502–512.
43. Rahmani M, Cruz RP, Granville DJ, McManus BM (2006) Allograft vasculopathy versus atherosclerosis. Circ Res 99: 801–815.
44. Babaev VR, Yancey PG, Ryzhov SV, Kon V, Breyer MD, et al. (2005) Conditional knockout of macrophage PPARgamma increases atherosclerosis in C57BL/6 and low-density lipoprotein receptor-deficient mice. Arterioscler Thromb Vasc Biol 25: 1647–1653.

Characterisation of the Xenogeneic Immune Response to Microencapsulated Fetal Pig Islet-Like Cell Clusters Transplanted into Immunocompetent C57BL/6 Mice

Vijayaganapathy Vaithilingam[1,3]⁹, Cherry Fung[1]⁹, Sabina Ratnapala[1], Jayne Foster[1], Vijesh Vaghjiani[2], Ursula Manuelpillai[2], Bernard E. Tuch[1,3]*

1 Diabetes Transplant Unit, Prince of Wales Hospital, School of Medical Sciences, University of New South Wales, Randwick, New South Wales, Australia, **2** Centre for Reproduction and Development, Monash Institute of Medical Research, Monash University, Clayton, Victoria, Australia, **3** Materials, Science and Engineering, Commonwealth Scientific and Industrial Research Organization, North Ryde, New South Wales, Australia

Abstract

Xenotransplantation of microencapsulated fetal pig islet-like cell clusters (FP ICCs) offers a potential cellular therapy for type 1 diabetes. Although microcapsules prevent direct contact of the host immune system with the xenografted tissue, poor graft survival is still an issue. This study aimed to characterise the nature of the host immune cells present on the engrafted microcapsules and effects on encapsulated FP ICCs that were transplanted into immunocompetent mice. Encapsulated FP ICCs were transplanted into the peritoneal cavity of C57BL/6 mice. Grafts retrieved at days 1, 3, 7, 14 and 21 post-transplantation were analysed for pericapsular fibrotic overgrowth (PFO), cell viability, intragraft porcine gene expression, macrophages, myofibroblasts and intraperitoneal murine cytokines. Graft function was assessed *ex vivo* by insulin secretion studies. Xenogeneic immune response to encapsulated FP ICCs was associated with enhanced intragraft mRNA expression of porcine antigens MIP-1α, IL-8, HMGB1 and HSP90 seen within the first two weeks post-transplantation. This was associated with the recruitment of host macrophages, infiltration of myofibroblasts and collagen deposition leading to PFO which was evident from day 7 post-transplantation. This was accompanied by a decrease in cell viability and loss of FP ICC architecture. The only pro-inflammatory cytokine detected in the murine peritoneal flushing was TNF-α with levels peaking at day 7 post transplantation. This correlated with the onset of PFO at day 7 implying activated macrophages as its source. The anti-inflammatory cytokines detected were IL-5 and IL-4 with levels peaking at days 1 and 7, respectively. Porcine C-peptide was undetectable at all time points post-transplantation. PFO was absent and murine intraperitoneal cytokines were undetectable when empty microcapsules were transplanted. In conclusion, this study demonstrated that the macrophages are direct effectors of the xenogeneic immune response to encapsulated FP ICCs leading to PFO mediated by a combination of both pro- and anti-inflammatory cytokines.

Editor: Kathrin Maedler, University of Bremen, Germany

Funding: This research was supported by Project Grant 455241 from the National Health and Medical Research Council (NHMRC) of Australia and Ursula Manuelpillai by 606473. Vijesh Vaghjiani and Ursula Manuelpillai are supported by the Victorian Government's Operational Infrastructure Support Program. The funders had no role in study design, data collection and analysis, decision to publish, or preparation of the manuscript.

Competing Interests: The authors have declared that no competing interests exist.

* E-mail: bernie.tuch@csiro.au

⁹ These authors contributed equally to this work.

Introduction

Porcine islet xenotransplantation offers a potential treatment for type 1 diabetes and a partial solution to the problem of human donor tissue shortage. Sources of porcine tissue include adult porcine islets, neonatal porcine pancreatic cell clusters (NPCCs) and fetal pig islet-like cell clusters (FP ICCs). Although adult porcine islets and NPCCs have been extensively studied in varied transplantation settings [1–3], FP ICCs have received less attention. As with NPCCs, FP ICCs are easily isolated [4], and are relatively resistant to hypoxia and attack by the pro-inflammatory cytokines that destroy adult β cells [5,6]. A disadvantage of using FP ICCs is the low proportion of mature insulin-producing β cells at the time of transplantation compared to adult pig islets. However, as with NPCCs, following transplantation, most of the primitive duct cells differentiate into insulin-producing β cells [4]. Preclinical studies from our group have shown that FP ICCs can normalize blood glucose levels (BGLs) of diabetic recipients both when transplanted beneath the renal capsule of immunodeficient mice [7] and when allografted into an immunosuppressed pig [8]. Human trials with FP ICCs implanted into immunosuppressed diabetic recipients conferred neither a confirmed functional benefit nor any adverse consequences with some cells staining positive for insulin [9,10]. One of the major problems facing the use of porcine islet tissue is the xenograft rejection by the host immune system and the need for chronic immunosuppression to prolong graft survival.

Encapsulation of porcine tissue using alginate hydrogels has been widely used to overcome immune rejection and prevent the need for anti-rejection drugs [11]. Previous studies from our group and others have shown that encapsulation of FP ICCs or NPCCs in alginate microcapsules enhanced graft survival and normalised BGLs when transplanted into the peritoneal cavity of SCID or nude diabetic mice [12,13]. Despite these promising results in immunodeficient animals, data from immunocompetent animals have been inconsistent. Some investigators have shown that encapsulated porcine islets contained within barium-alginate or calcium-alginate microcapsules functioned in mice and non-human primates [14–16], whereas others have observed poor graft survival [17,18]. Further, a human trial with microencapsulated NPCCs did not offer a major clinical benefit with only a slight reduction in the recipient's daily insulin requirements despite the microcapsules remaining intact for at least 9.5 years post-transplantation and there being a small number of glucose-responsive islets at this time [19]. Although microencapsulation prevents direct interaction of the graft and the host immune system, leakage of xenoantigens from the encapsulated cells may provoke an inflammatory and/or immune response [17]. A greater understanding of the host immune response to xenografted encapsulated FP ICCs is required before it might be considered for application clinically. This study aimed to examine the xenogeneic immune response to microencapsulated FP ICCs and effect on graft survival and function when transplanted into the peritoneal cavity of immunocompetent C57BL/6 mice. Our results suggest macrophages and myofibroblasts as direct effectors of the xenogeneic immune response to encapsulated FP ICCs leading to PFO and graft failure which is mediated by a combination of both pro- and anti-inflammatory cytokines.

Materials and Methods

Source of FP ICCs and mice

A total of 18 large White Landrace fetal pigs with an average gestational age of 78 days as determined by the crown rump length obtained from QAF Meats (Corowa, NSW, Australia) were used as the source of ICCs. Immunocompetent, normoglycemic male C57BL/6 mice (n = 20) were used as the transplantation recipients. All animal work was approved by the Animal Care and Ethics Committee of the University of New South Wales.

Isolation of FP ICCs

Pancreata were removed from the fetal pigs under sterile conditions and placed in a 30 mm petri dish containing phosphate-buffered saline (PBS). Briefly, 1 g of pancreatic tissue was finely minced and then enzymatically digested using Collagenase P (3 mg/ml; Boehringer-Mannheim, Mannheim, Germany) following a previously published protocol [12]. Isolated cells were then cultured in modified RPMI-1640 medium (Gibco, Mulgrave, VIC, Australia) supplemented with 10% fetal calf serum (FCS) (Sigma, St Louis, MO) at 37°C in 5% CO_2 for 3 days to allow the cells to round up and form ICCs.

Encapsulation

On day three post-isolation, ICCs were washed with 0.9% NaCl and centrifuged at 40× *g* for 5 min. After removal of supernatant, the ICCs were suspended in highly purified 2.2% alginate (60:40 guluronic acid: mannuronic acid; UP MVG Pronova, FMC Biopolymer, Sandvika, Norway) solution in a 1:6 ratio. The microcapsule formation was carried out in an air-driven droplet generator (Steinau, Berlin, Germany) as described previously [12] with an air flow rate of 8 l/min at a pressure of 100 kPa. The barium alginate microcapsules were then washed thrice in 0.9% saline with subsequent removal of the supernatant in between each washing to sieve off the smaller microcapsules which take a longer time to settle. The average diameter of the barium alginate microcapsules was found to be 244.9±13.9 μm (Figure S1). Encapsulated FP ICCs were then cultured overnight in a modified RPMI-1640 medium (Gibco) at 37°C in a humidified atmosphere with 5% CO_2 and air.

Viability

The viability of encapsulated FP ICCs was assessed using the fluorescent dyes 6-carboxyfluorescein diacetate (6-CFDA; Sigma) and propidium iodide (PI; Sigma). The percentage of cells with green fluorescence (live) to red (dead cells) was assessed to evaluate viability (n = 100 capsules, for each time point and preparation). Samples were analysed under a fluorescent microscope (Axioskop 2, Zeiss, Berlin, Germany and using Axiovision LE software).

Insulin secretion and content

To measure the insulin content and secretion ability of FP ICCs, static stimulation in response to a stimulus *in vitro* was performed. Unlike adult β cells, fetal β cells are immature and do not secrete insulin in response to glucose. Instead, potassium chloride (KCl) was used as the stimulus since it has the ability to depolarise cell membranes of both immature and mature β cells, leading to an influx of calcium and stimulate insulin secretion [20]. Aliquots of encapsulated FP ICCs were randomly hand picked and washed with HEPES-buffered Earles Medium (Gibco) containing 0.2% bovine serum albumin (Sigma) (HBEM-BSA). Approximately 100 encapsulated FP ICCs were either exposed to basal HBEM-BSA medium or stimulatory medium containing 20 mM KCl in HBEM-BSA (n = 3; for both basal and stimulus and each containing 100 encapsulated FP ICCs) for 1 h at 37°C with gentle agitation. After 1 h, the supernatant was collected and stored at −80°C for the measurement of secreted insulin by radioimmunoassay (RIA) (Linco, St. Charles, MI). The cell pellet was washed in Hanks Balanced Salt Solution (HBSS; Sigma) followed by the addition of cold acid ethanol and vortexed vigorously to enhance cell lysis. The cell extract was kept at 4°C overnight and supernatant collected the following day and stored at −20°C for measurement of insulin content by RIA.

Transplantation of microencapsulated FP ICCs

Approximately 8000 microencapsulated FP ICCs with a graft volume of 400 μl were transplanted into the peritoneal cavity of each immunocompetent normoglycemic C57BL/6 mouse (n = 20). Briefly, the mice were anaesthetised with pentobarbitone (70 mg/kg) and the encapsulated FP ICCs were infused into the peritoneal cavity using a 14-gauge catheter *via* a 3 ml syringe. The catheter was flushed twice with 1 ml of 0.9% sterile saline to transfer all remaining microcapsules, then removed and the peritoneum closed by a purse-string suture and the skin stapled. Controls consisted of mice (n = 4) transplanted with an equivalent number of empty microcapsules (400 μl) into the peritoneal cavity.

Graft retrieval and collection of peritoneal fluid

At days 1, 3, 7, 14 and 21 post-transplantation, four recipient mice were killed at each of these time-points. Beating heart blood was collected from recipient mice, centrifuged at 15,000× *g* for 5 min and serum stored at −80°C until analysis by RIA for porcine C-peptide. Capsules were retrieved by flushing the peritoneal cavity with 5 ml HBSS containing 0.06% BSA, 1% penicillin and streptomycin, 2 mM L-glutamine and 10 mM HEPES (Sigma), at pH 7.4. The microcapsules were removed from the peritoneal lavage fluid by gravity separation. The resulting peritoneal fluid was then spun at 3000 rpm to remove immune cells and debris, and then frozen at −80°C for future analysis of chemokines/cytokines. The peritoneal cavity was flushed with 0.9% NaCl and subsequently examined for any remaining capsules. The packed cell volume of the graft recovered was recorded. Empty capsules were retrieved from control mice (n = 4) at day 21 post-transplantation. A random aliquot of microcapsules were then taken for morphological assessment, viability, static stimulation with KCl, real-time PCR and histological analysis.

Morphological assessment of retrieved graft

Retrieved capsules (n = 100) from each recipient mouse were examined under a light microscope for the degree of cellular/fibrotic overgrowth using a scoring system as described previously [21] where score 0 = no overgrowth, score 1 = <25% of overgrowth, score 2 = 25–50%, score 3 = 51–75% and score 4 = >75% of overgrowth.

Decapsulation and RNA extraction

Aliquots of encapsulated ICCs were decapsulated using a solution containing 0.5 M EDTA (Gibco) and 1 M HEPES. RNA extraction was undertaken using the RNeasy Mini Kit (Qiagen, Valencia, CA), following manufacturer's protocols. Following RNA integrity testing, the RNA was converted to cDNA using the Superscript First-Strand synthesis system (Invitrogen) in a Myocycler ® thermal cycler (Bio-Rad, Hercules, CA) and stored at −20°C for later quantitative real-time RT-PCR analysis.

Real-time PCR

cDNA samples from ICCs retrieved at 3, 7, 14 and 21 days after transplantation were analysed by quantitative real-time PCR using TaqMan fluorescent (FAM)-labelled probes and primers (Sigma-Genosys, Sydney, Australia). The probe/primer pair sequences are shown in Table S1. All primers used were desalted and all probes were purified by HPLC. The probe/primer sets were designed using Primer Express (Applied Biosystems, Carlsbad, CA). The PCR reactions contained 0.25 μl of 10 μM forward and reverse primers, 0.25 μl of 10 μM appropriate TaqMan probe, 12.5 μl of 2× universal buffers, and 5 μl of 0.2 μg/μl cDNA in a total reaction volume of 25 μl. To verify the quality of the cDNA, samples from each time point were run with porcine glyceraldehyde-3 phosphate dehydrogenase (GAPDH) primers. Real time analysis was done using the ABI Prism 7700 Sequence Detection System® (Applied Biosystems). The PCR conditions were as follows: 50 °C for 2 min, 95°C for 10 min, 95°C for 15 sec, then 60°C for 1 min. Expression of target genes was normalized to GAPDH and expressed as a fold change.

Histological analyses

Haematoxylin & Eosin staining. Microencapsulated FP ICCs were washed twice in PBS and incubated in 10% neutral buffered formalin overnight. Capsules were washed again in PBS and suspended in 2% agarose and embedded in paraffin. These were cut into 5 μm sections using (820 Spencer Microtome, Labequip, Ontario, Canada). Sections were stained with haematoxylin and eosin (H&E) using a Shandon Varistain 24-4 staining machine® (Thermo Scientific, Kalamazoo, MI) to examine the morphology of FP ICCs.

Insulin staining. Paraffin embedded capsules, prepared as for H&E staining, were cut into 5 μm thick sections and stained for insulin. Sections were deparaffinised and rehydrated followed by guinea pig anti-insulin antibody (1:500; Dako, Glostrup, Denmark). The secondary antibody rabbit anti-guinea pig tetramethyl rhodamine isothiocyanate (TRITC) conjugated immunoglobulins (1:1000 dilution; Sigma) was used to detect the bound primary antibody. Cell nuclei were stained with 4,6-diamidino-2-phenylindole (DAPI) (1:10000 dilution; Molecular Probes, Carlsbad, CA). Sections were viewed under a fluorescent microscope (Axioskop 2, Zeiss using Axiovision LE software).

Collagen staining. Paraffin embedded capsules, prepared as for H&E staining, were cut into 5 μm thick sections and stained for collagen. Briefly, the sections were deparaffinised and rehydrated followed by nuclear staining with haematoxylin. The sections were then washed for 10 min in running tap water and stained with picro-sirius red for 1 h. After two washes in acidified water, sections were dehydrated in three changes of 100% ethanol followed by a final wash in xylene. The sections were then mounted and viewed under a bright field microscope (Olympus IX81, Center Valley, PA).

Immunostaining for macrophages and myofibroblasts. Paraffin embedded capsules were cut into 5 μm thick sections. The sections were dewaxed and rehydrated. Macrophages were detected with rat anti-mouse F4/80 (1:4000; Abcam; Cambridge, UK) and myofibroblasts with mouse anti-human α-smooth muscle actin (α-SMA) antibody which cross reacts with mouse (1:5000; Sigma-Aldrich). Endogenous peroxidase was quenched with 0.6% H_2O_2 and non specific binding blocked with CAS block (Invitrogen; Camarillo, CA). Primary antibodies were incubated at 4 °C overnight (F4/80) or 30 min at room temperature (α-SMA). Primary antibodies were omitted from negative controls. After three washes, sections were incubated with biotinylated goat anti-mouse IgG (Vector Laboratories, Burlingame, CA; 1:200; α-SMA) or biotinylated rabbit anti-rat IgG (Dako; Glostrup, Denmark; 1:150; F4/80). Antibody binding was detected using the ABC kit (Vector Laboratories) followed by DAB (Sigma-Aldrich) as chromagen. Slides were counter stained with haematoxylin, dehydrated and mounted with DPX (Sigma-Aldrich).

Porcine C-peptide assay

Frozen samples of murine serum were thawed and levels of C-peptide were quantified using a commercial porcine C-peptide RIA kit (Linco) according to supplier's protocol. Centrifugation was performed at 4200×*g* for 40 min to prevent pellet loss while decanting the supernatant. Serum from mice that did not undergo transplantation was used as the negative control.

Quantification of mouse cytokines

Frozen samples (1.5 ml) of mouse peritoneal fluid were thawed and concentrated at 250×*g* for 1.5 h at 40°C using a MiVac Duo Concentrator centrifuge (Genevac, Gardiner, NY). This was followed by further centrifugation at 250×*g* for 1 h at 45°C to further concentrate the samples to 100 μl (15× concentrated). Mice transplanted with empty capsules served as controls. Concentrated samples were analysed using a commercial multiplex bead-based immunoassay kit for mouse IL-1β, IL-2, IL-4, IL-5, IL-10, IL-12, TNF-α and IFN-γ (Linco), according to supplier's protocols. HBSS was used as the matrix solution. Mouse peritoneal cytokines were then quantified using a Bio-plex (Bio-Rad) suspension array system. Data were analysed from the standard curves generated by Bio-plex manager v4.1.1 (Bio-Rad).

Statistical analysis

All data are presented as mean ± standard error of mean (SEM). Differences between two groups were analysed by the two-tailed Student's t-test and of more than two groups by one-way ANOVA with *post-hoc* Tukey-Kramer Multiple-Comparison test. The software NCSS 2004 (NCSS, Kaysville, UT) was used to perform the statistical data analysis. Significant differences among data groups were assigned when $p<0.05$.

Results

Graft retrieval

Graft recovery decreased with time post-transplantation. Empty microcapsules retrieved at day 21 post-transplantation remained round and intact with no fibrosis or

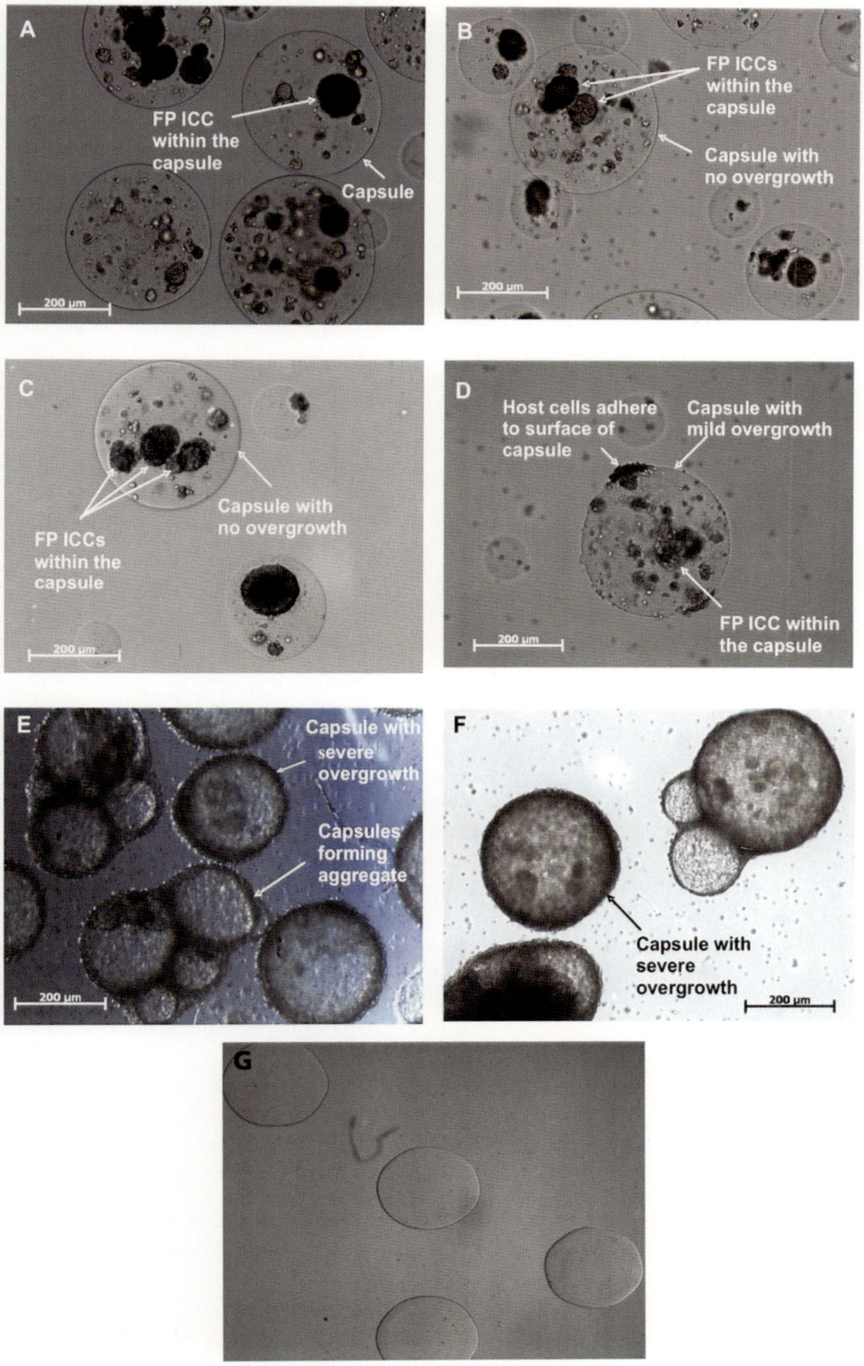

Figure 1. Light micrographs of microencapsulated FP ICCs. (A) Microencapsulated FP ICCs pre-transplantation, (B) day 1 post-transplantation, (C) day 3 post-transplantation, (D) day 7 post-transplantation, (E) day 14 post-transplantation and (F) day 21 post-transplantation. No capsule overgrowth was observed at days 1 and 3 post-transplantation (panels B and C). Capsule overgrowth was evident at days 7 to 21 post-transplantation (panels D to F), with an example of mild overgrowth (score =1) shown in panel (D), and examples of severe overgrowth (score =4) shown in panels (E and F). (G) Empty microcapsules explanted at day 21 post-transplantation had no fibrotic overgrowth (score =0).

Table 1. Assessment of the degree of PFO.

Time post-transplantation	Median overgrowth score*	Capsule overgrowth score (% of capsules examined)				
		0	1	2	3	4
Day 1	0	100±0	0±0	0±0	0±0	0±0
Day 3	0	100±0	0±0	0±0	0±0	0±0
Day 7	1	34±12	17±4	22±5	16±1	11±2
Day 14	4	10±4	4±1	1±0	2±1	84±4
Day 21	4	6±2	1±1	2±1	0±0	90±3

*0 = no overgrowth, 1 = <25% of overgrowth, 2 = 25–50% of overgrowth, 3 = 51–75% of overgrowth and 4 = >75% of overgrowth. Values are mean ± SEM (n = 4 mice for each time point).

capsule breakage (Figure 1G). This indicates that the barium-alginate microcapsules were biocompatible and were not degraded in the recipient. With morphologies similar to the pre-transplantation controls, no pericapsular fibrotic overgrowth (PFO) was observed on the surface of capsules containing FP ICC at days 1 and 3 post-transplantation (Figures 1A–C; Table 1) However, at day 7 post-transplantation, PFO was observed, with scores ranging from 0 to 4. About half of the capsules had either no or only mild overgrowth (Figure 1D). At days 14 and 21 post-transplantation, over 80% of the capsules examined had an overgrowth score of 4, indicating severe PFO. The majority of the capsules had host cells covering the whole surface of the capsule and some of the capsules had formed aggregates (Figures 1E&F). The PFO at days 7 to 21 post-transplantation correlated with the decrease in graft recovery at these times. Only free floating capsules were recovered from the flushing of the peritoneal cavity by modified HBSS. Compared to days 1 and 3, at day 7 post-transplantation, the graft recovery rate was only 66±13% and this decreased further to 56±6% by day 21 (Table 2). The decrease in graft recovery may have been due to the attachment of the capsules with PFO to abdominal organs. The graft recovery rate was 100% for empty microcapsules retrieved at day 21 post-transplantation due to the absence of PFO (Figure 1G).

Graft viability decreased with time post-transplantation. The viability of encapsulated FP ICCs was assessed using 6-CFDA and PI staining. The viability prior to transplantation was 84±1%. Once transplanted into C57BL/6 mice viability was reduced to 80±1% at day 1 post-transplantation and cell death increased further especially at days 14 to 21 post-transplantation, with viability declining to a nadir of 20±4% at day 21 (Figures 2A&B). The low viabilities seen at days 14 and 21 post-transplantation correlated with severe PFO overgrowth (Table 1), which would be expected to block the passage of nutrients to the encapsulated cells.

Loss of FP ICC architecture by day 7 post-transplantation. Paraffin sections of encapsulated FP ICCs were examined for their morphology with H&E staining to assess graft survival. Similar to the pre-transplantation controls (Figure 3A), encapsulated FP ICCs retrieved at days 1 and 3 post-transplantation (Figures 3B&C) were healthy and had intact islet structure with no host cells adherent to the surface of the recovered microcapsules. Smaller FP ICCs were observed from days 7 to 21 post-transplantation, with loss of islet architecture (Figures 3D–F). At day 21 post-transplantation cellular debris was observed without nuclear staining. Several layers of PFO were observed at days 14 to 21 post-transplantation (Figures 3E&F).

Intragraft porcine transcript expression

Analysis of the cDNA synthesised from decapsulated FP ICCs recovered at various time points post-transplantation revealed an increase in the expression of pro-inflammatory factors macrophage inflammatory protein-1 alpha (MIP-1α) and interleukin-8 (IL-8) especially at days 7 and 14 compared to day 3 (Figure 4). A similar expression pattern was observed with the chaperone heat shock protein 90 (HSP90) and the high mobility group B1 (HMGB1) with levels peaking at days 7 and 14, respectively. Levels of porcine MIP-1α, IL-8, HSP90 and HMGB1 were very low in FP ICCs recovered 3 days post-transplantation, and returned to low values in those recovered 21 days post-transplantation. In contrast, levels of interferon gamma-induced protein 10 (IP10) and heat shock protein 72 (HSP72) remained low at all time points examined. The increased expression of the pro-inflammatory factors MIP-1α and IL-8 by FP ICC are consistent with the inflammatory response associated with mild to severe PFO and decrease in cell viability seen on days 7 and 14 post-transplantation respectively (Table 1 & Figure 2).

Table 2. Graft recovery rates.

Time post-transplantation	Volume of graft recovered (μl)	Graft recovery (%)
Day 1	380±10	94±3
Day 3	390±5	96±1
Day 7	260±50	66±13
Day 14	240±24	59±6
Day 21	230±25	56±6

The grafts were retrieved at different time points post-transplantation and the recovered graft volume recorded. Values are mean ± SEM (n = 4 mice for each time point).

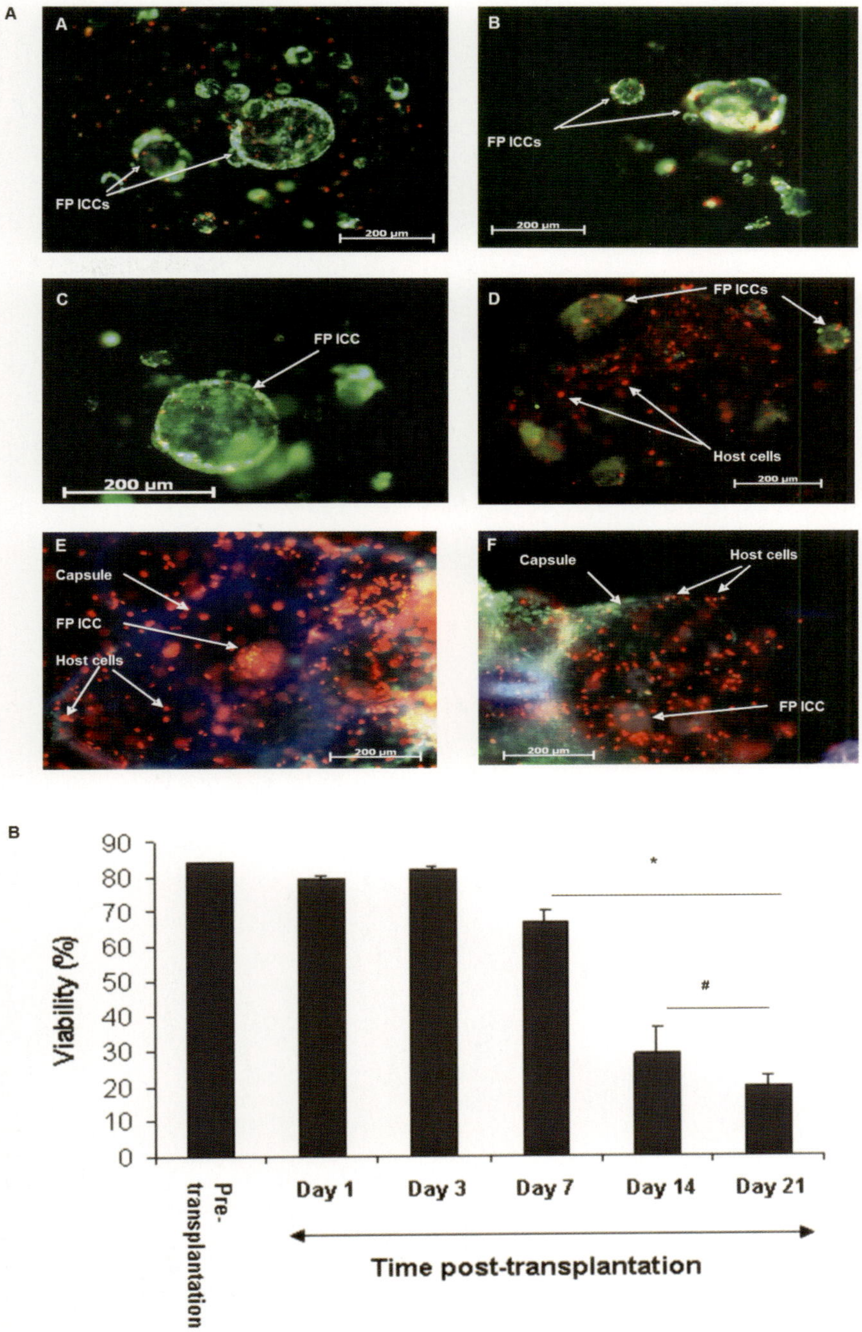

Figure 2. Viability of microencapsulated FP ICCs decreased with time post-transplantation. A) Fluorescent images of encapsulated FP ICCs stained with 6-CFDA for viable cells (green) and PI for non-viable cells (red) to assess viability at (A) pre-transplantation, (B) day 1, (C) day 3, (D) day 7, (E) day 14 and (F) day 21 post-transplantation. B) Viability decreased with time post-transplantation. Values are mean ± SEM (n = 100 microcapsules/mice for each time point); *p<0.05 viability for days 7 to 21 when compared to pre-transplantation control and days 1 and 3 post-transplantation; #p<0.05 viability for days 14 and 21 when compared to day 7 post-transplantation (one-way ANOVA with post-hoc Tukey-Kramer Multiple-Comparison test).

Host immune cells and cytokines associated with PFO formation

Fibroblasts and macrophages are seen within the PFO. H&E staining revealed the attachment of host cells and fibrosis on the surface of the capsules (Figure 3). We investigated the types of host cells within the PFO. Macrophages and fibroblasts appeared to be the dominant cell types that constituted the PFO from days 7 to 21 post-transplantation. This was shown by positive staining for F4/80 which is specific for macrophages (Figure 5A), and alpha-smooth muscle actin staining for myofibroblasts (Figure 5B). The presence of collagen was confirmed with picro-sirius red staining as shown in Figure 5C.

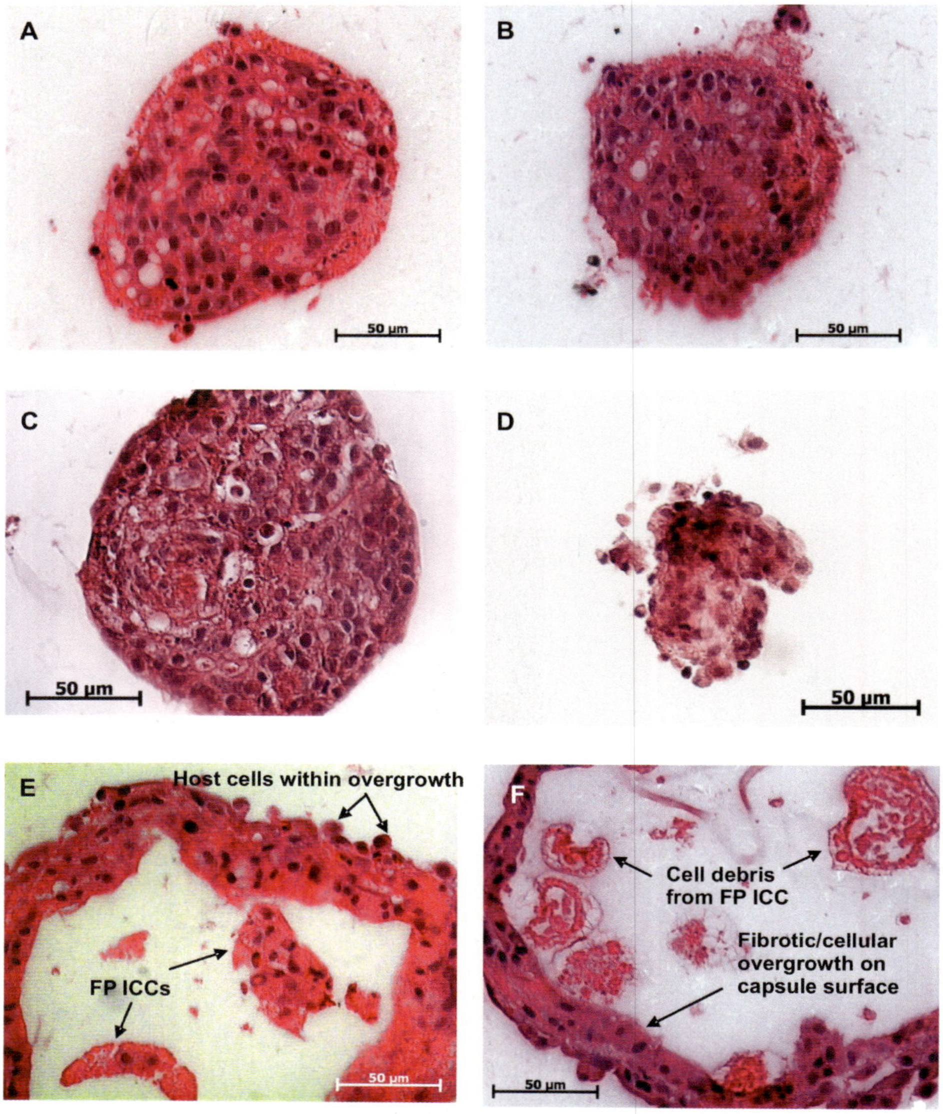

Figure 3. Histological analysis of microencapsulated FP ICCs. Microencapsulated FP ICCs at (A) pre-transplantation, (B) day 1, (C) day 3, (D) day 7, (E) day 14 and (F) day 21 post-transplantation. Morphology of encapsulated FP ICCs at days 1 and 3 was similar to pre-transplantation controls. Loss of FP ICC architecture and PFO was evident from days 7 to 21 indicating cell death associated with presence of cellular debris.

Intraperitoneal cytokines TNF-α, IL-4 and IL-5 are associated with PFO formation. As the fibrotic/cellular overgrowth was evident by day 7 post-transplantation, we explored which cytokines were associated with the PFO. The peritoneal fluid was collected from mice transplanted with empty microcapsules at day 21 post-transplantation and those transplanted with encapsulated FP ICCs at days 1, 3, 7, 14 and 21 respectively. The peritoneal fluid was subsequently concentrated and analysed for both pro- and anti-inflammatory cytokines. The only pro-inflammatory cytokine detected in the peritoneal fluid was TNF-α with levels peaking significantly at days 7 and 14 post-transplantation (Figure 6A) when mild to severe PFO was evident (Table 1). The levels of TNF-α decreased subsequently and reached basal levels at day 21 post-transplantation. A similar pattern was also seen with the multifunctional cytokine IL-4 with protein levels peaking at days 7 and 14 and subsequently reaching basal levels by day 21 (Figure 6B). However, other pro-inflammatory cytokines such as IL-1β, IL-2, IL-12 and IFN-γ were undetectable at all time points post-transplantation. On the other hand, levels of the anti-inflammatory cytokine IL-5 increased significantly one day after grafting, but declined thereafter to basal levels by day 21 post-transplantation (Figure 6C). The anti-inflammatory cytokine IL-10 was undetectable at all time points post-transplantation.

Effect of the host xenogeneic immune response on graft function

Few insulin-positive cells were observed. To investigate whether there were insulin-positive cells in the encapsulated FP ICCs, paraffin sections of the retrieved graft were stained for insulin. A small number of insulin-positive cells were identified in encapsulated FP ICC pre-transplantation, but the number of insulin-positive cells was less than the positive control, non-encapsulated adult pig pancreas (Figures 7A&B). Few insulin-

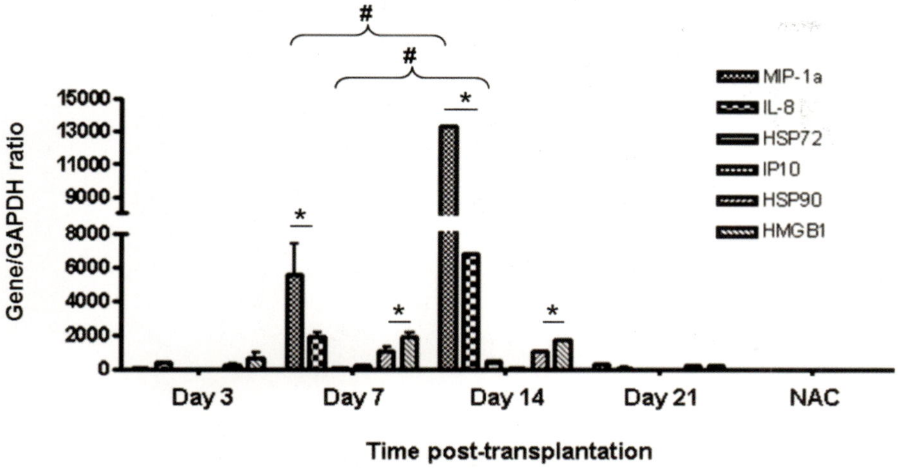

Figure 4. Intragraft porcine transcript expression in encapsulated FP ICCs. Increased intragraft transcript expression of porcine MIP-1α, IL-8, HSP90 and HMGB1 were seen within the first two weeks post-transplantation. The gene/GAPDH ratios were multiplied by 10,000 for clarity purposes. NAC (non-amplification control) represents the negative-RT sample analysed. Values are mean ± SEM (n = 4 mice for each time point); *$p<0.05$ for MIP-1α, IL-8, HSP90 and HMGB1 expression levels on days 7 and 14 when compared to days 3 and 21 post-transplantation (one-way ANOVA with post-hoc Tukey-Kramer Multiple-Comparison test); #$p<0.05$ for MIP-1α and IL-8 expression levels when compared between days 7 and 14 post-transplantation (Student's t-test).

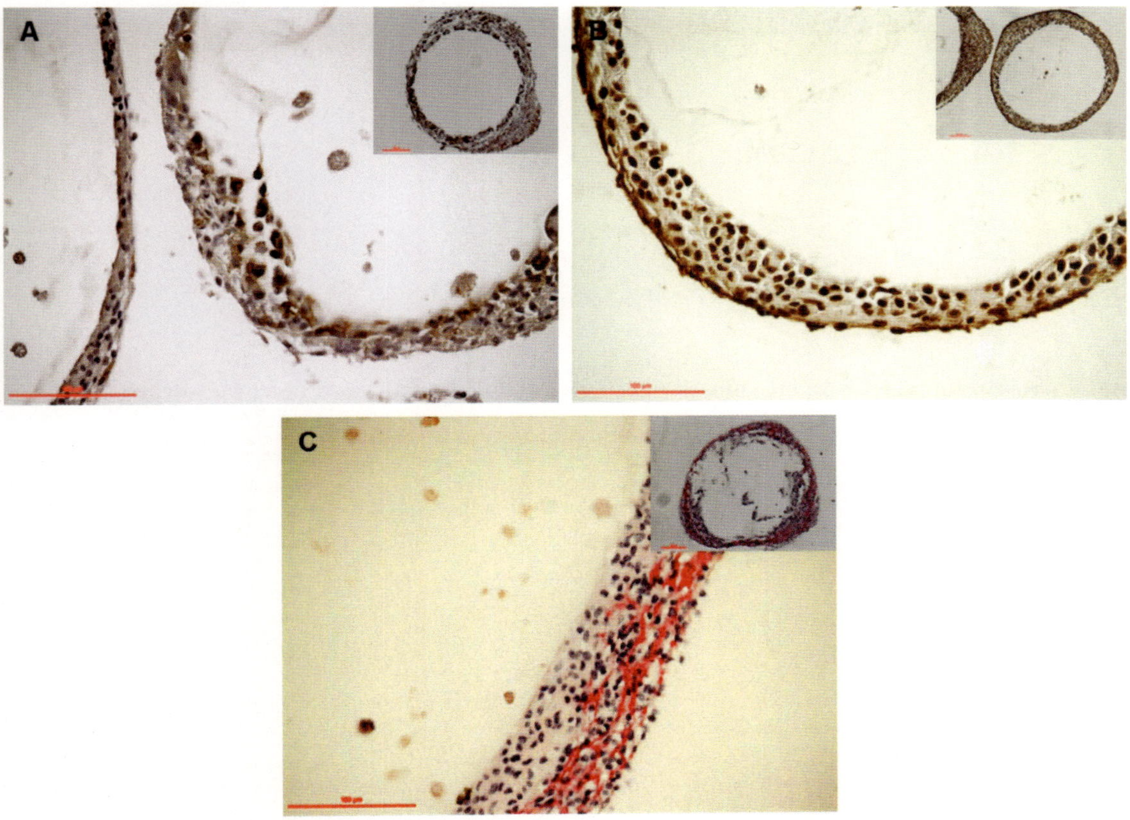

Figure 5. Immunohistological analysis of host immune cells associated with PFO. (A) Macrophages (F4/80+ cells) and (B) myofibroblasts (α-smooth muscle actin+ cells) were present in the PFO. (C) Positive picro-sirius red staining indicating the presence of collagen matrix. Micrographs are representative of grafts retrieved at day 21 post-transplantation.

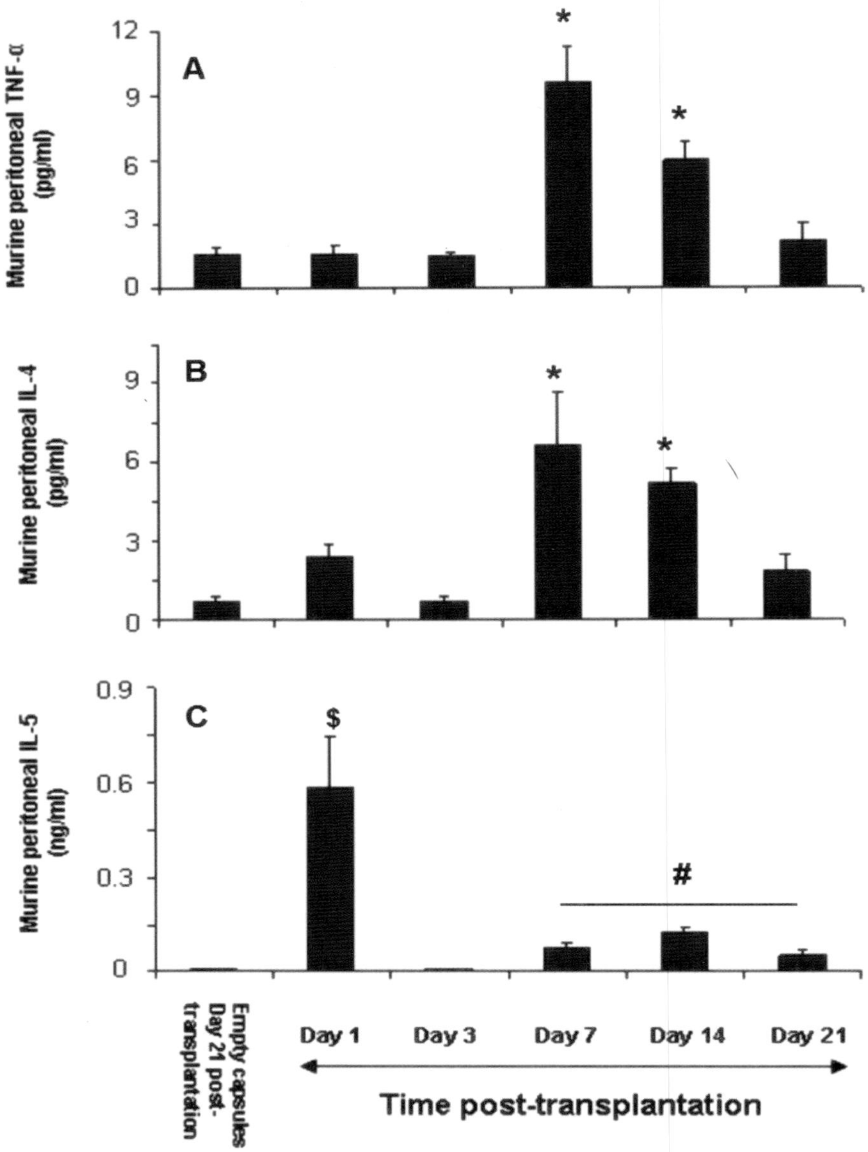

Figure 6. Determination of murine pro- and anti- inflammatory cytokines. Among the cytokines analysed, the only pro-inflammatory cytokine detected in the mouse peritoneal fluid was A) TNF-α and the anti-inflammatory cytokines detected were B) IL-4 and C) IL-5. Values are mean ± SEM (n = 4; for each time point); *$p<0.05$ for TNF-α and IL-4 levels on days 7 & 14 when compared to days 1, 3, 21 post-transplantation and empty capsules retrieved on day 21 post-transplantation; $$p<0.05$ for IL-5 levels on day 1 when compared to days 3, 7, 14, 21 post-transplantation and empty capsules retrieved on day 21 post-transplantation; #$p<0.05$ for IL-5 levels on days 7, 14 and 21 when compared to day 3 and empty capsules retrieved on day 21 post-transplantation (one-way ANOVA with post-hoc Tukey-Kramer Multiple-Comparison test).

positive cells were observed in FP ICCs at days 1 to 3 post-transplantation (Figures 7C&D), and this decreased between days 7 and 14 post-transplantation (Figures 7E&F), as PFO commenced. Insulin positive cells were absent in the small FP ICCs by day 21 post-transplantation which had a massive PFO (Figure 7G).

Insulin secretion and content of retrieved graft decreased post-transplantation. As insulin staining showed the presence of few insulin-positive cells within the encapsulated FP ICCs, ability of the grafts to secrete insulin ex vivo was analysed. Encapsulated FP ICCs recovered from grafted mice were exposed to the insulinogenic stimulus 20 mM KCl and secreted insulin levels were measured. Encapsulated FP ICCs prior to transplantation secreted 1.7±0.02 ng/100 ICCs/h insulin after exposure to KCl and this level declined significantly to 0.28±0.04 ng/100 ICCs/h in FP ICCs recovered one day after transplantation (Figure 8A). Levels continued to decline thereafter reaching low levels by day 21 post-transplantation. The insulin content of FP ICCs followed a similar trend. Levels were 88±10 ng/100 ICCs prior to transplantation, declining to 8±0.1 ng/100 ICCs on day 1 and 1 ng/100 ICCs on day 21, respectively (Figure 8B).

Lack of graft function as evident by non-detectable porcine C-peptide levels. To determine if PFO might affect graft function, the level of porcine C-peptide in the host mouse sera was measured. This hormone was undetectable at all time points both before and after onset of PFO on day 7; suggesting that immaturity of the tissue [22], rather than blockage of nutrient

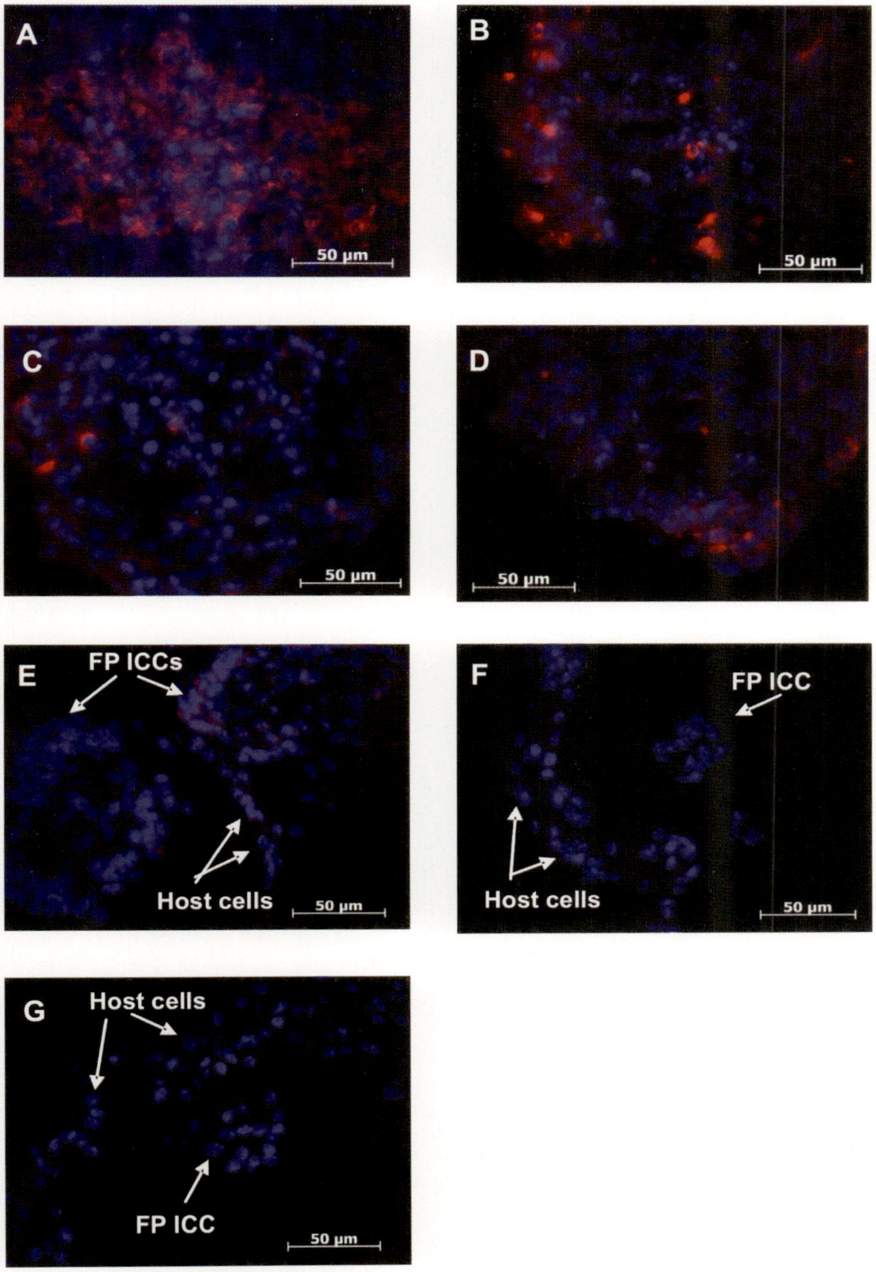

Figure 7. Immunofluorescent insulin staining of microencapsulated FP ICCs. (A) Insulin staining in adult pig pancreas (positive control), (B–G) microencapsulated FP ICCs at (B) pre-transplantation, (C) day 1, (D) day 3, (E) day 7, (F) day 14 and (G) day 21 post-transplantation. Insulin was stained with TRITC (in red) and nuclei stained with DAPI (in blue).

supply was the reason. The controls, sera from mice transplanted with empty microcapsules, similarly had non-detectable levels of porcine C-peptide.

Discussion

Previous studies with non-encapsulated FP ICCs transplanted into immunocompetent mouse recipients demonstrated heavy infiltration of $CD4^+$ T cells and macrophages within day 5 post-transplantation and complete graft rejection within 8 to 14 days [23–25]. However, in our study encapsulated FP ICCs experienced no PFO by day 3 post-transplantation and only a slight fibrotic overgrowth by day 7 (Table 1). The extent of PFO correlated well with cell viability. This improved survival of FP ICCs may be attributed to the alginate microcapsules acting as a physical barrier to prevent direct contact of the FP ICCs with host immune cells. Although the alginate microcapsule improved graft survival, it can only offer a partial protection as the graft viability decreased with marked PFO which is evident even by day 14 post-transplantation. This is consistent with previous findings which showed a negative correlation between the PFO and cell viability with anti-porcine antibodies being detected in mouse sera within 5 to 14 days post-transplantation [14,17]. The possibility that an

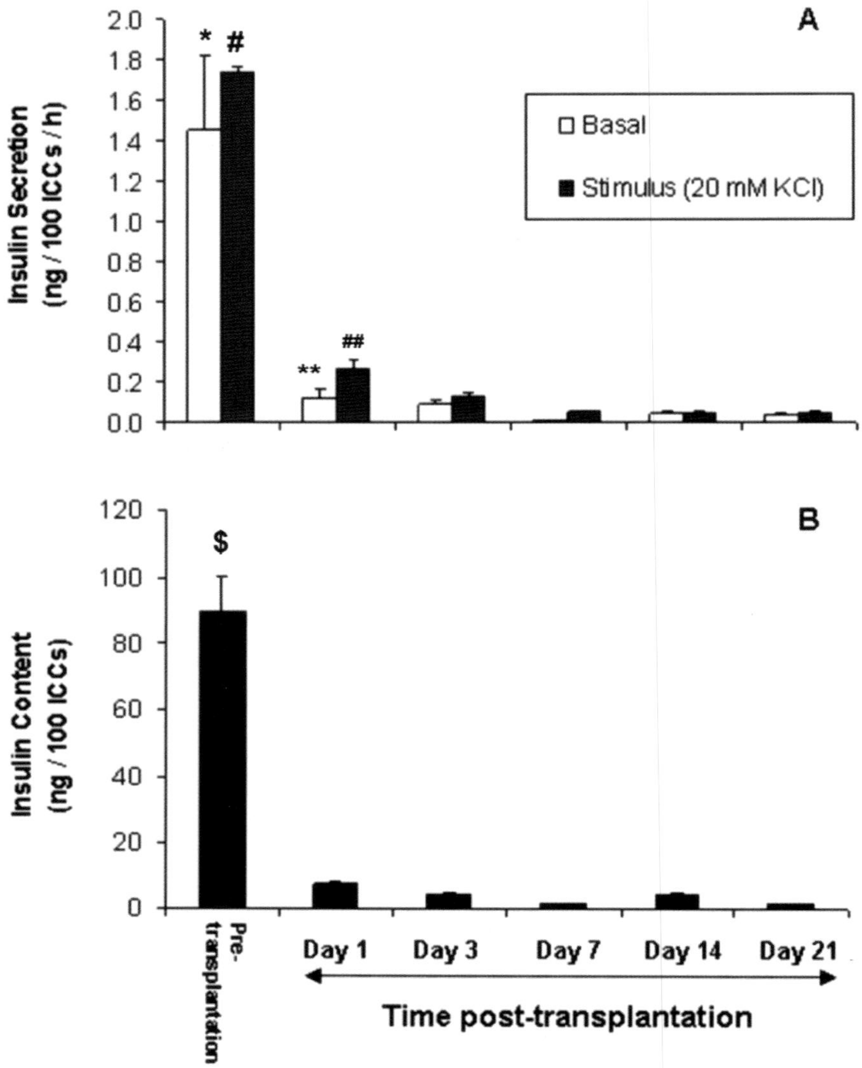

Figure 8. Insulin secretion from and insulin content of encapsulated FP ICCs. A) Recovered microencapsulated FP ICCs were stimulated ex vivo with a stimulus of 20 mM KCl in basal media (black bars) or with control basal media alone (white bars) to measure their insulin secretion. B) Ex vivo insulin content measurements on recovered microencapsulated FP ICCs after static stimulation. Values are mean ± SEM (n = 3 for pre-transplantation control and each time point post-transplantation); *,#p<0.05 for basal and stimulated insulin secretion levels of pre-transplantation controls when compared to all time points post-transplantation; **p<0.05 for basal insulin secretion level on day 1 compared to days 7, 14 and 21 post-transplantation; ##p<0.05 for stimulated insulin secretion level on day 1 compared to days 3, 7, 14 and 21 post-transplantation; $p<0.05 for insulin content level of pre-transplantation controls when compared to all time points post-transplantation (one-way ANOVA with post-hoc Tukey-Kramer Multiple-Comparison test).

immune response is not elicited against the alginate material itself can be ruled out as empty barium alginate microcapsules retrieved at 21 days post-transplantation were free of PFO consistent with our earlier studies [21,26]. These findings suggest that xenoantigens and cytokines permeating through the porous alginate microcapsules lead to inflammation and the PFO. We have previously determined that the pore size of these alginate microcapsules would allow the trafficking of proteins up to ~250 kDa in size [26]. The increased intragraft mRNA expression of porcine MIP-1α, IL-8, HMGB1 and HSP90 seen at days 7 and 14 post-transplantation suggest that small xenoantigens such as these could diffuse through the microcapsule pores and initiate an immune response which correlates with the appearance of PFO seen at day 7.

Macrophages are key players in chronic inflammation because of their ability to produce varied biologically active products and are known to be involved in immune responses against xenotransplanted microencapsulated islets [27,28]. Siebers *et al.*, demonstrated that xenografting microencapsulated adult pig islets into the peritoneal cavity of rats resulted in the recognition of xenoantigens by the host macrophages with subsequent activation of them [27]. Similarly, in our study macrophages were seen within the PFO as part of the inflammatory reaction towards the xenografted encapsulated FP ICCs. This host xenogeneic immune response towards the encapsulated FP ICCs might be a delayed hypersensitivity response (DHR), which does not require T cells, but does involve macrophages and natural killer cells [29,30]. The increase in the intragraft mRNA expression of MIP-1α at days 7 and 14 is consistent with a previous finding [31], and the role of this chemokine in recruiting macrophages to initiate the inflammatory process resulting in PFO seen on days 7 and 14, respectively. Previously, it has been shown that heat shock proteins (HSP) which are released upon cell death can activate macrophages as part of the innate immune response and stimulate them to secrete cytokines [32,33]. In our study, although the protein levels were not measured, we found increased intragraft mRNA expression of HSP90 which correlated with a significant decrease in cell viability and appearance of PFO by day 7. Increased HSP90 expression seen at day 7 might have activated the peritoneal macrophages by an innate immune response and led to cytokine production. This possibility is further supported by the murine TNF-α protein levels measured in the peritoneal fluid with levels peaking at day 7 post-transplantation. It is known that the effects of activated macrophages are mediated by the production of pro-inflammatory cytokines such as TNF-α and reduced levels in serum has been correlated with macrophage depletion [34,35]. In our study the increase in murine TNF-α levels seen at day 7 post-transplantation correlates with the onset of PFO and this is consistent with activated macrophages being an important source of this pro-inflammatory cytokine.

The cytokines, other than TNF-α which are detectable in the mouse peritoneal fluid and are involved in the xenogenic immune response leading to PFO, were IL-4 and IL-5. This observation is similar to previous studies where predominant changes in the expression of anti-inflammatory cytokines have been observed from days 4 to 8 post-transplantation [36–38]. It is known that activated immune cells release various cytokines such as IL-4, IL-5, IL-6, IL-10 and IL-13 and an immune response is elicited by increased levels of IL-4 [39]. In our study we found that the IL-5 and IL-4 levels peaked at days 1 and 7 respectively post-transplantation and their levels decreased with time thereafter. This is similar to a previous study where enhanced expression of IL-4 and IL-5 transcripts were seen within the first few days postransplantation (days 4 to 8) in pig proislet xenografts [40]. Interestingly, the anti-inflammatory cytokine IL-10, a potent suppressor of macrophage function and inhibitor of pro-inflammatory cytokine synthesis, was undetectable at any time post-transplantation. This might explain the presence of macrophages and the proinflammatory cytokine TNF-α leading to PFO seen at days 7 to 21 post-transplantation. Our findings are consistent with a previous study [41] where marked expression of IL-5 and TNF-α was observed but not IFN-γ in the pig pro-islet xenografts within the first few days following transplantation. Further, TNF-α is also involved in the chronic inflammatory process inducing fibroblast proliferation thereby producing extracellular matrix proteins such as collagen, proteoglycans and glycoproteins [42]. Indeed, we found that the PFO associated with chronic inflammation stained strongly for α-smooth muscle actin, a marker of activated myofibroblasts and collagen. This correlated well with the increase in intraperitoneal TNF-α on day 7 suggesting the possibility of TNF-α induced proliferation of active pericapsular fibroblasts leading to PFO. Based on the above evidence, it can be postulated that the macrophages are direct effectors of the xenorejection of encapsulated FP ICC leading to PFO mediated by a combination of both pro-and anti-inflammatory cytokines.

The PFO associated with an inflammatory response is likely to hinder graft function from day 7 post transplantation as passage of nutrients becomes impaired. However, immaturity of the tissue appears to be the key factor as we were unable to detect porcine C-peptide at any stage during the 3 weeks post transplantation. We have previously demonstrated that it took at least a month for encapsulated FP ICCs to fully differentiate into insulin producing cells and normalise blood glucose levels when transplanted into immunocompromised diabetic recipients [12]. Moreover, when fetal pig pancreatic tissue was grafted into non-diabetic immunodeficient mice, porcine C-peptide was detectable in mouse serum only after 3 weeks [43]. The low levels of insulin secretion from and graft content of *ex vivo* encapsulated ICCs at days 1 and 3 post transplantation, as compared to levels obtained pre-transplantation, can best be explained as a response to a recent change in environmental conditions. Viability of the grafts was high at this time and pro-inflammatory cytokines were not detectable in mouse peritoneal fluid. Even if they had, fetal pig β cells [44], as compared to adult β cells [45,46], have been shown to be resistant to the adverse effect of these cytokines.

In conclusion, our findings have further characterised the mechanism of xenogeneic immune response in terms of the intraperitoneal cytokines and immune cells involved in the rejection of microencapsulated FP ICCs. Encapsulated FP ICC xenograft rejection was associated with enhanced intragraft transcript expression of porcine antigens MIP-1α, IL-8, HMGB1 and HSP90 seen on days 7 to 14 post-transplantation. This pattern was consistent with the recruitment of macrophages and infiltration of activated myofibroblasts leading to PFO and loss of viability of the graft. This study also demonstrates that microencapsulation with barium alginate beads is not sufficient by itself to prevent the xenograft rejection of FP ICCs transplanted into the peritoneal cavity of immunocompetent mice. Strategies such as temporary macrophage depletion by clodronate and inhibition of co-stimulatory pathways by anti-LFA-1/anti-CD154 antibodies have resulted in prolonged survival of encapsulated porcine tissue [18,47]. Thus, future research exploring the combination of microencapsulation and immunosuppressive strategies to overcome xenograft rejection will advance the possibility of using encapsulated FP ICCs as a treatment for insulin-dependent diabetes.

Acknowledgments

The authors are grateful to the volunteers from Diabetes Australia for the transport of fetal pigs from the abattoir at Corowa to Albury airport for transit to Sydney.

Author Contributions

Conceived and designed the experiments: V. Vaithilingam CF SB JF BT. Performed the experiments: V. Vaithilingam CF SB JF V. Vaghjiani. Analyzed the data: V. Vaithilingam CF SB JF V. Vaghjiani UM BT. Contributed reagents/materials/analysis tools: UM BT. Wrote the paper: V. Vaithilingam CF JF UM BT.

References

1. Bottino R, Balamurugan AN, Smetanka C, Bertera S, He J, et al. (2007) Isolation outcome and functional characteristics of young and adult pig pancreatic islets for transplantation studies. Xenotransplantation 14: 74–82.
2. Korbutt GS, Elliott JF, Ao Z, Smith DK, Warnock GL, et al. (1996) Large Scale Isolation, Growth, and Function of Porcine Neonatal Islet Cells. J. Clin. Invest. 97: 2119–2129.
3. Trivedi N, Hollister-Lock J, Lopez-Avalos MD, O'Neil JJ, Keegan M, et al. (2001) Increase in β-Cell Mass in Transplanted Porcine Neonatal Pancreatic Cell Clusters Is Due to Proliferation of β-Cells and Differentiation of Duct Cells. Endocrinology 142: 2115–2122.
4. Korsgren O, Jansson L, Eizirik D, Andersson A (1991) Functional and morphological differentiation of fetal porcine islet-like cell clusters after transplantation into nude mice. Diabetologia 34: 379-386.
5. Bai L, Tuch BE, Hering B, Simpson AM (2002) Fetal pig beta cells are resistant to the toxic effects of human cytokines. Transplantation 73: 714–722.
6. Bai L, Maedler K, Donath M, Tuch BE (2004) Expression of Fas but not Fas ligand on fetal pig β cells. Xenotransplantation 11: 426–435.
7. Tu J, Khoury P, Williams L, Tuch BE (2004) Comparison of fetal porcine aggregates of purified beta-cells versus islet-like cell clusters as a treatment of diabetes. Cell Transplant 13: 525–534.
8. Vo L, Tuch BE, Wright DC, Keogh GW, Roberts S, et al. (2001) Lowering of blood glucose to nondiabetic levels in a hyperglycemic pig by allografting of fetal pig islet-like cell clusters. Transplantation 71: 1671–1677.
9. Groth CG, Korsgren O, Tibell A, Tollemar J, Moller E, et al. (1994) Transplantation of porcine fetal pancreas to diabetic patients. Lancet 344: 1402–1404.
10. Reinholt FP, Hultenby K, Tibell A, Korsgren O, Groth CG (1998) Survival of fetal porcine pancreatic islet tissue transplanted to a diabetic patient: Findings by ultrastructural immunocytochemistry. Xenotransplantation 5: 222–225.
11. Lanza RP, Jackson R, Sullivan A, Ringeling J, McGrath C, et al. (1999) Xenotransplantation of cells using biodegradable microcapsules. Transplantation 67: 1105–1111.
12. Foster JL, Williams G, Williams LJ, Tuch BE (2007) Differentiation of transplanted microencapsulated fetal pancreatic cells. Transplantation 83: 1440–1448.
13. Rayat GR, Rajotte RV, Ao Z, Korbutt GS (2000) Microencapsulation of neonatal porcine islets: protection from human antibody/complement-mediated cytolysis in vitro and long-term reversal of diabetes in nude mice. Transplantation 69: 1084–1090.
14. Duvivier-Kali VF, Omer A, Lopez-Avalos MD, O'Neil JJ, Weir GC (2004) Survival of Microencapsulated Adult Pig Islets in Mice In Spite of an Antibody Response. Am J Transplant. 4: 1991–2000.
15. Omer A, Duvivier-Kali VF, Trivedi N, Wilmot K, Bonner-Weir S, et al. (2003) Survival and maturation of microencapsulated porcine neonatal pancreatic cell clusters transplanted into immunocompetent diabetic mice. Diabetes 52: 69–75.
16. Sun Y, Ma X, Zhou D, Vacek I, Sun AM (1996) Normalization of Diabetes in Spontaneously Diabetic Cynomologus Monkeys by Xenografts of Microencapsulated Porcine Islets without Immunosuppression. J. Clin. Invest. 98: 1417–1422.
17. Kobayashi T, Harb G, Rajotte RV, Korbutt GS, Mallett AG, et al. (2006) Immune mechanisms associated with the rejection of encapsulated neonatal porcine islet xenografts. Xenotransplantation 13: 547–559.
18. Kobayashi T, Harb G, Rayat GR (2005) Prolonged survival of microencapsulated neonatal porcine islets in mice treated with a combination of anti-CD154 and anti-LFA-1 monoclonal antibodies. Transplantation 80: 821–827.
19. Elliott RB, Escobar L, Tan PLJ, Muzina M, Zwain S, et al. (2007) Live encapsulated porcine islets from a type 1 diabetic patient 9.5 yr after xenotransplantation. Xenotransplantation 14: 157–161.
20. Weinhaus AJ, Tabiin MT, Poronnik P, Palma CA, Cook DI, et al. (2003) Insulin secretagogues, but not glucose, stimulate an increase in [Ca2+]i in the fetal human and porcine beta-cell. J Clin Endocrinol Metab. 88: 2753–2759.
21. Vaithilingam V, Oberholzer J, Guillemin GJ, Tuch BE (2010) The humanized NOD/SCID mouse as a preclinical model to study the fate of encapsulated human islets. Rev Diabet Stud. 7: 62–73.
22. Tuch BE, Tabiin MT, Casamento FM, Yao M, Georges P, et al. (2001) Role of pancreatic polypeptide as a marker of transplanted insulin-producing fetal pig cells. Cell Transplant. 10: 285–93
23. Solomon MF, Kuziel WA, Mann DA, Simeonovic CJ (2003) The role of chemokines and their receptors in the rejection of pig islet tissue xenografts. Xenotransplantation 10: 164–177.
24. Koulmanda M, Laufer TM, Auchincloss H, Smith RN (2004) Prolonged survival of fetal pig islet xenografts in mice lacking the capacity for an indirect response. Xenotransplantation 11: 525–530.
25. Krook H, Hagberg A, Song Z, Landegren U, Wennberg L, et al. (2002) A Distinct Th1 Immune Response Precedes the Described Th2 Response in Islet Xenograft Rejection. Diabetes 51: 79–86.
26. Vaithilingam V, Kollarikova G, Qi M, Lacik I, Oberholzer J, et al. (2011) Effect of prolonged gelling time on the intrinsic properties of barium alginate microcapsules and its biocompatibility. J Microencapsul. 28: 499–507.
27. Siebers U, Horcher A, Brandhorst H, Brandhorst D, Hering B, et al. (1999) Analysis of the cellular reaction towards microencapsulated xenogeneic islets after intraperitoneal transplantation. J Mol Med. 77: 215–218.
28. Weber CJ, Zabinski S, Koschitzky T, Wicker L, Rajotte R, et al. (1990) The role of CD4+ helper T cells in the destruction of microencapsulated islet xenografts in nod mice. Transplantation 49: 396–404.
29. Candinas D, Belliveau S, Koyamada N, Miyatake T, Hechenleitner P (1996) T cell independence of macrophage and natural killer cell infiltration, cytokine production, and endothelial activation during delayed xenograft rejection. Transplantation 62: 1920–1927.
30. Lin Y, Vandeputte M, Waer M (1997). Natural killer cell- and macrophage-mediated rejection of concordant xenografts in the absence of T and B cell responses. J Immunol 158: 5658–5667.
31. Solomon MF, Kuziel WA, Mann DA, Simeonovic CJ (2003) The role of chemokines and their receptors in the rejection of pig islet tissue xenografts. Xenotransplantation 10: 164–177.
32. Basu S, Binder RJ, Suto R, Anderson KM, Srivastava PK (2000) Necrotic but not apoptotic cell death releases heat shock proteins, which deliver a partial maturation signal to dendritic cells and activate the NF-kappa B pathway. Int Immunol 12: 1539–1546.
33. Byrd CA, Bornmann W, Erdjument-Bromage H, Tempst P, Pavletich N (1999) Heat shock protein 90 mediates macrophage activation by Taxol and bacterial lipopolysaccharide. Proc Natl Acad Sci 96: 5645–5650.
34. El-Ouaghlidi A, Jahr H, Pfeiffer G, Hering BJ, Brandhorst D et al. (1999) Cytokine mRNA expression in peripheral blood cells of immuno-suppressed human islet transplant recipients. J Mol Med 77: 115–117.
35. Bottino R, Fernandez LA, Ricordi C, Lehmann R, Tsan MF et al. (1998) Transplantation of allogeneic islets of Langerhans in the rat liver. Diabetes 47: 316–323.
36. Simeonovic CJ, Townsend MJ, Morris CF, Hapel AJ, Fung MC, et al. (1999) Immune mechanisms associated with the rejection of fetal murine proislet allografts and pig proislet xenografts: comparison of intragraft cytokine mRNA profiles. Transplantation 67: 963–971.
37. Morris CF, Simeonovic CJ, Fung MC, Wilson JD, Hapel AJ (1995) Intragraft expression of cytokine transcripts during pig proislet xenograft rejection and tolerance in mice. J Immunol 154: 2470–2482.
38. Kovarik J, Koulmanda M, Mandel TE (1997) The role of cytokines during rejection of foetal pig and foetal mouse pancreas grafts in nonobese diabetic mice. Transpl Immunol 5: 307–314.
39. Zamorano J, Rivas MD, Perez G (2003) Interleukin-4: A multifunctional cytokine. Immunologia 22: 215–224.
40. Simeonovic CJ, Townsend MJ, Morris CF, Hapel AJ, Fung MC (1999) Immune mechanisms associated with the rejection of fetal murine proislet allografts and pig proislet xenografts: comparison of intragraft cytokine mRNA profiles. Transplantation 67: 963–971.
41. Morris CF, Simeonovic CJ, Fung MC, Wilson JD, Hapel AJ (1995) Intragraft expression of cytokine transcripts during pig proislet xenograft rejection and tolerance in mice. J Immunol. 154: 2470–2482.
42. Vilcek J, Palombella VJ, Henriksen-DeStefano D, Swenson C, Feinman R, et al. (1986) Fibroblast growth enhancing activity of tumor necrosis factor and its relationship to other polypeptide growth factors. J Exp Med 163: 632–643.
43. Amaratunga A, Tuch BE, Han XG, Georges P, Dean SK, Scott H (2001) Secretion of pancreatic icosapeptide from porcine pancreas. Endocrinology 12: 4314–4319.
44. Bai L, Tuch BE, Hering B, Simpson AM (2002) Fetal pig β cells are resistant to the toxic effects of human cytokines. Transplantation 73: 714–722.
45. Cole DR, Waterfall M, McIntyre M, Baird JD (1992) Microencapsulated islet grafts in the BB/E rat: a possible role for cytokines in graft failure. Diabetologia 35: 231–237.
46. King A, Sandler S, Andersson A (2001) The effect of host factors and capsule composition on the cellular overgrowth on implanted alginate capsules. J Biomed Mater Res 57: 374–383.
47. Omer A, Keegan M, Czismadia E, de Vos P, van Rooijen N, et al. (2003) Macrophage depletion improves survival of porcine neonatal pancreatic cell clusters contained in alginate macrocapsules transplanted into rats. Xenotransplantation 10: 240–251.

Standardization of the Teratoma Assay for Analysis of Pluripotency of Human ES Cells and Biosafety of Their Differentiated Progeny

Michal Gropp[1,❡], Vitali Shilo[2,❡], Gilad Vainer[3], Miri Gov[2], Yaniv Gil[1], Hanita Khaner[1], Limor Matzrafi[2], Maria Idelson[1], Juri Kopolovic[3], Naomi B. Zak[2], Benjamin E. Reubinoff[1]*

1 The Hadassah Human Embryonic Stem Cell Research Center, The Goldyne Savad Institute of Gene Therapy and Department of Gynecology, Hadassah-Hebrew University Medical Center, Jerusalem, Israel, **2** CellCure NeuroSciences Ltd., Jerusalem, Israel, **3** The Department of Pathology, Hadassah-Hebrew University Medical Center, Jerusalem, Israel

Abstract

Teratoma tumor formation is an essential criterion in determining the pluripotency of human pluripotent stem cells. However, currently there is no consistent protocol for assessment of teratoma forming ability. Here we present detailed characterization of a teratoma assay that is based on subcutaneous co-transplantation of defined numbers of undifferentiated human embryonic stem cells (hESCs) with mitotically inactivated feeder cells and Matrigel into immunodeficient mice. The assay was highly reproducible and 100% efficient when 100,000 hESCs were transplanted. It was sensitive, promoting teratoma formation after transplantation of 100 hESCs, though larger numbers of animals and longer follow-up were required. The assay could detect residual teratoma forming cells within differentiated hESC populations however its sensitivity was decreased in the presence of differentiated cells. Our data lay the foundation, for standardization of a teratoma assay for pluripotency analysis. The assay can also be used for bio-safety analysis of pluripotent stem cell-derived differentiated progeny.

Editor: Dimas Tadeu Covas, University of Sao Paulo - USP, Brazil

Competing Interests: BR is the CSO and holds shares in CellCure Neurosciences Ltd. VS, M. Gov, LM and NBZ were employees of CellCure Neurosciences Ltd. when the study was performed. M. Gropp was funded for this study by CellCure Neurosciences Ltd.

* E-mail: benjaminr@ekmd.hugi.ac.il

❡ These authors contributed equally to this work.

Introduction

Human embryonic stem cells (hESCs) are pluripotent cells derived from preimplantation embryos. These cells can self-renew for long periods, and have the potential to differentiate into any cell type [1,2]. Hence they may be exploited for applications in regenerative medicine, drug discovery and basic research of early human development.

When transplanted into immune-deficient mice at growth-permissive sites, hESCs form teratoma-like masses containing differentiated progeny representing the three germ layers [1–4]. Formation of cells from all three germ layers within a teratoma is considered as an essential criterion to define the pluripotent potential of a hESC line [5]. In the consensus guidance for the banking, testing and distribution of hESC lines, published by the International Stem Cell Banking Initiative (ISCBI), the teratoma formation assay is defined as the "gold standard" for pluripotency [6]. In accordance with these guidelines many publications on the derivation of new hESC lines include characterization of the line's pluripotency by a teratoma formation assay. In addition, the teratoma assay is considered by many as a criterion that should be fulfilled in order to ascertain that a genuine induced pluripotent stem (iPS) cell line has been obtained [7]. However, the methods that different research groups use to induce teratomas differ in important parameters such as cell preparation, number of transplanted cells, mode of transplantation, site of transplantation, and the length of time that animals are monitored for tumor formation. Moreover, the pathological analysis of tumors and the report of experimental data are often incomplete and highly variable. If the teratoma assay is regarded as the "gold standard" for defining pluripotency, standardization of the assay is invaluable. Indeed, recently Mueller and colleagues published a call for the standardization of the teratoma formation assay [8].

Standardization of the teratoma assay is not important only for assessing hESC pluripotency but also for evaluating the tumorigenic potential of hESC-derived progeny. The field of hESCs is moving rapidly towards clinical applications, with the first spinal injury patient being recently transplanted with hESC derived cells [9]. A key hazard in the implementation of hESC-based cell therapy is potential tumor formation caused by the presence of pluripotent hESCs within the transplanted cell preparations. A standardized sensitive teratoma assay to detect low numbers of tumor forming cells within a therapeutic cell preparation would be highly valuable.

Previous studies reported inconsistent detection sensitivities of various teratoma assays. The sensitivities ranged from 1×10^4 hESCs after intra-testicular [10], or intra-muscular [11] transplantation, 1×10^3 after injection into human fetal tissue grafts in SCID mice [12], and 245 hESCs after intra-muscular co-injection of hESCs with their feeder fibroblasts [13].

In view of the importance of standardizing the teratoma assay, we present here a detailed characterization of an efficient, quantitative, sensitive and easy-to-perform teratoma assay. Our data lay the foundation, for the standardized use of this assay for the analysis of pluripotency of hESC and iPS cell lines. We further demonstrate the use of the assay for safety analysis of the tumorigenic potential of hESC-derived differentiated populations intended for the clinic.

Results

Key Features of the Teratoma Assay

To establish a teratoma assay that is sensitive, quantitative, easy to perform and to monitor, we included the following components in our protocol:

(1) Quantification of the number of transplanted cells. Prior to inoculation, hESC colonies were dissociated into single cell suspensions, to enable transplantation of defined numbers of cells.

(2) Characterizing the phenotype and genotype of transplanted cells. Prior to transplantation, we quantified by FACS the percentage of cells expressing pluripotency-associated cell surface markers (Tra-1-60, Tra-1-81, and SSEA-4). We also confirmed that the karyotype of the transplanted cells was normal.

(3) The mode and site of transplantation. To increase the sensitivity of the assay, hESCs were co-transplanted with mitotically inactivated human foreskin- fibroblast-feeders. The beneficial effect of co-transplantation of hESCs with their own feeders was observed by Hentze *et al* [13]. To further increase the sensitivity, the transplanted cells were also mixed with Matrigel. The cells were injected subcutaneously (s.c.) since transplantation to this site is easy to perform, does not involve an invasive surgical procedure, and allows simple monitoring of teratoma development. Subcutaneous transplantation of hESCs with Matrigel was reported to induce teratomas with high efficiency [14].

(4) Recipient animals. To minimize the risk of immune rejection, the cells were transplanted into NOD/SCID mice. These mice were previously shown to tolerate hESC grafts well in comparison to immune-competent mice [15]. Since NOD/SCID mice have a tendency to develop spontaneous tumors, and to rule out the unlikely formation of tumors by the co-transplanted feeders, in each experiment we included a control group of mice transplanted with mitotically-inactivated feeders.

(5) Duration of monitoring of tumor formation. We monitored the development of tumors in the transplanted animals for a period of 30 weeks. The prolonged follow-up increased the sensitivity of the assay by allowing the detection of late appearing tumors that developed from a small number of cells.

(6) Defined histological criteria for teratoma. We defined a tumor as a teratoma only if it contained tissues representing all three germ layers. The histological analysis was performed by a pathologist.

We adhered to these guidelines throughout the study. We characterized the sensitivity of detection and the time course of tumor formation with this teratoma assay protocol by transplanting various numbers of hESCs, ranging from 5×10^5 to 1×10^1. We also studied whether the efficiency and sensitivity of the assay could be improved by supplementing the transplanted cell preparation with the p-160-Rho-associated coiled-coil kinase (ROCK) inhibitor, Y-27632. This inhibitor was shown to enhance hESC survival under unfavorable conditions [16]. We thus hypothesized that its addition to the dissociated hESCs prior to transplantation might have a beneficial effect on their survival and improve the efficiency of teratoma formation from a small number of transplanted hESCs.

Evaluation of the Assay with a Relatively Large Number of Transplanted Cells

In initial experiments we evaluated the assay by transplantation of relatively large numbers of undifferentiated hESCs (5×10^5 and 1×10^5). Prior to transplantation we confirmed that the transplanted hESCs (HES-1 cell line; [2]) carried a normal karyotype (46, XX). FACS analyses, performed on the day of transplantation, showed that the majority of transplanted cells expressed high levels of cell surface markers associated with undifferentiated hESCs (Tra-1-60, Tra-1-81, and SSEA-4: Fig. S1A). Five week old NOD/SCID mice (n = 10) were transplanted subcutaneously with 5×10^5 hESCs combined with 5×10^5 mitomycin (MMC)-treated foreskin cells, and Matrigel, in the presence or absence of the ROCK inhibitor Y-27632 (5 animals in each group). In all transplanted animals, tumors were observed 3–4 weeks after transplantation. By 8–10 weeks the tumors were larger than 1 cm^3 (average tumor volume of 2.2 ± 0.4 cm^3) and the animals were sacrificed (Fig. 1). Macroscopic analysis of the tumors revealed that they were encapsulated, and sometimes cystic. Assessment of the peritoneal cavity, liver, spleen and lungs tissues of the sacrificed animals did not show additional sites of tumor formation. Histological analysis of each of the tumors revealed the presence of cells and structures representing the three germ layers. The three germ layer structures were randomly arranged within the teratomas (Fig. 2 A–C). In contrast, none of the control animals (n = 10) transplanted with 1×10^6 MMC-treated foreskin fibroblasts, either in the presence or absence of ROCK inhibitor, developed tumors. Notably, the addition of ROCK inhibitor had no effect on the length of time from injection to tumor detection, nor did it promote the development of larger teratomas (Fig. S2).

Transplantation of 1×10^5 hESCs gave similar results. All animals (n = 15) transplanted with hESCs developed teratomas while none of the control animals (n = 6) developed tumors. The tumors were first observed 3–5 weeks after transplantation and reached volumes larger than 1 cm^3 by 8–9 weeks (average tumor volume of 1.3 ± 0.1 cm^3) (Fig. 1). Addition of ROCK inhibitor had no effect on the timing of tumor detection or on its size (Fig. S2).

Transplantation of 1×10^5 hESCs from a different line (HES-2, [2]) also gave rise to teratomas in all animals (n = 3) (Table S1).

These results demonstrated that subcutaneous transplantation of 5×10^5 or 1×10^5 undifferentiated hESCs, combined with their feeders and Matrigel, into NOD/SCID mice was highly efficient, leading to teratoma formation in 100% of the transplanted mice. Moreover, tumor progression was rapid, as shown by the detection of tumors in all animals within 3.7 ± 0.3 weeks, and the development of teratomas to a size larger than 1 cm^3 within 9.0 ± 0.2 weeks after transplantation.

Determination of Assay Sensitivity

After demonstrating that our assay could efficiently promote teratoma formation from relatively large numbers of hESCs, we sought to evaluate the sensitivity of the assay. For this purpose we transplanted decreasing numbers of undifferentiated HES-1

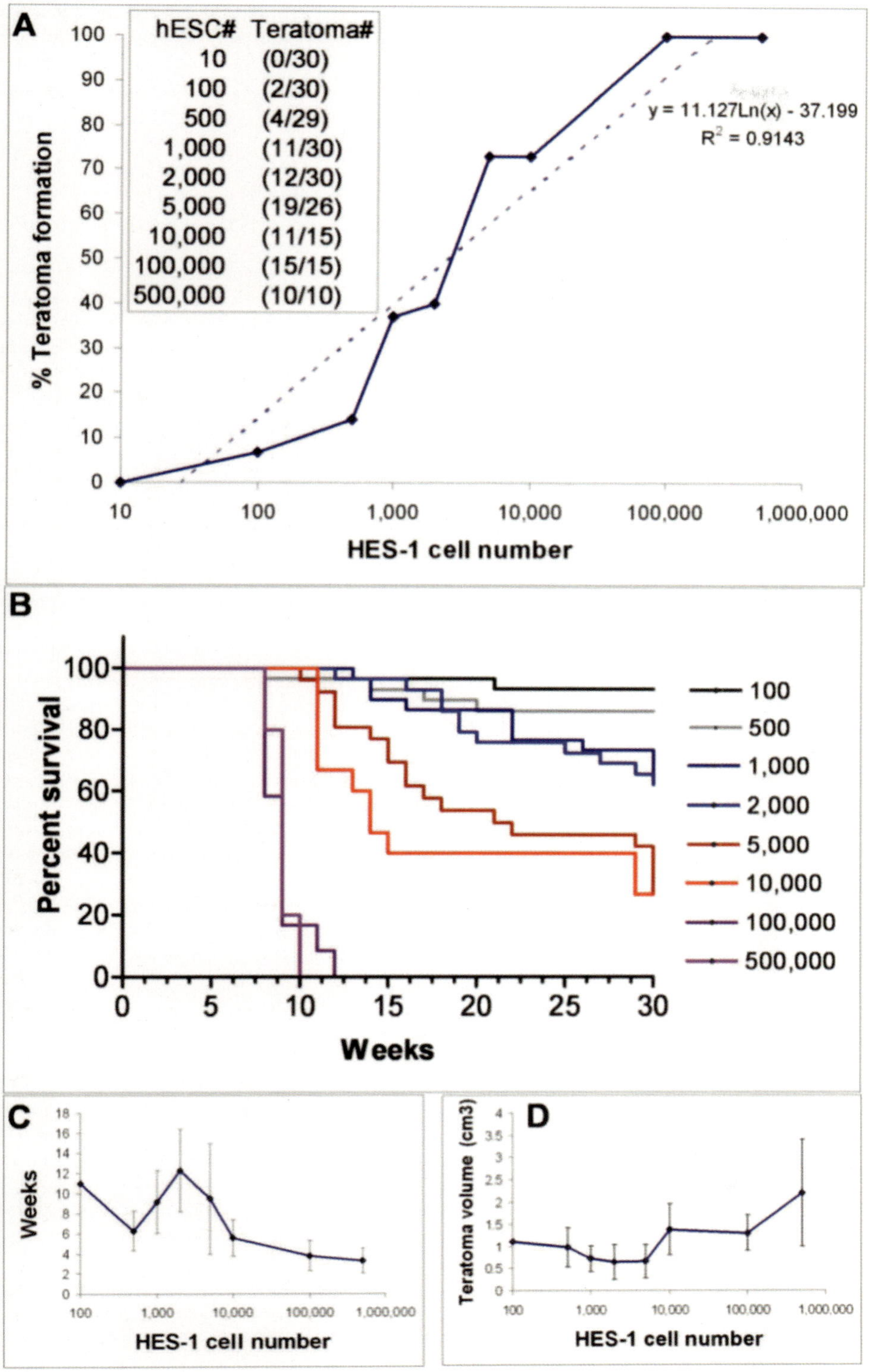

Figure 1. Kinetics of Teratoma Formation after Transplantation of Various Specific Numbers of Undifferentiated HES-1 Cells. Specific numbers of undifferentiated HES-1 cells were mixed with MMC-treated foreskin fibroblasts (to a total of 1×10^6 cells) and Matrigel, and transplanted s.c. into NOD/SCID mice. The transplanted animals were monitored weekly for the appearance of tumors, and for the progression of tumor size. The endpoint of the experiments was when the tumors reached a size of $\geq$ 1 cm^3 or 30 weeks after transplantation. (**A**): Efficiencies of teratoma tumor formation after transplantation of decreasing numbers of undifferentiated HES-1 cells. The trendline is depicted in dotted line. (**B**): A Kaplan-Meier plot showing the percentage of surviving mice transplanted with decreasing numbers of hESCs, at various time-points (1 W–30 W) during the transplantation experiments. The mice were sacrificed when the tumors reached a volume of $\geq$ 1 cm^3. (**C**): The average time interval between transplantation and the detection of tumors. (**D**): The average volume of the teratomas at the time of animal sacrifice. All data relate to animals that developed teratomas. Data presented as mean $\pm$ SEM.

cells (1×10^4, 5×10^3, 2×10^3, 1×10^3, 5×10^2, 1×10^2, and 1×10^1) using the transplantation method described above. Since we expected lower efficiencies of teratoma formation after transplantation of decreased numbers of hESCs, we increased the size of the transplanted animal groups (15–30 animals/group) per each specific number of hESCs. In addition, in each transplantation experiment, we included f a positive control of a mouse transplanted with 1×10^5 hESCs. In accordance with our protocol, we first confirmed that the majority of transplanted hESCs expressed high levels of pluripotency associated cell surface markers (Fig. S1B) and had a normal karyotype. All the positive control animals (n = 6), transplanted with 1×10^5 hESCs, rapidly developed teratomas, while we did not observe tumors in any of the negative control animals (n = 30), transplanted with 1×10^6 feeders cells (in the presence; n = 15 and absence; n = 15 of ROCK inhibitor). As the number of transplanted hESCs decreased we observed lower efficiencies of teratoma formation (Fig. 1A). The smallest number of undifferentiated HES-1 cells that could still generate teratomas in our assay was 100 hESCs (Fig. 2 D–G). We did not observe tumor formation in animals transplanted with 10 hESCs. When we subjected the data in Fig. 1A to a regression analysis, a trendline with a high R squared value (R^2 = 0.91) was obtained. This analysis revealed that the predicted detection limit of the assay is 28 hESCs (Fig. 1A). Decreased numbers of transplanted hESCs affected not only teratoma formation efficiency but also the kinetics of teratoma formation. When lower numbers of hESCs were transplanted, the time intervals for tumor detection were prolonged (Fig. 1C). A Kaplan-Meier analysis of the fraction of the animals that survived at different time points along the experiment (1 W–30 W) revealed a significant increase in the fraction of surviving animals ($p < 0.0001$) as the number of transplanted hESCs decreased (Fig. 1B). Moreover, when 5,000 or less hESCs were transplanted in many animals the tumors did not reach a volume of 1 cm^3 by 30 weeks (Fig. 1D). In addition, histological analysis showed that with low numbers of transplanted hESC (≤5,000 cells) some small tumors (8 tumors with average volume of 0.3 ± 0.12 cm^3) did not include derivatives of all three germ layers, and therefore did not meet the histological criteria of a teratoma tumor. These non-teratoma tumors were excluded from the analysis.

We confirmed with an additional line (HES-2) that the efficiency of teratoma formation decreases with the reduction of the number of transplanted cells, and that transplantation of 100 cells could give rise to teratoma formation (Table S1).

These results demonstrate that the assay is highly sensitive, promoting and detecting teratoma formation by as few as 100 undifferentiated hESCs.

Effect of ROCK Inhibitor on Teratoma Formation

As mentioned above, for each experimental group with a specific number of hESC, cells were transplanted in the presence or absence of ROCK inhibitor. Given the improved survival of dissociated hESCs in the presence of ROCK inhibitor *in vitro* [16], we tested whether its supplementation would improve the efficiency of teratoma formation, in particular when a small number of hESCs are transplanted. We did not observe any beneficial effect of ROCK inhibitor supplementation, neither on tumor formation efficiency nor on tumor growth (Fig. S2). Since the ROCK-inhibitor did not increase the sensitivity of the assay we did not include it in the following experiments.

Using the Assay to Detect Teratoma Forming Cells within hESC-derived Differentiated Cell Populations

We next analyzed the capability of the assay to evaluate the tumorigenic potential of hESC-derived differentiated populations. We evaluated the assay with two types of differentiated cell populations that differed with regard to their contamination by undifferentiated hESCs.

A population of differentiated cells enriched for neural progenitors (NPs) was derived from hESCs (HES-1) as previously described [17]. Routine FACS analysis performed after 6 weeks of differentiation showed that the majority of cells (94.6 ± 1.5%) expressed the early neural marker PSA-NCAM, while a minority of the cells (3.2 ± 0.8%) expressed the pluripotent stem-cell marker Tra-1-81. Following transplantation of 5×10^5 cells from 7 W NPs enriched population, mixed with 5×10^5 feeders, 1 out of 4 mice (25%) developed a teratoma. These results confirmed the ability of the assay to detect residual pluripotent stem cells within differentiated progeny of hESCs.

We next transplanted RPE cells that were derived from HES-1 cells according to our previously published protocol [18]. FACS analyses, performed on the day of transplantation, showed that the majority of transplanted cells (99%) expressed high levels of CD81, a cell surface marker associated with RPE cells [19], while cells expressing Tra-1-60 and Tra-1-81 were not detected. 15 animals were transplanted s.c., in two separate experiments, with 5×10^5 hESC-derived RPE cells, mixed with 5×10^5 MMC-treated foreskin fibroblasts, and Matrigel. After an observation period of 30 weeks, we did not detect teratomas in any of the transplanted animals. The transplanted RPE cells remained at the site of transplantation as small grafts that could be visualized due to their pigmentation (Fig. 3A). Histological analysis of the RPE-grafts revealed that they contained pigmented cells (Fig. 3B). Imunofluorescence staining of a representative RPE-graft showed that the majority of the cells within the graft expressed high levels of Bestrophin (Fig. 3C) and RPE65 (Fig. 3D), markers specific for RPE cells. Thus the transplanted RPE cells survived at the site of transplantation, and in line with the FACS analysis that did not show residual pluripotent stem cells, teratoma tumors were not observed.

We further performed a spiking study to analyze the sensitivity of the assay to detect pluripotent stem cells within the RPE population. We spiked decreasing numbers of undifferentiated HES-1 cells into 5×10^5 HES1-derived RPE cells mixed with 5×10^5 MMC-treated foreskin fibroblasts. Spiking of 1×10^4 undifferentiated HES-1 cells into 5×10^5 RPE cells promoted teratoma formation adjacent to a small RPE graft (Fig. 4A–B) in 2 out of 5 transplanted animals. Spiking of lower numbers of hESCs (5×10^3, 1×10^3, and 1×10^2) did not generate teratomas (Fig. 4C), and the transplanted RPE cells generated only the small pigmented grafts.

Thus, the sensitivity of the assay was lower when pluripotent hESCs were transplanted in the presence of RPE cells.

Discussion

The field of pluripotent stem cells is rapidly evolving concomitant with the establishment of multiple new hES and iPS cell lines worldwide. Defining uniform standards for the assessment of the pluripotency of new putative pluripotent stem cell lines is of major importance. The teratoma assay is considered by many as one of the minimal criteria that should be fulfilled in order to determine pluripotency [7,8,20]. However, currently there is lack of consistency in the performance and analysis of the assay in different laboratories.

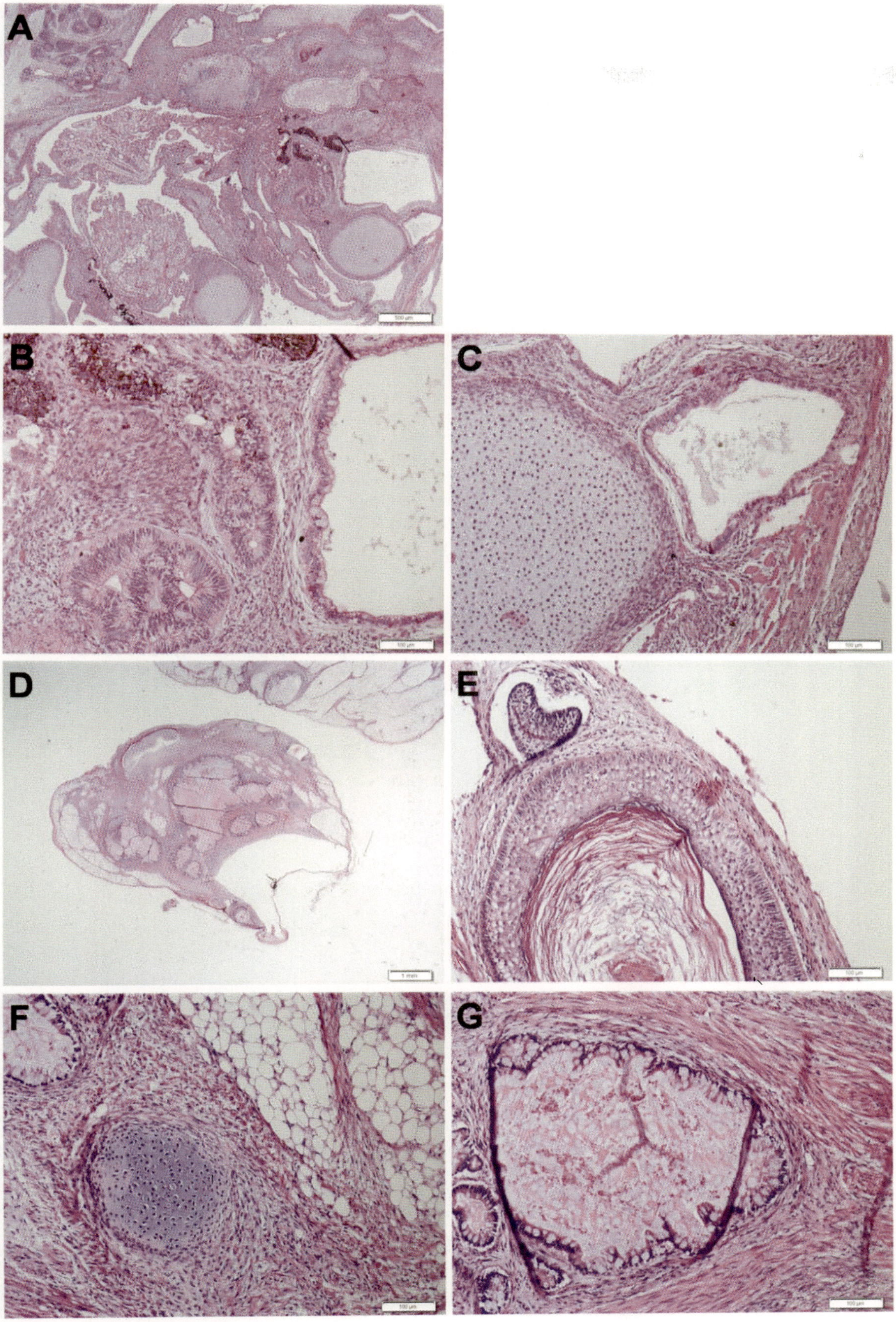
A
B
C
D
E
F
G

Figure 2. Histological Analysis of Teratomas Formed after Transplantation of undifferentiated HES-1 Cells. Images of sections of teratomas, formed after s.c. transplantation of undifferentiated hESCs with their feeders and Matrigel into NOD/SCID mice. (**A–C**): A teratoma formed from transplantation of 5×10^5 hESCs. (A) A lower magnification ($\times$ 4) of a section of a teratoma showing derivatives of all three germ layers. (B–C) A higher magnification ($\times$ 20) of regions of (A) showing ectodermal, and endodermal structures (B) and mesodermal and endodermal structures (C). (**D–G**): A teratoma formed from transplantation of 100 hESCs. (D) A lower magnification ($\times$ 1.25) of a section of a teratoma showing derivatives of all three germ layers (E–G) a higher magnification ($\times$ 20) of regions of (D) showing ectodermal structures (E), mesodermal structures (F) and endodermal structures (G).

Here we present a quantitative analysis of a teratoma assay in which defined numbers of characterized hESCs were co-transplanted subcutaneously with feeders and Matrigel into NOD/SCID mice. We show that the assay was highly reproducible and 100% efficient when $1\times10^5-5\times10^5$ hESCs were transplanted, with decreasing efficiency when smaller numbers of hESCs were transplanted. We further show that the assay is sensitive down to 1×10^2 hESCs. Importantly, we demonstrate the potential usefulness of this assay for bio-safety detection of residual teratoma forming cells within differentiated cell populations, albeit with a lower sensitivity than when pure hESCs are transplanted. Our data pave the way towards standardization of the teratoma assay for analysis of pluripotency and for analysis of residual teratoma forming ability in therapeutic cell populations during product development.

In the design of the assay we specifically addressed parameters which we considered important for standardization of the teratoma assay. These included characterization of the transplanted stem cells, quantification of the number of engrafted cells, the mode and site of transplantation, monitoring of tumor formation and growth, and its pathological analysis. The assay was designed on the basis of pooled published data with emphasis on the approach that it should be easy to perform and monitor and consistently promote efficient formation of teratomas.

The phenotype and genotype of the transplanted cells may affect the results of the teratoma assay. hESC cultures are most commonly heterogeneous with variable levels of background differentiation. Transplantation of relatively homogenous pluripotent stem cell populations is expected to promote higher efficiencies of teratoma formation. Therefore, since the goal of this study was standardization of the assay, we confirmed that the

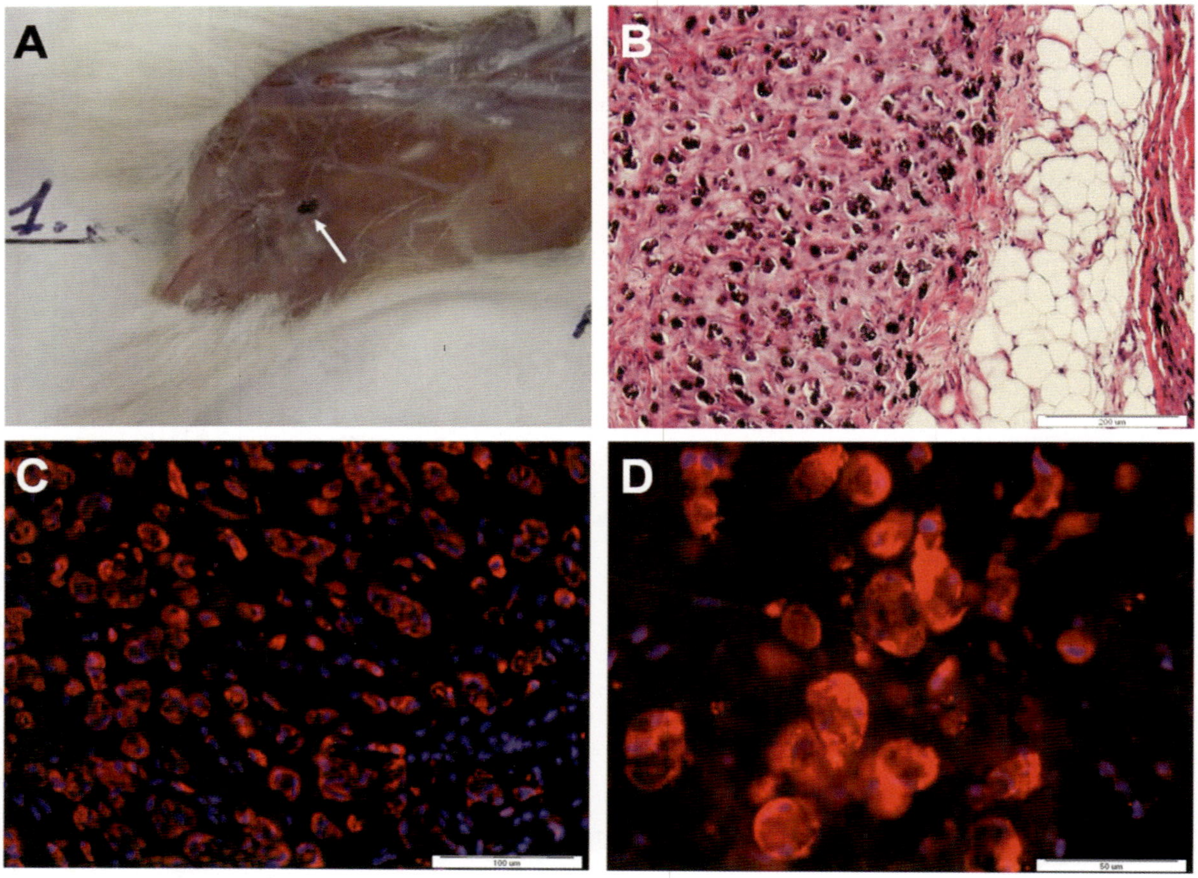

Figure 3. Analysis of HES-1-derived RPE Cell Grafts. Following transplantation of 5×10^5 HES-derived differentiated RPE cells, the transplanted cells remained as small RPE-grafts at the site of injection. (**A**): The grafts could be visualized because RPE cells are pigmented. The arrow indicates the pigmented graft. (**B**): H&E staining of a section of a RPE-graft revealed pigmented cells. (**C–D**): Immunofluorescence staining of a section of the graft for markers specific for RPE cells, Bestrophin (C, red), and RPE65 (D, red), together with DAPI (blue) showed that the majority of cells within the graft expressed these markers.

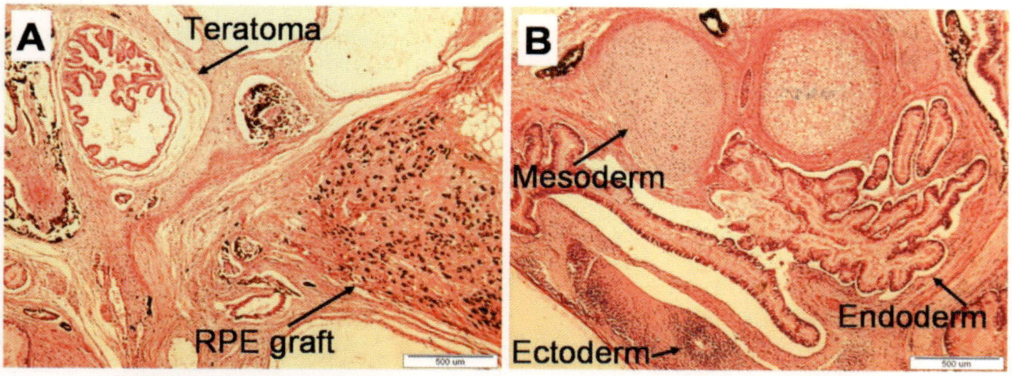

C

RPE cell number	hESC number	Transplanted animals number	Teratoma number
5 x 10^5	1 x 10^4	5	2
5 x 10^5	5 x 10^3	4	----
5 x 10^5	1 x 10^3	5	----
5 x 10^5	1 x 10^2	5	----

Figure 4. Histological Analysis of Teratomas formed after Transplantation of RPE Cells Spiked with Undifferentiated HES-1 Cells. (**A–B**): H&E staining of a section of a teratoma and an RPE graft generated after transplantation of 5×10^5 HES-1-derived RPE cells spiked with 1×10^4 undifferentiated HES-1 cells. (**C**): Efficiency of teratoma formation after transplantation of 5×10^5 HES-1-derived RPE cells spiked with decreasing numbers of undifferentiated HES-1 cells.

vast majority of transplanted cells in the various experimental groups expressed pluripotency-associated cell-surface markers. Quantitative analysis by FACS of the percentage of undifferentiated cells within transplanted cell preparations should be routinely included as part of the teratoma assay. Prior to transplantation we also confirmed the normal karyptype of the transplanted cells. During prolonged propagation in culture hESC and iPS cell lines were shown to acquire chromosomal abnormalities of which some are similar to those observed in their malignant counterparts, embryonal carcinoma (EC) cells [21–24]. Similar to EC cells, karyotypically abnormal hESCs and iPS cells may generate teratocarcinomas that contain undifferentiated cells [24,25] and show more limited differentiation capacity. Hence, it is essential to ascertain that stem cells that are evaluated by the teratoma assay carry a normal diploid karyotype.

Immune deficient NOD/SCID mice were used in our assay since they tolerate hESC grafts and support the development of teratoma tumors [2,15]. A potential disadvantage of NOD/SCID mice is their tendency to develop thymus tumors. However, within ten weeks of follow up, none of the transplanted mice developed these tumors. Moreover, none of the control mice that were grafted only with fibroblasts developed tumors. These data support the suitability of this animal model for the standardized teratoma assay of pluripotency.

A qualitative histological analysis of the tumors was performed by a certified pathologist. This ensured accurate identification of progeny representing the three germ layers.

As part of assay development, we determined the sensitivity of the assay that included all the above parameters. We carried out quantitative analysis of the ability to detect teratomas after transplantation of decreasing hESC numbers. We show that transplantation of $1\times10^5-5$ hESCs reproducibly gave rise to teratoma tumors that developed into a size of 1 cm^3 within 10 weeks in all transplanted animals. Given the 100% reproducibility of the assay with this cell number, if the number of cells to be transplanted is within or above this range, a limited number of animals may be used for the analysis of pluripotency.

Based on the data presented, Figure 5 shows our recommendations for a standard teratoma assay for pluripotency.

The standardized assay presented here is based on s.c. injection and is easy to perform and monitor. It is highly sensitive, allowing the detection of as few as 1×10^2 undifferentiated hESCs. A quantitative limiting dilution analysis of the data in Fig. 1A suggested that the detection limit of the assay is 28 hESCs. This sensitivity is higher than the reported sensitivity in previous publications [11–13] and may be attributed to the site of transplantation as well as the inclusion of both feeders [13] and Matrigel [14] in the transplanted cell-mixture. In light of the low number of hESCs that generated teratomas in our xenograft transplantation assay, the possibility that even a lower number of residual pluripotent cells may give rise to teratomas in an autologous iPS transplantation should be considered. In the mouse ES cell system, the minimal number of ES cells that could generate teratomas was reported to be 2 cells [26]. The higher sensitivity of the mESC assay could be due to a higher tumorigenic potential of mESCs [24], or due to a higher survival rate of mESCs as single cells. The fact that the inclusion of ROCK inhibitor in the transplants did not increase the appearance of tumors, suggests that the former may be the more likely reason.

Assessment of the bio-safety of stem cell-based products for clinical studies and future therapy is of major importance, and several publications have proposed guidelines for the design of

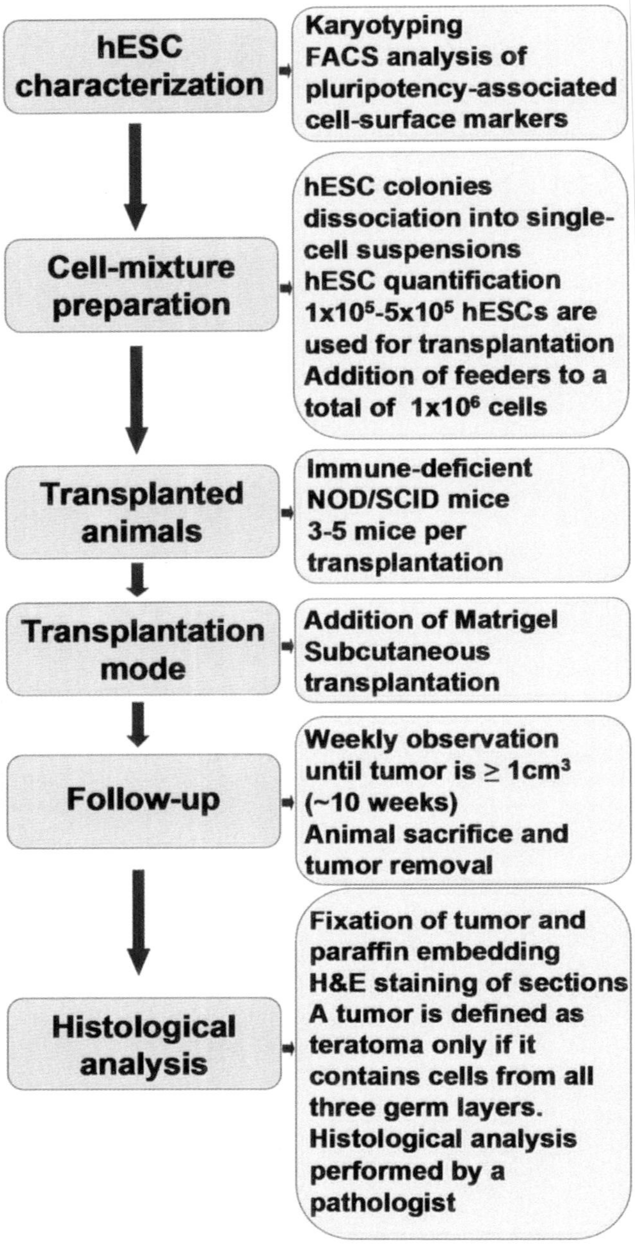

Figure 5. Proposed protocol for a standardized teratoma assay of pluripotency. The scheme describes our recommendations for the performance and analysis of a standardized teratoma assay of pluripotency.

safety assays in animal models [27,28]. It is largely accepted that safety analysis should include evaluation of the tumorigenic potential of the cells after transplantation into the intended site of clinical transplantation, using methods of delivery that mimic, as best as possible, the planned clinical study [27]. Nonetheless, a universal, sensitive, quantitative and easy to perform teratoma assay such as described here may be highly valuable for on-line assessment of the tumorigenic potential of hESC-derived differentiated cell preparations during the course of product development. Indeed, we found a good correlation between the ability or inability of differentiated populations of NP or RPE, respectively, to bring about teratoma formation under these assay conditions and other characteristics of each population pointing to the presence, or absence, of pluripotent cells.

Our data show that tumors arising from the transplantation of low numbers of undifferentiated hESC may be detected after a prolonged monitoring period and at relatively low frequencies. Therefore, long-term follow-up, and expanded animal experimental groups are needed to detect low numbers of undifferentiated tumor forming cells within differentiated cell preparations. Several lines of evidence indicate that the potential of undifferentiated hESCs to give rise to teratoma tumors was reduced when they were transplanted in the presence of a mixture of differentiated cells and feeders compared to feeders only. This was observed for the residual, about 3%, undifferentiated hESCs present within a cell population enriched for NPs. In this experiment the efficiency of tumor formation by about 15,000 hESCs among the 5×10^5 NP cells (25%) was lower than anticipated (about 70%). It was further observed in the RPE spiking experiments in which the presence of 1×10^4 undifferentiated hESCs added to 5×10^5 RPE cells gave rise to teratoma formation in 40% of the cases but the presence of a smaller number of hESCs, such as 5×10^3, did not yield any teratomas. The reduced potential of the hESC present in largely differentiated populations to form teratomas could be due to signals arising from the differentiated cells leading to hESC death or differentiation and may be an additional important consideration in the assessment of the safety of these populations. In the two cases above the decrease in sensitivity appears to be of a similar magnitude However, it is possible that the sensitivity of the assay may vary depending on the specific differentiated cell population that is being analyzed and hence should be specifically determined for various differentiated cell populations.

In conclusion, we have presented detailed characterization of a quantitative, sensitive, easy-to-perform and monitor teratoma assay. Our results may serve as a basis for a standardized and uniform teratoma assay for the analysis of pluripotency. The assay may be also used for preclinical bio-safety analysis of pluripotent stem cell-derived differentiated therapeutic populations during the course of their development.

Materials and Methods

Cell Culture

hESC lines HES-1 and HES-2 [2] were cultured on human foreskin feeders in serum free medium as described [29]. The cells were passaged routinely as small clusters by treatment with 1 mg/ml collagenase type IV (Invitrogen, Carlsbad, CA). Foreskin fibroblasts [29] were cultured in 90% DMEM (Invitrogen) supplemented with 10% Fetal Calf Serum (FCS, Biological industries), 0.2 mM L-glutamine, 50 U/ml penicillin, and 50 μg/ml streptomycin. The cells were inactivated by treatment with 10 microgram/ml mitomycin C (MMC), dissociated into a single cell suspension with 0.05% trypsin-EDTA (Invitrogen), and frozen. HES-1 derived retinal pigment epithelium (RPE) cells were cultured as previously described [18].

Characterization of Transplanted hESCs

Prior to transplantation a cell-sample was collected for karyotype analysis. In addition, FACS analyses were performed for detection of cell surface markers that are expressed in undifferentiated hESCs, using the following antibodies: Tra-1-60 (mouse monoclonal, clone MAB4360, Chemicon, Temecula, CA, 1:100), Tra-1-81 (mouse monoclonal, clone MAB4381, Chemicon, 1:100), and SSEA-4 (mouse monoclonal, clone MAB4304, Chemicon, 1:100).

Preparation of hESCs for Transplantation

On the day of transplantation hESCs were harvested and dissociated into a single cell suspension using 0.05% EDTA (Biological Industries, Beit-Haemek, Israel) .To ensure a single cell suspension the cells were filtered through a sterile filter. The filtered cells were centrifuged and the pellet was re-suspended in PBS (Invitrogen). To determine the number of viable cells, an aliquot of the hESCs was counted. Frozen MMC-treated foreskin fibroblasts were thawed and centrifuged. The pellet was re-suspended in PBS (Invitrogen), and viable cells were counted. For transplantation, various numbers of hESCs were combined with MMC-treated foreskin cells to a total of 1×10^6. The cell-mixture was centrifuged and the pellet was re-suspended in PBS to a total volume of 50 μl. For negative controls, 1×10^6 MMC-treated foreskin cells were transplanted. When the ROCK inhibitor Y-27632 (Calbiochem, Darmstadt, Germany) was included in the experiment, it was added to the cell mixture to a final concentration of 10 μM. The cells were kept for a minimal period at room temperature and transferred to the animal facility. The cell-mixture was combined with 50 μl undiluted cold Matrigel Basement membrane matrix (BD #354234, NJ, USA) immediately before transplantation. Pre-cooled pipettes, tips and syringes were used.

Transplantation and Animal Observation

Five week old immune-deficient NOD/SCID mice were used for transplantation. They were maintained under non-specific pathogen-free (SPF) conditions, at the Hadassah Animal Facility. The cell-Matrigel mixture (100 μl) was injected into the subcutis of the right hind leg of the mice. The transplanted animals were observed routinely once a week, and tumor growth was measured with a caliper. They were sacrificed after development of tumors larger than 1 cm^3 or following an observation period of 30 weeks. The sacrificed animals were subjected to general inspection. When tumors were observed at the injection site, they were collected. In addition, the liver, lungs and spleen tissues of the all animals were inspected for tumor invasion into other organs.

Histological Analysis

The tumor containing tissues were fixed in 4% PFA, embedded in paraffin and serially sectioned into 6 micron sections. Every other section was mounted on slides (2–3 sections per slide, and 20 slides for each tumor). 4 slides, containing 8–12 sections from various parts of the tumor (slides #3, 8, 13 and 18) were stained with hematoxylin and eosin, and subjected to histological analysis by a certified pathologist. Large tumors were cut into halves before fixation, and the two halves were placed in the paraffin block so that the central parts of tumor (with the larger surface area) were faced up. To enable analysis of the different parts of large tumors, the sectioning was performed from the upper part of the paraffin block, containing the central parts of both halves of the tumor, towards the tumor's edges.

Statistical Analysis

Data is presented as mean ± SEM (standard error of mean). Kaplan-Meier analysis was performed using the GraphPad PRISM version 4.0 software.

Ethics Statement

This study was performed in accordance with the recommendations of the Authority for Biological and Biomedical Models of the Hebrew University, Jerusalem. The protocol was approved by the Committee on the Ethics of Animal Experiments (Permit Number: MD-09-11663-4).

Supporting Information

Figure S1 Expression of pluripotency-associated cell surface markers in transplanted HES-1 cells. (A): A representative FACS analysis of the expression levels of pluripotency-associated cell-surface markers, Tra-1-60, Tra-1-81, and SSEA-4 in transplanted HES-1 cells. **(B):** Average expression levels of Tra-1-60, Tra-1-81, and SSEA-4 in transplanted HES-1 cells from twelve transplantation experiments. Data presented as mean ± SEM.

Figure S2 Effect of the ROCK-inhibitor Y-27632 on Teratoma Formation. Kinetics of teratoma formation after transplantation of decreasing numbers of undifferentiated HES-1 cells in the presence (dark gray) or absence (light gray) of the ROCK-inhibitor Y-27632. **(A):** Efficiency of teratoma formation **(B):** The average volume of the teratomas at the time of animals sacrifice. **(C):** The average time interval between transplantation and the detection of tumors. **(D):** The average time interval between transplantation and the experiment endpoint. Data presented as mean ± SEM.

Table S1 Teratoma Formation Kinetics after Transplantation of Various Defined Numbers of Undifferentiated HES-2 Cells. Various numbers of undifferentiated HES-2 cells were mixed with MMC-treated foreskin fibroblasts (to a total of 1×10^6 cells) and Matrigel, and transplanted s.c. into NOD/SCID mice. The transplanted animals were weekly monitored for the appearance of tumors, and for the progression of tumor size. The endpoint of the experiments was when the tumors reached a size of ≥ 1 cm^3 or 30 weeks after transplantation. Data presented as mean ± SEM.

Author Contributions

Conceived and designed the experiments: Michal Gropp BER NBZ. Performed the experiments: Michal Gropp VS Miri Gov YG. Analyzed the data: Michal Gropp VS GV JK NBZ BER. Contributed reagents/materials/analysis tools: HK LM MI. Wrote the manuscript: Michal Gropp BER.

References

1. Thomson JA, Itskovitz-Eldor J, Shapiro SS, Waknitz MA, Swiergiel JJ, et al. (1998) Embryonic stem cell lines derived from human blastocysts. Science 282: 1145–1147.
2. Reubinoff BE, Pera MF, Fong CY, Trounson A, Bongso A (2000) Embryonic stem cell lines from human blastocysts: somatic differentiation in vitro. Nat Biotechnol 18: 399–404.
3. Lensch MW, Ince TA (2007) The terminology of teratocarcinomas and teratomas. Nat Biotechnol 25: 1211.
4. Blum B, Benvenisty N (2008) The tumorigenicity of human embryonic stem cells. Adv Cancer Res 100: 133–158.
5. Brivanlou AH, Gage FH, Jaenisch R, Jessell T, Melton D, et al. (2003) Stem cells. Setting standards for human embryonic stem cells. Science 300: 913–916.
6. (2009) Consensus guidance for banking and supply of human embryonic stem cell lines for research purposes. Stem Cell Rev 5: 301–314.
7. Maherali N, Hochedlinger K (2008) Guidelines and techniques for the generation of induced pluripotent stem cells. Cell Stem Cell 3: 595–605.
8. Muller FJ, Goldmann J, Loser P, Loring JF (2010) A call to standardize teratoma assays used to define human pluripotent cell lines. Cell Stem Cell 6: 412–414.
9. Mayor S (2010) First patient enters trial to test safety of stem cells in spinal injury. Bmj 341: c5724.

10. Werbowetski-Ogilvie TE, Bosse M, Stewart M, Schnerch A, Ramos-Mejia V, et al. (2009) Characterization of human embryonic stem cells with features of neoplastic progression. Nat Biotechnol 27: 91–97.
11. Lee AS, Tang C, Cao F, Xie X, van der Bogt K, et al. (2009) Effects of cell number on teratoma formation by human embryonic stem cells. Cell Cycle 8: 2608–2612.
12. Shih CC, Forman SJ, Chu P, Slovak M (2007) Human embryonic stem cells are prone to generate primitive, undifferentiated tumors in engrafted human fetal tissues in severe combined immunodeficient mice. Stem Cells Dev 16: 893–902.
13. Hentze H, Soong PL, Wang ST, Phillips BW, Putti TC, et al. (2009) Teratoma formation by human embryonic stem cells: Evaluation of essential parameters for future safety studies. Stem Cell Res 2: 198–210.
14. Prokhorova TA, Harkness LM, Frandsen U, Ditzel N, Burns JS, et al. (2008) Teratoma Formation by Human Embryonic Stem Cells is site-dependent and enhanced by the presence of Matrigel. Stem Cells Dev 18: 47–54.
15. Drukker M, Katchman H, Katz G, Even-Tov Friedman S, Shezen E, et al. (2006) Human embryonic stem cells and their differentiated derivatives are less susceptible to immune rejection than adult cells. Stem Cells 24: 221–229.
16. Watanabe K, Ueno M, Kamiya D, Nishiyama A, Matsumura M, et al. (2007) A ROCK inhibitor permits survival of dissociated human embryonic stem cells. Nat Biotechnol 25: 681–686.
17. Cohen MA, Itsykson P, Reubinoff BE (2007) Neural differentiation of human ES cells. Curr Protoc Cell Biol Chapter 23: Unit 23 27.
18. Idelson M, Alper R, Obolensky A, Ben-Shushan E, Hemo I, et al. (2009) Directed differentiation of human embryonic stem cells into functional retinal pigment epithelium cells. Cell Stem Cell 5: 396–408.
19. Chang Y, Finnemann SC (2007) Tetraspanin CD81 is required for the alpha v beta5-integrin-dependent particle-binding step of RPE phagocytosis. J Cell Sci 120: 3053–3063.
20. Daley GQ, Lensch MW, Jaenisch R, Meissner A, Plath K, et al. (2009) Broader implications of defining standards for the pluripotency of iPSCs. Cell Stem Cell 4: 200–201; author reply 202.
21. Draper JS, Smith K, Gokhale P, Moore HD, Maltby E, et al. (2004) Recurrent gain of chromosomes 17q and 12 in cultured human embryonic stem cells. Nat Biotechnol 22: 53–54.
22. Baker DE, Harrison NJ, Maltby E, Smith K, Moore HD, et al. (2007) Adaptation to culture of human embryonic stem cells and oncogenesis in vivo. Nat Biotechnol 25: 207–215.
23. Spits C, Mateizel I, Geens M, Mertzanidou A, Staessen C, et al. (2008) Recurrent chromosomal abnormalities in human embryonic stem cells. Nat Biotechnol 26: 1361–1363.
24. Blum B, Benvenisty N (2009) The tumorigenicity of diploid and aneuploid human pluripotent stem cells. Cell Cycle 8: 3822–3830.
25. Andrews PW, Matin MM, Bahrami AR, Damjanov I, Gokhale P, et al. (2005) Embryonic stem (ES) cells and embryonal carcinoma (EC) cells: opposite sides of the same coin. Biochem Soc Trans 33: 1526–1530.
26. Lawrenz B, Schiller H, Willbold E, Ruediger M, Muhs A, et al. (2004) Highly sensitive biosafety model for stem-cell-derived grafts. Cytotherapy 6: 212–222.
27. Fink DW Jr (2009) FDA regulation of stem cell-based products. Science 324: 1662–1663.
28. Goldring CE, Duffy PA, Benvenisty N, Andrews PW, Ben-David U, et al. Assessing the safety of stem cell therapeutics. Cell Stem Cell 8: 618–628.
29. Ben-Dor I, Itsykson P, Goldenberg D, Galun E, Reubinoff BE (2006) Lentiviral vectors harboring a dual-gene system allow high and homogeneous transgene expression in selected polyclonal human embryonic stem cells. Mol Ther 14: 255–267.

Permissions

All chapters in this book were first published in PLOS ONE, by The Public Library of Science; hereby published with permission under the Creative Commons Attribution License or equivalent. Every chapter published in this book has been scrutinized by our experts. Their significance has been extensively debated. The topics covered herein carry significant findings which will fuel the growth of the discipline. They may even be implemented as practical applications or may be referred to as a beginning point for another development.

The contributors of this book come from diverse backgrounds, making this book a truly international effort. This book will bring forth new frontiers with its revolutionizing research information and detailed analysis of the nascent developments around the world.

We would like to thank all the contributing authors for lending their expertise to make the book truly unique. They have played a crucial role in the development of this book. Without their invaluable contributions this book wouldn't have been possible. They have made vital efforts to compile up to date information on the varied aspects of this subject to make this book a valuable addition to the collection of many professionals and students.

This book was conceptualized with the vision of imparting up-to-date information and advanced data in this field. To ensure the same, a matchless editorial board was set up. Every individual on the board went through rigorous rounds of assessment to prove their worth. After which they invested a large part of their time researching and compiling the most relevant data for our readers.

The editorial board has been involved in producing this book since its inception. They have spent rigorous hours researching and exploring the diverse topics which have resulted in the successful publishing of this book. They have passed on their knowledge of decades through this book. To expedite this challenging task, the publisher supported the team at every step. A small team of assistant editors was also appointed to further simplify the editing procedure and attain best results for the readers.

Apart from the editorial board, the designing team has also invested a significant amount of their time in understanding the subject and creating the most relevant covers. They scrutinized every image to scout for the most suitable representation of the subject and create an appropriate cover for the book.

The publishing team has been an ardent support to the editorial, designing and production team. Their endless efforts to recruit the best for this project, has resulted in the accomplishment of this book. They are a veteran in the field of academics and their pool of knowledge is as vast as their experience in printing. Their expertise and guidance has proved useful at every step. Their uncompromising quality standards have made this book an exceptional effort. Their encouragement from time to time has been an inspiration for everyone.

The publisher and the editorial board hope that this book will prove to be a valuable piece of knowledge for researchers, students, practitioners and scholars across the globe.

List of Contributors

Chaoyang Lv, Yao Zhang, Shunmei He, Mengjuan Xue, Mingxiang Yu and Xin Gao
Department of Endocrinology and Metabolism, Zhongshan Hospital, Fudan University, Shanghai, P.R. China

Ming Xu and Tongyu Zhu
Department of Urology, Zhongshan Hospital, Fudan University, Shanghai Key Laboratory of Organ Transplantation, Shanghai, P.R. China

Jian Gao
Evidence Base Medicine Center, Zhongshan Hospital, Fudan University, Shanghai, P.R. China

Minling Chen
Department of Endocrinology and Metabolism, Zhongshan Hospital, Fudan University, Shanghai, P.R. China
Department of Endocrinology and Metabolism, People's Hospital Affiliated to Fujian University of Traditional Chinese Medicine (The People's Hospital of Fujian Province), Fuzhou, P.R. China

Guiping Xu
Department of Endocrinology and Metabolism, Zhongshan Hospital, Fudan University, Shanghai, P.R. China
Department of Cadre's Ward, Fujian Provincial Hospital, Fujian Medical University, Fuzhou, Fujian, P.R. China

Izabela Nowak, Agnieszka Kowal, Maciej Miazga, Marta Wagner, Wanda Niepiekło-Miniewska, Andrzej Wiśniewski, Edyta Majorczyk, Wioleta Łuszczek and Piotr Kuśnierczyk
Aboratory of Immunogenetics and Tissue Immunology, Department of Clinical Immunology, Ludwik Hirszfeld Institute of Immunology and Experimental Therapy, Polish Academy of Sciences, Wrocław, Poland

Maria Magott-Procelewska and Marian Klinger
Department and Clinic of Nephrology and Transplant Medicine, Faculty of Medicine, Medical University of Wroclaw, Wrocław, Poland

Małgorzata Kamińska
Health Care Center at the Ludwik Hirszfeld Institute of Immunology and Experimental Therapy, Wrocław, Poland

Andrzej Pawlik
Department of Pharmacokinetics and Therapeutic Drug Monitoring, Pomeranian Medical University, Szczecin, Poland

Rafał Płoski
Department of Medical Genetics, Centre of Biostructure Research, Medical University of Warsaw, Warsaw, Poland

Ewa Barcz
1st Chair and Clinic of Obstetrics and Gynecology, Medical University of Warsaw, Warsaw, Poland

David Senitzer
City of Hope Comprehensive Cancer Center, Duarte, California, United States of America

Christopher J. Scarlett, Emily K. Colvin, Mark Pinese, Elizabeth A. Musgrove, Marina Pajic, Susan M. Henshall and Robert L. Sutherland
Cancer Research Program, Garvan Institute of Medical Research, Darlinghurst, Sydney, Australia

Andrew V. Biankin and David K. Chang
Cancer Research Program, Garvan Institute of Medical Research, Darlinghurst, Sydney, Australia
Division of Surgery, Bankstown Hospital, Eldridge Road, Bankstown, Sydney, Australia

Adrienne L. Morey
Department of Anatomical Pathology, St Vincent's Hospital, Darlinghurst, Australia

Minoti Apte
South Western Sydney Clinical School, The University of New South Wales, Sydney, Australia

James G. Kench
Cancer Research Program, Garvan Institute of Medical Research, Darlinghurst, Sydney, Australia
Department of Anatomical Pathology, Royal Prince Alfred Hospital, Camperdown, Sydney, Australia

Shuzi Zhang, Hehua Dai, Ni Wan, Yolonda Moore and Zhenhua Dai
Department of Microbiology and Immunology, Center for Biomedical Research, University of Texas Health Science Center, Tyler, Texas, United States of America

Xiao Li, Jun-Jie Li, De-Sheng Wang, Wei Zhao, Wen-Jie Song, Wei-Min Li, Jian-Feng Wang, Wei Han, Zhuo-Chao Zhang, Yong Yu, Da-Yong Cao and Ke-Feng Dou
Department of Hepatobiliary Surgery, Xijing Hospital, Fourth Military Medical University, Xi'an, Shaanxi Province, China

Jing-Yue Yang
Department of Clinical Oncology, Xijing Hospital, Fourth Military Medical University, Xi'an, Shaanxi Province, China

Lucile Drujont, Laura Carretero-Iglesia, Laurence Bouchet-Delbos, Gaelle Beriou, Emmanuel Merieau, Marcelo Hill, Maria Cristina Cuturi and Cedric Louvet
ITUN, Inserm UMR_S 1064, Center for Research in Transplantation and Immunology, Nantes, France

Yves Delneste
UMR Inserm 892 CNRS 6299, Université d'Angers, CHU Angers, Laboratoire d'Immunologie et Allergologie, Angers, France

Zhu Li, Juan Chen, Xue-Hua Li, Zhi-Heng Liu, Gui-Jie Liu, Yan-Chao Gao, Xue-Li Zhang and Hiu-Dong Sun
Department of Hepatobiliary Surgery, Liaocheng People's Hospital, Liaocheng, Shandong, China

Li Li and Jiang-Hua Ran
The First People's Hospital of Kunming, Kunming, Yunnan, China

Yaojun Wang, Zhao Zheng, Yunchuan Wang, Jiaqi Liu, Na Li, Xiaolong Hu, Fu Han, Yang Liu and Dahai Hu
Department of Burns and Cutaneous Surgery, Xijing Hospital, Fourth Military Medical University, Xi'an, Shaanxi Province, China

Vijayaganapathy Vaithilingam and Bernard E. Tuch
Diabetes Transplant Unit, Prince of Wales Hospital, School of Medical Sciences, University of New South Wales, Randwick, New South Wales, Australia
Materials, Science and Engineering, Commonwealth Scientific and Industrial Research Organization, North Ryde, New South Wales, Australia

Vitali Shilo, Miri Gov, Naomi B. Zak and Limor Matzrafi
CellCure NeuroSciences Ltd., Jerusalem, Israel

Gilad Vainer and Juri Kopolovic
The Department of Pathology, Hadassah-Hebrew University Medical Center, Jerusalem, Israel

Tatiana Jofra, Angela Stabilini and Manuela Battaglia
San Raffaele Diabetes Research Institute, San Raffaele Scientific Institute, Milan, Italy

Nicola Gagliani
San Raffaele Diabetes Research Institute, San Raffaele Scientific Institute, Milan, Italy
San Raffaele Telethon Institute for Gene Therapy, San Raffaele Scientific Institute, Milan, Italy
Vita-Salute San Raffaele University, Milan, Italy

Silvia Gregori
San Raffaele Telethon Institute for Gene Therapy, San Raffaele Scientific Institute, Milan, Italy

Maria Grazia Roncarolo
San Raffaele Telethon Institute for Gene Therapy, San Raffaele Scientific Institute, Milan, Italy
Vita-Salute San Raffaele University, Milan, Italy

Andrea Valle
San Raffaele Diabetes Research Institute, San Raffaele Scientific Institute, Milan, Italy
Vita-Salute San Raffaele University, Milan, Italy

David M. Rothstein
Starzl Transplantation Institute, University of Pittsburgh Medical Center, Pittsburgh, Pennsylvania, United States of America

Mark Atkinson
Department of Pathology, The University of Florida, Gainesville, Florida, United States of America

Dolores Wolfram, Nadine Eberhart and Gerhard Pierer
Department of Plastic, Reconstructive and Aesthetic Surgery, Innsbruck Medical University, Innsbruck, Austria

Ravi Starzl
Language Technologies Institute, Carnegie Mellon University, Pittsburgh, Pennsylvania, United States of America

Hubert Hackl
Division of Bioinformatics, Biocenter, Innsbruck Medical University, Innsbruck, Austria

Derek Barclay and Yoram Vodovotz
Department of Immunology, University of Pittsburgh, Pittsburgh, Pennsylvania, United States of America

Theresa Hautz and Johann Pratschke
Department of Visceral, Transplant and Thoracic Surgery, Innsbruck Medical University, Innsbruck, Austria

Bettina Zelger
Department of Pathology, Innsbruck Medical University, Innsbruck, Austria

Gerald Brandacher and W. P. Andrew Lee
Department of Plastic and Reconstructive Surgery, Johns Hopkins University School of Medicine, Baltimore, Maryland, United States of America

Stefan Schneeberger
Department of Visceral, Transplant and Thoracic Surgery, Innsbruck Medical University, Innsbruck, Austria
Department of Plastic and Reconstructive Surgery, Johns Hopkins University School of Medicine, Baltimore, Maryland, United States of America

Ali Xiong, Lihua Duan, Jie Chen, Zhigang Fan, Fang Zheng and Zheng Tan
Department of Immunology, Tongji Medical College, Huazhong University of Science and Technology, Wuhan, Hubei, China

Feili Gong and Min Fang
Department of Immunology, Tongji Medical College, Huazhong University of Science and Technology, Wuhan, Hubei, China
Key Laboratory of Organ Transplantation, Ministry of Education, Wuhan, Hubei, China
Key Laboratory of Organ Transplantation, Ministry of Health, Wuhan, Hubei, China

Jennifer R. Zitzner, Josetta Houlihan, Nancy Herrera, Luting Xu, Joshua Miller, James M. Mathew and Anat R. Tambur
Comprehensive Transplant Center, Northwestern University Feinberg School of Medicine, Chicago, Illinois, United States of America

Yuming Yu
Comprehensive Transplant Center, Northwestern University Feinberg School of Medicine, Chicago, Illinois, United States of America
Department of Organ Transplantation, Nanfang Hospital, Southern Medical University, Guangzhou, Guangdong, China

Xunrong Luo
Comprehensive Transplant Center, Northwestern University Feinberg School of Medicine, Chicago, Illinois, United States of America
Department of Medicine, Northwestern University Feinberg School of Medicine, Chicago, Illinois, United States of America

Michaela Kaldenbach, Francisco Javier Cubero, Stephanie Erschfeld, Christian Liedtke, Christian Trautwein and Konrad Streetz
Department of Internal Medicine III, University Hospital, RWTH Aachen, Aachen, Germany

Jun Araki, Makoto Mihara and Isao Koshima
Department of Plastic Surgery, University of Tokyo, Tokyo, Japan

Yuji Nishizawa and Tatsuo Nakamura
Department of Bioartificial Organs, Institute for Frontier Medical Science, Kyoto University, Kyoto, Japan

Tomoyuki Sato
Saitama Shinkaibashi Clinic, Saitama, Japan

Munekazu Naito
Department of Anatomy, Tokyo Medical University, Tokyo, Japan

Satoshi Fujii
Pathology Division, Research Center for Innovative Oncology, National Cancer Center Hospital East, Chiba, Japan

Shoba Amarnath, Jason E. Foley, Carliann M. Costanzo and Daniel H. Fowler
Experimental Transplantation and Immunology Branch, National Cancer Institute, National Institutes of Health, Bethesda, Maryland, United States of America

Hao Chen
Critical Care Medicine, Clinical Center, National Institutes of Health, Bethesda, Maryland, United States of America
Department of Cardiac Surgery, Huadong Hospital, Fudan University, Shanghai, China

Joel D. Sennesh
Department of Pathology, Inova Fairfax Hospital, Fairfax, Virginia, United States of America

Michael A. Solomon
Critical Care Medicine, Clinical Center, National Institutes of Health, Bethesda, Maryland, United States of America
Cardiovascular and Pulmonary Branch, National Heart, Lung and Blood Institute, National Institutes of Health, Bethesda, Maryland, United States of America

Daxu Li, Julia Y. S. Tsang, Jiao Peng, Jiang Zhu, Vincent C. H. Lui and Paul K. H. Tam
Paediatric Surgery Division, Department of Surgery, The University of Hong Kong, Hong Kong SAR, China

Yan Chen
Paediatric Surgery Division, Department of Surgery, The University of Hong Kong, Hong Kong SAR, China
Department of Chemistry, The University of Hong Kong, Hong Kong SAR, China

Derek H. H. Ho
Department of Chemistry, The University of Hong Kong, Hong Kong SAR, China

Yee Kwan Chan
School of Biological Science, The University of Hong Kong, Hong Kong SAR, China

Aimin Xu
Department of Medicine, The University of Hong Kong, Hong Kong SAR, China

Jonathan R. Lamb
Division of Cell and Molecular Biology, Faculty of Natural Sciences, Imperial College London, London, United Kingdom

Fang Xiao, Liang Ma, Vincenzo Mirenda, Anthony Dorling, Robert Lechler and Giovanna Lombardi
Medical Research Council (MRC) for Transplantation, King's College London, London, United Kingdom

Min Zhao and Guocai Huang
Department of Diabetes and Endocrinology, King's College London, London, United Kingdom

Chloe L. Rackham, Peter M. Jones and Aileen J. F. King
Diabetes Research Group, Division of Diabetes and Nutritional Sciences, School of Medicine, King's College London, London, United Kingdom

Vikram Mathews, Biju George, Auro Viswabandya, Aby Abraham, Rayaz Ahmed, Abhijeet Ganapule, Eunice Sindhuvi, Kavitha M. Lakshmi and Alok Srivastava
Department of Haematology, Christian Medical College, Vellore, India

Kristin Mussar, Andrew Tucker, Linsey McLennan, Addie Gearhart, Antonio J. Jimenez-Caliani, Vincenzo Cirulli and Laura Crisa
Department of Medicine, Institute of Stem Cell and Regenerative Medicine, University of Washington, Seattle, Washington, United States of America

Ryuichi Nishimura, Satoshi Sekiguchi, Keisei Fujimori, Noriaki Ohuchi and Susumu Satomi
Division of Advanced Surgical Science and Technology, Tohoku University, Sendai, Japan

Sho Nishioka, Ikuma Fujisawa and Hitoshi Shiku
Graduate School of Environmental Studies, Tohoku University, Sendai, Japan

Miki Shimada
Department of Pharmaceutical Sciences, Tohoku University Hospital, Sendai, Japan

Akira Ushiyama
Department of Environmental Health, National Institute of Public Health, Wako, Japan

Tomokazu Matsue
WorldPremier InternationalResearch Center Initiative Advanced Institute for Materials Research, Tohoku University, Sendai, Japan

Masafumi Goto
Division of Advanced Surgical Science and Technology, Tohoku University, Sendai, Japan
New Industry Creation Hatchery Center, Tohoku University, Sendai, Japan

Agnes Trabucco, Katherine Hamill, Erick Marangos, Hannah Gilligan, Elizabeth A. Pomfret, James J. Pomposelli and Mary A. Simpson
Department of Transplant Surgery, Lahey Clinic Medical Center, Burlington, Massachusetts, United States of America

Monica Grafals
Department of Transplant Surgery, Lahey Clinic Medical Center, Burlington, Massachusetts, United States of America
Department of Medicine, Georgetown University, Washington, D.C., United States of America

Brian Smith, Jamil Azzi and Leonardo V. Riella
Transplantation Research Center, Renal Division, Brigham and Women's Hospital, Harvard Medical School, Boston, Massachusetts, United States of America

Naoka Murakami
Department of Medicine, Beth Israel Medical Center, New York, New York, United States of America

Nader Najafian
Transplantation Research Center, Renal Division, Brigham and Women's Hospital, Harvard Medical School, Boston, Massachusetts, United States of America
Department of Nephrology, Cleveland Clinic Florida, Weston, Florida, United States of America

Shusen Zheng, Changhai Jin, Haiyang Xie, Lin Zhou, Penghong Song and Wenfeng Song
Key Laboratory of Combined Multi-organ Transplantation of Ministry of Public Health, First Affiliated Hospital, School of Medicine, Zhejiang University, Hangzhou, China

Xiaosun Liu
Department of Surgery, First Affiliated Hospital, School of Medicine, Zhejiang University, Hangzhou, China

Biguang Tuo
Department of Gastroenterology, Affiliated Hospital of Zunyi Medical College, Zunyi, China

Xiaofan Huang, Lingyun Ren, Chao Cheng, Jie Wu, Yuan Sun and Zheng Liu
Department of Cardiovascular Surgery, Union Hospital, Tongji Medical College, Huazhong University of Science and Technology, Wuhan, People's Republic of China

Ping Ye
Department of Cardiology, Central Hospital of Wuhan, Wuhan, People's Republic of China

Sihua Wang
Department of Thoracic Surgery, Union Hospital, Tongji Medical College, Huazhong University of Science and Technology, Wuhan, People's Republic of China

Aini Xie
Division of Diabetes, Endocrinology and Metabolism, Department of Medicine, Baylor College of Medicine, Houston, Texas, United States of America

Jiahong Xia
Department of Cardiovascular Surgery, Union Hospital, Tongji Medical College, Huazhong University of Science and Technology, Wuhan, People's Republic of China
Department of Cardiovascular Surgery, Central Hospital of Wuhan, Wuhan, People's Republic of China

Cherry Fung, Sabina Ratnapala and Jayne Foster
Diabetes Transplant Unit, Prince of Wales Hospital, School of Medical Sciences, University of New South Wales, Randwick, New South Wales, Australia

Vijesh Vaghjiani and Ursula Manuelpillai
Centre for Reproduction and Development, Monash Institute of Medical Research, Monash University, Clayton, Victoria, Australia

Michal Gropp, Yaniv Gil, Hanita Khaner, Maria Idelson and Benjamin E. Reubinoff
The Hadassah Human Embryonic Stem Cell Research Center, The Goldyne Savad Institute of Gene Therapy and Department of Gynecology, Hadassah-Hebrew University Medical Center, Jerusalem, Israel

Index

R

S

T

V

X